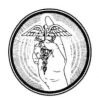

**Developed by the
American Society for
Surgery of the Hand**

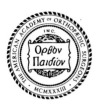

**Published by the
American Academy of
Orthopaedic Surgeons**

D1400566

Hand Surgery Update 2

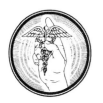

**Developed by the
American Society for
Surgery of the Hand**

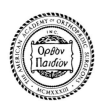

**Published by the
American Academy of
Orthopaedic Surgeons**

American Society for Surgery of the Hand

Edited by
Terry R. Light, MD

Dr. William M. Scholl
Professor and Chair
Department of Orthopaedic Surgery
and Rehabilitation
Loyola University Chicago
School of Medicine
Maywood, Illinois

Hand Surgery Update 2

Published 1999
by the American Academy of Orthopaedic Surgeons™
6300 North River Road
Rosemont, Illinois 60018
1-800-626-6726

First Edition

Copyright © 1999
by the American Society for Surgery of the Hand

The material presented in *Hand Surgery Update 2* has been made available by the American Society for Surgery of the Hand for educational purposes only. This material is not intended to present the only, or necessarily best, methods or procedures for the medical situations discussed, but rather is intended to represent an approach, view, statement, or opinion of the author(s) or producer(s), which may be helpful to others who face similar situations.

Some drugs or medical devices demonstrated in ASSH or AAOS courses or described in ASSH or AAOS print or electronic publications have not been cleared by the Food and Drug Administration (FDA) or have been cleared for specific uses only. The FDA has stated that it is the responsibility of the physician to determine the FDA clearance status of each drug or device he or she wishes to use in clinical practice.

Any statements about commercial products are solely the opinion(s) of the author(s) and do not represent an Academy endorsement or evaluation of these products. These statements may not be used in advertising or for any commercial purpose.

ISBN: 0-89203-233-2

Library of Congress Cataloging-in-Publication Data:

Hand Surgery Update 2/edited by Terry R. Light; developed by
the American Society for Surgery of the Hand.—2nd ed.

    p. cm.

    Rev. ed. of: Hand Surgery Update/developed by
the American Society for Surgery of the Hand. c1994.

    Includes bibliographical references and index.

    ISBN 0-89203-233-2 (soft cover)

    1. Hand—Surgery. I. Title: Hand surgery update two. II. Light, Terry R.
III. American Society for Surgery of the Hand.

    [DNLM: 1. Hand—surgery. 2. Hand injuries—surgery. WE 830 H2335 1999]

    RD559. H35994 1999
    617.5'75059 21—dc21

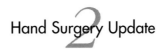

Acknowledgments

American Society for Surgery of the Hand Council, 1998-99

Vincent R. Hentz, MD, President

Terry S. Axelrod, MD

William P. Cooney, MD

Marybeth Ezaki, MD

Richard H. Gelberman, MD

Steven Z. Glickel, MD

Terry R. Light, MD

Dean S. Louis, MD

Andrew K. Palmer, MD

William C. Pederson, MD

Dennis B. Phelps, MD

Peter J. Stern, MD

Robert M. Szabo, MD

Joan F. Wright, MD

Mark C. Anderson, Executive Director

American Academy of Orthopaedic Surgeons Publications Department Staff

Marilyn L. Fox, PhD, Director

Karen Danca

Bruce Davis

Geraldine Dubberke

Loraine Edwalds

Pamela Hutton Erickson

Sharon O'Brien

Jana Ronayne

Jackie Shadinger

David Stanley

Sophie Tosta

Vanessa Villarreal

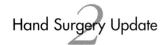

Contributors

Edward Akelman, MD
Professor and Vice Chair,
Department of Orthopedics
Brown University Medical School
Providence, Rhode Island

Peter C. Amadio, MD
Professor, Orthopedic Surgery
Mayo Clinic
Rochester, Minnesota

Pat L. Aulicino, MD
Professor of Orthopaedic Surgery
Eastern Virginia Graduate School of Medicine
Norfolk, Virginia

Terry S. Axelrod, MD, MSc, FRCS(C)
Associate Professor and Chief,
Division of Orthopaedic Surgery
University of Toronto
Toronto, Ontario, Canada

Michael S. Bednar, MD
Associate Professor,
Department of Orthopaedic Surgery
  and Rehabilitation
Stritch School of Medicine,
Loyola University Chicago
Maywood, Illinois

Richard A. Berger, MD, PhD
Associate Professor of Orthopedic Surgery
  and Anatomy
Division of Hand Surgery,
Department of Orthopedic Surgery
Mayo Clinic
Rochester, Minnesota

Richard E. Brown, MD
Clinical Associate Professor and
  Hand Fellowship Director
Division of Plastic Surgery
Southern Illinois University
Springfield, Illinois

Thomas M. Brushart, MD
Professor of Orthopaedic Surgery,
  Plastic Surgery and Neurology
Johns Hopkins
Baltimore, Maryland

Ronald C. Burgess, MD
Associate Clinical Professor, Orthopaedic Surgery
University of Kentucky
Lexington, Kentucky

Mark S. Cohen, MD
Associate Professor,
Department of Orthopaedic Surgery
Director, Hand and Elbow Program
Rush-Presbyterian-St. Lukes Medical Center
Chicago, Illinois

Paul Dell, MD
Professor and Chief of Hand and Microsurgery
Department of Orthopaedics
University of Florida
Gainesville, Florida

Edward Diao, MD
Associate Professor and Chief
Division of Hand, Upper Extremity
  and Microvascular Surgery
University of California
San Francisco, California

Marybeth Ezaki, MD
Director of Hand Surgery
Texas Scottish Rite Hospital for Children
Dallas, Texas

Thomas J. Fischer, MD
Associate Clinical Professor of
 Orthopaedic Surgery
Indiana University School of Medicine
Indianapolis, Indiana

Waldo E. Floyd III, MD
Clinical Professor of Surgery (Hand),
Mercer University School of Medicine
Clinical Assistant Professor of
 Orthopaedic Surgery,
Emory University School of Medicine
Macon, Georgia

Thomas J. Graham, MD
Director, The Hand and Upper Extremity Center
Department of Orthopaedic Surgery
The Cleveland Clinic Foundation
Cleveland, Ohio

Jeffrey A. Greenberg, MD, MS
Clinical Assistant Professor
Indiana University School of Medicine
Indianapolis, Indiana

Vincent R. Hentz, MD
Professor of Functional Restoration
 (Hand Surgery)
Stanford University Medical School
Stanford, California

Neil Ford Jones, MD
Professor and Chief of Hand Surgery
Department of Orthopaedic Surgery and
Division of Plastic and Reconstructive Surgery
University of California
Los Angeles, California

Jesse B. Jupiter, MD
Professor of Orthopaedic Surgery
Harvard Medical School
Boston, Massachusetts

Michael W. Keith, MD
Professor, Orthopaedics and
 Biomedical Engineering
Case Western Reserve University
Cleveland, Ohio

William B. Kleinman, MD
Clinical Professor of Orthopaedic Surgery
Indiana University Medical Center
Indianapolis, Indiana

L. Andrew Koman, MD
Professor and Vice Chair,
Department of Orthopaedic Surgery
Wake Forest University
Winston-Salem, North Carolina

William G. Kraybill, MD
Chief, Soft Tissue-Melanoma and Bone Service
Associate Professor of Surgery,
Surgical Oncology Division
State University of New York
Buffalo, New York

John O. Kucan, MD
Professor of Surgery
Division of Plastic and Reconstructive Surgery
Southern Illinois University
Springfield, Illinois

Stephen J. Leibovic, MD, MS
Clinical Assistant Professor,
Department of Orthopedic Surgery and
Division of Plastic Surgery
Medical College of Virginia
Richmond, Virginia

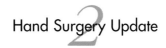

L. Scott Levin, MD
Associate Professor,
Orthopaedic and Plastic Surgery and Chief
Division of Plastic Surgery
Duke University
Durham, North Carolina

Terry R. Light, MD
Dr. William M. Scholl Professor and Chair
Department of Orthopaedic Surgery
 and Rehabilitation
Loyola University Chicago School of Medicine
Maywood, Illinois

Gary M. Lourie, MD
Assistant Clinical Professor,
Department of Orthopaedics
Emory University School of Medicine
Atlanta, Georgia

Susan E. Mackinnon, MD
Shoenberg Professor of Surgery and Chief,
Division of Plastic and Reconstructive Surgery
Washington University School of Medicine
St. Louis, Missouri

Paul R. Manske, MD
Professor, Orthopedic Surgery
Washington University
St. Louis, Missouri

Steven J. McCabe, MD, FRCS(C)
Hand Surgeon, Division of Hand Surgery,
Department of Surgery
University of Louisville
Louisville, Kentucky

Brian E. McGrath, MD
Attending Orthopedic Surgeon
Division of Orthopedic Oncology
State University of New York
Buffalo, New York

William J. Morgan, MD
Professor and Chief,
Upper Extremity Service
Department of Orthopedics
 and Physical Rehabilitation
UMASS Memorial Medical Center
Worcester, Massachusetts

David T. Netscher, MD
Associate Professor and Chief
 of Plastic Surgery and Hand Surgery,
Veterans Affairs Medical Center
Division of Plastic Surgery,
Baylor College of Medicine
Houston, Texas

Dennis P. Orgill, MD, PhD
Associate Chief,
Department of Surgery,
Division of Plastic Surgery
Brigham and Women's Hospital
Boston, Massachusetts

Elizabeth Anne Ouellette, MD
Professor, Division of Hand Surgery,
Department of Orthopedics
University of Miami School of Medicine
Miami, Florida

Clayton A. Peimer, MD
Professor of Orthopaedic Surgery
 and Clinical Associate Professor
 of Anatomical Sciences
University at Buffalo,
State University of New York
Buffalo, New York

Keith B. Raskin, MD
Clinical Associate Professor,
Department of Orthopaedic Surgery
New York University Medical Center
New York, New York

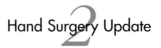

x

Ghazi M. Rayan, MD
Clinical Professor of Orthopedic Surgery and
Director, Hand Surgery Fellowship Program
University of Oklahoma Health Sciences Center
Oklahoma City, Oklahoma

W. Bradford Rockwell, MD
Chairman and Associate Professor
Division of Plastic Surgery
University of Utah
Salt Lake City, Utah

Douglas M. Rothkopf, MD
Associate Professor and Director,
 Hand Surgery Service
Division of Plastic Surgery
University of Massachusetts Medical Center
Worcester, Massachusetts

Lawrence H. Schneider, MD
Director, Division of Hand Surgery
Jefferson Medical College
Philadelphia, Pennsylvania

William H. Seitz, Jr, MD
Associate Clinical Professor
 in Orthopaedic Surgery
Case Western Reserve University
 School of Medicine
Cleveland, Ohio

Saleh M. Shenaq, MD
Professor and Chief,
Division of Plastic Surgery
Baylor College of Medicine
Houston, Texas

Randy Sherman, MD
Professor and Chief,
Division of Plastic and Reconstructive Surgery
University of Southern California
Los Angeles, California

Peter J. Stern, MD
Professor and Chairman,
Department of Orthopaedic Surgery
University of Cincinnati College of Medicine
Cincinnati, Ohio

Robert M. Szabo, MD, MPH
Professor of Orthopaedic and Plastic Surgery and
Chief, Hand and Upper Extremity Service
University of California, Davis
Sacramento, California

John S. Taras, MD
Clinical Assistant Professor,
Division of Hand Surgery
Jefferson Medical College of
 Thomas Jefferson University
Philadelphia, Pennsylvania

Thomas E. Trumble, MD
Professor and Chief,
Division of Hand and Microvascular Surgery
University of Washington
Seattle, Washington

Arnold-Peter C. Weiss, MD
Professor of Orthopaedics
Brown University School of Medicine
Providence, Rhode Island

Robert Lee Wilson, MD
Clinical Lecturer, Orthopedic Surgery
University of Arizona
Director, Phoenix Integrated Hand Fellowship
 Program
Pheonix, Arizona

R. Christie Wray, Jr, MD
Professor of Surgery
Chief, Hand and Upper Extremity Surgery
Medical College of Georgia
Augusta, Georgia

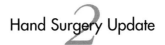
Table of Contents

Section 1
Hand Fractures and Joint Injuries

Section Editor

Jesse B. Jupiter, MD

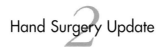

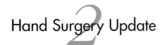

<table>
<tr><td>

Section 4

Nerves

Section Editor

Thomas M. Brushart, MD

</td><td>

Section 5

Skin and Soft-Tissues

Section Editor

R. Christie Wray, Jr, MD

</td></tr>
</table>

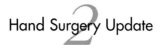

Section 6

Vascular

Section Editor

Saleh M. Shenaq, MD

Section 7

Arthritis

Section Editor

Robert Lee Wilson, MD

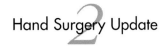
Section 8

Tumors

Section Editor

Clayton A. Peimer, MD

Section 9

Pediatric Hand

Section Editor

Marybeth Ezaki, MD

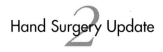

Section 10

Other Conditions

Section Editor

Peter J. Stern, MD

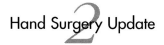

Preface

This volume is intended as an update, ideal for those seeking an understanding of the state of the art of hand surgery at the end of the twentieth century. References are principally drawn from work published after the first edition of *Hand Surgery Update* in 1994.

The expansion of knowledge in the field of hand surgery has been so vast that a text of this length cannot hope to be complete. Each chapter is structured to provide sufficient background to understand the importance of recent developments. Supplementation by the first volume of *Hand Surgery Update* or a standard hand surgery text is recommended.

The publication of this book has only been possible through the dedicated efforts of many individuals. The 45 chapters have been authored by a carefully selected group of physicians. Most are members of the American Society for Surgery of the Hand. All are busy, experienced clinicians able to critically sift through the literature to identify the most useful articles in recent years. The ten section editors each quite ably provided overview and organization to assure balanced presentation of controversies and to minimize overlap.

I am also grateful for the support and guidance of ASSH Executive Directors Jeryl Hough and Mark Anderson. Stephanie Kyte of the ASSH staff beautifully catalogued and organized materials. Finally, the American Academy of Orthopaedic Surgeons publications department staff, especially Sharon O'Brien, provided the editorial expertise and professional guidance necessary to bring this important project to the printed page.

Terry R. Light, MD

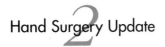

Section I
Hand Fractures and Joint Injuries

Chapter 1
Phalangeal Fractures

Chapter 2
Metacarpal Fractures

Chapter 3
Intra-articular Fractures

Chapter 4
Thumb Injuries

Chapter 5
Reconstruction of Finger Deformities

American Society for Surgery of the Hand

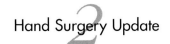
Chapter 1
Phalangeal Fractures

William J. Morgan, MD

Introduction

Phalangeal fractures, one of the most common fracture types in the skeletal system, occur in all age groups. The highest incidence occurs in men aged 40 to 69 years, as a result of machine-related accidents. The second most common occurrence is in ages 10 to 29 years, with fractures related to sports injuries. In the age group 70 years and older, most fractures result from accidental falls. Phalangeal fractures are often viewed as trivial injuries; this could result in suboptimal care.

Given the similar skeletal anatomy as well as similar fracture pattern presentation and treatment modalities, the management of proximal phalangeal and middle phalangeal injuries will be considered together, followed by discussion of distal phalanx injuries.

General Principles

Many phalangeal fractures are nondisplaced and/or stable fractures that will respond well to protective splinting and early controlled range of motion. Some fractures, however, will have displacement and comminution and may remain unstable following a closed manipulative reduction. Indications for surgical management include (1) failure to achieve or maintain a stable anatomic reduction; (2) intra-articular fractures that are displaced; (3) associated soft-tissue injury requiring fracture stability for soft-tissue rehabilitation; (4) open fractures with or without bone loss; and (5) fractures with associated polytrauma, when surgery will facilitate overall upper limb rehabilitation.

Treatment options should be based on the geometry of the fracture (transverse, oblique, spiral, and degree of comminution), fracture location (diaphyseal, periarticular, or articular), and presenting deformity (malrotation, malangulation, or shortening). Accurate assessment of associated soft-tissue injuries is critical. With higher impact injuries there will be increasing degrees of soft-tissue disruption and a greater likelihood of postoperative stiffness and loss of motion. Other associated soft-tissue injuries may include a

digital compartment syndrome secondary to crush, in which decompression may be necessary.

Additional factors influencing functional outcome include the patient's age, associated systemic diseases, socioeconomic status, compliance, and the surgeon's experience.

Diagnosis

Diagnosis of a phalangeal fracture is based on the clinical examination and radiographic findings. Knowledge of the mechanism of the injury is of utmost importance in determining the degree of associated soft-tissue injury and the prognosis.

Examination

The examination must include a detailed inventory of the injured structures. From 30% to 50% of phalangeal fractures present as open fractures. In some, the injury will also include disruption of tendon, nerve, artery, and/or joint capsule.

Care must be taken to recognize any degree of shortening, angulation, or rotation secondary to the fracture. Angular deformity is best assessed with the fingers in extension, and the injured digits should be compared to the associated uninjured digits as well as to the digits of the contralateral uninjured hand. Rotational deformity, however, is more accurately determined with flexion so that the nail plates can be observed (Fig. 1). The nail plates should normally align in a parallel fashion. The examiner must carefully observe the contralateral uninjured hand in partial flexion, because there may be some degree of rotation or angulation of the index or small fingers with respect to the long finger that can be misinterpreted as malrotation. Fracture stability should be assessed under digital block anesthesia with gentle manipulation, preferably under fluoroscopy. Radiographic evaluation should always include anteroposterior, oblique, and true lateral images.

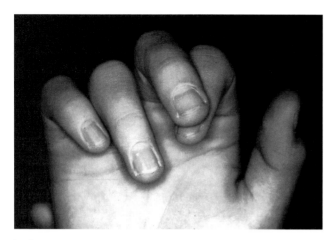

Figure 1

Examination for malrotation of a phalangeal fracture should be performed with the fingers in flexion. In a normal alignment, the nail plates should be parallel with no crossover of digits. Abnormal alignment is indicated by malrotation of the index finger. (Reproduced with permission from Breen TF: Sport-related injuries of the hand, in Pappas AM, Walzer J (eds): *Upper Extremity Injuries in the Athlete.* New York, NY, Churchill Livingstone, 1995, pp 451–496.)

Treatment

Treatment will be predicated on the assessment of skeletal and soft-tissue injury. A stable, closed, well-aligned fracture without associated soft-tissue injury may be treated by protective immobilization and early range of motion. Those fractures that are unstable or have significant soft-tissue injury may require internal fixation.

The type of implant used for fixation of the fracture will depend on the fracture type, location, comminution, and degree of soft-tissue injury. Fixation choices include closed reduction with percutaneous pin or screw fixation, open reduction and internal fixation with pin fixation, tension band and interosseus wiring, and internal fixation by mini- and microscrew and plating systems. Extensive bony comminution and/or severe soft-tissue disruption may require definitive treatment with an external fixation device.

Proximal and Middle Phalangeal Fractures

Diaphyseal Injuries

Diaphyseal fractures may present as transverse, oblique, spiral, or markedly comminuted fractures. When assessing the fracture pattern, the associated soft tissues (eg, the flexor tendon sheath, the pulley mechanism, and the osteocutaneous liga-

ments of Grayson and Cleland) may become interposed in the fracture. These structures may impact the degree of displacement as well as the potential ease or difficulty of reduction. Reduction becomes difficult or impossible if the tip of an oblique or spiral fracture becomes entrapped in a cord of Grayson's or Cleland's ligaments or if the flexor or extensor tendon or sheath becomes entrapped in the fracture site.

Unstable transverse fractures of the proximal phalanx will characteristically present with the apex of the fracture in a volar direction. The proximal fragment is flexed by the insertion of the volar interosseous tendon to the base of the proximal phalanx. The deformity is further accentuated by the pull of the central slip of the extensor mechanism on the base of the middle phalanx (Fig. 2). A similar situation is found with a displaced fracture of the middle phalanx located distal to the attachment of the flexor digitorum sublimis. A fracture of the middle phalanx located proximal to the insertion of the flexor digitorum sublimis will result in dorsal angulation of the fracture apex (Fig. 3). Recognition of these deforming forces is instrumental in achieving a manipulative reduction and maintaining the reduction in a splint or cast.

Stability of a fracture is related to the degree of energy causing the fracture. Low-energy injuries usually do not damage the periosteal sleeve and associated soft-tissue structures, and remain stable. High-energy injuries, however, will strip periosteum and soft-tissue structures at the area of the fracture, resulting in instability. When displaced fractures cannot be readily reduced, soft-tissue interposition should be suspected.

Closed Reduction Closed reduction of displaced fractures should be considered in situations in which reduction is

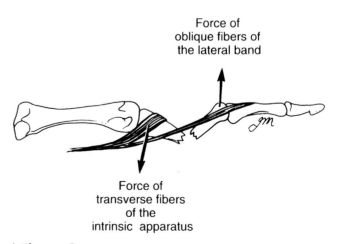

Force of
oblique fibers of
the lateral band

Force of
transverse fibers
of the
intrinsic apparatus

Figure 2

Deforming forces cause volar apex angulation of the proximal phalanx. (© Joy Marlowe, 1995.)

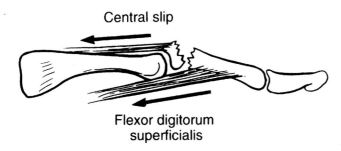

Central slip

Flexor digitorum
superficialis

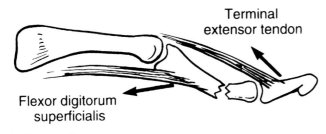

Terminal
extensor tendon

Flexor digitorum
superficialis

Figure 3

Deforming forces of middle phalangeal fracture. A proximal fracture will angulate the apex dorsally, and distal fractures will angulate the apex volarly. (© Joy Marlowe, 1995.)

likely to result in a stable fracture complex. This includes most transverse fractures and Salter II metaphyseal fractures. Reduction of oblique, spiral, or intra-articular fractures may be attempted, but it is unlikely that these will be maintained without percutaneous or open fixation. Closed reduction of phalangeal fractures is best accomplished with anesthesia at the level of the metacarpal heads or with wrist block anesthetics. Hematoma block or a "ring block" can result in increased swelling at the fracture site, which may make closed reduction more difficult.

Fracture reduction is obtained by axial traction, followed by reversal of the clinical deformity. When available, fluoroscopic control will be an asset. Following reduction the patient can actively flex the digits as a more accurate control for clinical alignment; passive manipulation can force the digits into a false position of "normal" alignment. Radiographs should be obtained immediately after reduction and repeated in 3 to 7 days, depending on the clinical stability of the fracture. If fracture stability is equivocal, the fractured digit may be buddy-taped to the adjacent normal digit to prevent subsequent shortening or malrotation. Caution must be exercised when buddy-taping an injured digit to an adjacent one in order to prevent angular or rotational forces and subsequent loss of reduction. Phalangeal fractures are immobilized in an ulnar or radial gutter splint with the

metacarpophalangeal joints flexed to 70° and the proximal interphalangeal joints in extension. The wrist should be immobilized in 20° of extension to limit the deforming forces of the tenodesis effect of the flexor and extensor tendons with wrist motion. Immobilization should continue for 3 weeks in most fractures.

It has been shown that digital performance deteriorated when active range of motion was delayed longer than 3 weeks. Stability of the fracture can be assessed at 3 weeks under fluoroscopy. If no motion is apparent, a removable gutter splint can be fabricated and active assisted range of motion exercises initiated. If there is continued failure to regain motion, the addition of passive range of motion and dynamic splinting may be initiated when fracture stability is ensured, usually by 4 to 5 weeks after injury.

Closed Reduction and Percutaneous Fixation   In unstable phalangeal fractures, stability may be achieved with the addition of percutaneous pin or screw fixation. Percutaneous fixation is desirable because it minimizes any further soft-tissue disruption during open fracture fixation. Percutaneous fixation may be provided through several types of implants, including smooth Kirschner wires (K-wires), absorbable polyglycolic or polylactic acid pins and screws, and metal screw fixation. K-wires may be used as intermedullary devices or provide fracture fixation by transfixing opposing cortices. In the case of an unstable transverse or minimally oblique fracture, a 0.045 K-wire may be used as an intramedullary device in proximal phalangeal fractures by placing the wire into the proximal phalanx tangential to the metacarpal head or by placing it through the metacarpal head and into the proximal phalanx. If the latter technique is used, the metacarpophalangeal joint should be flexed to 70° to avoid causing an extension contracture. Wires should be placed with the use of a power driver, and pins should be placed with the augmentation of a drill guide to prevent soft-tissue injury.

In cases of long oblique or spiral fractures, once the fracture has been reduced, the reduction may be held using percutaneous sharp bone-reducing forceps. The pins are best placed in a midaxial position to avoid injury to the extensor or flexor mechanism. The initial starting point in pin direction should be confirmed, preferably under fluoroscopy, to minimize multiple passes that may weaken the fracture fragments or cause further soft-tissue injury. In long spiral or oblique fractures, fixation can often be obtained with a percutaneous placement of a 1.5- or 2.0-mm screw. This can be accomplished through a midaxial incision and is enhanced with fluoroscopy. When compared biomechanically, a single compression screw provided superior fracture fixation to that of a pin. A percutaneous screw clamp was recently developed to help maintain and align the proper orientation for screw placement (Fig. 4).

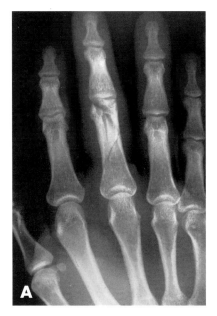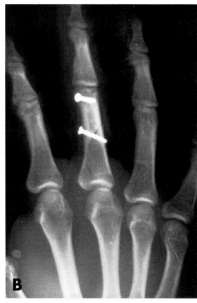

Figure 4

A, Comminuted oblique butterfly fragments of the proximal phalanx. **B,** Fracture fragment repaired with interfragmentary screw technique. (Reproduced with permission from Breen TF: Sport-related injuries of the hand, in Pappas AM, Walzer J (eds): *Upper Extremity Injuries in the Athlete.* New York, NY, Churchill Livingstone, 1995, pp 451–496.)

If rigid fixation is obtained by percutaneous screw fixation, a removable protective gutter splint can be fabricated for the patient, and early active assisted range of motion exercises can be initiated.

Open Reduction and Internal Fixation Open reduction and internal fixation should be considered if stable reduction cannot be obtained by closed means, the expected force of soft-tissue rehabilitation exceeds the stability of the fracture, or there is a high degree of comminution or segmental defects necessitating maintenance of length by bone graft replacement (and usually plate fixation). Methods available for internal fixation include smooth wire fixation; interosseous and tension band wire techniques; interfragmentary lag screw fixation; plate fixation techniques (eg, tension band, lag screw and plate, neutralization plate, buttress plate, spanning plate, and condylar plate); or intramedullary fixation devices other than K-wires.

The choice of fixation device is determined by the character of the fracture and the degree of associated soft-tissue injury. The goal is to achieve maximal rigid fixation with minimal soft-tissue disruption and minimal prominence of the fixation device.

Each technique requires a learning curve to understand potential tricks, traps, and pitfalls that may be encountered.

The proximal and middle phalanges can be approached through either a midline dorsal skin incision, a midaxial incision, or a combination thereof (Fig. 5). The proximal phalanx may be approached with a midline splitting incision through the extensor tendon or by retraction of the extensor mechanism with partial incision of the transverse retinacular ligament and parasagittal fibers. Dorsally placed implants may impede normal excursion of the extensor mechanism, and bulky implants should be avoided. Laterally placed implants such as the condylar plate will avoid interference with the gliding of the extensor mechanism. Lag screws should be countersunk to avoid prominence of the screw head. The implant size should complement the skeletal size of the phalanx and the expected forces of rehabilitation.

In cases of significant bone loss, length and alignment can be maintained with a bridge plate and the use of a corticocancellous bone graft. This should provide adequate stability for early motion. Stability must be assessed intraoperatively and subsequent rehabilitation adjusted accordingly.

External Fixation Indications for external fixation of phalangeal diaphysis fractures include grossly contaminated open fractures; soft-tissue disruption or loss requiring subsequent reconstruction; and segmental defects in which digital length needs to be preserved and open reduction and internal fixation with bone graft should be delayed. External fixation devices may provide temporary stability or may provide definitive fracture care. Most fixators are small enough to allow early active assisted range of motion of the injured and associated uninjured digits. Care must be taken during application of the external fixation device to avoid injury to tendon and neurovascular structures. Maintenance of fracture alignment should be monitored by weekly radiographs so that remanipulation can be achieved if necessary. The fixation device can be removed in 3 to 6 weeks, based on evidence of clinical and radiographic fracture healing.

Periarticular Fractures

Periarticular fractures of the proximal and middle phalanges are frequently unstable and require percutaneous or internal fixation to maintain stability. These metaphyseal fragments

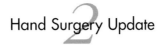

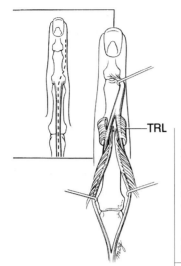

Figure 5

Surgical approaches to fractures of the proximal and middle phalanges. TRL = transverse retinacular ligament. (Reproduced with permission from Stern PJ: Fractures of the metacarpals and phalanges, in Green DP, Hotchkiss RN (eds): *Operative Hand Surgery*. New York, NY, Churchill Livingstone, 1993, vol 1, pp 695–758.)

are usually small, difficult to reduce, and difficult to hold by closed means. The risk of adjacent joint stiffness is high.

Displaced neck fractures are more common in young children and may present as subtle fractures; these require a high index of suspicion. These fractures are difficult to manipulate into position and hold and frequently yield poor results with closed treatment. Reduction is accomplished by proximal interphalangeal or distal interphalangeal joint flexion. In this position, percutaneous pins may be applied along the lateral condyle and into the proximal shaft. This type of pin fixation will necessitate fixation of the adjacent collateral ligaments and consequently interfere with the ability to proceed with early motion.

The pins can be removed in 3 to 4 weeks and successful rehabilitation achieved. As in diaphyseal fractures, a careful clinical and radiographic check for malrotation and malangulation must be performed. Angulated Salter-Harris fractures of the proximal phalanx to the small finger (extra octave fractures) are commonly seen in children. This fracture can be reduced by manipulating the metacarpophalangeal joint into full flexion, which will stabilize the proximal fragment through the collateral ligaments. Angular reduction can be corrected by manipulation of the distal fragment. The use of mechanical devices such as a pencil between the digits as a lever is discouraged because of the potential for digital nerve injury. Clinical and radiographic assessments are conducted after reduction. The small finger is taped to the ring finger and splinted in an ulnar gutter splint for 3 weeks.

Open Reduction and Internal Fixation If periarticular fractures cannot be reduced or held by closed means, open

reduction and internal fixation may be necessary. Frequently soft tissue may be interposed at the fracture site, necessitating open reduction, or impaction could necessitate an open disimpaction to manipulate the fragments into anatomic position. Care must be taken to minimize soft-tissue disruption during internal fixation to minimize further loss of motion due to iatrogenic causes. Periarticular fractures are usually amenable to fixation with minicondylar plates or interosseous wiring techniques. They provide good fixation into cancellous bone, but have little bulk and low profile to minimize interference with the function of the extensor mechanism.

External Fixation The indications for external fixation in periarticular fractures are similar to those of diaphyseal fractures. In periarticular fractures, however, the external fixation device frequently is placed across the joint, providing fixation through the associated collateral ligaments. The usual indication in periarticular fractures is a temporary one, with subsequent internal fixation being provided once tissue equilibrium has been established.

Complications

In fractures associated with significant soft-tissue injury, such as crush injury, resultant adhesions of the extensor and flexor mechanisms occur relatively frequently, particularly in fractures immobilized for more than 3 weeks. In cases of proximal phalangeal fractures that are treated by percutaneous pins and gutter immobilization, the distal interphalangeal joint should be left free to allow active and passive range of motion to minimize adhesions of the flexor profundus. Adhesions of the extensor and flexor mechanism that do not respond to dynamic splinting and intensive hand therapy may require tenolysis with subsequent immediate active range of motion.

Distal Phalanx Fractures

Although fractures of the distal phalanx are the most common type of hand fracture, the vast majority can be treated by closed means. Tuft fractures generally occur secondary to a crushing injury and frequently are associated with disruption of the nail matrix. Painful subungual hematomas should be decompressed. In nondisplaced tuft fractures with subungual hematoma, decompression through the nail plate is all that is required. In displaced fractures of the tuft with a subungual hematoma, nail plate removal and repair of the nail matrix should be considered. Tuft fractures are protected with a stack splint, which allows proximal interphalangeal joint motion, and should be treated symptomatically (generally 10 to 14 days). Radiographically, these fractures frequently fail to unite, but they remain stable by way of a fibrous union. Once symptoms resolve, the patient may resume normal activity.

Shaft fractures in the distal phalanx are usually transverse or longitudinal. Nondisplaced fractures are usually stabilized by the associated soft tissues and can be treated by 3 or 4 weeks of immobilization. Displaced transverse fractures will frequently be associated with a subluxation of the nail plate out of the eponychial fold, with damage to the sterile or germinal matrix. Reduction may be difficult to hold because of opposing flexor and extensor forces. Frequently, reduction is best maintained with a longitudinally placed K-wire. The germinal and sterile matrix should be repaired in conjunction with fixation. Displaced longitudinal fractures are usually secondary to a crushing injury; if widely displaced, they should be reduced with a sharp bone-reducing forceps and held with a K-wire or a micro-lag screw.

Annotated Bibliography

Complications

Creighton JJ Jr, Steichen JB: Complications in phalangeal and metacarpal fracture management: Results of extensor tenolysis. *Hand Clin* 1994;10:111–116.

This retrospective review is an analysis of 56 patients who underwent extensor tenolysis following management of metacarpal and phalangeal fractures. Extensor lag decreased in digits requiring only extensor tenolysis, while extensor lag tended to increase in those digits requiring dorsal capsulotomy in addition to extensor tenolysis. Time from injury to tenolysis did not appear to influence results.

Diaphyseal Injury Management

Oxford KL, Hildreth DH: Fracture bracing for proximal phalanx fractures. *J Hand Ther* 1996;9:404–405.

To allow early mobilization of stable proximal phalanx fractures, a circumferential fracture brace is fabricated and the patient begins active range of motion. The guidelines for use and instructions for fabrication are presented.

Internal and External Fixation

Bischoff R, Buechler U, De Roche R, Jupiter J: Clinical results of tension band fixation of avulsion fractures of the hand. *J Hand Surg* 1994;19A:1019–1026.

This review of 100 cases of tension band wiring included 8 fractures of the lateral phalangeal base and 3 avulsion fractures of the base of the dorsal aspect of the middle phalanx. Physical and radiographic evidence showed excellent or satisfactory results in 9 of the 11 phalangeal fractures.

Fitoussi F, Ip WY, Chow SP: External fixation for comminuted phalangeal fractures: A biomechanical cadaver study. *J Hand Surg* 1996;21B:760–764.

A biomechanical model was used to assess the rigidity obtained by external fixation versus lateral plate and crossed K-wires in the management of comminuted phalangeal fractures. Lateral plating provided the best rigidity against apex palmar bending and compression, and external fixation provided the best rigidity in torque testing.

Gonzalez MH, Hall RF Jr: Intramedullary fixation of metacarpal and proximal phalangeal fractures of the hand. *Clin Orthop* 1996;327:47–54.

The use of flexible intramedullary rods for fixation of unstable transverse and short oblique diaphyseal fractures is discussed, and a new spacer with proximal and distal locking screws to control length and rotation is demonstrated. The techniques provide fracture stabilization, allowing for immediate mobilization.

Gonzalez MH, Igram CM, Hall RF: Intramedullary nailing of proximal phalangeal fractures. *J Hand Surg* 1995;20A:808–812.

This article presents a retrospective review of 25 patients with phalangeal fractures fixed with flexible intramedullary nails. Average follow-up was 10 months. Flexible rodding of selected proximal phalangeal fractures gave excellent results and low complication rates. Proper selection and surgical technique are needed to avert complications.

Lu WW, Furumachi K, Ip WY, Chow SP: Fixation for comminuted phalangeal fractures: A biomechanical study of five methods. *J Hand Surg* 1996;21B:765–767.

This study compared the rigidity of 5 different fixation techniques—4 K-wire, lateral plating with 6 screws, lateral plating for the triangular butterfly fragment defect, 2 screws, and 2 crossed intramedullary K-wires. Lateral plating with 6 screws provided the most rigid fixation, followed by the 4 K-wire method of fixation.

Matloub HS, Jensen PL, Sanger JR, Grunert BK, Yousif NJ: Spiral fracture fixation techniques: A biomechanical study. *J Hand Surg* 1993;18B:515–519.

A cadaver model was used to compare the mechanical strengths of 5 fixation techniques used for spiral fractures—crossed K-wires, interosseous loops, dorsal miniplate, single compression screw, and K-wire plus cerclage wire. A single compression screw provided the best overall fixation for the proximal phalanx.

Ouellette EA, Freeland AE: Use of the minicondylar plate in metacarpal and phalangeal fractures. *Clin Orthop* 1996;327:38–46.

A retrospective review of 53 consecutive patients treated with 1.5-mm or 2-mm minicondylar plates for unstable intra-articular and periarticular phalangeal and metacarpal fractures is presented. Minicondylar plates provide secure fixation and allow adequate function for the management of these fractures when less invasive methods cannot restore stability.

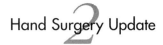
Pelto-Vasenius K, Hirvensalo E, Rokkanen P: Absorbable pins in the treatment of hand fractures. *Ann Chir Gynaecol* 1996; 85:353–358.

In this review of 32 hand fractures (including 12 phalangeal fractures) treated with absorbable devices, the absorbable implants generated good results for management of intra-articular fractures in the phalanges.

Vandenberk P, De Smet L, Fabry G: Finger fractures in children treated with absorbable pins. *J Pediatr Orthop* 1996;5B:27–30.

In this study of the use of biodegradable PDS rods for the management of phalangeal neck fractures in children, the implants maintained fracture reduction and allowed early mobilization of surrounding joints.

Etiology of Phalangeal Fractures

De Jonge JJ, Kingma J, van der Lei B, Klasen HJ: Phalangeal fractures of the hand: An analysis of gender and age-related incidence and aetiology. *J Hand Surg* 1994;19B:168–170.

Etiology and age of 6,857 patients with phalangeal fractures were analyzed. Sports injury was the main cause of fractures in the 10- to 29-year age group, and accidental falls were the leading cause in the 70+ age group. The highest incidence occurred in men aged 40 to 69 years; machinery was the cause of fracture.

Outcomes

Weiss AP, Hastings H II: Distal unicondylar fractures of the proximal phalanx. *J Hand Surg* 1993;18A:594–599.

This retrospective review of 38 patients with phalangeal fractures presents 4 classes of fracture patterns, as well as fracture management and patient outcome.

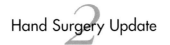

Chapter 2
Metacarpal Fractures

Terry S. Axelrod, MD, MSc, FRCS(C)

Introduction

Metacarpal fractures account for approximately 30% to 40% of all hand fractures. The outer areas of the hand are the most commonly affected; fractures of the neck of the fifth metacarpal account for 10% of all hand fractures. The highest incidence of metacarpal fractures occurs in men from 10 to 29 years of age, with a life-time expected occurrence of 2.5%. Transport accidents, bicycle and otherwise, were responsible for most fractures in this age group. In the lower incidence groups, those 9 years old and younger and those older than 50 years of age, falls accounted for most of the fractures.

Over the past 5 years, since the first publication of this update, there have been developments in the understanding of the biomechanics of metacarpal fractures, in the nonsurgical management of these fractures, and in the use of implants for surgically stabilizing these injuries.

Biomechanics

From a functional standpoint, it is apparent that shortening of the metacarpals is generally well tolerated. There are no clearly defined limits to this, although it is believed that up to 3 to 4 mm of shortening can be tolerated. Metacarpals from cadaver specimens were serially shortened to define the extent of extensor lag created at the metacarpophalangeal joint. For every 2 mm of shortening, 7° of extensor lag results. Functionally, compensatory mechanisms exist to balance the skeletal deformity, thus disability may be less noticeable.

Several laboratory studies have compared the strengths and failure rates for simulated metacarpal fractures. Fatigue strength was tested in bending, torsion, and axial loading. Dorsal plating with a lag screw proved to be superior in all modes of testing, followed by lag screws alone, Kirschner wire (K-wire) tension banding, and intramedullary K-wire fixation, which was the weakest. Fatigue life of the plate was significantly greater than that of lag screws alone.

Comparative studies of micro- and miniplating systems indicate that for metacarpal fractures tested in apex dorsal 3- or 4-point bending that the larger minisystems applied dorsally provide the greatest rigidity. The newer 3-dimensional plate designs afford increased rigidity, as does increasing the thickness of the linear, traditional plate designs.

Self-tapping miniscrews used for metacarpal fixation show the same failure rates as traditional pretapped screws when tested for shear stress and axial stress during torsional loading and cantilevered bending of spiral metacarpal fracture models.

Resorbable internal fixation devices have been compared to the standard metallic implants, both biomechanically and with a cost analysis. The resorbable polyglycolic acid (PGA) and poly (L-lactic acid) (PLLA) plates compared favorably in apex dorsal rigidity to the titanium systems, yet were inferior in torsional testing. The use of self-reinforced polyglycolide (SR-PGA) rods as fixation for metacarpal fractures indicates that the initial bending stiffness is only 60% of that of traditional K-wire techniques. When subjected to a saline bath, the material totally lost its stability by 4 weeks. The use of such devices for diaphyseal fixation is not recommended.

Cost Analysis: Bioresorbable Implants

One of the reasons that resorbable implants are being considered for use for metacarpal fractures is to reduce or eliminate the need for secondary surgery to remove the implants. A cost minimization study, which includes the direct medical costs of the procedures and the costs of time lost from work, indicates that there are financial savings with these absorbable implants. However, not all metallic implants are routinely removed. If fewer than 19% of metallic implants used for metacarpal fracture fixation are removed, no cost savings are to be expected with the resorbable implants. Above this rate, some savings are projected.

Metacarpal Neck Fractures

These fractures are among the most common hand fractures. Historically, there has been a fair amount of discussion about the degree of acceptable deformity, levels of impairment, and functional outcomes. Rotational deformity is unacceptable and must be corrected, either through closed reduction and splinting or with internal fixation.

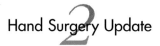

Angular deformity of up to 70° has not been shown to be associated with functional loss.

A randomized trial comparing 3 different forms of treatment for displaced metacarpal neck fractures, including an ulnar plaster cast from the proximal interphalangeal joint to the elbow, a functional brace around the wrist, or an elastic bandage, indicated no difference in the level of patient satisfaction. The functional brace provided equal pain relief to the plaster cast, and better pain relief than the elastic bandage. Mobilization was faster with the brace than the cast, and occurred at the same rate as with the elastic bandage alone. The authors recommend the use of the brace as an effective treatment for these fractures.

The use of a custom thermoplastic fracture-brace has been shown to be as effective as a cast in reducing initial fracture angulation deformity (reduced by one half) in the treatment of isolated fifth metacarpal neck fractures. The brace did not result in the initial stiffness of the wrist and fingers that occurred with the use of an ulnar gutter splint. The brace is not sufficient to allow heavy immediate use of the hand.

An advance in surgical treatment of these fractures has been the use of intramedullary fixation. Access is through a window created at the base of the metacarpal; intramedullary K-wires are advanced distally into the metacarpal head to maintain the reduction. The fracture is splinted for 1 week, followed by free movement of the digit and hand. Results seem to be excellent, with good correction of deformity and free digit motion.

Nonsurgical management remains the standard for the vast majority of metacarpal neck fractures. The use of functional custom thermoplastic hand fracture-braces seems to provide adequate stability to allow pain relief and early light functional use of the hand. In addition, it is effective in maintaining at least a 50% correction of the deformity. If rotational deformity cannot be held with closed means, or if surgery is indicated for other reasons, such as multiple metacarpal fractures, open fractures, and so forth, it would be reasonable to use the intramedullary techniques. These methods are less likely to cause the problems of extensor lag, and they lessen the need for protracted rehabilitation.

Metacarpal Shaft Fractures

Nonsurgical Treatment

Nonsurgical treatment remains the mainstay for the vast majority of metacarpal fractures. The use of closed reduction and splinting has been shown to be effective in maintaining the reduction and allowing an excellent functional result in most patients.

It is generally agreed that the degree of acceptable angulation ranges from 10° for the radial 2 rays to 30° to 40° for the ulnar digits. The ulnar digits have more mobility at the carpometacarpal joints to allow compensation for the deformity. There have been no recent publications to document an outcomes correlation between the level of functional impairment and the angulation deformity present at fracture union. Rotational deformity is less well tolerated and must be addressed either with closed treatment or surgical intervention.

Currently, there is substantial interest in the use of custom thermoplastic functional cast-braces for the hand as an alternative to the larger below elbow plaster casts or plastic splints. These hand-based splints will maintain a fracture reduction and allow earlier functional use of the hand. Whichever method of treatment is used, most patients will achieve normal mobility and grip strength at 3 months after injury, with the brace group recovering somewhat faster. A specific commercial brace, previously reported to be associated with skin breakdown complications, was studied in comparison with a dorsal/ulnar plaster splint. Only 42% of the patients with the commercial brace completed treatment; 60% were excluded because of complications with the brace. It appears that at this time the commercial brace does not have a role in the nonsurgical treatment of metacarpal fractures.

Surgical Treatment

The indications for surgical treatment of metacarpal shaft fractures include failure to obtain or maintain a satisfactory closed reduction, particularly with rotation; open fractures requiring surgical wound care; multiple fractures of the hand; replantation; complex injuries; displaced or unstable intraarticular fractures; and fractures with extensive soft-tissue injury requiring the support of a stable skeletal element.

The methods used for surgical fixation of metacarpal fractures have been refined over the past 5 years, with more versatility of the implants, use of bioabsorbable devices, and ease of application. The goal remains, as with all forms of stable internal fixation, early mobilization and functional use of the extremity.

In general, plates and screws, relatively bulky implants, are far better tolerated with metacarpal fractures than with phalangeal fractures. The associated complications, in particular tendon adherence, are readily dealt with by implant removal and extensor tenolysis after the fracture has healed. The functional results of surgical management are generally excellent.

Percutaneous Pinning Techniques

Transverse percutaneous pinning techniques are a valuable tool in the management of displaced, isolated metacarpal shaft and neck fractures. In this technique, K-wires are passed transversely proximal and distal to the fracture site

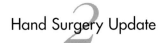

across into the adjacent intact metacarpal (Fig. 1). The metacarpal is best held with 2 K-wires distally to maintain the reduction and prevent rotation of the distal segment and loss of reduction. The advantages of this technique include the closed nature of the procedure, the lack of exposure of the fracture hematoma, the avoidance of tendon irritation or impalement, early functional aftercare, and ease of implant removal. As the fracture becomes more complex and the fragments smaller or more angulated, this technique becomes less applicable.

Intramedullary pinning using modifications of the Hall technique have gained in popularity. Modifications of the technique, such as prebending the ends of the wires to achieve an improved fracture reduction, have been reported. This modification has resulted in anatomic reduction of 50 of 62 fractures in 1 series over a 6-year period.

The use of flexible intramedullary nailing provides consistent, reproducible results over time. A series of 98 metacarpal fractures, including 2 open fractures, revealed that all fractures went on to heal. Three complications occurred, 2 of rod bending and 1 of rods backing out. This technique is recommended for short oblique and transverse fractures; it is contraindicated in long oblique and comminuted fractures because the rotational stability and length control may not be sufficient. (Fig. 2)

A new intramedullary spacer device has been designed to allow for length and rotational control with locking screws. This is preliminary and, as such, the indications and results to be expected are yet to be determined.

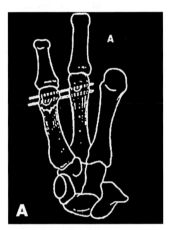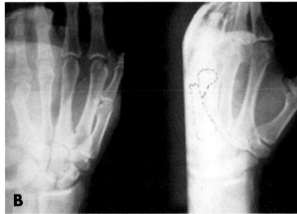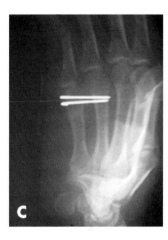

Figure 1

A, Closed percutaneous transverse pinning. B, A closed, palmarly displaced fracture of the fifth metacarpal neck in the dominant hand of a 38-year-old accountant. Closed reduction failed to reduce the palmar displacement and rotational malalignment. C, Three weeks following closed reduction and percutaneous transverse pinning to the adjacent metacarpal. There was full return of function by 6 weeks after surgery.

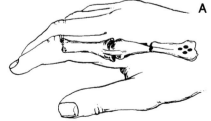
A Placement of drill holes, dorsal cortex

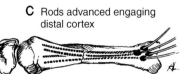
C Rods advanced engaging distal cortex

Figure 2

Technique of closed intramedullary Kirschner wire (K-wire) fixation of the fifth metacarpal. A small window is made at the base of the metacarpal using a drill or a small awl. Prebent 0.8-mm K-wires are manually advanced distally into the metacarpal head. Attempts are made to diverge the wires distally to improve rotational control. (Reproduced with permission from Gonzalez MH, Ingram CM, Hall RF Jr: Flexible intramedullary nailing for metacarpal fractures. *J Hand Surg* 1995;20A:382–387.)

Plates and Screws

Titanium has gained increasing popularity as a material used for plates and screws for hand fractures. The theoretical advantages include greater biocompatibility with fewer allergic reactions, less soft-tissue reaction, and, thus, less scarring and less tendon adherence. A multicenter study reviewed the use of titanium versus stainless steel plates and screws in 133 patients. No significant difference was found with respect to any parameters. The titanium had some soft-tissue staining in 1 case. The use of the more expensive titanium implants remains of debatable benefit.

Plate designs also have evolved. There are now many commercial hand plate sets with implants of varying sizes. Biomechanical studies indicate that the 3-dimensional plating systems provide increased rigidity with lower implant profile. The use of these designs may involve more soft-tissue stripping and devascularization of the bone. The dorsal plates are extremely versatile and remain the mainstay of rigid internal fixation for metacarpal fractures.

The AO/ASIF minicondylar plate is used for periarticular metacarpal fractures, and its use can be extended to some diaphyseal fractures. The plate can be applied laterally to avoid interference with the extensor mechanism. The plate's design adds stability to the fracture fixation in complex fractures (Fig. 3). The implant is not strong in bending and needs to be used in conjunction with a compression-stable opposite cortex, either established directly or with the use of a compression-resistant bone graft. Complex and combined injury metacarpal fractures treated with this device have achieved a reasonably high level of excellent results.

In an additional study of the use of miniplates and screws in complex injuries, the authors report that although wiring techniques may be of use with these problems, the use of miniplates and screws is indicated in situations that require stable and rigid internal fixation (Fig. 4).

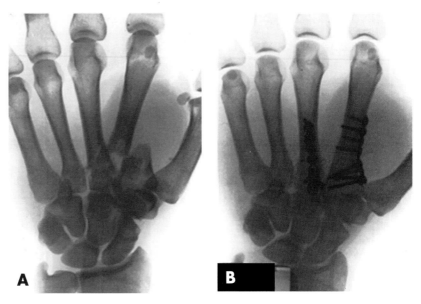

Figure 3

A, Closed multiple juxta-articular fractures in the dominant hand of a 40-year-old man. The displacement is evident. **B,** Open reduction and stable internal fixation was performed using the 2.0-mm minicondylar plates. The fracture location and pattern were ideally suited to the design of these implants.

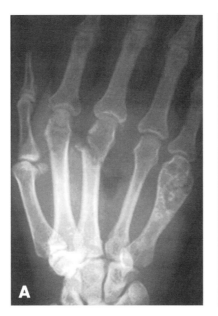 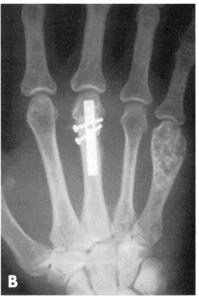

Figure 4

A, Crush injury resulting in an open complex fracture to the distal diaphysis of the third metacarpal. Associated injuries were complete transection of the extensor tendon, flexor tendons, radial digital nerve, and artery. Note the incidental enchondroma of the fifth metacarpal neck. **B,** Following debridement of the soft-tissue defect, immediate stability was provided with the use of two 2.0-mm lag screws with the complex neutralized by a 2.0-mm miniplate. All soft-tissue repairs could then be completed on a stable skeletal scaffold.

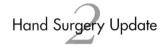
External Fixation of Metacarpal Fractures

The use of mini external devices has been reported for complex hand fractures with severe soft-tissue injuries. In one study, the devices had an associated patient satisfaction rate of 84% and complications occurred in approximately one third of patients. Loss of reduction did occur in some patients.

The stability conferred by external fixation is less than that with current plate designs. The pins interfere with the soft-tissue elements. External fixation for metacarpal fractures should probably be reserved for complex fractures with major soft-tissue injuries and defects and/or grossly contaminated wounds. In some select cases, external fixation may have a temporary role, allowing skeletal stabilization during appropriate soft-tissue management, followed by definitive internal fixation. These devices may prove to be invaluable for dealing with gunshot wounds or septic complications of metacarpal fractures.

In dealing with complex, multisystem injuries to the hand, it is imperative that stable skeletal fixation be achieved. It is this stable skeleton that provides the scaffolding on which to reconstruct the soft-tissue elements of the hand. If stability is achieved at the initial surgery, the rehabilitation of the soft-tissue elements can begin immediately. Plates and screws provide the most stable, biomechanically rigid construct available and should still be considered the mainstay of treatment for complex injuries.

Reconstruction After Surgical Management of Metacarpal Fractures

Extensor tendon adherence and joint contracture are fairly common complications after hand fractures. These problems are associated with the use of open reduction and fixation of fractures. The bulk of the implants and the dorsal location of placement leads to the development of adhesions between the extensor mechanism and the underlying plate and screw heads. Lower profile plate and screw designs may reduce the incidence of this problem.

In dealing with this complication, the fracture is allowed to heal and then the plate is removed. At the time of implant removal, a careful tenolysis is performed, freely mobilizing the tendon well proximal and distal to the zone of surgery. Use of local anesthesia is ideal in allowing the surgeon to determine the range of active digital motion achieved. Associated capsulotomy may be required, particularly of the metacarpophalangeal joint, to achieve full digital motion. Because the results of extensor tenolysis are favorable, tenolysis should be considered in dealing with the stiff digit after internal fixation of metacarpal fractures.

Annotated Bibliography

Introduction

de Jonge JJ, Kingma J, van der Lei B, Klasen HJ: Fractures of the metacarpals: A retrospective analysis of incidence and aetiology and a review of the English-language literature. *Injury* 1994;25:365–369.

The incidence and etiology of 3,858 metacarpal fractures in a series of 235,427 patients were studied. Males aged 10 to 29 years had the highest incidence of fractures (2.5%). Accidental fall was the dominant cause in the young and older age groups. Transport accidents, particularly bicycle-related, were frequent causes in all age groups.

Hove LM: Fractures of the hand: Distribution and relative incidence. *Scand J Plast Reconstr Surg Hand Surg* 1993; 27:317–319.

In a series of 1,000 consecutive hand fractures in Bergen, Norway, metacarpal, phalangeal, and carpal bones accounted for 36%, 46%, and 18% of the fractures, respectively.

Biomechanics

Firoozbakhsh KK, Moneim MS, Howey T, Castaneda E, Pirela-Cruz MA: Comparative fatigue strengths and stabilities of metacarpal internal fixation techniques. *J Hand Surg* 1993;18A:1059–1068.

One hundred five human cadaveric metacarpals were cyclically tested in bending, torsion, and axial loading after oblique osteotomies and internal fixation. Methods of internal fixation tested were dorsal plate with lag screw, 2 dorsal lag screws, crossed K-wire tension banding, and intramedullary K-wire fixation. The fatigue life of the plate fixation was significantly longer in bending, torsion, and axial loading than that of the second strongest fixation, the dorsal lag screws.

Maruyama T, Saha S, Mongiano DO, Mudge K: Metacarpal fracture fixation with absorbable polyglycolide rods and stainless steel K wires: A biomechanical comparison. *J Biomed Mater Res* 1996;33:9–12.

Self-reinforced polyglycolide rods (SR-PGA) were used to stabilize a human metacarpal cortical fracture. The construct was compared to K-wires at time zero and after being immersed in a buffered saline solution for 4 weeks. At initial fixation, the stiffness of the SR-PGA rod constructs was 61% that of the K-wire model, yet after 4 weeks in the saline, the specimens lost all of their mechanical stability.

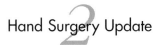
Prevel CD, Eppley BL, Ge J, et al: A comparative biomechanical analysis of resorbable rigid fixation versus titanium rigid fixation of metacarpal fractures. *Ann Plast Surg* 1996;37:377–385.

Linear flat Lactosorb plate and screws had apex dorsal rigidity equal to all but 2 of the titanium plates (3D). In torsional testing, the 3D-flat Lactosorb plate had the highest torsional rigidity of the resorbable systems, but it was only moderately rigid compared to the titanium plating systems.

Prevel CD, Eppley BL, Jackson JR, Moore K, McCarty M, Sood R: Mini and micro plating of phalangeal and metacarpal fractures: A biomechanical study. *J Hand Surg* 1995;20A:44–49.

A cadaveric metacarpal fracture model was used to test a dorsal miniplate, a dorsal microplate, and bilateral microplates in a 3-point bending model with both dorsal and palmar apex loading. This study confirms that a dorsally applied miniplate provides the greatest rigidity to a dorsal apex load.

Prevel CD, McCarty M, Katona T, et al: Comparative biomechanical stability of titanium bone fixation systems in metacarpal fractures. *Ann Plast Surg* 1995;35:6–14.

Eleven different mini- and microplating systems were tested for apex bending and torsional rigidity in a cadaveric human metacarpal model. Increasing plate thickness and 3-dimensional design were associated with increased rigidity.

Prevel CD, Morgan R, Molnar J, Eppley BL, Moore K: Biomechanical testing of titanium self-tapping versus pretapped lag screw fixation of spiral metacarpal fractures. *Ann Plast Surg* 1996;37:34–40.

The authors studied the effects of varying screw design and size in biomechanical testing of a spiral oblique metacarpal fracture model. Statistical analysis revealed no significant differences in shear stress or axial stress with increasing screw size or with self-tapping versus pretapped screw designs.

Strauch RJ, Rosenwasser MP, Lunt JG: Metacarpal shaft fractures: The effect of shortening on the extensor tendon mechanism. *J Hand Surg* 1998;23A:519–523.

Nine fresh cadaver hands were used to create a metacarpal shaft model in the second and fifth rays. Sequential shortening in 2-mm increments up to 10 mm was performed to assess the extensor lag created at the metacarpophalangeal joint. Results indicated 7° of extensor lag for every 2 mm of shortening.

Cost Analysis

Bostman OM: Metallic or absorbable fracture fixation devices: A cost minimization analysis. *Clin Orthop* 1996;329:233–239.

The authors provide a cost-minimization analysis of bioresorbable implants based on a clinical series of 994 patients treated with resorbable implants and 1,173 patients treated with conventional metallic implants. The cost savings for resorbable implants is to be found in time lost from work and direct medical costs from the second surgery. However, not all implants are routinely removed. For metacarpal fractures, cost savings would be realized only if more than 19% of implants are routinely removed.

Metacarpal Neck Fractures

Hansen PB, Hansen TB: The treatment of fractures of the ring and little metacarpal necks: A prospective randomized study of three different types of treatment. *J Hand Surg* 1998;23B:245–247.

This randomized trial looks at 3 different methods for treatment of metacarpal neck fractures: dorsal-ulnar plaster cast, functional brace around the wrist, or elastic bandage wrap. The authors found that the functional brace was superior to the other 2 in that it provided pain relief equal to that of the plaster cast, yet allowed early mobilization of the digits, preventing the stiffness of the plaster cast.

Jones AR: Reduction of angulated metacarpal fractures with a custom fracture-brace. *J South Orthop Assoc* 1995;4:269–276.

A thermoplastic fracture-brace was compared to closed reduction and ulnar gutter splinting in the treatment of 38 isolated metacarpal neck fractures with angulation of greater than 40°. Both treatments allowed for maintenance of the fracture reduction with union at one half of the initial angulation. The fracture-brace allowed early hand usage and was not associated with the early stiffness of the ulnar gutter splint. The difference resolved by 3 months posttreatment.

Larkin G, Bruser P, Safi A: Possibilities and limits of intramedullary Kirschner wire osteosynthesis in treatment of metacarpal fractures (German). *Handchir Mikrochir Plast Chir* 1997;29:192–196.

Thirty-three patients with 37 fractures of the fifth metacarpal were treated with intramedullary K-wire fixation using access from the base of the metacarpal. The results were excellent with few complications, anatomic healing, and full mobility of all digits.

Metacarpal Shaft Fractures: Nonsurgical Treatment

Sorensen JS, Freund KG, Kejla G: Functional fracture bracing in metacarpal fractures: The Galveston metacarpal brace versus a plaster-of-Paris bandage in a prospective study. *J Hand Ther* 1993;6:263–265.

One hundred thirty-three patients with fractures of the second through fifth metacarpals were randomized to treatment with either a functional brace (Galveston) or a dorsal/ulnar plaster cast. Only 42% of the patients with the brace completed treatment in contrast to 81% in the plaster group. Brace complications accounted for 60% of the exclusions.

Metacarpal Shaft Fractures: Surgical Treatment

Chen SH, Wei FC, Chen HC, Chuang CC, Noordhoff S: Miniature plates and screws in acute complex hand injury. *J Trauma* 1994;37:237–242.

Complex hand injuries were treated with skeletal stabilization using miniplates and screws in 72 fractures in 36 patients. The overall results were good in 46%, fair in 32%, and poor in 21%. The rigid

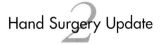

fixation provided by these implants has definite benefits in dealing with complex hand injuries.

Gonzalez MH, Hall RF Jr: Intramedullary fixation of metacarpal and proximal phalangeal fractures of the hand. *Clin Orthop* 1996;327:47–54.

The technique of intramedullary fixation of metacarpal fractures is described. Expansion of the technique to include multifragmentary fractures using locking screws and intramedullary spacers is reported.

Gonzalez MH, Igram CM, Hall RF Jr: Flexible intramedullary nailing for metacarpal fractures. *J Hand Surg* 1995;20A:382–387.

Ninety-eight metacarpal fractures were treated with closed flexible intramedullary nailing. Three minor complications were encountered. All fractures healed. The authors recommend the method for short oblique and transverse metacarpal fractures and believe it is contraindicated in long oblique and bicortical comminuted fractures.

Ouellette EA, Freeland AE: Use of the minicondylar plate in metacarpal and phalangeal fractures. *Clin Orthop* 1996; 327:38–46.

The authors report on the use of this plate for 53 patients with 68 fractures. Many of the fractures were open with soft-tissue defects. There were no nonunions or malunions. Metacarpal fractures had a significantly higher percentage of excellent results than did the phalangeal fractures. This implant provides secure fixation and can result in adequate function, even in the presence of severe combined injuries.

Paul AS, Kurdy N, Kay PR: Fixation of closed metacarpal shaft fractures: Transverse K-wires in 22 cases. *Acta Orthop Scand* 1994;65:427–429.

Twenty-two patients with closed displaced metacarpal shaft fractures were treated with transverse percutaneous K-wire fixation. The results in patients in which a single wire was used distally were unsatisfactory because of pivoting of the distal fragment on the wire with consequent deformity. When 2 wires were used distally, the reduction position was maintained.

Pfeiffer KM, Brennwald J, Buchler U, et al: Implants of pure titanium for internal fixation of the peripheral skeleton. *Injury* 1994;25:87–89.

One hundred thirty-three patients in 7 centers were operated on using titanium implants. The opinion of the surgeons regarding the qualities and effectiveness of titanium were evaluated. The outcome of the internal fixations was the same for titanium as for steel implants. There was more screw breakage and 1 case of soft-tissue staining with the titanium implants.

Schlageter M, Winkel R, Porcher R, Haas HG: Intramedullary osteosynthesis of distal metacarpal fractures with curved wires (German). *Handchir Mikrochir Plast Chir* 1997;29:197–203.

Anatomic reduction was obtained using prebent K-wires with the intramedullary technique in 50 of 62 displaced metacarpal fractures. The authors believe the prebend allows for better fracture reduction.

External Fixation for Metacarpal Fractures

Drenth DJ, Klasen HJ: External fixation for phalangeal and metacarpal fractures. *J Bone Joint Surg* 1998;80B:227–230.

Thirty-three patients with 29 phalangeal and 7 metacarpal fractures were treated over a 6-year period with a mini-Hoffmann device. The fractures all healed; there were 10 complications overall, 2 requiring repositioning of the fixator. Twenty-eight patients were satisfied with the result. Metacarpal fractures did better overall with this technique than the phalangeal fractures.

Reconstruction Following Surgical Management of Metacarpal Fractures

Creighton JJ Jr, Steichen JB: Complications in phalangeal and metacarpal fracture management: Results of extensor tenolysis. *Hand Clin* 1994;10:111–116.

The common complications of extensor tendon adherance and joint contracture after hand fractures are discussed with respect to the role of tenolysis and dorsal capsulotomy.

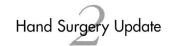

Chapter 3
Intra-articular Fractures

19

Stephen J. Leibovic, MD

Articular fractures in the hand can represent complex management problems. Articular incongruencies and deficiencies are poorly tolerated in such small mobile joints whose function is critical to dexterity and strength. Joints rendered unstable by intra-articular fractures or ligament injury must be stabilized so that postoperative rehabilitation can proceed. If such stability cannot be achieved, failure is likely. The small size of the joints, and the complex interdependence of closely applied tendons and ligaments in such confined spaces, can make surgery perilous.

Articular injury should be suspected with any significant trauma to the hand. Visible deformity is occasionally present, but cannot be relied on to predict the presence of articular injury. Examination must proceed in a logical manner, including inspection and palpation of all involved bones and joints, and ligamentous stability should be tested. Localized pain and swelling will often be the best guide for radiography, which is essential for accurate diagnosis. In the unresponsive patient, localized swelling or instability must be investigated. Because of the dearth of thick soft-tissue covering much of the fingers and hand, dislocation will usually present with clinically apparent deformity. Sometimes massive swelling, particularly over the dorsum of the hand, will obscure this observation.

Radiographs must be carefully scrutinized. Posteroanterior and true lateral views of the fingers represent the minimum requirement for investigating digital injury. On a true lateral view of a finger, the 2 condyles of the proximal and middle phalanges will be superimposed. If they are not, there is an obliquity to the image, and it should be repeated. Oblique views may be helpful in defining the fracture anatomy.

For injury at the metacarpal and carpal levels, radiologic technologists should be advised of the area of interest. Radiologic inspection of the metacarpals requires different exposure parameters than inspection of the phalanges in lateral projection. Brewerton views (taken with the dorsum of the fingers against the X-ray plate, the metacarpophalangeal (MCP) joints flexed 60°, and the incident beam angled at 15°, ulnar to radial) are helpful for identifying MCP joint injury. In addition to posteroanterior and lateral views of the hand, splay lateral views are often useful. They should be performed in a standardized manner, with the fingers cascaded in a defined order. True laterals of all the fingers cannot be seen in this fashion; if one or more of the fingers is in a true lateral, some or all of the other fingers are often slightly oblique. The carpus and wrist, however, should be viewed in true lateral projection.

Fractures of the small bones of the hand require specialized types of hardware as well as surgical techniques that are different from those used in large bones. Kirschner wires (K-wires) are commonly used for fixation of small articular fragments as well as shaft fractures. They are relatively easy to insert and occupy little space in such small fragments, but the fixation they afford is at times tenuous. They do not allow compression between adjacent fragments, and fragments may slide back and forth on the wire allowing redisplacement. Tension bands and intraosseous wiring allow compression, while minimizing the risk of further fragmentation of small fragments. They require significantly more soft-tissue dissection than K-wires. Small interfragmentary screws can be very useful in articular fractures, but demanding techniques for their use require practice and skill. Newly available screws with diameters as small as 1.0 mm to 1.2 mm can be used with small fracture fragments previously unsuitable for lag-screw fixation. Combined with plates of the same sizes, they can be used in the presence of considerable comminution.

Articular fractures range from simple nondisplaced avulsion fractures to complex comminuted articular destruction. Treatment of each type varies.

Avulsion Fractures of the Base of the Phalanges

Lateral forces on the MCP, proximal interphalangeal (PIP), or distal interphalangeal (DIP) joints can result in avulsion fractures of the corresponding joint. If the ligament is sufficiently strong, the bone will fail in tension at the site of ligament attachment. If the articular involvement is less than 20% to 25%, the displacement is small, and the joint is stable, these fractures are treated with protective splints for 2 to 3 weeks followed by mobilization. If joint stability is compromised, surgical treatment may be necessary for larger fragments. Pull-out wires, intraosseous wiring, or lag-screw

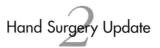

fixation are appropriate. If surgical intervention is anticipated, care must be taken to preserve the soft-tissue attachments of the small bony fragment (Fig. 1). If adjacent articular surfaces are impacted, reconstruction of the articular impaction may require supporting bone graft.

Dorsal avulsion fractures at the base of the middle phalanx (P2) often result from volar PIP dislocation. The central tendon's attachment to the dorsal base of the phalanx is maintained, but volar displacement of the phalanx results in bone failure under tension. This has the potential of becoming a boutonnière deformity if displacement persists. Accordingly,

if the articular fragment is of any significant size, it should be fixed with pull-out wires, intraosseous wiring, or lag-screw fixation (Fig. 2).

Volar avulsion fractures from the base of the P2 are extremely common. They are often the only radiologic finding after a painful hyperextension injury. Soft-tissue constraints at the IP joints can be thought of as a 3-sided box, with collateral ligaments on each side and the palmar plate on the bottom. The central tendon over the dorsum of the joint protects against volar subluxation but is not as stout a structure as the collateral ligaments or palmar plate. With hyperextension injury, the palmar plate is placed under tension, and often avulses a small articular fragment from the base of P2. The fragment is usually less than 1 mm in diameter and displaced less than 2 mm, and is best thought of as a radiologic marker for palmar plate injury. Recommended treatment is buddy-taping or dorsal block splinting of the joint in about 30° of flexion for 2 to 3 weeks. Scar contracture of the injured palmar plate can result in flexion contractures at the joint, however, so dorsal block splinting should not be prolonged.

Fractures and Dislocations of the Proximal Interphalangeal and Distal Interphalangeal Joints

Proximal Interphalangeal Fractures and Dislocations

Sprains and dislocations at the PIP joint are the most common ligament injuries in the hand. Sprains, indicating

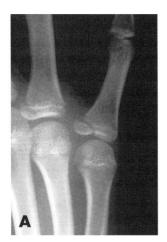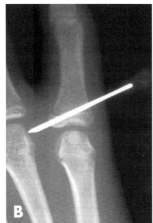

Figure 1

A, Lateral stress combined with axial loading resulted in a Salter type 2 avulsion fracture. The bone fragment was pulled off by the attached collateral ligament. **B,** Fixation with a single K-wire was sufficient.

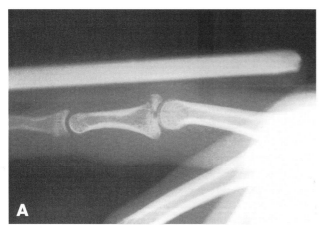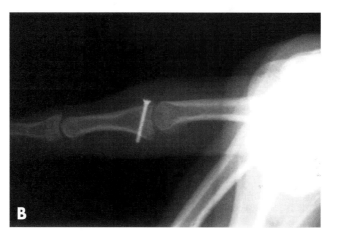

Figure 2

A, In this bony boutonnière-type fracture, the disruption of the central slip attachment to the base of the middle phalanx resulted in a typical boutonnière deformity. **B,** If the detachment is with a large enough bony fragment, secure fixation can be obtained with a lag screw.

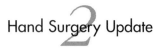
stretched or partly torn ligaments, are very common and do not result in joint instability; however, they can lead to significant tenderness and pain for months. Passive tests of joint stability, particularly lateral stress to the joints in 10° to 15° of flexion, may produce pain without indicating instability in these injuries.

Similar mechanisms of injury can produce collateral ligament tears. In these cases, lateral stress to the anesthetized joints in 10° to 15° of flexion produces large angular displacement. If such displacement is 20° more than the contralateral side, collateral ligament tear is generally assumed. These tears warrant surgical reconstruction, with either direct repair of the ligament, reattachment through bone tunnels or suture anchor techniques, or ligament replacement with palmaris longus tendon graft.

Proximal IP joint dislocations are usually the result of hyperextension forces combined with axial compression. The middle phalanx most commonly dislocates dorsal to the proximal phalanx (Fig. 3). The 3-sided box consisting of the collateral ligaments and palmar plate stabilizing the IP joints is disrupted in joint dislocation, which requires damage to at least one of these 3 structures. Most often the palmar plate becomes detached from its insertion at the volar base of P2, with or without a bony avulsion fragment. The avulsion fragment may be small, as in simple PIP hyperextension injury without dislocation, or large (> 35% to 40% of the articular surface). In rare instances, the palmar plate can become detached proximally at its origin behind the condyles of the proximal phalanx (P1). With this proximal injury, the palmar plate is more likely to become interposed in the joint, preventing reduction.

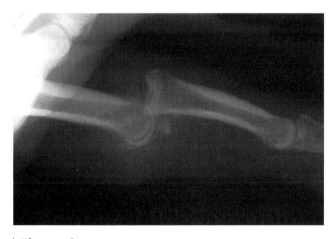

Figure 3

This dorsal proximal interphalangeal dislocation left a typical comminuted volar fragment at the base of the middle phalanx. Reduction was simple, and a dorsal blocking pin afforded stability while allowing motion through a protected arc.

In the absence of interposed soft tissue, reduction is usually simple. Postreduction stability must be carefully checked. With small or no bony injury, stability is usually afforded with slight flexion of the joint. Maintenance in a dorsal block splint for 2 weeks in 30° to 40°of flexion, with further flexion encouraged within the confines of the splint, may be followed by straightening the splint to 10° to 15° for an additional 10 to 14 days. Alternately, the joint can be flexed sufficiently to maintain stability of the reduction and then splinted in this position. Lateral radiographs confirm the adequacy of reduction. Over a period of 2 to 4 weeks, the extension block splint is gradually straightened, with periodic radiographic checks to ensure that the reduction remains congruent. Stability may not be achieved by flexion alone, especially if the volar P2 fragment is large or comminuted. Lateral images must confirm that the condyles of P1 and the base of P2 are precisely congruent. Widening of the joint space dorsally signifies an inadequate reduction.

If the P2 fragment is single and sufficiently large, open reduction and fixation of this fragment (to which the palmar plate and part or all of the collateral ligaments remain attached) ensures stability. Lag-screw fixation with 1.0 or 1.2 mm screws is technically difficult, but will lead to the best results if the articular surface is perfectly restored. Alternately, a steel or Prolene pull-out suture can be passed from the dorsum of the phalanx through the fracture site, into the fragment and back to the dorsum of the phalanx. The suture can be tied either directly over the bone, or over a button on the skin. Comminution of the P2 fracture may preclude open reduction and internal fixation; in this situation, palmar plate arthroplasty may result in stability, congruent joint reduction, and acceptable motion.

The primary complication of closed treatment of PIP dislocations is flexion contracture. The trade-off between maintenance of a dorsal block splint for stability and free unrestricted motion must be carefully considered. A residual flexion contracture of 10° to 20° is not uncommon. The joint frequently remains enlarged, because scar in the collateral ligaments and around the joint is poorly disguised by the thin soft-tissue covering. Patients may complain about residual swelling, when in fact the enlargement is not edema but more permanent scar. Rings should generally not be resized until 1 year after injury—some of this enlargement will recede as the scar matures.

Untreated PIP dislocations that are reduced but not splinted can sometimes lead to chronic hyperextension deformity if the palmar plate fails to reattach and provide restraint against hyperextension. Late reattachment of the palmar plate varies in effectiveness, often resulting in chronic flexion contracture.

Infrequently, the middle phalanx (P2) can dislocate laterally or volarly with respect to the proximal phalanx. Lateral dislocations are usually stable after reduction and can be treated with a dorsal block splint for 2 to 3 weeks. Volar dislocations are sometimes irreducible. Longitudinal compression and rotatory force are usually responsible for the deformity, and the condyle of P1 can buttonhole through a rent between the central slip and lateral band. The extensor mechanism will then be caught in the joint, and axial traction in a reduction attempt may tighten the extensor mechanism buttonhole, preventing reduction. Gentle traction with MCP and PIP flexion, combined with a rotational force, can sometimes unlock the buttonholed extensor mechanism from around the proximal phalangeal condyle. If this maneuver fails, however, open reduction is often necessary. The approach is through a midaxial or dorsal incision, and the interposed soft tissue is removed from the joint. Because the disruption is primarily of the extensor mechanism, immobilization should be in extension (Fig. 4).

Distal Interphalangeal Fractures and Dislocations

DIP joint dislocation is less common than PIP dislocation, and is usually more stable after reduction. The moment arm acting on the joint is short, and the collateral ligaments stout. The attachment of the flexor digitorum profundus provides additional stability. The dislocated distal phalanx is most often displaced dorsally or laterally. Because the skin at the DIP joint adheres tightly to surrounding structures, the dislocation is often open and appropriate measures should be taken to cleanse the joint. Reduction is generally achieved

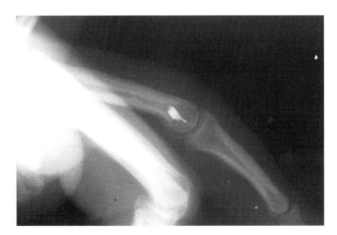

Figure 4

Less common than the dorsal dislocation, proximal interphalangeal dislocations can occur in the volar direction. This case required open reduction because the head of the proximal phalanx buttonholed through a rent between the lateral band and the central slip, preventing reduction. After open reduction, the joint was unstable due to a complete tear of the collateral ligament. The ligament was reattached with the aid of a suture anchor.

by closed manipulation. Flexor tendon avulsions can occur with or without bony fragments, as classified by Leddy and Packer. In type I injuries, the flexor tendon retracts into the palm and both vinculae of the flexor are ruptured. Vascularity, usually provided through vinculae, is impaired and results are poor. Type II injuries are more common when the long vinculum remains intact and the tendon retracts only to the PIP joint. A type III injury involves the largest bone fragment, which precludes retraction of the tendon beyond the A4 pulley. Surgical repair of the tendon avulsion with a steel or Prolene pull-out suture over a button should be performed. If the bony fragment is large (type III), lag-screw fixation is most effective. On rare occasions, a type III fracture is combined with a flexor avulsion from the fragment (type IIIA); repair must include both the fracture and the tendon avulsion.

Axial impaction injury at the DIP joint can result in comminution of the articular surfaces. This commonly occurs in sports activity when a baseball impacts the end of the finger ("baseball finger" injury). This situation sometimes requires open reduction and internal fixation with bone graft.

P1 and P2 Fractures Extending into the Phalangeal Bases

Shaft fractures that extend into the base of P1 and P2 can be associated with articular incongruity. Spiral fractures of the phalanges can cause rotational and angular deformity of the digit as well as articular step-off. Nondisplaced fractures can be treated by 3 weeks of cast or splint immobilization. Safe position splinting (MCP joints flexed 80° to 90°, IP joints extended), followed by supervised mobilization, will generally result in excellent function. Radiographs must be obtained weekly to check for displacement; if displacement occurs, rapid surgical intervention is needed.

Reduction and fixation are necessary if deformity exists. In the absence of articular comminution, fixation technique is generally dictated by the type of shaft fracture. In a typical spiral oblique phalangeal fracture, if the length of the fracture line is greater than 3 times the diameter of the bone, lag-screw fixation with 2 or 3 well-placed lag screws usually suffices. This has historically been an open procedure, but with the advent of various targeting devices fixation can sometimes be performed percutaneously. If the length of the fracture line is less than 2 times the diameter of the bone, plate fixation may be required. Screws of 1.2, 1.3, 1.5, 1.7, or 2.0 mm are generally used in the middle and proximal phalanges. Appropriate overdrilling of a gliding hole for the screw affords maximal compression with lag-screw techniques, which can be employed with or without plates (Fig. 5).

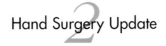

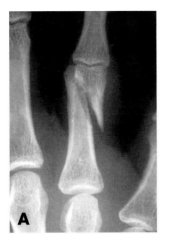
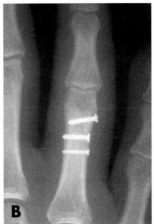

Figure 5

Oblique phalangeal shaft fractures may extend into the adjacent joints. **A,** In this case, the obliquity was over 3 times the length of the phalangeal diameter. **B,** Lag-screw fixation was secure and sufficient.

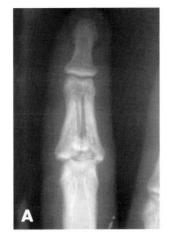
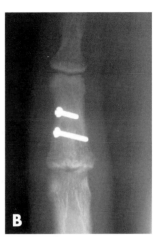

Figure 6

A, In this comminuted pilon fracture of the base of the phalanx, peripheral fragments were large enough to allow lag-screw fixation. Bone graft from the distal radius was packed into the void left after reduction of the central depressed articular fragment, and the bone graft helped prevent overcompression by the lag screws. **B,** Secure fixation was achieved, allowing early protected motion.

Pilon and Comminuted Base Fractures of P1 and P2

Injury due to an axial compression force can result in impaction and comminution of the base of the phalanx. Pilon-type fractures present with volar and dorsal articular rims of the base of the phalanx split away from the shaft, and central depression of comminuted articular fragments. These injuries can be extremely difficult to reconstruct. Small central depressed fragments may not be amenable to secure fixation. Bone graft is useful in supporting articular fragments from behind, but must be combined with some form of stabilizing fixation. Lag-screw fixation must be used carefully; with extensive comminution, it can lead to compression of adjacent sides of the articular surface through the area of bone void (Fig. 6).

Step-by-step reduction and interfragmentary fixation of the shaft components can sometimes help reestablish the articular surface. Some form of traction and early motion is usually the best treatment for these difficult fractures. A number of methods of external traction have been described. Traction can be achieved with a transverse pin through P1 for base of P1 injuries, or through P2 for base of P2 injuries. The pin is attached by rubber bands to an outrigger Schenk-type splint carefully constructed so that the center of rotation is appropriately placed and protected motion can be achieved with traction. Alternatives are force couple splints or a mobile external fixator (Fig. 7). These are particularly appropriate at the PIP joint. If carefully applied,

they permit active and passive mobilization, which has been shown to benefit cartilage healing, while maintaining traction at the joint. With central articular fragment depression or with wide divergence of articular rim fragments, open reduction and internal fixation combined with traction is useful. When an axially directed force produces the fracture, fragments around the circumference of the bone may be relatively large and central fragments small. In this circumstance, cerclage wiring may be effective, with 24-gauge stainless steel wire providing circumferential containment of the fragments. Significant dissection is necessary, however, and postoperative stiffness is often severe.

Studies have shown that remodeling of the joint surface is possible, and is enhanced by early motion. Although radiographic results can be quite worrisome with clearly widened articular surfaces, acceptable clinical results can be achieved if overall congruity of the joint margins is maintained without subluxation. One group found that, while anatomic joint surface reduction has been shown to be important in larger joints, good results can be achieved after PIP joint pilon fractures without such anatomic reconstruction of the articular surface so long as joint subluxation is eliminated. With persistent joint subluxation, however, glide of P2 around the condyles of P1 cannot be congruent, and pain and disability result. Early protected motion of the injured joint must be initiated as soon as possible, particularly if the joint surface is not anatomically reconstructed. This motion is usually initiated with application of some form of traction.

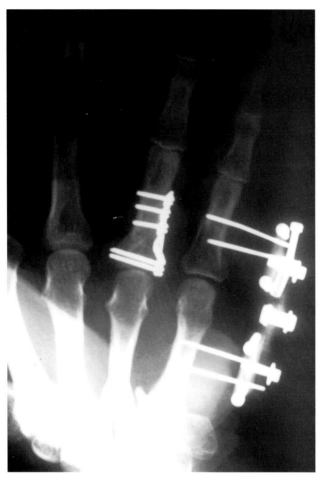

Figure 7

Comminution at the bases of the proximal phalanges of ring and small fingers make fixation difficult. A condylar plate secured the ring finger, while a mobile external fixator was used for the small finger. Early motion was facilitated.

Metacarpophalangeal Joint Injuries

The moment arm acting on the MCP joints is greater than that on the PIP or DIP joints by virtue of the additional length of the finger. However, the MCP joints are stabilized by the intermetacarpal ligaments and the adjacent MCP joints so that dislocation is less common than in the more distal joints. The sagittal bands of the extensor hood also provide stability that is absent in the more distal

joints. The border joints of the index and small fingers are more often dislocated than the central joints. Forced hyperextension of the joint usually produces rupture of the palmar plate at its attachment to the metacarpal. The cartilaginous palmar plate then often becomes interposed between the articular surfaces. The lumbrical muscles and flexor tendons, and the abductor digiti quinti tendon in the small finger may impede reduction.

Reduction should be attempted by flexing the wrist to relax the flexor tendons and applying pressure directly over the proximal phalanx, trying to slide it into a more volar position. The prominence of the metacarpal head can be felt in the palm when the proximal phalanx is displaced dorsally. If this closed reduction technique fails, open reduction is necessary through either a dorsal or a volar approach. A safe dorsal approach can be made to the joint and the palmar plate found interposed. If the palmar plate is split longitudinally, it can be extracted from the joint and replaced in its native position. A volar approach allows direct observation and treatment of the volar structures blocking reduction; however, this approach puts the neurovascular bundle, which is draped tightly over the volarly displaced metacarpal head, at risk. Release of the A1 pulley facilitates extraction of the metacarpal head from the noose of soft-tissue blocking reduction.

Metacarpal head fractures have been classified by McElfresh as epiphyseal, ligamentous avulsion, osteochondral, oblique sagittal, vertical coronal, horizontal transverse, and comminuted. The second metacarpal had the highest incidence of head fracture, followed by the small finger—both border digits. For a noncomminuted displaced intra-articular metacarpal head fracture, open reduction and internal fixation with lag screws or tension band wiring may provide satisfactory results. Bone stock is usually of reasonable quality to allow purchase of screws. A dorsal approach splitting the extensor tendon affords exposure. Particularly for horizontal transverse fractures, the incidence of osteonecrosis is very high. Surgical fixation of comminuted head fractures is often futile. Fragments can be very small, and the head can fragment like an egg shell. Often, the overall contour of the head is maintained. A short period of immobilization for 2 weeks in MCP flexion followed by aggressive therapy may provide acceptable results. Skeletal traction can allow immediate mobilization and may reduce stiffness. Traction can be afforded by a Schenk-type splint, or a mobile external fixator in the case of a border digit (Fig. 8). Stiffness is the most common complication of metacarpal head fractures.

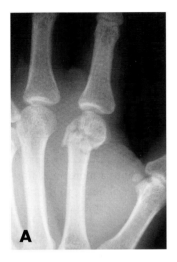

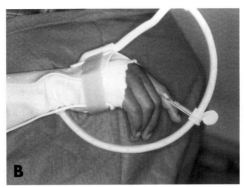

Figure 8

A, Fragmentation of the metacarpal head precluded open reduction and internal fixation in this comminuted head fracture. **B,** Traction was provided with a transverse pin through the middle phalanx and a Schenk-type splint. Early motion was permitted and an excellent result achieved.

Uni- and Bicondylar Fractures of the Proximal and Middle Phalanges

London classified condylar fractures as stable nondisplaced (type I), unstable unicondylar (type II), and bicondylar (type III). Unicondylar (types I and II) fractures were further classified by Weiss and Hastings as volar, sagittal, or coronal. Often overlooked, these fractures can lead to significant disability. Unicondylar fractures that are initially undisplaced will frequently displace over the course of immobilization. Such displacement can lead to angular deformity of the finger and articular incongruity. Posteroanterior, lateral, and often oblique radiographs should be obtained to rule out such injury.

Type I fractures can be treated closed with immobilization if frequent radiographs are taken. Surgical intervention must be considered at the first sign of displacement. Type II fractures (all displaced fractures in the Weiss and Hastings classification) can be treated by compression fixation with lag screws, or K-wires with or without lag screws. Exacting technique is necessary; these fractures can be quite difficult to fix well. Occasionally, percutaneous reduction and fixation can be achieved under fluoroscopic control, but an imperfect reduction is not acceptable. Open reduction is

achieved through a gently curved dorsal incision favoring the ulnar or radial side. For sagittal split and dorsal coronal fractures, the approach to the proximal phalangeal condyles can usually be made between the central slip and lateral band, to prevent detachment of the central slip. The fractured condyle remains attached to the collateral ligament, through which it receives much of its blood supply; detachment from the collateral ligament must be avoided. In direct vision, the fracture can be reduced and held in place with provisional bone clamps. Lag screws provide the most secure fixation when 2 screws can be inserted (Fig. 9). If 2 screws of 1.0 or 1.2 mm diameter cannot be used, one screw and a K-wire will suffice. If the bony interdigitations are sufficiently interlocked with compression, one screw may be sufficient.

Type III fractures are more complex. Closed reduction and immobilization will not provide stability to displaced fragments. If the condylar fractures are asymmetric, lag-screw fixation of both condyles to each other and to the shaft of the phalanx can be achieved. If they are symmetric and the fracture line between the shaft and the condyles is relatively transverse, plate fixation is usually needed. The condylar plate is ideally suited to these fractures, but its application is technically quite demanding. Exposure must be sufficient to allow reduction and fixation without devascularizing the fragments. Usually one condyle is first reduced and fixed to the other, and then the reduced head fragment is secured to the shaft. Occasionally, in the presence of comminution, bone graft should be used to prevent overcompression of the condyles or shortening of the shaft.

Carpometacarpal Dislocations

Up to 70% of carpometacarpal (CMC) dislocations of the fingers occur at the fifth metacarpal–hamate junction. The relative mobility of the fifth CMC joint, its border position, and the inclination of the junction with the base of the hamate all contribute to this high occurence. An axial compression force is usually responsible for the fracture-dislocation. Because the fourth metacarpal base also articulates with the hamate, both

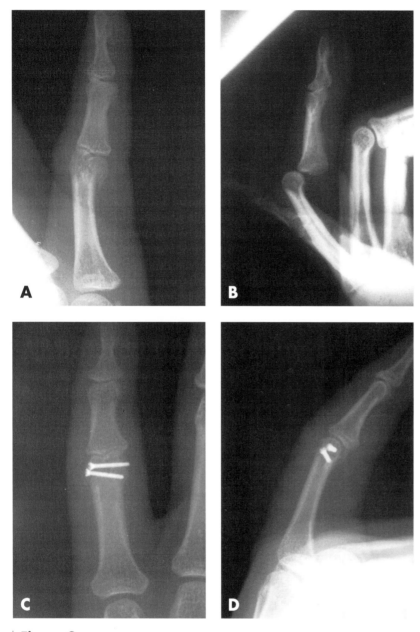

ture). The pull of the flexor and extensor carpi ulnaris and the abductor digiti minimi contribute to the proximal displacement of the metacarpal (Fig. 10).

Diagnosis may be elusive. Perfectly positioned posteroanterior and lateral views of the hand are mandatory; oblique views are sometimes needed. The tendency of X-ray technicians to accept less than perfect positioning can lead to errors in diagnosis. Often the wrist remains slightly dorsiflexed and the MCP and IP joints slightly flexed with a painful, swollen hand. This obscures the CMC junctions and precludes accurate diagnosis. Similarly, if the attempted lateral view is just slightly oblique, subtle dorsal displacement of the metacarpal base may be missed because it can be obscured by adjacent bony structures. Occasionally, computed tomographic scans may provide definitive diagnosis and elucidation of fracture patterns at the base of the metacarpal.

The fifth CMC junction is the most mobile of the 4 fingers. Articular irregularities are more prone to generate symptoms here than in the less mobile index or middle finger CMC junction.

Although reduction is generally easily achieved, it is often not easily maintained. In the case of simple dislocation without fracture, stability is assessed after reduction; if adequate, cast immobilization for 3 to 4 weeks allows stabilization of the ligamentous supports. Frequent radiographs must be taken, however, as redisplacement is common. If instability exists, percutaneous pinning from the fifth metacarpal base to either the hamate or the adjacent fourth metacarpal base stabilizes the dislocation. Fluoroscopy assists in the reduction and pin fixation. The dorsal sensory branch of the ulnar nerve is at risk in fourth and fifth CMC dislocations, and the dorsal sensory branch of the radial

Figure 9

This type II unicondylar fracture was effectively treated with 2 small (1.2-mm) lag screws. Accurate joint reduction without detachment of the collateral ligament ensures the best results. **A** and **B,** Preoperative posteroanterior and lateral radiographs. **C** and **D,** Postoperative views.

intermetacarpal ligaments as well as volar and dorsal ligaments between the metacarpal base and the hamate help stabilize the joint. The radial side of the fifth metacarpal base often remains attached to the hamate and fourth metacarpal base by these ligaments as the ulnar portion of the base and shaft displace (reverse Bennett's-type fifth metacarpal frac-

nerve is at risk in second and third CMC dislocations. If comminution exists at the base of the metacarpal or the carpus and the fragments are large enough, accurate open reduction and fixation should be performed. Otherwise, molding of the articulation can occur and healing may proceed to allow a reasonably functional joint, but pain may be

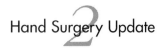

Fracture dislocations at the PIP joint are reviewed. Three types of fracture-dislocations are identified—palmar lip fractures with dorsal subluxation, dorsal lip fractures with palmar subluxation, and pilon fractures with central depression. Dorsal and palmar lip fractures are further classified into stable, tenuous, and unstable. Reduction of any associated subluxation is critical to a good result, but anatomic restoration of the articular surface is not. Use of a mobile PIP fixator allows early motion and provides stability to the joint in otherwise unstable injuries. This technique can be used in combination with open reduction and internal fixation or palmar plate arthroplasty. Guidelines for acceptable treatment of these difficult injuries are discussed.

Krakauer JD, Stern PJ: Hinged device for fractures involving the proximal interphalangeal joint. *Clin Orthop* 1996;327:29–37.

Twenty patients had a mobile PIP external fixator applied in conjunction with closed or open reduction of an articular injury of the PIP joint. In the acute fractures, postoperative range of PIP motion was 9° to 82°; in a group of chronic injuries, the range was 21° to 77°. The fixator was found to be an excellent device for treatment of these complex injuries.

Rawes ML, Oni OO: Swan-neck deformity as a complication of the Agee technique. *J Hand Surg* 1995;20B:255–257.

This case report demonstrates one of the pitfalls of application of the Agee force-couple splint.

Weiss AP, Hastings H II: Distal unicondylar fractures of the proximal phalanx. *J Hand Surg* 1993;18A:594–599.

Unicondylar fractures are classified as oblique volar, long sagittal, dorsal coronal, or volar coronal. This is a more detailed classification than provided by London, and is a subset of his type I and type II fractures. Treatment was not stratified by fracture classification, and results did not differ significantly by classification. Thirty-six of 38 fractures required surgical intervention. Average extension was 13°, and flexion 85°. Selection and placement of fixation devices is discussed in relation to fracture type.

Distal Interphalangeal Fractures and Dislocations

Lubahn JD, Hood JM: Fractures of the distal interphalangeal joint. *Clin Orthop* 1996;327:12–20.

This review article summarizes etiology and treatment of mallet fingers, flexor digitorum profundus avulsions, and condylar fractures of the middle phalanx.

Takami H, Takahashi S, Ando M, Masuda A: Flexor digitorum profundus avulsion with associated fracture of the distal phalanx. *Acta Orthop Trauma Surg* 1997;116:504–506.

Two case reports of flexor digitorum profundus avulsion combined with distal phalanx (P3) fractures are cited; neither fits into the Leddy and Packer classification. In one acute case, the P3 fracture was extra-articular but otherwise similar to a type IV injury as classified by Smith. In another chronic case treated 20 months after injury, only tenolysis of the pseudotendon was performed. Despite this approach, 10° of DIP flexion was obtained in a pain-free finger with normal grip strength.

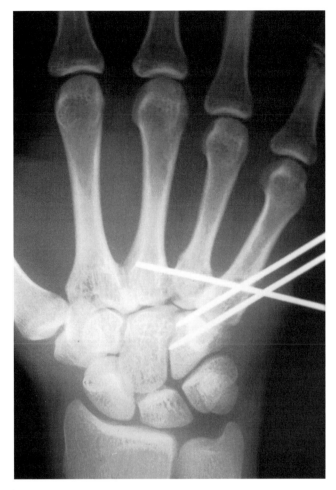

Figure 10

Dislocation of both the fourth and fifth metacarpals from the hamate often leads to instability. While reduction is generally easily accomplished, there may be a tendency to redislocate. Percutaneous pins between the fifth, fourth, and third metacarpals, and from the fifth metacarpal to the hamate, secured this dislocation.

persistent. In such cases, CMC fusion can be performed; however, the loss of motion at the fourth or fifth CMC junction is potentially more disabling than at the less mobile second or third CMC junction.

Annotated Bibliography

Proximal Interphalangeal Fractures and Dislocations

Kiefhaber TR, Stern PJ: Fracture dislocations of the proximal interphalangeal joint. *J Hand Surg* 1998;23A:368–380.

P1 and P2 Fractures Extending into the Phalangeal Bases

Allison DM: Fractures of the base of the middle phalanx treated by a dynamic external fixation device. *J Hand Surg* 1996;21B:305–310.

Fourteen patients with pilon or dorsal fracture dislocations of the PIP joint were treated with a spring-loaded external fixator that allowed active motion and provided distraction. All fractures were treated within 25 days of injury. Final postoperative range of motion of the PIP joint was 9° to 86°. Most patients had no pain or mild pain with use.

Pilon and Comminuted Base Fractures of P1 and P2

Seno N, Hashizume H, Inoue H, Imatani J, Morito Y: Fractures of the base of the middle phalanx of the finger: Classification, management and long-term results. *J Bone Joint Surg* 1997;79B:758–763.

Middle phalangeal base fractures were treated in 140 fingers. A new classification system based on radiologic and surgical findings established 5 main fracture types, 4 of which were intra-articular. Types 1 and 2 correspond to the traditional volar and dorsal avulsion fractures of the PIP joint, and type 3 was the pilon fracture. Computer modeling may be useful in predicting the fracture type based on mechanism of injury. Fifty-five percent of the fractures were treated nonsurgically, and 45% surgically. Damaged collateral ligaments or palmar plates were also repaired intraoperatively. Type 1 and 2 fractures had better overall results than types 3, 4, or 5. While poor radiologic results tended to correlate with poor clinical results, no single radiologic parameter predicted poor clinical results.

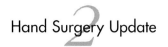

Chapter 4
Thumb Injuries

Thomas J. Fischer, MD

The unique anatomic and functional role of the thumb creates an environment of injury unto itself. The protective influences of adjacent stable rays are diminished by both distance and orientation. For the purpose of this review, both the nature of thumb injuries and their treatment are considered separately from other metacarpal, phalangeal, and intra-articular injuries of the digits. Included is a distinct section on carpometacarpal (CMC) joint injuries. This review will be divided into 5 categories of injury to anatomic structures—phalangeal (P1, P2) injuries, thumb interphalangeal (IP) joint injuries, metacarpal injuries, metacarpophalangeal (MCP) joint injuries, and CMC joint injuries.

The major role of the thumb dictates its treatment principles. Stability associated with power grasp and pinch is important to achieving acceptable outcomes. Restoration of complete and untethered range of motion of the distal 2 joints of the thumb is not essential in quantitative studies of the outcome of repair. However, full restoration of the first web space is a desired outcome when evaluating the basic hand functions of grasp, pinch, and hook grasp.

Phalangeal Injuries

Fractures of the thumb phalanges have no distinct differences in diagnosis and treatment from phalanges of other digits. One exception to this generalization lies in the use of intramedullary Kirschner wires (K-wires). For proximal phalanx fractures of the index through small finger rays, surgeons avoid transfixing the proximal interphalangeal joint and opt for an antegrade pin placement. Access to the intramedullary canal of the P1 (proximal) phalanx in the thumb is readily available across the forgiving IP joint of the thumb. Hence intramedullary pins for proximal phalanx fractures can be applied retrograde from the thumb tip for the treatment of unstable fractures not amenable to closed treatment. Indications for thumb phalangeal fracture treatment with internal fixation include: failure of closed reduction to maintain rotation, length, or angular alignment; intra-articular fractures in which joint incongruity will compromise small joint function; and unstable

fractures associated with significant soft-tissue injury, where fracture instability precludes the normal soft-tissue rehabilitation program (ie, flexor tendon rehabilitation).

The thumb position relative to the hand allows ready access for percutaneous K-wire fixation. All 3 periarticular areas of diaphysis are anatomically accessible to percutaneous application of K-wires. As with other digits, subcondylar fractures can be particularly unstable.

Interphalangeal Joint Injuries

Mallet bony avulsions or soft-tissue injuries occur less frequently in the thumb than in other digits. A report of 51 bony mallet fractures that were repaired with tension band looped wire or suture fixation included only 4 involving the thumb IP joint. Closed treatment remains appropriate unless the joint is subluxated.

Dislocation of the IP joint is treated (as with any small joint dislocation) by gentle reduction with adequate anesthesia. Bursting laceration of the palmar skin surface may give rise to open dislocation. These injuries are particularly common with thrown or batted balls. A recent review documents the irreducible IP dislocation with similar soft-tissue/tendon interposition preventing reduction. As with other IP joints of the hand, if the reduction is stable then pin fixation is unnecessary.

Metacarpal Fractures

Adjacent metacarpal soft-tissue attachments fail to provide the support for the thumb metacarpal that the index through little metacarpals provide for each other. Fractures that are often stable in the finger metacarpals, by virtue of the intermetacarpal ligaments and stable CMC joints, may prove unstable in the thumb. Manipulative reduction may obtain but not maintain anatomic alignment because of the pull of the adductor pollicis and thenar muscle. Typically, apex dorsal or apex radial deformities occur with fractures in the proximal quarter of the metacarpal. Extension of the thumb through the CMC joint coupled with retropulsion may place the thumb in a reduced position. Maintenance of this nonphysiologic position is not sustainable or tolerable with casts or splints. Percutaneous pinning can be used to maintain fracture alignment without splints or casts exerting undue pressure on the thumb MCP joint and proximal phalanx. Angulation of 20° to 25° at the fracture site is acceptable because of available compensatory motion at the CMC joint. In addition to loss of radial abduction with angular deformity, a loss of thenar muscle length and the mechanical advantage of the thenar muscle compromise MCP joint function. After reduction, angular deformity may recur due to medial comminution of a fracture at the base of the metacarpal.

Metacarpophalangeal Joint Injuries

The MCP joint is still the most frequently injured, and commands the largest share of scientific analysis and published work on the thumb. The injury patterns can be divided into 4 categories—hyperextension injuries/capsular injuries, articular fractures (without ligamentous avulsion), dislocations, and collateral ligament injuries.

Combinations of the above categories occur. Pure capsular injuries rarely occur in the absence of collateral ligament sprain. Fractures may involve a large bony fragment still attached to a collateral ligament. A stable pain-free thumb MCP joint is essential to the many activities of daily living requiring power pinch. Because pain inhibits pinch, a painful but stable arthrosis of the MCP or CMC joint is as disabling as an unstable MCP or CMC joint complex resulting from subluxation or ligament instability.

Hyperextension injuries result from forces applied by activity, including sport and industrial injury. Dorsal dislocation with volar plate avulsion and fracture of the sesamoid bones occur acutely. Late sequelae of untreated or unstable injuries to these structures can present as locking or subluxation. The palmar protrusion of the metacarpal head allows extension from a neutral position but blocks MCP flexion. In these cases, the metacarpal head may be protruding through a gap created by a band of radial accessory collateral ligament, radial sesamoid bone, and volar plate.

Sesamoid fractures were seen in 7 of 26 patient studied with MCP extension injuries. Acute treatment yielded good results while late treated sesamoid fractures resulted in MCP joint pain. Insertion of the strong thenar muscle onto the volar plate via the sesamoids appears to stabilize the volar plate. Disruption of this tendon-fibrocartilage-tendon complex may lead to volar structural instability.

Sesamoid degeneration is treated with excision. Injury to the ulnar sesamoid is more common than injury to the radial sesamoid. Closed treatment is the method of choice for stable injuries, with some splinting or taping of the joint to prevent further injury.

Dorsal radial capsular tears of the thumb MCP joint can occur in the absence of gross radial collateral ligament (RCL) or ulnar collateral ligament (UCL) injury. Pain, swelling, and local tenderness are the clinical findings. Focal dorsal tenderness in the absence of both tenderness at the RCL and pain with stress of the collateral ligaments remain the hallmark for diagnosis of dorsal capsular tears. Loss of active extension may be apparent. Initial treatment consists of immobilization with radiographic confirmation of thumb alignment in the cast or splint.

Metacarpophalangeal Joint Collateral Ligament Injuries

The bulk of injuries creating patient disability as well as both diagnostic and therapeutic dilemmas are MCP joint collateral ligaments. Acute and chronic injuries can occur to either the RCL or the UCL. Although UCL injuries have been more widely discussed, the RCL sprain can be equally disabling. Operative treatment of either is indicated if the ligament avulsion results in a bone fragment that has a significant portion of articular surface attached to it. Studies are unclear as to the amount of articular surface involvement or displacement that requires surgical fixation. Fragment size from 15% to 30% of the joint surface has been suggested as a threshold.

Little controversy exists for treating partial ligament injuries. In those nonoperative cases, the joint is reduced, the injury is a closed injury, and a definite end-point is felt on stress testing of the ligament. Ligament stress testing is done at 30° of MCP flexion to isolate the function of the UCL from the volar plate (Fig. 1). Radial deviation of 30° or more is considered diagnostic of complete rupture when the anesthetized injured joint is stressed in radial deviation. When the stress test is compared to the normal side, a difference of 20° is considered diagnostic. The presence of laxity of the UCL accessory collateral ligament is demonstrated when laxity is noted on testing with the joint in extension. If laxity is detected in both flexion and extension, the likelihood of a Stener lesion has been suggested to be as high as 80%.

It is here that the diagnostic dilemma presents itself. Do bony lesions with rotation or minimal displacement behave clinically like the pure soft-tissue counterpart? Does the presence of a Stener lesion constitute an indication for surgery? How many Stener lesions will be found in complete ruptures? Does a complete rupture displace enough without a true Stener configuration to warrant surgical correction? Finally, what diagnostic tools provide the best image and detection of a Stener lesion?

In cases of bony avulsion with minimal displacement or rotation, persistent pain can occur in a high percentage of patients despite appropriate immobilization. In those cases, surgical treatment yields satisfactory results in pain relief, strength, and mobility. In a series of 40 unstable thumbs treated with splint immobilization, all 12 bony avulsions healed. The majority had no pain, but 15% went on to late operative treatment. Late operative treatment has had less desirable results than acute treatment when pain, motion, stability, and strength are documented.

The incidence of a Stener lesion at surgical repair has been reported from 14% to 87%. This wide variability may reflect preselection bias of the cohorts based on clinical findings. Most agree that the physical examination and stress test can detect the majority of complete ruptures, yet detection of the Stener lesion has a high false negative rate by physical examination. Several studies now report the accuracy of ultrasound (US), magnetic resonance imaging (MRI), and MRI-enhanced arthrography to be superior to arthrography alone. Ultrasound has been shown as highly accurate in the hands of experienced examiners both with static and dynamic imaging. MRI and MRI-enhanced arthrography have been demonstrated to have greater sensitivity and greater specificity compared to US. The T2-weighted image of MRI is most useful. Ultrasound and MRI may be indicated in cases in which the stress test is positive or unclear and the patient wants to minimize the time for return to normal activities. An accurate early diagnosis can result in a shorter time to treatment, eliminating ineffective immobilization. Surgical repair of UCL tears has shown uniformly good results. Accurate anatomic repair (Fig. 2) and postoperative immobilization for 4 weeks is followed by initiation of active range of motion at 4 weeks; splinting is discontinued at 6 weeks. This compares favorably to nonsurgical treatment plans that require 8 to 12 weeks of cast or splint immobilization.

An understanding of "accurate anatomic repair" is enhanced by the knowledge that small changes in the proximal and distal origins of the UCL will substantially influence joint motion. Significant losses in flexion and ulnar stability occur in the laboratory with nonanatomic repair. Furthermore, the UCL is subjected to the least strain when the MCP joint is immobilized in extension. Strain is significantly greater in the 0° to 25° arc of motion of MCP flexion. No single method of repair or fixation using pull-out wires, drill holes through bone, tension

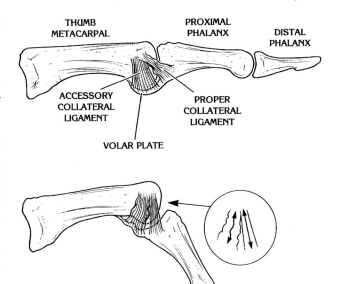

Figure 1

Anatomical relation of collateral ligament in flexion and extension (© Manus).

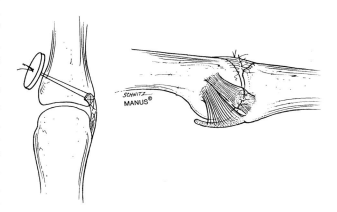

Figure 2

Interstitial repair and enthesis repair (© Manus).

band wires, K-wire fixation, arthroscopic reduction, or suture anchor attachment of ligament to bone has been shown to be superior to other methods. Authors do not agree on the amount of displacement of bony avulsion fracture fragments that constitute an indication for reduction. Good results with closed treatment have been reported in fractures with fragments smaller than 30% of

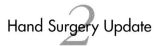

the articular surface and less than 1.5 mm of displacement. One series of patients with complete tears confirmed by stress testing underwent arthroscopic evaluation and reduction of displaced Stener lesions and pin fixation of the joint; good results equal to those of open repair were obtained. This method uses a small (1.7 mm) arthroscope. Good results with operative repair have been reported with and without the use of postoperative K-wire immobilization of the joint (Fig. 3).

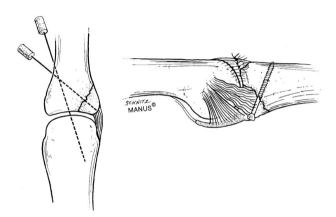

Figure 3

Avulsion fracture repair with and without joint fixation (© Manus).

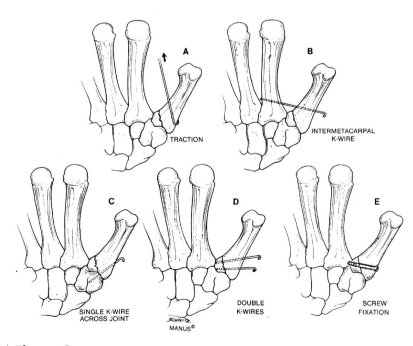

Figure 4

Methods of Bennett's fracture fragment fixation (© Manus).

MCP fusion remains an effective and functional salvage operation for cases of failed or painful joint repair.

Carpometacarpal Joint Injuries

The CMC joint facilitates the thumb's unique function as an opposable digit. Because of the complex shape of the articular surface and its unique soft-tissue support, the trapeziometacarpal (TMC) joint has a distinct set of injury patterns. Joint reactive forces at this joint are 10 to 12 times the force applied to the thumb tip in pinch and the thumb ray in grasp. Three basic injuries to the CMC joint can occur—dislocation of the TMC joint with soft-tissue avulsion, fracture/dislocation of the Bennett type, and comminuted fractures of the base of the metacarpal with intra-articular extension (Rolando fracture).

The ligamentous support for the TMC joint has 4 components. The dorsoradial ligament is most important in preventing dorsal subluxation. In experimental settings, the TMC joint did not dislocate with this ligament intact. In extension, the anterior oblique ligament prevented subluxation, but failed to give adequate support with any degree of TMC flexion. The intermetacarpal ligament and the posterior oblique ligament allowed complete dislocation in 20% of cases when these ligaments remained intact and all others sectioned. In TMC dislocations treated among historic cohorts, closed reduction and pinning resulted in a higher incidence of late subluxation when compared to early ligament reconstruction of the TMC joint with tendon graft. Degenerative changes were apparent and associated with symptoms of weakness and pain in those joints treated with closed reduction. Open reduction may demonstrate debris in the joint space. Eaton's stabilization technique uses distally based flexor carpi radialis tendon passed through the volar aspect of the first metacarpal to reconstruct the dorsoradial and anterior oblique ligaments.

Long-term evaluation of surgical treatment of Bennett's fracture has not had the same length of follow-up as closed treatment methods. Studies at 10 years after surgery demonstrate osteoarthritic changes in the TMC joint that correlate to the quality of initial joint reduction. Despite correlation of joint reduction

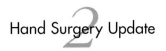
and osteoarthritic changes, symptoms of joint pain do not correlate with radiographic findings.

Displacement of articular surface fragments should be reduced to displacement of 1 mm or less. Bennett's fracture fragments can be held to the displaced shaft and joint surface with K-wires across the fracture, or across the joint indirectly stabilizing the fracture. Screw interfragmentary fixation can be used with larger fragments (Fig. 4). In highly comminuted fractures, screw and plate fixation is not obtainable. Reduction of the joint surface is obtained with K-wires and bone graft. An external fixator that maintains the relationship between the first and second metacarpal and first metacarpal to TMC joint is an effective means of fixation. In this fracture treatment technique, the external fixator serves to neutralize the deforming forces on the joint. The K-wires and bone graft serve to establish articular surface reduction, protected by the positioning of the external fixator (Fig. 5). In cases of multiple fragments of diaphysis and metaphysis, screw fixation can be used to lag the larger fragments together to reconstitute the joint and fixators used to align these coaptated fragments to the shaft.

Complex soft-tissue injuries with bone loss occur infrequently in the first web space. In many cases, fracture or instability to the base of the thumb accompany soft-tissue injury. An external fixator applied to the first and second metacarpals provides a means for controlling thumb position, affords access for soft-tissue wound care, and provides a stable platform that allows functional rehabilitation of unaffected digits.

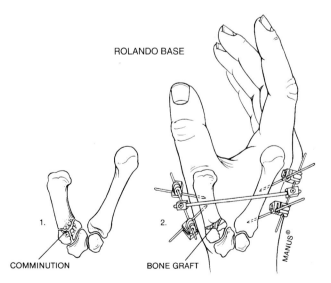

ROLANDO BASE

1.

COMMINUTION

2.

BONE GRAFT

MANUS®

Figure 5

Small frame external fixator used as a neutralization device (© Manus).

Annotated Bibliography

Metacarpophalangeal Joint Injuries

Adams BD, Muller DL: Assessment of thumb positioning in the treatment of ulnar collateral ligament injuries. *Am J Sports Med* 1996;24:672–675.

UCL strain was examined in a laboratory study to determine optimum position for immobilization or early motion. Strain increases readily from 0° to 25° of MCP flexion. Early motion will increase strain in the ligament with only small degrees of flexion.

Ahn JM, Sartoris DJ, Kang HS, et al: Gamekeeper thumb: Comparison of MR arthrography with conventional arthrography and MR imaging in cadavers. *Radiology* 1998;206:737–744.

High field strength MR arthrography was 100% accurate in assessing the presence of a tear in 14 surgically treated torn collateral ligaments. Displacement of the torn UCL was likewise detected with MR arthrography in 100% of specimens.

Bean CH, Tencer AF, Trumble TE: The effect of thumb metacarpophalangeal ulnar collateral ligament attachment site on joint range of motion: An in vitro study. *J Hand Surg* 1999;24A: 283–287.

This laboratory study demonstrates that joint flexion is decreased when the UCL is repaired with the distal insertion on the phalanx advanced distally. Flexion was diminished when the ligament was repaired to an extra-anatomic palmar location on P1.

Bischoff R, Buechler U, De Roche R, Jupiter J: Clinical results of tension band fixation of avulsion fractures of the hand. *J Hand Surg* 1994;19A:1019–1026.

Tension band stabilization of 38 displaced bony avulsions of the UCL were performed in 2 departments. Postoperative splints were used instead of K-wire transfixation of the MCP joint in all but one case. Thirty-one patients had excellent results with no pain; the other 7 patients had satisfactory results with occasional pain, stiffness, and cold-related ache. One patient had an asymptomatic nonunion. The authors describe surgical technique.

Dinowitz M, Trumble T, Hanel D, Vedder NB, Gilbert M: Failure of cast immobilization for thumb ulnar collateral ligament avulsion fractures. *J Hand Surg* 1997;22A:1057–1063.

Persistent thumb pain was found in 9 patients with small, minimally displaced bony avulsions at the base of the P1 phalanx. Despite prompt treatment and compliance with immobilization, pain persisted. Relief of signs and symptoms without alteration in motion resulted from late surgical intervention and bone fixation.

Dong PR, Seeger LL, Shapiro MS, Levere SM: Fractures of the sesamoid bones of the thumb. *Am J Sports Med* 1995; 23:336–339.

Fractures of the thumb sesamoid were detected with oblique radiographs in 8 cases. Dislocation was associated with one case. All were treated with immobilization for 2 to 3 weeks, which resulted in pain-free outcomes 2 months after injury.

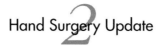

34　Thumb Injuries

Hergan K, Mittler C: Sonography of the injured ulnar collateral ligament of the thumb. *J Bone Joint Surg* 1995;77B:77–83.

Ultrasonographic examination of 30 patients was followed by surgical documentation of the lesion. Rupture and rupture with displacement of the ligament (Stener lesion) were correctly detected. Early examination with US improved diagnostic accuracy.

Hergan K, Mittler C, Oser W: Ulnar collateral ligament: Differentiation of displaced and nondisplaced tears with US and MR Imaging. *Radiology* 1995;194:65–71.

MRI of the torn UCL of 17 patients was more effective than US in differentiating displaced tears (Stener lesions). The T2-weighted sequence for scanning was used.

Hoglund M, Tordai P, Muren C: Diagnosis by ultrasound of dislocated ulnar collateral ligament of the thumb. *Acta Radiol* 1995;36:620–625.

Ultrasound was found to be effective in detecting a Stener lesion in 32 out of 39 operated patients. Scans were done both in a longitudinal and transverse orientation.

Jackson M, McQueen MM: Gamekeeper's thumb: A quantitative evaluation of acute surgical repair. *Injury* 1994;25:21–23.

Subjective and objective findings are compared for surgically treated UCL tears in 19 patients out of 44 who were treated from 1985 to 1988. Pain, subjective weakness, range of motion, and pinch and grip strength were documented in a standard manner. Subjective findings did not always correlate with objective measurements.

Kozin SH, Bishop AT: Tension wire fixation of avulsion fractures at the thumb metacarpophalangeal joint. *J Hand Surg* 1994;19A:1027–1031.

Rotation or displacement of avulsed UCL ligament fragments constituted indication for internal fixation with tension band wiring. Casting followed open reduction and internal fixation for 3 to 6 weeks. Tension band wire provides an excellent fixation method for stabilization of small fragments. Subjective and objective data suggest predictable good outcomes for accurate fracture reduction.

Krause JO, Manske PR, Mirly HL, Szerzinski J: Isolated injuries to the dorsoradial capsule of the thumb metacarpophalangeal joint. *J Hand Surg* 1996;21A:428–433.

Repair of the dorsoradial capsule in 7 of 11 symptomatic patients resulted in pain relief. Extension lag was found in 2 out of 7 patients despite pin fixation for 3 to 4 weeks. Ligamentous laxity may protect the collateral ligaments and allow capsular tears.

Kuz JE, Husband JB, Tokar N, McPherson SA: Outcome of avulsion fractures of the ulnar base of the proximal phalanx of the thumb treated nonsurgically. *J Hand Surg* 1999; 24A:275–282.

In this retrospective review of 30 patients who sustained bony avulsion fractures of the UCL insertion, none had surgery. All 30 answered a questionnaire, and 20 were examined. Three of 20 patients had instability and 25% had a nonunion. Effective outcomes were routinely achieved in the 30 patients manifest by their minimal symptoms and return to work and recreational activities.

Landsman JC, Seitz WH Jr, Froimson AI, Leb RB, Bachner EJ: Splint immobilization of gamekeeper's thumb. *Orthopedics* 1995;18:1161–1165.

Immobilization for 8 to 12 weeks was used to treat 39 patients with acute complete UCL tears. At an average follow-up of 2.4 years, 85% of patients had no significant pain, stiffness, arthrosis, or instability. Six patients were treated with late repair, and none had any bony avulsions. A satisfactory outcome was reported in these late repairs despite loss of motion and weakness of pinch; late repairs have been described by others as having diminished results when compared to acute repair.

Murphey SL, Hashimoto BE, Buckmiller J, Kramer D, Wiitala L: Ultrasonographic stress testing of ulnar collateral ligament injuries of the thumb. *J Ultrasound Med* 1997;16:201–207.

Real-time ultrasonography during stress testing was used to evaluate 25 patients with UCL injuries. Findings were confirmed surgically in 14 patients. Of the 11 patients treated in a cast, all healed without signs and symptoms. Two lesions determined by surgical findings were missed in the ultrasonographic evaluation.

Ryu J, Fagan R: Arthroscopic treatment of acute complete thumb metacarpophalangeal ulnar collateral ligament tears. *J Hand Surg* 1995;20A:1037–1042.

Arthroscopic reductions of displaced ulnar collateral ligaments were obtained in 8 surgically treated thumbs. Reduction of the joint was maintained with a K-wire. Reduction of the ligament to the avulsed bony bed was confirmed arthroscopically.

Weiland AJ, Berner SH, Hotchkiss RN, McCormack RR Jr, Gerwin M: Repair of acute ulnar collateral ligament injuries of the thumb metacarpophalangeal joint with an intraosseous suture anchor. *J Hand Surg* 1997;22A:585–591.

Suture anchors were successfully used to reapproximate the avulsed ligament to bone in 30 patients treated surgically for complete ruptures.

Carpometacarpal Joint Injuries

Simonian PT, Trumble TE: Traumatic dislocation of the thumb carpometacarpal joint: Early ligamentous reconstruction versus closed reduction and pinning. *J Hand Surg* 1996;21A:802–806.

CMC instability resultant of trauma may cause recurrent dislocation or subluxation and early posttraumatic degenerative joint disease. Two groups were studied, with similar ages and timing of treatment. Closed reduction and percutaneous pinning resulted in recurrent subluxation in 50% of cases. In the group of 9 patients treated with early ligament reconstruction with tendon graft, no recurrent subluxation occurred and clinical results were acceptable.

Strauch RJ, Behrman MJ, Rosenwasser MP: Acute dislocation of the carpometacarpal joint of the thumb: An anatomic and cadaver study. *J Hand Surg* 1994;19A:93–98.

The strongest restraint to dorsal dislocation of the CMC joint when tested with applied laboratory loads is the dorsoradial ligament.

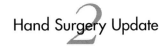

Chapter 5
Reconstruction of Finger Deformities

Keith B. Raskin, MD

Introduction

Deformities and posttraumatic arthritis affecting the small joints of the fingers can limit a wide range of hand functions depending on the specific affected digit, associated pain, loss of motion, and postural malalignment. Both posttraumatic and arthritic changes of the digits can create disability due to pain or loss of function. Although arthrodeses of the interphalangeal (IP) and metacarpophalangeal (MCP) joints alleviate pain, the cost is restricted motion. Advances in surgical techniques for arthrodeses of the hand ensure a more reliable, rapid union rate. The quest to achieve pain relief while preserving digit motion has led to advances in arthroplasty design, surgical procedures, and postoperative management. The use of osteochondral autograft reconstruction from a lower demand articular region of the hand or foot has expanded the options for treatment of the traumatized digit. Periarticular injuries of the digit can result in both complex articular damage and disruption of the surrounding supportive soft tissue. The palmar plate arthroplasty technique has evolved, along with awareness of the role of collateral ligament contractures in flexion deformities of the proximal interphalangeal (PIP) joint.

Proximal phalangeal diaphyseal malunions can be devastating injuries because of pain, motion limitation, loss of strength, tendon imbalance, and hand dysfunction secondary to a scissoring overlap to the adjacent digit. Improved understanding of malunion pathoanatomy has led to more predictable osteotomies with the possibility of restored hand function.

Arthrodesis

Arthrodesis of the small joints of the hand remains the mainstay of treatment for painful or deformed digital articulation. The distal interphalangeal (DIP) joints that are most adversely affected by osteoarthritis are effectively treated by compression arthrodesis techniques, because pinch and grasp strength depend more on distal phalangeal stability than motion. The optimal position of fusion varies from 10°

to 20°, with increasing flexion posture for the ulnar digits. In contrast, the sacrifice of motion of the PIP joint for the relief of pain, correction of angular deformity, or restoration of stability must be weighed when evaluating a digit for arthrodesis instead of arthroplasty. The index and middle fingers are more appropriate for arthrodesis because they must have lateral stability for lateral pinch. The ring and small finger PIP joints are more often considered for arthroplasty to preserve flexion motion's contribution to grasp, eliminate pain, and maintain maximum function.

Although the thumb carpometacarpal (CMC) joint non-implant arthroplasty has gained popularity with trapezial excision and soft-tissue reconstruction, the MCP and IP joints are dependably treated by arthrodesis. The commonly affected thumb MCP joint is well-suited for fusion in approximately 15° of flexion. Careful evaluation of the IP and CMC joints is essential in the comprehensive management of thumb MCP joint arthritis, because concomitant conditions may affect the patient's ability to adapt to the loss of metacarpal joint motion.

Recent advances in implant arthroplasty design, surgical technique, and postoperative management are challenging the concept of fusion of the PIP and MCP joints in the treatment of the common arthropathies.

Finger Interphalangeal Joints

Of the recent advances in fusion of the small joints of the hand, none have stimulated a greater interest than current compression arthrodesis techniques. Although the technology has expanded to provide new equipment and implants, not all treatment modalities have been confirmed as beneficial.

In a recent cadaveric study, DIP joints were stabilized with either Herbert screw fixation or tension band wire arthrodesis. Mechanical testing revealed a significantly increased anteroposterior bending strength and greater torsional rigidity in the Herbert screw specimens. A substantial majority of specimens (10 of 15 males and 15 of 15 females) demonstrated distal phalangeal fractures, thread penetration at the tip, and nailbed disturbance with the Herbert screw. Although increased rigidity can be obtained with this technique, it may not be well suited for smaller diameter (< 3.9 mm) distal phalanges (Fig. 1).

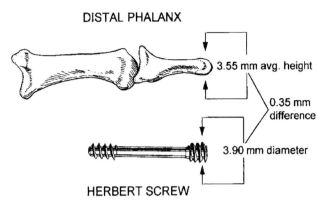

DISTAL PHALANX

3.55 mm avg. height

0.35 mm difference

3.90 mm diameter

HERBERT SCREW

Figure 1

The difference in diameter between the distal phalanx and Herbert compression screw can lead to thread penetration and nailbed disturbance in distal interphalangeal arthrodesis. (Reproduced with permission from Wyrsch B, Dawson J, Aufranc S, Weikert D, Milek M: Distal interphalangeal joint arthrodesis comparing tension-band wire and Herbert screw: A biomechanical and dimensional analysis. *J Hand Surg* 1996;21A:438–443.)

In another review of 224 PIP joint arthrodeses, Herbert screw fixation demonstrated superior results when compared to other fusion techniques. Herbert screw fixation resulted in a lower nonunion rate than Kirschner wires (K-wires), tension band wires, or plate fixation. Attention was directed to precise surgical technique. Iatrogenic fracture was avoided during insertion of the Herbert screw by accurate proximal placement of the starting drill hole away from the arthrodesis site along the dorsal surface of the proximal phalanx. Clinical fusion was apparent at an average of 7 weeks while radiographic confirmation was noted by 10 weeks regardless of technique. Segmental bone loss and comminution are contraindications to Herbert screw fusion.

Tension band arthrodesis continues to be popular due to the simplicity of the surgical technique and the paucity of related complications (Fig. 2). Of 290 tension band fusions of the PIP and MCP joints, only 10 required treatment for failure of union. Nine percent required removal of hardware. Long-term complications were avoided in the vast majority of patients. It has been suggested that postoperative external splinting can be avoided in the cooperative patient, a significant benefit for the rheumatoid patient

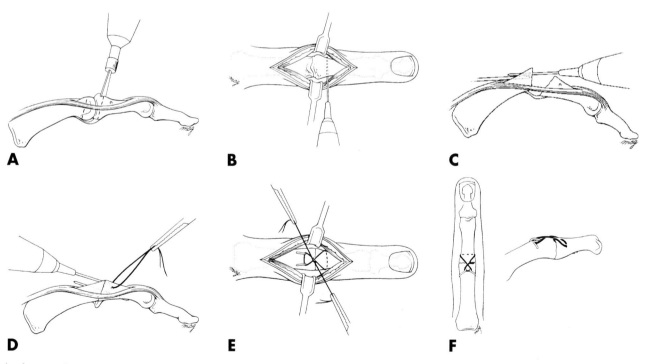

A   **B**   **C**

D   **E**   **F**

Figure 2

Surgical technique of proximal interphalangeal tension band arthrodesis. **A,** Phalangeal osteotomy at desired angle with oscillating saw. **B,** Preparation for 25- or 26-gauge stainless steel wire. **C,** Retrograde insertion of K-wires. **D,** Wire advancement into anterior cortex of middle phalanx. **E,** Figure-of-eight tension band. **F,** Final views after completion of procedure. (Reproduced with permission from Stern PJ, Gates NT, Jones TB: Tension band arthrodesis of small joints in the hand. *J Hand Surg* 1993;18A:194–197.)

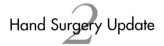
undergoing simultaneous MCP joint implant arthroplasty requiring postoperative extension outrigger splint.

Regardless of the technique of internal fixation of arthrodesis of the hand, the attainment of fusion still depends on complete crossbridging across the intended fusion site. Maximal cancellous bone surface contact is a major contributing factor to strong union. The various techniques include flat cuts, chevron cuts, and the cup and cone technique. In one recent series using K-wire fixation of chevron cuts, successful union was achieved in all 98 joints within an average of 9 weeks. Only one malunion and 2 minor infections were noted. The apex of the chevron is proximal. Precise bone cuts are required to achieve the appropriate degree of flexion.

Thumb Metacarpophalangeal Joint

Arthritic degeneration as well as posttraumatic chronic instability resulting in weakness, pain, and functional limitations can affect the thumb MCP joint. Due to its unique role in opposition and critical involvement in hand functions, instability or arthritis of the MCP joint of the thumb can be disabling.

Hyperextension injuries of the thumb often result in restoration of pain-free motion after a prolonged period of healing of the volar plate and surrounding soft tissue. Residual hyperextension deformity of the MCP joint secondary to trauma or as a result of concomitant CMC arthritis can limit strength and function. Hyperextension deformities of the thumb MCP joint are also seen in patients with cerebral palsy. Sesamoid arthrodesis to the thumb metacarpal has been suggested as treatment of the hyperextended MCP joint of the thumb in both the cerebral palsy patient and arthritic CMC joint patient (Fig. 3). In a review of 42 patients, hyperextension deformity was prevented in all but

3 patients with cerebral palsy and 1 patient with basal joint arthroplasty. There was an average loss of only 8° of MCP flexion compared to preoperative motion; however, a range of 5° to 70° of flexion was preserved. This technique provides an alternative to MCP arthrodesis in patients with more than 30° of preoperative flexion of the MCP joint.

Advances in bioabsorbable implants have led to their use in arthrodesis of the thumb MCP joint in an effort to avoid complications of hardware and the need for implant removal. High molecular weight polylactic acid rods and pins were evaluated in experimental and clinical settings for arthrodesis. Histologic studies showed resorption of the implant beginning at 4 months and completing within 3 years without symptomatic inflammation. Of 13 thumb MCP joints fused by either 1 rod or 1 to 2 pins, complete uncomplicated arthrodesis occurred at 6 to 8 weeks. Further research into bioabsorbable implants will improve understanding of the optimal material for joint fusion and perhaps fracture fixation.

Arthroplasty-Implant

Metacarpophalangeal Joints

MCP implant arthroplasties continue to provide reliable treatment of painful, deviated, disrupted joints commonly seen in rheumatoid arthritis. Improvements in implant design, surgical technique, and postoperative therapy have expanded the indications for implant arthroplasties beyond the low-demand hand and suggested application in PIP joint replacement.

A comprehensive search for literature on long-term complications of Swanson silicone finger joint implants identified 70 pertinent articles evaluating over 15,000 small joint implants.

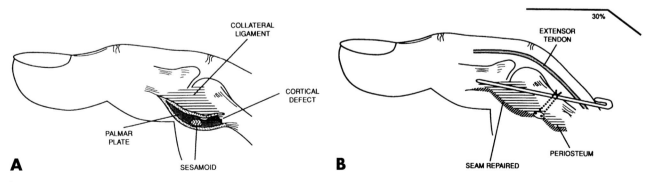

Figure 3

A, Sesamoid arthrodesis is prepared through the interval of accessory collateral ligament and volar plate. **B,** The sesamoid is advanced into a prepared cortical defect in the metacarpal head–neck junction. The joint is stabilized in 30° of flexion, and soft tissue is repaired. (Reproduced with permission from Tonkin MA, Beard AJ, Kemp SJ, Eakins DF: Sesamoid arthrodesis for hyperextension of the thumb metacarpophalangeal joint. *J Hand Surg* 1995;20A:334–338.)

Seven categories of complications were identified—synovitis, lymphadenopathy, bone change, implant fracture, implant loosening, infection, and implant removal. Each of the complications occurred in 1% or less, except for implant fracture (2%) and bone changes (4%). There were no reported cases of systemic or immunologic effects associated with the use of silicone implants.

Although most authors have described success with the Swanson MCP joint implant arthroplasties, not all results have been satisfactory. In a retrospective review of 168 Sutter silicone MCP joint arthroplasties for rheumatoid arthritic patients, 45% demonstrated implant fracture within 3 years after surgery. This correlated with recurrence in ulnar drift, but not with patient satisfaction. The authors switched to the Swanson design as a result of their findings even though there was no measurable difference in patient outcome.

In an attempt to avoid the complications associated with the silicone implants, isoelastic implant arthroplasties have been performed and evaluated by a group in the Netherlands. Sixty-eight rheumatoid MCP joints were replaced and followed for an average of more than 3 years. As with many forms of silicone implants, patient satisfaction was high with decreased pain and improved cosmesis; however, function did not significantly improve. Due to increased rigidity, there were no implant fractures; however, osteolysis around the implant and proximal metacarpal migration were of concern. The authors concluded that soft-tissue rebalancing, which decreases the demands placed upon the implant, is critical to successful long-term recovery.

Equally important to patient selection and intraoperative surgical technique is the method proposed for treatment of the digits after implant arthroplasty. Refinements to early protected motion with dynamic splinting and active assistive exercises continue to be made, due to improved splinting material and a better understanding of a safe protocol that promotes tendon gliding without compromise of the stability of the reconstructed joint. The common deformities of ulnar deviation, volar subluxation, and pronation deformity are addressed with appropriate metacarpal bone resection, measurement of the optimal implant size, and soft-tissue rebalancing of the intrinsic and extrinsic tendons and collateral ligaments. Dynamic splinting protects soft-tissue repair during the early recovery period while permitting motion.

Continuous passive motion has been compared to the dynamic splint protocol in rheumatoid arthritic patients who had MCP implant arthroplasties. In a prospective randomized study, 100 MCP joint arthroplasties in 25 hands were managed postoperatively either with dynamic splinting or with continuous passive motion. Improved arc of motion and greater strength was documented in the group managed with standard dynamic splinting. Although a slight decrease in ulnar drift was noted for the continuous passive motion group, it was not enough to justify the additional costs.

Proximal Interphalangeal Joints

Over the past several years, investigators have attempted to determine whether implant arthroplasty could provide long-term success comparable to arthrodesis. Forty proximal implant arthroplasties in patients with inflammatory arthritis were evaluated at an average of 94 months. All procedures were performed through a dorsal approach, and 26 fingers had concurrent or previous MCP implant arthroplasties. Overall results were 12 good, 18 fair, and 10 poor; improvement in pain relief or motion restoration was inconsistent. Swan neck and boutonnière deformities recurred in over 80% of the patients, with the greatest functional loss in the digits with swan neck deformities. This study emphasized the importance of MCP joint correction in fingers with boutonnière deformity. This correction restores balance between the extrinsic and intrinsic musculotendinous forces.

Other groups have reported the impact of changes in surgical approach and product design on outcome of PIP joint arthroplasty. The palmar approach to the PIP joint for implant arthroplasty allows for immediate progression of active motion because there is no extensor tendon disturbance. In one series of 36 patients, 69 PIP joint silicone implant arthroplasties accomplished through a palmar approach were reviewed at an average of 3.4 years after surgery. The middle and ring fingers were the most common digits treated by this method. Pain relief was consistently achieved, and patients reported improved hand function. The lack of improvement in range of motion and ulnar deviation deformity have been attributed more to implant design than surgical approach. The dorsal approach is still recommended for PIP implant arthroplasty treatment of swan neck and boutonnière deformities.

An alternative PIP joint implant design has been developed, using an unconstrained surface replacement arthroplasty consisting of a CoCr proximal component and an ultra-high molecular weight polyethylene distal component. Sixty-six implants were evaluated after a mean follow-up of 4.5 years. Results varied from good to poor, with a variety of complications. Poor results are associated with the more severe conditions, and the authors' growing experience has led to improvement in final recovery. They have adopted the dorsal approach in lieu of previously used midaxial and palmar approaches. The implant has demonstrated superior results for painful degenerative arthritic conditions.

Use of dynamic splinting to facilitate early range of motion for PIP implant arthroplasty will depend on the surgical approach and the preservation of the central slip extensor tendon. The lateral and volar approaches allow earlier active digital motion as the critical extensor mechanism remains intact.

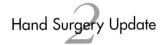
Arthroplasty-Nonimplant

Motion-preserving procedures for treatment of posttraumatic arthritis of the MCP and PIP joints have had a guarded prognosis due to the poor results associated with implant arthroplasties, related soft-tissue pathology, and functional loss. Osteochondral autograft replacement of intra-articular finger joint defects has been proposed as a motion-preserving alternative to arthrodesis in these devastating injuries.

One author described 5 patients ranging in age from 23 to 60 years who underwent insertion of metatarsophalangeal autografts into MCP defects. All patients had sustained a saw injury to the index finger and were surgically managed with the same technique (Fig. 4). All but one patient had radiographic union without osteonecrosis. Articular step-off of 1 mm or less was uniformly achieved, and all patients regained a functional range of motion without significant pain or weakness.

A similar surgical procedure has been advocated for proximal and distal IP joint posttraumatic articular deformities. The ipsilateral second or third CMC joint provided the donor osteochondral graft in 10 cases that were reviewed after 2 years. Slight improvement in range of motion and angular deformity was achieved without donor morbidity. The procedure was recommended for children with articular injuries of less than 50% of the IP joint surface that do not affect the growth plates.

More extensive injuries of the hand involving the PIP joint can be salvaged by either free or island-vascularized joint transfer, thereby avoiding the need for arthrodesis. In one study, follow-up results were presented for 27 vascularized joints transferred for PIP joint reconstruction. These procedures were performed in cases of severe digital trauma with substantial periarticular bone loss. The critical prerequisite for vascularized joint transfer is an intact flexor tendon system. When island joint transfer is selected, a patent digital artery is required. Despite successful union in the majority of cases, patients achieved limited motion recovery; the toe transfer joints had the most guarded prognosis. Unique to this series is the homodigital island DIP joint transfer, which sacrifices the distal IP joint for the more essential proximal articulation. Although these various techniques provide compound tissue transfer, rapid bone union, good lateral stability, growth potential, and cartilage preservation, improvements in recovery of motion will require further research.

Periarticular Soft-Tissue Reconstruction

Posttraumatic arthritis of the PIP joint is of particular concern when a jammed finger results in fracture subluxation

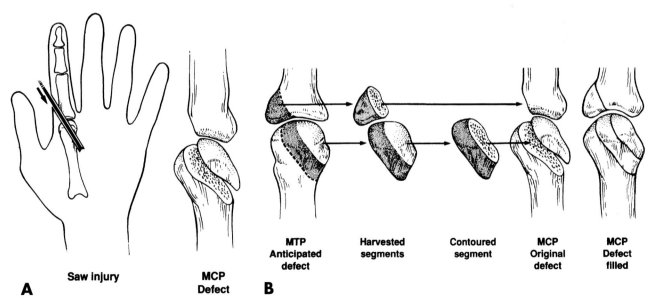

MTP Anticipated defect   **Harvested segments**   **Contoured segment**   **MCP Original defect**   **MCP Defect filled**

Saw injury   **MCP Defect**

A   **B**

Figure 4

Osteochondral metatarsophalangeal (MTP) graft for metacarpophalangeal (MCP) articular defect. **A,** Saw injury to index finger with articular defect. **B,** Reconstruction with MTP joint donor segments replacing defect in MCP joint. (Reproduced with permission from Boulas HJ, Herren A, Buchler U: Osteochondral metatarsophalangeal autografts for traumatic articular metacarpophalangeal defects: A preliminary report. *J Hand Surg* 1993;18A:1086–1092.)

secondary to volar plate avulsion and middle phalangeal comminution. If left untreated, this injury will likely cause permanent joint pain, loss of motion, and angular deformity. Palmar plate arthroplasty has gained increasing acceptance for surgical management of these complex injuries. In a modification of this procedure, 2 separate sutures are used to secure the ends of the palmar plate. The sutures are tied beneath the skin of the dorsum of the middle phalanx (rather than over the skin as a pull-out stitch). The complication of resubluxation is more often seen in injuries with severe volar comminution extending beyond the articular region of the phalanx, and in cases with incomplete reduction.

Trauma to the PIP joint can result in loss of motion and pain without articular damage. Joint contracture secondary to collateral ligament scarring can be a challenging condition. Total collateral ligament excision has been demonstrated to yield reproducible results (Fig. 5). Active range of motion increased from an average of 38° to 78° in 16 patients treated with this method; average follow-up was 66 months. Supplemental tenolyses and palmar plate release were required in the majority of patients. No PIP joint instability was reported despite the total elimination of the collateral ligamentous structures.

In a subsequent study, magnetic resonance imaging revealed neocollateral ligament formation after total excision of the PIP collateral ligaments. The early postoperative thickening along the region of the excised collateral ligaments with maintained stability has stimulated investigation of the potential soft-tissue formation of neocollateral ligaments. In one series, 10 contracted PIP joints were treated by total collateral ligament excision. In postoperative MRI, newly formed soft tissue was identified in the position of the collateral ligaments with the same low-signal intensity band bridging the proximal to middle phalanges. Consistent tissue contour, distribution, and density were found in all patients. Although the ultrastructure of this tissue has yet to be determined, clinical and imaging studies were similar to that of normal collateral ligamentous tissue.

Malunion Corrective Osteotomy

Malunions of the phalanges and metacarpals can result in pain due to distortion of the joints, loss of active range of motion due to imbalance of the intrinsic and extrinsic tendons, crossing or scissoring of the fingers, and weakness of grip. These conditions are also commonly associated with joint contractures and tendon adhesions. Corrective osteotomies have been advocated for correction either at the original fracture site or proximal to the fracture at the metacarpal base.

In one cohort study of 59 phalangeal malunions, corrective osteotomies were completed through various combinations of rotation, angulation, and length correction with the use of rigid internal fixation. Tenocapsulolysis of the adjacent tendons and capsules was required in 50% of the patients. Bone union was achieved in all patients; good to excellent recovery was reported in 96% of the patients with bone involvement alone, and in 64% of malunions involving multiple surrounding structures. The authors attribute this success to comprehensive preoperative planning, meticulous surgical technique, and intensive aftercare. Adjunct soft-tissue procedures are a key element of recovery, and can be performed in a single stage when rigid fixation is achieved.

In situ osteotomy for proximal phalangeal malunions was explored in a recent series of 11 patients with extra-articular deformities. All patients underwent in situ osteotomies, stabilized by dorsal plate fixation; early postoperative active and passive motion exercises were initiated. All patients healed the osteotomy site in an average of 7 weeks, with correction of the angular and rotation deformity eliminating the scissoring effect with finger flexion. Results were superior to step-cut osteotomies with respect to time to union and active range of motion.

Another group described single osteotomy combining both rotation and angulation correction. This procedure was used in 6 patients with various congenital and acquired deformities of the digits. The authors recommend sterilizing a cork during the operation to replicate the deformity and act as a template to determine the degree of correction

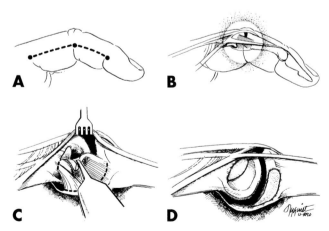

Figure 5

Total collateral ligament excision technique. **A,** Midaxial incision. **B,** Relation of extensor mechanism to collateral ligament. **C,** Extensor mechanism mobilization allowing for proximal and distal dissection of collateral ligament. **D,** Final appearance of proximal interphalangeal joint after excision. (Reproduced with permission from Diao E, Eaton RG: Total collateral ligament excision for contractures of the proximal interphalangeal joint. *J Hand Surg* 1993;18A:395–402.)

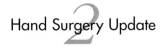

required before completing the osteotomy. The more oblique the osteotomy, the greater the ratio of angulation to rotation correction. All 6 patients healed with satisfactory results and no complications.

Nonunion/Bone Loss Reconstruction

Nonunion of the digit is an unusual occurrence, often related to the magnitude of the initial fracture displacement and associated soft-tissue trauma. Most phalangeal and metacarpal fractures unite in approximately 4 to 6 weeks. The true definition of nonunion of the digits has yet to be established; however, most physicians agree that after 16 weeks of delayed or incomplete union, the prognosis for fracture healing is poor.

The predominant factor in nonunions of the hand and digits is the degree of initial trauma and fracture displacement. Open fractures have the highest incidence of delayed union and nonunion. Other factors predisposing to nonunion include diabetes, thyroid disease, immunocompromise, and smoking.

Two basic types of nonunion of the digits dictate the appropriate surgical management. Hypertrophic, reactive nonunions are often in need of improved skeletal fixation. After the abundant callus bone is excised along with the nonunion site, malalignment of the phalanx or metacarpal is corrected and stabilization afforded with lag screws, plate fixation, or various K-wire support. Intraoperative assessment of correction of the rotation and angular deformity is important. Fluoroscopic evaluation of the osteotomy site may be helpful. The more rigid the fixation, the more quickly the patient can resume range of motion exercises of the fingers.

Atrophic nonunion requires supplemental cancellous bone graft along with techniques of rigid fixation similar to those described for the hypertrophic nonunions. Although there are no comparative studies at this time, allograft and bone substitutes have been gaining popularity in the surgical treatment of nonunions, delayed unions, and malunions of the hand and upper extremity.

Although healing of the nonunion site is the primary concern, equally challenging is reestablishment of active finger motion after prolonged immobilization. Follow-up surgical procedures, such as tenolysis, capsulectomy, and collateral ligament release, may be required after successful union if occupational therapy fails to restore an acceptable range of motion.

Substantial bone loss of the phalanx or metacarpal as a result of open trauma is an uncommon condition and difficult to manage. Concurrent open wounds and associated soft-tissue trauma add to the complexity of these conditions. Although early bone grafting and stable internal fixation are desirable, the potential for contamination and possible infection warrant caution. Treatment priorities are elimination of nonviable tissue; provision of suitable soft-tissue coverage with skin grafts, pedicle flaps, or free tissue transfers; and establishment of primary skeletal fixation. Once the soft tissue is covered, the bone loss can be safely addressed through bone grafting and definitive internal or external fixation. The timing of intervention remains controversial; some advocate immediate bone grafting at the time of soft-tissue coverage, and others prefer delayed staged surgical procedures. Phalangeal bone loss is of greater consequence than metacarpal bone loss due to the independence of each digit as well as the demands placed on the PIP joint from tendon and ligament involvement. A wider range of treatment options is available for metacarpal bone loss injuries; crossbridging of the bone graft to the adjacent metacarpals along with tendon grafts or tendon transfers will often provide satisfactory results.

Annotated Bibliography

Arthrodesis

Leibovic SJ, Strickland JW: Arthrodesis of the proximal interphalangeal joint of the finger: Comparison of the use of the Herbert screw with other fixation methods. *J Hand Surg* 1994;19A:181–188.

In this retrospective review of 224 PIP joint arthrodeses with various techniques, the authors recommend Herbert screw fixation based on low complication and high union rates.

Pribyl CR, Omer GE, McGinty L: Effectiveness of the chevron arthrodesis in small joints of the hand. *J Hand Surg* 1996; 21A:1052–1058.

Ninety-eight joints were successfully fused by chevron arthrodesis, with very few complications. Precise surgical bone preparation, increasing the contact surface of the arthrodesis, is emphasized.

Stern PJ, Gates NT, Jones TB: Tension band arthrodesis of small joints in the hand. *J Hand Surg* 1993;18A:194–197.

Two hundred ninety fusions of the MCP and PIP joints were performed using the tension band technique. Only 14 attempted fusions failed to unite. External splinting may be unnecessary in the cooperative patient.

Tonkin MA, Beard AJ, Kemp SJ, Eakins DF: Sesamoid arthrodesis for hyperextension of the thumb metacarpophalangeal joint. *J Hand Surg* 1995;20A:334–338.

Forty-two sesamoid-metacarpal arthrodeses were reviewed for correction of thumb MCP joint hyperextension. This procedure is recommended for patients with cerebral palsy and as an adjunct in basal joint arthroplasty for arthritis.

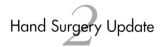

Voche P, Merle M, Membre H, Fockens W: Bioabsorbable rods and pins for fixation of metacarpophalangeal arthrodesis of the thumb. *J Hand Surg* 1995;20A:1032–1036.

Thirteen thumbs in 12 patients were arthrodesed, employing bioabsorbable rods and pins. All fused in 6 to 8 weeks without complications. This material is recommended to eliminate the need for hardware removal.

Wyrsch B, Dawson J, Aufranc S, Weikert D, Milek M: Distal interphalangeal joint arthrodesis comparing tension-band wire and Herbert screw: A biomechanical and dimensional analysis. *J Hand Surg* 1996;21A:438–443.

Thirty cadaveric DIP joints were prepared with either Herbert screw or tension band wire to simulate arthrodesis. Although additional strength was identified with the Herbert screw, numerous phalangeal fractures and instances of screw penetration were observed.

Arthroplasty-Implant

Adamson GJ, Gellman H, Brumfield RH Jr, Kuschner SH, Lawler JW: Flexible implant resection arthroplasty of the proximal interphalangeal joint in patients with systemic inflammatory arthritis. *J Hand Surg* 1994;19A:378–384.

Forty PIP implants in 19 patients were reviewed after an average of 94 months. Digits with boutonnière and swan neck deformities did not demonstrate significant improvement in range of motion. Boutonnière deformities that were managed with concurrent MCP implant arthroplasty demonstrated better results than those undergoing only PIP implant arthroplasty.

Bass RL, Stern PJ, Nairus JG: High implant fracture incidence with Sutter silicone metacarpophalangeal arthroplasty. *J Hand Surg* 1996;21A:813–818.

This retrospective review of 168 Sutter implants in 34 patients with rheumatoid arthritis identified a 20% implant fracture rate at an average follow-up of 27 months. The fracture rate increased to 45% in patients followed longer than 3 years. The authors have abandoned use of the Sutter implant.

Foliart DE: Swanson silicone finger joint implants: A review of the literature regarding long-term complications. *J Hand Surg* 1995;20A:445–449.

Foliart presents a review of 70 pertinent articles covering 15,556 small joint implants, and summarizes long-term complications. Few complications were identified; no reports of immunologic reactions, connective tissue disease, or other systemic effects related to the small joint silicone implants were found.

Kirkpatrick WH, Kozin SH, Uhl RL: Early motion after arthroplasty. *Hand Clin* 1996;12:73–86.

The authors describe an implant arthroplasty surgical technique and postoperative management with early controlled range of motion. Forms of active assisted motion and dynamic splinting are also covered.

Lin HH, Wyrick JD, Stern PJ: Proximal interphalangeal joint silicone replacement arthroplasty: Clinical results using an anterior approach. *J Hand Surg* 1995;20A:123–132.

Sixty-nine PIP joint silicone implants were inserted through a palmar approach in 36 patients, and reviewed at an average follow-up of 3.4 years. Pain relief was the most consistent finding. No significant improvement in total active motion or correction of coronal deformity was noted.

Linscheid RL, Murray PM, Vidal MA, Beckenbaugh RD: Development of a surface replacement arthroplasty for proximal interphalangeal joints. *J Hand Surg* 1997;22A:286–298.

Sixty-six surface replacement PIP prostheses consisting of a CoCr proximal component and ultra-high molecular weight polyethylene distal component, were evaluated over a 14-year period. Good results were seen in approximately half the patients. The authors attribute good results to a dorsal approach, as well as improved surgical technique and experience.

Ring D, Simmons BP, Hayes M: Continuous passive motion following metacarpophalangeal joint arthroplasty. *J Hand Surg* 1998;23A:505–511.

In a prospective randomized trial, standard dynamic splint protocol was compared to continuous passive motion for rehabilitation after MCP joint implant arthroplasty. In the 25 hands studied, at 6 months no significant improvement was identified among hands treated with continuous passive motion. Although there was less ulnar deviation of the digits with continuous passive motion, the dynamic splinting group had greater strength and arc of motion.

Vermeiren JA, Dapper MM, Schoonhoven LA, Merx PW: Isoelastic arthroplasty of the metacarpophalangeal joints in rheumatoid arthritis: A preliminary report. *J Hand Surg* 1994;19A:319–324.

Sixty-eight rheumatoid patients who had isoelastic implant arthroplasties of the MCP joints were followed for an average of 3+ years. Subjective scoring improved postoperatively; however, functional results were not significantly improved. The rigidity of the implant helps prevent ulnar deviation, but osteolysis around the ends of the implant has been identified.

Arthroplasty-Nonimplant

Boulas HJ: Autograft replacement of small joint defects in the hand. *Clin Orthop* 1996;327:63–71.

The author describes an attempt to prevent posttraumatic arthritis through osteochondral autograft replacement of the articular surface to the MCP joints. Follow-up at 33 months revealed restoration of functional range of motion, with maintenance of articular congruity.

Foucher G, Lenoble E, Smith D: Free and island vascularized joint transfer for proximal interphalangeal reconstruction: A series of 27 cases. *J Hand Surg* 1994;19A:8–16.

Proximal interphalangeal joint reconstruction with homodigital island, heterodigital island, free heterodigital, or free second toe PIP joint transfer was performed in 27 cases. Follow-up revealed the poorest results in the second toe free-joint transfer, with 33° mean active range of motion.

Ishida O, Ikuta Y, Kuroki H: Ipsilateral osteochondral grafting for finger joint repair. *J Hand Surg* 1994;19A:372–377.

The CMC articulation site provided the osteochondral graft for reconstruction of the interphalangeal joints of the ipsilateral hand in

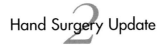
10 patients. After greater than 2-year follow-up, a significant improvement in angular deformity was noted. This procedure is specifically recommended for children with articular damage.

Periarticular Soft-Tissue Reconstruction

Bilos ZJ, Vender MI, Bonavolonta M, Knutson K: Fracture subluxation of the proximal interphalangeal joint treated by palmar plate advancement. *J Hand Surg* 1994;19A:189–195.

The authors describe a modification of the palmar plate advancement for PIP subluxation. A 2-suture technique is employed, tying deep to the skin over the dorsum of the middle phalanx. Eleven patients were followed long-term with good functional recovery.

Diao E, Eaton RG: Total collateral ligament excision for contractures of the proximal interphalangeal joint. *J Hand Surg* 1993;18A:395–402.

A significant increase in active range of motion was observed in 16 patients treated by total collateral ligament excision for flexion contractures. Instability was not encountered during the postoperative period.

Eaton RG, Sunde D, Pang D, Singson R: Evaluation of "neocollateral" ligament formation by magnetic resonance imaging after total excision of the proximal interphalangeal collateral ligaments. *J Hand Surg* 1998;23A:322–327.

MRI evaluation of PIP joints after total collateral ligament excision for flexion contracture revealed neocollateral ligaments by scar tissue in 10 joints. Although the ultrastructure of the newly formed tissue has yet to be determined, stability of the joint was maintained in all cases.

Malunion Corrective Osteotomy

Buchler U, Gupta A, Ruf S: Corrective osteotomy for post-traumatic malunion of the phalanges in the hand. *J Hand Surg* 1996; 21B:33–42.

Fifty-nine corrective osteotomies were performed during a 12-year period for rotational, deviation, shortening deformity, or a combination. Tenocapsulolysis was required in half of the cases. Satisfactory results were achieved in 76% of patients.

Evans DM, Gateley DR, Telfer JR: Rotation-angulation osteotomy in the hand. *J Hand Surg* 1996;21B:43–46.

A single osteotomy for the simultaneous correction of rotation and angulation deformity is described. The results of 6 patients managed with this technique are reviewed.

Trumble T, Gilbert M: In situ osteotomy for extra-articular malunion of the proximal phalanx. *J Hand Surg* 1998;23A:821–826.

Eleven patients with proximal phalangeal extra-articular malunion underwent in situ osteotomies without complications. The rotational and angular deformities were corrected, and were associated with an increased range of motion. Isolated rotational and combined rotational and angular deformity correction techniques are described.

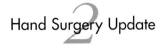
Section II
Distal Radius and Carpus

American Society for Surgery of the Hand

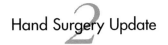
Chapter 6
The Anatomy and Biomechanics of the Wrist and Distal Radioulnar Joint

Richard A. Berger, MD, PhD

Introduction

The wrist is not isolated from the distal radioulnar joint (DRUJ), nor is it isolated from the hand. Each joint in the upper extremity forms a true linkage between contiguous joints and the interposed bones. The wrist should be conceptualized as a weightbearing joint, even though humans spend but a fraction of their normal existence in a quadrupedal posture. The concept of weightbearing stems from the direction of physiologic loading of the musculotendinous units motoring the hand and wrist. All but one of these musculotendinous units cross the wrist without insertions, thus transmitting load proximally across the wrist to the forearm with every action of the hand.

Anatomy of the Wrist

Vascular Anatomy

Blood Supply of the Distal Radius The arterial blood supply of the distal radius has been documented in detail, to facilitate development of predictable, pedicled vascularized bone grafts. On the anterior surface of the radius, deep to and just distal to the pronator quadratus, the palmar carpal and palmar metaphyseal arches provide variable nutrient vessels to the radius. The more commonly recognized vessels are found dorsally (Fig. 1). The nomenclature of these vessels is based on their relationship with the extensor retinaculum. Each named vessel has a proximal origin with either the radial artery or the posterior division of the anterior interosseous artery or the ulnar artery, and forms anastomoses distally with those arteries or one of 3 transverse arches—supraretinacular, radiocarpal, or intercarpal. Four dorsal vessels have a practical application to vascularized bone grafts. The 2 most radial vessels are the 1,2 intercompartmental supraretinacular artery (ICSRA) and the

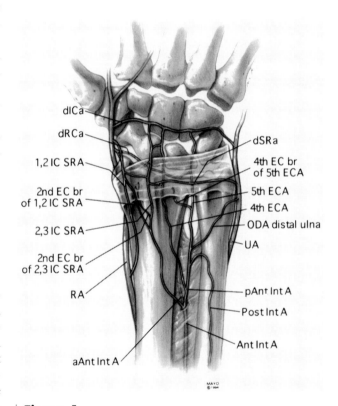

Figure 1

The extraosseous blood supply of the distal radius and carpus from a dorsal perspective. The longitudinally anastomosing vessels are named relative to the extensor compartments, and are either found between adjacent compartments on the supraretinacular surface (ICSRA) or within an extensor compartment (ECA). RA = radial artery, UA = ulnar artery, Ant Int A = anterior interosseous artery, pAnt Int A = posterior division of anterior interosseous artery, dRC = dorsal radiocarpal arch, dICa = dorsal intercarpal arch, dSRa = dorsal supraretinacular arch. (Reproduced with permission from the Mayo Foundation, Rochester, MN.)

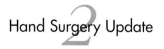
2,3 ICSRA. These vessels are found between the respective extensor compartments designated by the numbers, and are, therefore, intercompartmental and supraretinacular in location. The ulnarmost vessels are the 4th extensor compartmental artery (ECA) and the 5th ECA. These vessels are typically found within the extensor compartment proper, although the 5th ECA may be located within the septum separating the 4th and 5th extensor compartments. Understanding of this vascular anatomy has led to the development of pedicled, retrograde-flow, vascularized bone grafts, useful for transporting viable bone regionally to treat conditions such as Kienböck's disease, scaphoid nonunions, and Preiser's disease.

The most commonly used graft for the treatment of scaphoid nonunion, osteonecrosis of the proximal pole of the scaphoid secondary to a scaphoid fracture, and Preiser's disease has been based upon the 1,2 ICSRA. A corticocancellous graft is elevated on the pedicle of the 1,2 ICSRA, maintaining the distal anastomosis with either the dorsal radiocarpal arch or the radial artery proper. Although smaller in caliber, the 2,3 ICSRA is a useful alternative, and can be harvested by elevating Lister's tubercle on the vessel, maintaining its distal anastomosis with the dorsal radiocarpal arch. For the treatment of Kienböck's disease, the 4th ECA has been shown to have a rich nutrient contribution to the distal radial metaphyseal bone, but has a scant distal anastomotic connection with the dorsal carpal arches. The 5th ECA has a large diameter and reliable distal anastomosis, but lacks any contribution to the nutrient supply of bone in the distal radius. Consequently, a combined graft has been developed—the "4 on 5" graft. A corticocancellous graft is harvested from the 4th extensor compartment floor based on the 4th ECA, which is dissected proximally until it anastomoses with the posterior division of the anterior interosseous artery. The 5th ECA, also anastomosing with the interosseous artery system, is dissected distally through the 5th extensor compartment until its anastomosis with the dorsal radiocarpal arch is reached. The posterior division of the anterior interosseous artery is ligated proximal to the origins of the 4th and 5th ECAs, creating a graft that is dependent on retrograde flow from the dorsal radiocarpal arch through the 5th ECA and antegrade flow through the 4th ECA.

Extraosseous Blood Supply The carpus receives its blood supply through branches from 3 dorsal and 3 palmar arches supplied by the radial, ulnar, anterior interosseous, and posterior interosseous arteries (Fig. 2). The 3 dorsal arches are named (proximal to distal) radiocarpal, intercarpal, and basal metacarpal transverse arches. Anastomoses are often found between the arches, between radial and ulnar arteries, and within the interosseous artery system. The palmar arches are named (proximal to distal) radiocarpal, intercarpal, and deep palmar arches.

Intraosseous Blood Supply With the exception of the pisiform, all carpal bones receive their blood supply through dorsal and palmar entry sites—usually through more than 1 nutrient artery. A number of small-caliber penetrating vessels are usually present in addition to the major nutrient vessels. Intraosseous anastomoses can be found in 3 basic patterns: a direct anastomosis can occur between 2 large-diameter vessels within the bone; anastomotic arcades may form with similar-sized vessels, often entering the bone from different areas; and in a rare third pattern, a diffuse arterial network virtually fills the bone.

Although the intraosseous vascular patterns of each carpal bone have been defined in detail, studies of the lunate, capitate, and scaphoid are particularly germane, due to their tendency to develop clinically important vascular problems. The lunate has only 2 nonarticular surfaces available for vascular penetration—dorsal and palmar. From the dorsal and palmar vascular plexuses, 2 to 4 penetrating vessels enter the lunate through each surface. Three consistent patterns of intraosseous vascularization have been identified, based on the pattern of anastomosis. When viewed in the sagittal plane, the anastomoses form either a Y, X, or I pattern, with arborization of small-caliber vessels stemming from the main branches. The proximal subchondral bone is consistently the least vascularized. The capitate is supplied by both the palmar and dorsal vascular plexuses; however, the palmar supply is more consistent and from larger caliber vessels. Just distal to the neck of the capitate, vessels chiefly from the ulnar artery penetrate the palmar-ulnar cortex, while dorsal penetration occurs just distal to the midwaist level. The intraosseous vascularization pattern consists of proximally directed retrograde flow, with minimal anastomoses between dorsal and palmar vessels. When present, the dorsal vessels principally supply the head of the capitate, while the palmar vessels supply both the body and head of the capitate. The scaphoid typically receives its blood supply through 3 vessels originating from the radial artery—the lateral-palmar, dorsal, and distal arterial branches. The lateral-palmar vessel is believed to be the principal blood supply of the scaphoid. All vessels penetrate the cortex of the scaphoid distal to its waist, coursing in a retrograde fashion to supply the proximal pole. Although there have been reports of minor vascular penetrations directly into the proximal pole from the posterior interosseous artery, substantial risk for osteonecrosis of the proximal pole remains with displaced fractures through the waist of the scaphoid. The remaining carpal bones likely have multiple nutrient vessels penetrating their cortices from more than one side, hence reducing their risk of osteonecrosis by a substantial margin.

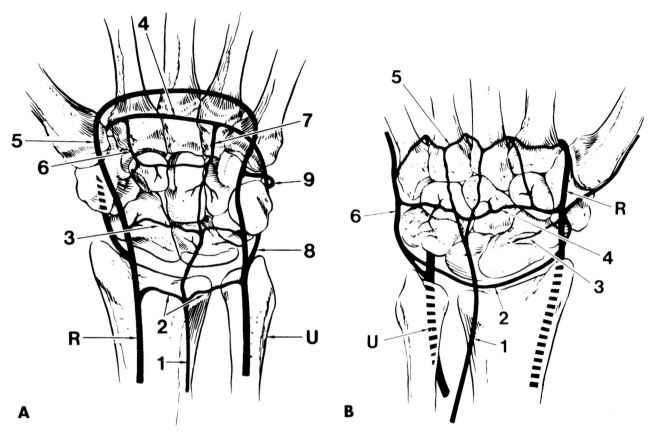

Figure 2

The common vascular patterns of the carpus. **A,** Anterior blood supply. R = radial artery, U = ulnar artery, 1 = anterior interosseous artery, 2 = palmar radiocarpal arch, 3 = palmar intercarpal arch, 4 = deep palmar arch, 5 = superficial palmar arch, 6 – 9 = anastomotic vessels. **B,** Posterior blood supply. 1 = posterior interosseous artery, 2 = dorsal radiocarpal arch, 4 = dorsal intercarpal arch, 5 = basal metacarpal arch. (Reproduced with permission from Gelberman RH, Panagis JS, Taleisnik J, Baumgaertner M: The arterial anatomy of the human carpus: Part I. The extraosseous vascularity. *J Hand Surg* 1983;8A:367–375.)

Joint Anatomy

Distal Radioulnar Joint The DRUJ is spatially related to wrist function kinematically and kinetically. The DRUJ is essentially a trochlear joint between the concave sigmoid notch forming the ulnar surface of the distal radius and the convex ulna head. The radii of curvatures of the articular surfaces forming this joint are dissimilar; the sigmoid notch has a greater radius of curvature than the ulna head. Approximately 130° of the ulna head's cylindrical surface are covered with articular cartilage. The distal surface of the ulna is composed of the slightly convex head, the styloid process of the ulna, and the fovea at its base. The styloid process is inconsistently covered with articular cartilage, varies in length from 3 to 6 mm, is on the posterior surface of the ulna, and often exhibits a variable radial curvature. The foveal region is devoid of articular cartilage and serves as an attachment for the triangular fibrocartilage. Under normal circumstances, the DRUJ is isolated from the radiocarpal joint by a competent triangular fibrocartilage. Degenerative changes and trauma may create perforations in the articular disk region of the triangular fibrocartilage, producing a direct communication between the 2 joints.

Radiocarpal Joint The radiocarpal joint is formed by the articulation of confluent surfaces of the concave distal articular surface of the radius and the triangular fibrocartilage with the convex proximal articular surfaces of the proximal carpal row bones. The secant of the concave distal articular surface of the radius is normally inclined palmarly from 10° to 15° and ulnarly 15° to 25° (Fig. 3). The distal articular surface of the radius is divided by a fibrocartilaginous ridge, the interfossal ridge, into a triangular-shaped scaphoid fossa and a quadrangular-shaped lunate fossa (Fig. 4, *A*). The triangular fibrocartilage normally forms a smooth and continuous surface with the distal articular surface of the radius. The prestyloid recess is located near the ulnar extent of the triangular fibrocartilage,

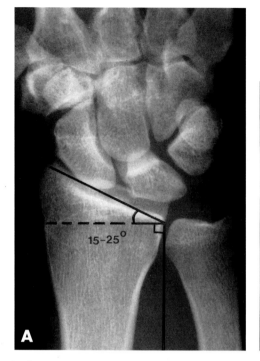

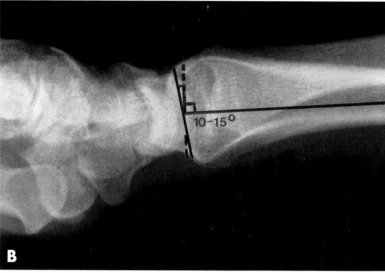

Figure 3

A, Posteroanterior wrist radiograph illustrating the normal range of ulnar inclination of the distal articular surface of the radius. **B,** Lateral view illustrating the normal range of palmar inclination of the distal articular surface of the radius. (Reproduced with permission from Berger RA: Anatomy and basic biomechanics of the wrist, in Manske PR (ed): *Hand Surgery Update.* Rosemont, IL, American Academy of Orthopaedic Surgeons, 1996, pp 47–62.)

and variably communicates with the ulnar styloid process. The central region of the triangular fibrocartilage is normally quite thin, often appearing translucent, but varies in thickness proportionately with the degree of length discrepancy of the distal radius and ulna. The radiocarpal joint is normally isolated from the DRUJ by the triangular fibrocartilage, and from the intercarpal joint by the proximal row interosseous ligaments. In approximately 70% of normal adults, there is a direct communication between the pisotriquetral joint and the radiocarpal joint. Age-related degenerative defects are commonly found in the central fibrocartilaginous regions of the triangular fibrocartilage and the proximal row interosseous ligaments.

Midcarpal Joint   The midcarpal joint is formed by the mutually articulating surfaces of the proximal and distal carpal rows. Communications are found between the midcarpal joint and the interosseous joint clefts of the proximal and distal row bones, as well as between the midcarpal joint and the second through fifth carpometacarpal (CMC) joints. Under normal circumstances, the midcarpal joint is isolated from the pisotriquetral, radiocarpal, and first CMC joints by intervening membranes and ligaments. The geom-

etry of the midcarpal joint is complex. Radially, the scaphoid-trapezium-trapezoid (STT) joint is composed of the slightly convex distal pole of the scaphoid articulating with the reciprocally concave proximal surfaces of the trapezium and trapezoid. The convex head of the capitate and the combined concave contiguous distal articulating surfaces of the scaphoid and the lunate form a structure much like a ball and socket joint. In 65% of normal adults, the hamate articulates with a medial articular facet at the distal ulnar margin of the lunate, which is associated with a higher rate of cartilage eburnation of the proximal surface of the hamate. The triquetrohamate region of the midcarpal joint is particularly complex; the mutual articular surfaces have both concave and convex regions, forming a helicoid-shaped articulation.

Carpometacarpal Joints   In their most elemental forms, the CMC joints can be classified as either fixed or mobile. The fixed CMC joints are the second and third; the first, fourth, and fifth CMC joints are mobile. The functional result of this arrangement allows the second and third metacarpals to form a stable buttress of the palm around which the first, fourth, and fifth metacarpals can rotate. This effectively deepens the palmar cusp and increases the prehensile ability of the fingers.

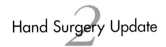

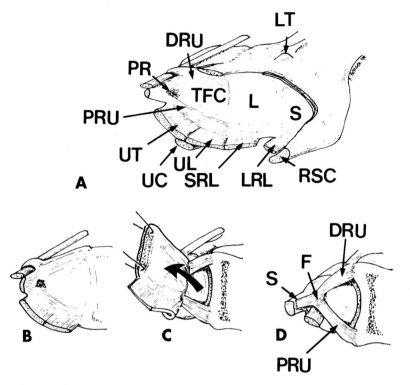

Figure 4

A, The proximal surface of the radiocarpal joint from a distal perspective. S = scaphoid fossa, L = lunate fossa, LT = Lister's tubercle, TFC = triangular fibrocartilage, PR = prestyloid recess. The capsular ligaments are seen in cross-section: RSC = radioscaphocapitate, LRL = long radiolunate, SRL = short radiolunate, UL = ulnolunate, UC ulnocapitate, UT = ulnotriquetral, DRU = dorsal radioulnar, PRU = palmar radioulnar. **B,** Focus on the distal surface of the TFCC. **C,** The distalmost surface of the TFCC is artificially dissected away, revealing the deep ligamentous anatomy of the TFCC. **D,** Deep ligamentous anatomy of the TFCC. DRU = dorsal radioulnar ligament, PRU = palmar radioulnar ligament, F = foveal attachment, S = styloid attachment.

ular interdigitation through basilar styloid processes on the second and third metacarpals and extensive ligamentous interconnections between the bases of the metacarpals, trapezoid, and capitate, and between the dorsal and palmar surfaces of the second and third CMC joints. Typically, the third metacarpal styloid process, stemming from the dorso-ulnar surface of the base of the metacarpal, is larger than the second metacarpal styloid process.

The fourth and fifth CMC joints are substantially less constrained than the second and third CMC joints. The geometry of the fourth CMC joint has been described as relatively planar in 86% of adults and somewhat conical in 14%. The base of the fourth metacarpal articulates with the capitate in 82% of normal adults. The fifth CMC joint is relatively planar, with only a slight concavity of the distal surface of the hamate matched by a slight convexity of the base of the fifth metacarpal. This results in an increased range of motion of the fourth and fifth CMC joints, averaging 10° to 20° of flexion, respectively, concurrent with a modest range of supination. This motion, however, remains constrained by the strong intermetacarpal and CMC ligaments, largely limited to the dorsal and palmar surfaces of the respective bones. Additionally, the fifth CMC joint capsule is reinforced by the insertions of the extensor carpi ulnaris tendon and the pisometacarpal ligament.

Interosseous Joints: Proximal Row The interosseous joints of the proximal row are relatively small and planar, allowing motion primarily in the flexion-extension plane between mutually articulating bones. The scapholunate joint has a smaller surface area than the lunotriquetral joint. A fibrocartilaginous meniscus extending from the membranous region of the scapholunate or lunotriquetral interosseous ligaments is often interposed into the respective joint clefts.

Interosseous Joints: Distal Row The interosseous joints of the distal row are more geometrically complex and allow substantially less interosseous motion than the proximal row joints (Fig. 6). The capitohamate joint is relatively planar, but the mutually articulating surfaces are only partially

The first (thumb) CMC joint is a diarthrodial saddle joint, with concavoconvex surfaces on both the base of the first metacarpal and the distal surface of the trapezium (Fig. 5). The axis of orientation of the convex surface of the distal trapezium is oriented in the anteroposterior plane of the first metacarpal, while the axis of orientation of the convex surface of the base of the first metacarpal is oriented in the medial-lateral plane of the first metacarpal. The first CMC joint is stabilized by a complex network of ligaments recently defined as the anterior and posterior oblique, ulnar collateral, dorso-radial, and intermetacarpal ligaments. The anterior oblique, posterior oblique, and intermetacarpal ligaments attach to the ulnar tubercle of the base of the first metacarpal, forming a force nucleus that stabilizes the intermetacarpal/CMC complex through a substantial range of circumduction.

The second and third CMC joints normally have little measurable motion. This is due to the combination of artic-

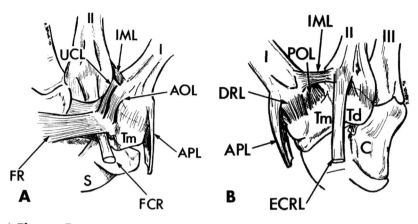

Figure 5

The first (thumb) carpometacarpal joint ligament complex. **A,** Anterior view. I = first metacarpal, II = second metacarpal, Tm = trapezium, S = scaphoid, FR = flexor retinaculum, FCR = flexor carpi radialis tendon, APL = abductor pollicis longus tendon, AOL = anterior oblique ligament, IML = intermetacarpal ligament, UCL = ulnar collateral ligament. **B,** Posterior view. III = third metacarpal, Td = trapezoid, ECRL = extensor carpi radialis longus tendon, DRL = dorsoradial ligament, POL = posterior oblique ligament. (Adapted with permission from Imaeda T, An K-N, Cooney WP III, Linscheid R: Anatomy of trapeziometacarpal ligaments. *J Hand Surg* 1993;18A:226–231.)

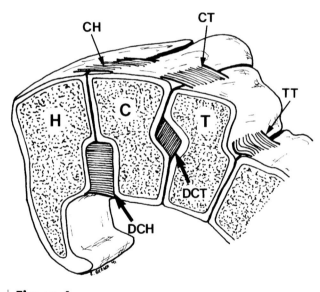

Figure 6

Cross-section of the distal carpal row from a distal and radial perspective. T = trapezoid, C = capitate, H = hamate, TT = dorsal trapeziotrapezoid ligament, CT = dorsal trapeziocapitate ligament, CH = dorsal capitohamate ligament, DCH = deep capitohamate ligament, DCT = deep trapeziocapitate ligament. (Reproduced with permission from An K-N, Berger RA, Cooney WP (eds): *Biomechanics of the Wrist Joint.* New York, NY, Springer-Verlag, 1991, p 15.)

covered by articular cartilage. The distal and palmar region of the joint space, occupied by the deep capitohamate interosseous ligament, is devoid of articular cartilage. Similarly, the central region of the trapeziocapitate joint surface is interrupted by the deep trapeziocapitate interosseous lig-

ament. The trapezium-trapezoid joint presents a small planar surface area with continuous articular surfaces.

Ligament Anatomy
The ligaments of the wrist have been described in a number of ways, creating confusion regarding various features of carpal ligaments. Several general principles have been identified to help simplify understanding of the ligamentous architecture of the wrist.

No ligaments of the wrist are extracapsular. Most can be anatomically classified as capsular ligaments with collagen fascicles clearly within the lamina of the joint capsule. The ligaments that are not entirely capsular, such as the interosseous ligaments between the bones within the carpal row, are intra-articular. This implies that they are not ensheathed in part by a fibrous capsular lamina. Ligaments may be classified as dorsal or palmar, intrinsic or extrinsic.

By convention, each ligament is named from the bones to which it attaches. If palmar is used as an adjective, existence of a dorsal counterpart to the same ligament is implied; lack of a dorsal or palmar designation implies that the structure is unique to one location in the wrist. Finally, the ligaments are named designating the most proximal or radial attachment first, followed by the distal or ulnar attachments.

The palmar capsular ligaments are more numerous than the dorsal, forming almost the entire palmar joint capsule of the radiocarpal and midcarpal joints. The palmar ligaments tend to converge toward the midline as they travel distally, forming an apex-distal V. The interosseous ligaments between the individual bones within a carpal row are generally short and transversely oriented; with certain exceptions, they cover the dorsal and palmar joint margins. Specific ligament groups are described below, and divided into capsular and interosseous groups.

Distal Radioulnar Ligaments The dorsal radioulnar (DRU) and palmar radioulnar (PRU) ligaments are the major stabilizers of the DRUJ. These ligaments form the dorsal and palmar margins of the triangular fibrocartilage complex (TFCC) in the region between the sigmoid notch of the radius and the styloid process of the ulna (Fig. 4). Attaching radially at the dorsal and palmar corners of the sigmoid notch, the ligaments are actually laminated coarsely into proximal and distal fibers. The most proximal fibers of the PRU and DRU ligaments converge ulnarly and firmly attach at the fovea, which is a depression at the base of the ulnar styloid process on the head of the ulna. From the fovea, the fibers continue across a zone free from ligament attachment to the ulnar styloid process, where a second insertion of the ligaments is found. The more dorsal fibers of the DRU ligament split to contribute to the proximal aspect of the extensor carpi ulnaris tendon subsheath. The distal fibers of the PRU ligament give rise to the disk-lunate and disk-triquetral ligaments.

Palmar Radiocarpal Ligaments The palmar radiocarpal ligaments arise from the palmar margin of the distal radius and course distally and ulnarly toward the scaphoid, lunate, and capitate (Fig. 7). Although the course of the fibers can be defined from an anterior view, the separate divisions of the palmar radiocarpal ligament are best appreciated from a dorsal view through the radiocarpal joint (Fig. 8). The palmar radiocarpal ligament can be divided into 4 distinct regions.

Beginning radially, the radioscaphocapitate (RSC) ligament originates from the radial styloid process, forms the radial wall of the radiocarpal joint, attaches to the scaphoid waist and distal pole, and passes palmar to the head of the capitate to interdigitate with fibers from the ulnocapitate ligament. Very few fibers from the RSC ligament attach to the capitate.

Just ulnar to the RSC ligament, the long radiolunate (LRL) ligament arises to pass palmar to the proximal pole of the scaphoid and the scapholunate interosseous ligament to attach to the radial margin of the palmar horn of the lunate. The interligamentous sulcus separates the RSC and LRL ligaments throughout their courses. The LRL ligament has historically been called the radiolunotriquetral ligament, but this label is misleading given the paucity of fibers continuing toward the triquetrum across the palmar horn of the lunate.

Ulnar to the origin of the LRL ligament, the radioscapholunate (RSL) ligament emerges into the radiocarpal joint space through the palmar capsule, and joins with the scapholunate interosseous ligament and the interfossal ridge of the distal radius (Fig. 9). Resembling a "mesocapsule" more than a true ligament, this structure is composed of small caliber blood vessels and nerves from the radial artery and anterior interosseous neurovascular bundle. Very little organized collagen is identified within this structure. The mechanical stabilizing effects of the RSL ligament have recently been shown to be minimal.

The final palmar radiocarpal ligament, the short radiolunate (SRL) ligament, arises as a flat sheet of fibers from the palmar rim of the lunate fossa, just ulnar to the RSL ligament. It courses immediately distally, to attach to the proximal and palmar margin of the lunate.

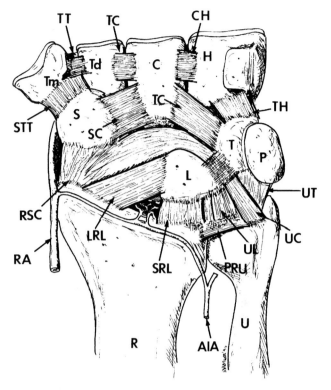

Figure 7

The palmar capsular ligaments from a palmar perspective. R = radius, U = ulna, S = scaphoid, L = lunate, P = pisiform, T = triquetrum, Tm = trapezium, Td = trapezoid, C = capitate, H = hamate, AIA = anterior interosseous artery, RA = radial artery. The ligaments are named: RSC = radioscaphocapitate, LRL = long radiolunate, SRL = short radiolunate, UL = ulnolunate, UC = ulnocapitate, UT= ulnotriquetral, TH = triquetrohamate, TC = triquetrocapitate, SC = scaphocapitate, STT = scapho-trapezio-trapezoid, TT = palmar trapeziotrapezoid, TC = palmar trapeziocapitate, PRU = palmar radioulnar, CH = palmar capitohamate. (Reproduced with permission from Berger RA: The ligaments of the wrist: A current overview of anatomy with considerations of their potential functions. *Hand Clin* 1997;13:63–82.)

Dorsal Radiocarpal Ligament The dorsal radiocarpal (DRC) ligament arises from the dorsal rim of the radius, equally distributed on either side of Lister's tubercle (Fig. 10). It courses obliquely distally and ulnarly toward the triquetrum, to which it attaches on the dorsal cortex. There are some deep attachments of the DRC ligament to the dorsal horn of the lunate. Loose connective and synovial tissue form the capsular margins proximal and distal to the DRC ligament.

Disk-Carpal Ligament The ulnocarpal ligament arises largely from the palmar margin of the TFCC, the PRU ligament and, in a limited fashion, the head of the ulna. It courses obliquely distally toward the lunate, triquetrum, and capitate (Figs. 4 and 7). The three divisions of the disk-carpal ligament are designated by their distal bony insertions. The disk-lunate ligament is essentially continuous with the SRL

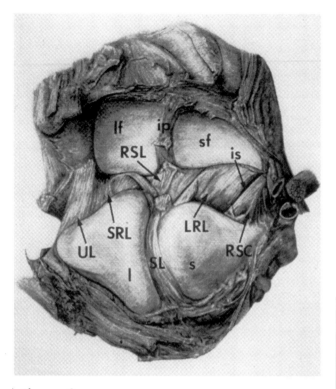

Figure 8

The radiocarpal joint from a dorsal and distal perspective, with the scaphoid (s) and lunate (l) palmarflexed via a dorsal capsulotomy. RSC = radioscaphocapitate ligament, LRL = long radiolunate ligament, RSL = radioscapholunate ligament, SRL = short radiolunate ligament, SL = scapholunate interosseous ligament, UL = ulnolunate ligament, sf = scaphoid fossa, lf = lunate fossa, ip = interfacet prominence. The RSC and LRL ligaments are separated by the interligamentous sulcus (is). (Reproduced with permission from Berger RA, Landsmeer JMF: The palmar radiocarpal ligaments: A study of adult and fetal human wrist joints. *J Hand Surg* 1990;15A:847–854.)

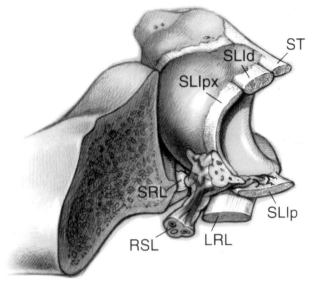

Figure 9

Scapholunate and radioscapholunate ligaments from a radial perspective, with the radial styloid process and scaphoid excised. RSL = radioscapholunate ligament, LRL = long radiolunate ligament, SRL = short radiolunate ligament, SLlp = palmar region, scapholunate ligament, SLlpx = proximal region, scapholunate ligament, SLld = dorsal region, scapholunate ligament, ST = dorsal scaphotriquetral ligament. (Reproduced with permission from Berger RA: The gross and histologic anatomy of the scapholunate interosseous ligament. *J Hand Surg* 1996;21A:170–178.)

ligament, forming a continuous palmar capsule between the TFCC and the lunate. Confluent with these fibers is the disk-triquetral ligament, connecting the TFCC and the palmar rim of the triquetrum. In approximately 90% of normal adults, a small orifice is found in the distal substance of the disk-triquetral ligament; this orifice leads to a communication between the radiocarpal and pisotriquetral joints. Just proximal and ulnar to the pisotriquetral orifice is the prestyloid recess, which is generally lined by synovial villi and variably communicates with the underlying ulnar styloid process. The ulnocapitate (UC) ligament arises from the foveal and palmar region of the head of the ulna, where it courses distally, palmar to the disk-lunate and disk-triquetral ligaments, and passes palmar to the head of the capitate; here the UC ligament interdigitates with fibers from the RSC ligament to form an arcuate ligament to the head of the capitate. Few fibers from the UC ligament insert to the capitate.

Midcarpal Ligaments The midcarpal ligaments on the palmar surface of the carpus are true capsular ligaments. They are generally short and stout, connecting bones across a single joint space (Fig. 7).

Beginning radially, the STT ligament forms a collateral ligament-like structure, particularly on the radial aspect of the scaphotrapezium joint. A vestigial ligament is found in the ulnar aspect of the scaphoid tubercle directed toward the trapezium. There is little ligamentous reinforcement on the palmar aspect of the joint, where the joint capsule serves a second role as the dorsal surface of the flexor carpi radialis tendon fibroosseous sheath.

The scaphocapitate (SC) ligament is a thick ligament coursing from the palmar surface of the distal pole of the scaphoid to the palmar surface of the body of the capitate. There are no strong ligamentous connections between the lunate and capitate, leaving these the only 2 contiguous carpal bones without interconnecting ligaments.

The triquetrocapitate (TC) ligament is analogous to the SC ligament. It is a thick ligament, passing from the palmar and radial corner of the distal margin of the triquetrum to the palmar surface of the body of the capitate. Immediately adjacent to the TC ligament, the triquetrohamate (TH) ligament

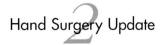
attaches to the palmar edge of the distal surface of the triquetrum, where it passes directly distally to attach to the body of the hamate. A distinct interligamentous sulcus can often be found coursing between the TC and TH ligaments.

The so-called arcuate ligament forms the bulk of the palmar midcarpal joint capsule, passing distal to the lunate and supporting the head of the capitate. It is formed primarily by interdigitation of fibers from the RSC, UC, and (when present) palmar scaphotriquetral ligaments.

The dorsal intercarpal (DIC) ligament, originating from the dorsal cortex of the triquetrum, crosses the midcarpal joint obliquely to attach to the dorsal and radial waist of the scaphoid and the dorsal cortex of the trapezoid (Fig. 10). The attachment of the DIC ligament to the triquetrum is confluent with the triquetral attachment of the DRC ligament.

A proximal thickened region of the joint capsule, roughly parallel to the DRC ligament, extends from the waist of the scaphoid across the distal margin of the dorsal horn of the lunate to the triquetrum. This band, called the dorsal scaphotriquetral ligament, forms a labrum that encases the head of the capitate, analogous to the RSC and UC ligaments palmarly.

Proximal Row Interosseous Ligaments The scapholunate (SL) and lunotriquetral (LT) interosseous ligaments form the interconnections between the bones of the proximal carpal row and share several anatomic features. Each ligament forms a barrier between the radiocarpal and midcarpal joints, connecting the dorsal, proximal, and palmar edges of the respective joint surfaces (Fig. 9). This leaves the distal edges of the joints without ligamentous coverage. The dorsal and palmar regions of the SL and LT interosseous ligaments are typical of articular ligaments, composed of collagen fascicles with numerous blood vessels and nerves. There are subtle differences as well; the dorsal region of the SL ligament is the thickest of the 3 regions, while the palmar region of the LT ligament is the largest. The proximal regions, however, are composed of fibrocartilage, devoid of vascularization and innervation, and without identifiable collagen fascicles. The RSL ligament merges with the SL interosseous ligament near the junction of the palmar and proximal regions. The UC ligament passes directly palmar to the LT interosseous ligament with substantial interdigitation and reinforcement of ligament fibers.

Distal Row Interosseous Ligaments The bones of the distal carpal row are rigidly connected by a complex system of interosseous ligaments. These ligaments are largely responsible for transforming the 4 distal row bones into a single kinematic unit. The trapeziotrapezoid, trapeziocapitate, and capitohamate joints are each bridged by palmar and

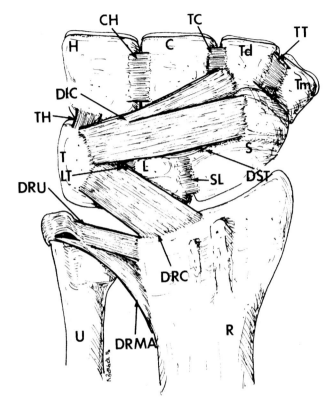

Figure 10

Dorsal wrist ligaments. R = radius, U = ulna, S = scaphoid, L = lunate, T = triquetrum, Tm = trapezium, Td = trapezoid, C = capitate, H = hamate. The dorsal radiocarpal ligament (DRC) and the dorsal intercarpal ligament (DIC) share a common attachment on the dorsal surface of the triquetrum. The dorsal radioulnar ligament (DRU) merges with the dorsal radial metaphyseal arcuate ligament (DRMA) and splits to form the extensor carpi ulnaris tendon subsheath. SL = scapholunate ligament, LT = lunotriquetral ligament, TT = trapeziotrapezoid ligament, TC = trapeziocapitate ligament, CH = capitohamate ligament. (Reproduced with permission from Berger RA: The ligaments of the wrist: A current overview of anatomy with considerations of their potential functions. *Hand Clin* 1997;13:63–82.)

dorsal interosseous ligaments (Figs. 6 and 7). These ligaments are composed of transversely oriented collagen fascicles and are covered superficially by the fibrous capsular lamina, which is also composed of transversely oriented fibers. This lamina gives the appearance of a continuous sheet of fibers spanning the entire palmar and dorsal surface of the distal row. The deep interosseous ligaments (Fig. 6) are unique to the trapeziocapitate and capitohamate joints. These 2 deep ligaments are entirely intra-articular, spanning the respective joint spaces between voids in the articular surfaces. Both are true ligaments with dense, collinear collagen fascicles, yet are also heavily invested with nerve fibers. The deep trapeziocapitate interosseous ligament, approximately 3 mm in diameter, is located midway between the palmar and dorsal limits of the joint, obliquely oriented from palmar-ulnar to dorsal-radial. The respective attachment sites of the trapezoid and capitate are angulated in the transverse plane to accommodate the orthogonal insertion of the ligament. The deep capitohamate interosseous ligament is found transversely oriented at the palmar and distal corner of the joint. It traverses the joint from quadrangular voids in the articular surfaces, and has a cross-sectional area of approximately 5 × 5 mm.

Selected Practical Applications of Wrist Anatomy

Surgical Approaches to the Wrist and Distal Radioulnar Joint Surgical approaches to the wrist and DRUJ have historically been made at the expense of the capsular ligaments. Because of concerns about stiffness and altered kinematics, fiber-splitting capsulotomies have been developed to preserve at least part of the native ligament anatomy, while allowing adequate exposure of the carpus for the designated task.

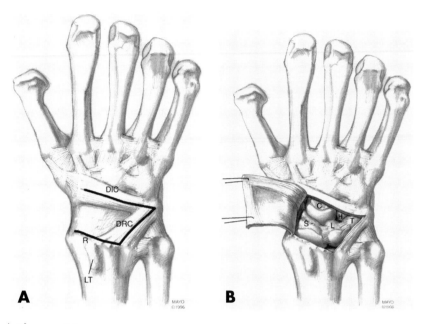

Figure 11

The radial capsulotomy technique. **A,** The incision lines in the dorsal wrist capsule are shown splitting the dorsal radio-carpal (DRC) and dorsal intercarpal (DIC) ligaments, extending radially along the dorsal margin of the distal radius (R). LT = Lister's tubercle. **B,** The radially based flap is elevated, exposing the scaphoid (S), lunate (L), triquetrum (T), capitate (C), and hamate (H). (Reproduced with permission from the Mayo Foundation, Rochester, MN.)

Dorsal Approaches to the Wrist The anatomic arrangement of the dorsal radiocarpal and intercarpal ligaments lends itself to the development of 2 dorsal approaches to the wrist. The most commonly employed approach splits the dorsal radiocarpal and dorsal intercarpal ligaments longitudinally, beginning at their mutual attachment on the triquetrum (Fig. 11). Proximally, the radial half of the DRC ligament is detached from the radius, and the capsulotomy is carried further along the dorsal rim of the radius to the radial styloid process. A capsular flap is then elevated radially, taking care to preserve the interosseous ligaments. This approach safely exposes the radial two thirds of the radiocarpal joint and the entire midcarpal joint, while preserving the integrity of the ulnar half of the DRC ligament and the distal half of the DIC ligament. To expose the ulnar third of the radiocarpal joint, the DRC ligament is split longitudinally from the radius to the triquetrum, and a proximodistally oriented capsulotomy is created in the interval between the 5th and 6th extensor compartments between the triquetrum and the DRU ligament (Fig. 12). A capsular flap is then elevated proximally, maintaining the integrity of the radial half of the DRC ligament and the entire DRU ligament.

Dorsal Approach to the Distal Radioulnar Joint After making a skin incision and exposing the deep antebrachial fascia, the fifth extensor compartment is unroofed, allowing translocation of the extensor digiti minimi tendon. The 6th extensor compartment should be left intact, if possible. The DRU ligament is palpated, and an L-shaped incision is made in the DRUJ capsule, with the transverse limb parallel to and just proximal to the DRU ligament, and the longitudinal limb parallel to the radial attachment of the DRUJ capsule at the sigmoid notch.

Volar Approach to the Distal Radioulnar Joint A longitudinal incision is made just radial to the termination of the flexor carpi ulnaris tendon. A careful dissection through the ulnar neurovascular bundle is made, or the entire bundle is retracted ulnarly to expose the superficial head of the pronator quadratus. The origin of the muscle is incised, leaving a short cuff of tendon for later repair. The muscle is elevated radially, exposing the palmar DRUJ capsule. The PRU ligament is palpated, and an L-shaped incision is made in the DRUJ capsule, with the transverse limb parallel to and just proximal to the PRU ligament, and the longitudinal limb parallel to the radial attachment of the DRUJ capsule at the sigmoid notch.

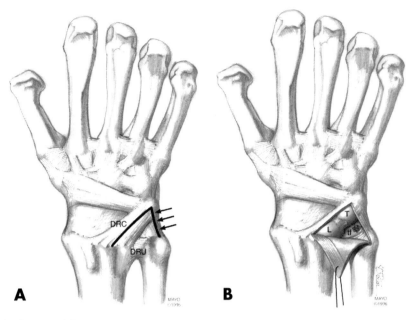

Figure 12

The ulnar capsulotomy technique. **A,** The incision lines in the dorsal wrist capsule are shown splitting the dorsal radiocarpal ligament (DRC) and the radial edge of the septum between the 5th and 6th extensor compartments. DRU = dorsal radioulnar ligament. **B,** The proximally based flap is carefully elevated, exposing the lunate (L), triquetrum (T), and triangular fibrocartilage (tf). (Reproduced with permission from the Mayo Foundation, Rochester, MN.)

Ulnar Approach to the Wrist A longitudinal incision is made along the ulnar margin of the wrist in the midlateral line. Great care is taken to identify and protect the dorsal sensory branch of the ulnar nerve coursing obliquely dorsally and distally just distal to the ulnar styloid process. The extensor retinaculum is incised anterior to the 6th extensor compartment, which should be left intact if possible. The free surface of the ulna is easily seen in the plane between the flexor and extensor carpi ulnaris tendons. This plane can then be incised sharply distally to a level just distal to the tip of the ulnar styloid process. This incision exposes the ulnar styloid process and the ulnocarpal joint by dividing the ulnar radiocarpal joint capsule in a fiber-splitting fashion.

Biomechanics of the Wrist and Distal Radioulnar Joint

Kinematics: Distal Radioulnar Joint
The overall motion of the DRUJ is rotation—the distal radius rotates about the head of the ulna, considered the fixed bone in this motion—combined with a modest degree of translation. The axes of rotation of the DRUJ pass roughly through the foveal region of the ulnar head at the base of the ulnar styloid process. Due to the differences in radii of curvature of the sigmoid notch and the ulnar head, translation occurs through the DRUJ such that the axes of rotation migrate volarly as pronation is reached and dorsally as supination is carried out. This implies that the radius translates volarly during pronation and dorsally during supination, allowing the ulnar head to appear more prominent dorsally during pronation than supination. Although the terms dorsal displacement and dorsal instability of the DRUJ are based upon the relative prominence of the ulnar head, in reality the position of the ulnar head is fixed; the distal radius is the mobile segment. Additionally, the degree of passive translation of the DRUJ is dependent on forearm rotation; the range of translation normally allowed in neutral rotation (5 to 6 mm) is significantly greater than the range of translation at the extremes of pronation and supination. This effect is created by a complex interaction of the ligaments of the DRUJ, the DRUJ joint capsule, and the interosseous membrane.

Motion through the proximal radioulnar joint is nearly perfectly rotational, with the axes of rotation passing through the geometric center of the radial head. Thus, the overall orientation of the axes of rotation of pronation and supination pass obliquely through the forearm, from the radial head proximally through the ulna head distally. This action results in the radius twisting about the ulna from supination (where the 2 bones are nearly collinear) to pronation (where the 2 bones are crossed), which leads to an apparent shortening of the distal projection of the radius relative to the ulna.

Kinematics: Overall Wrist Motion
The principal planes of motion of the wrist are the sagittal plane (flexion/extension) and the coronal plane (radial-ulnar deviation). Pronation and supination, occurring through the transverse plane, can also be measured. Most activities that require positioning the hand through the wrist involve a combination of rotations, such as circumduction, to properly position the hand in space. One commonly characterized combination of axes is called the "dart-throw axis."

Dorsiflexion is usually coupled with radial deviation, while palmar flexion is usually coupled with ulnar deviation.

The wrist has been characterized anatomically, as well as mechanically, to be composed of 2 rows of carpal bones. While there is certainly displacement of varying magnitude between the bones in each row, the majority of wrist motion stems from displacement through the radiocarpal and midcarpal joints. On average, the wrist enjoys approximately 75° to 90° of flexion, 75° to 90° of extension, 15° to 20° of radial deviation, and 25° to 40° of ulnar deviation. Passive rotation through the radiocarpal and midcarpal joints (distal to the forearm) in a relaxed examination averages a total arc of 40° pronation/supination, which reduces to less than 10° total arc of rotation in an active or resisted passive examination. The forearm typically rotates a total arc of 160° to 180° of pronation and supination, centered equally about the neutral forearm position (the position in a normal forearm in which the radial and ulnar styloid processes are mutually rotated as far from each other as possible). The so-called centers of rotation of the wrist have been estimated to be found passing through the head of the capitate for both radial/ulnar deviation and flexion/extension.

Kinematics: Individual Carpal Bone Motion

Although the carpus is most often thought of as having a proximal and distal row, this by no means invalidates the concepts of carpal columns. It is simply a way to reconcile the anatomic associations of the carpal bones within each row with the observed mechanics of those same bones. The bones within each row display kinematic behaviors that are more similar than behaviors observed between the 2 rows. Because the kinematic behaviors of the carpal bones are measurably different between flexion-extension and radioulnar deviation, these 2 arcs of motion will be considered separately.

Flexion-Extension   The metacarpals are pulled through the range of flexion and extension by the action of the extrinsic wrist motors inserting on their bases. The hand unit, composed of the metacarpals and phalanges, is securely associated with the distal carpal row through interlocking of articular surfaces and strong ligamentous connections of the second through fifth CMC joints. The trapezoid, capitate, and hamate undergo displacement with their respective metacarpals with no significant deviation of direction or magnitude of motion. Due to the strong interosseous ligaments, the trapezium generally tracks with the trapezoid, but remains under the influence of the mobile first metacarpal. The major direction of motion for this entire complex is flexion and extension, with little radioulnar deviation.

The proximal row bones generally follow the direction of motion of the distal row bones during flexion-extension of the wrist; however, the scaphoid, lunate and triquetrum are not as tightly secured to the hand unit as are the distal row bones. In addition, the interosseous ligaments between the proximal row bones allow substantial intercarpal motion. Thus there are measurable differences between the motions of the proximal and distal row bones, as well as between the individual bones of the proximal carpal row; this is most pronounced between the scaphoid and lunate. From the extreme of flexion to the extreme of extension, the scaphoid undergoes substantially more angular displacement than the lunate, primarily in the plane of hand motion. There are measurable out-of-plane motions between the scaphoid and lunate as well, as the scaphoid progressively supinates relative to the lunate as the wrist extends. The effect of the differential direction and magnitude of displacement between the scaphoid and lunate is to create a relative separation between the palmar surfaces of the 2 bones as extension is reached, and a coaptation of the 2 surfaces as flexion is reached. The extremes of displacement are checked by the twisting of the fibers of the interosseous ligaments. Once this limit is reached, the scaphoid and lunate will move as a unit through the radiocarpal and midcarpal joints. Although of lesser magnitude, similar behaviors occur through the lunatotriquetral joint. The lunate experiences the smallest magnitude of rotation of all carpal bones during flexion and extension. The radiocarpal and midcarpal joints contribute nearly equally to the range of extension and flexion of the wrist, when measured through the capitolunate/radiolunate joint column. In contrast, when measured through the radioscaphoid/STT joint column, more than two thirds of the range of motion occurs through the radioscaphoid joint.

Radioulnar Deviation   As with flexion and extension, the bones of the distal row move essentially as a unit—with themselves, as well as with the second through fifth metacarpals—during radial and ulnar deviation of the wrist. The proximal row bones, however, display a remarkably different kinematic behavior. As a unit, the proximal carpal row displays a reciprocating motion with the distal row, such that the principal motion during wrist radial deviation is flexion. Conversely, during wrist ulnar deviation, the proximal carpal row extends. In addition to the flexion-extension activity of the proximal carpal row, a less pronounced motion occurs, resulting in ulnar displacement during wrist radial deviation and radial displacement during wrist ulnar deviation. Additional longitudinal axial displacements occur between the proximal carpal row bones, as they do during flexion and extension. Although of substantially lower magnitude than the principal directions of rotation, these longitudinal axial displacements

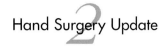
contribute to a relative separation between the palmar surfaces of the scaphoid and lunate in wrist ulnar deviation, and to a relative coaptation during wrist radial deviation, limited by the tautness of the scapholunate interosseous ligament. Once maximum tension is achieved, the 2 bones will displace as a single unit. As with flexion and extension, the lunate experiences the least rotation of all carpal bones during radial and ulnar deviation. The magnitude of rotation through the midcarpal joint is approximately 1.5 times greater than through the radiocarpal joint during radial and ulnar deviation.

Kinematics: Dissociative Instability of the Carpus

Scapholunate dissociation was the first carpal instability pattern to be studied clinically and in the laboratory. Believed to be the result of traumatic disruption of the scapholunate interosseous ligament, untreated scapholunate dissociation has been associated with the development of dorsiflexed (extended) intercalated segmental instability (DISI). Much like a coiled spring, the prestressed nature of the scapholunate joint is constrained by the scapholunate interosseous ligament. Division of this structure allows the lunate and triquetrum—the intercalated segments—to extend relative to the scaphoid, capitate, and radius. Several studies have attempted to measure kinematic changes with division of ligaments in cadaver specimens, but have been nonuniform and inconclusive in the reported results. Division of the RSL ligament has not been shown to contribute to scapholunate dissociation. The dorsal region of the scapholunate interosseous ligament is the key stabilizer of the scapholunate joint. Laboratory studies have confirmed that the greatest deviation from normal motion is seen with division of the dorsal region of the scapholunate ligament; repair of this region exhibits the greatest degree of restoration of normal kinematics.

Although not as common as scapholunate dissociation, volarflexion (flexion) intercalated segmental instability (VISI) is a condition in which the lunate tends to abnormally flex in the face of neutral alignment of the capitate relative to the radius. Division of the lunatotriquetral interosseous ligament alone will not produce substantial alterations of lunatotriquetral kinematics; however, division of both the lunatotriquetral and dorsal radiocarpal ligaments can lead to substantial instability and measurable flexion of the lunate and combined extension-supination of the triquetrum.

Kinematics: Limited Arthrodesis

Numerous laboratory studies have been conducted to evaluate the effect of limited intercarpal arthrodeses on carpal bone motion. These studies have substantially increased our understanding of the contributions of various intercarpal joints to global wrist motion. Arthrodesis of the midcarpal joint has been shown to decrease the range of wrist flexion by approximately 35%, while arthrodesis of the radiocarpal joint results in a loss of flexion of slightly over 60%. Both arthrodeses limit extension, with the greatest effect generated by arthrodesis of the radiocarpal joint. Arthrodeses between bones within the proximal row reduce wrist range of motion by 10% to 20%; intercarpal arthrodeses within the distal carpal row have little measurable effect on global wrist motion.

Kinetics

Force Analysis   Force analyses of the wrist have been attempted using a variety of methods—free body diagrams, rigid body spring models, and experimental methods employing force transducers, pressure-sensitive film, pressure transducers, and strain gauges. Due to the intrinsic geometric complexity of the wrist, the large number of carpal elements, the number of tissue interfaces to which loads are applied, and the large number of positions that the wrist can assume, these analyses have been difficult and are riddled with assumptions. Relative changes and trends in forces brought about by the introduction of experimental variables are generally more useful than absolute values.

Normal Joint Forces   Experimental and analytical studies of force transmission across the wrist in the neutral position are in general agreement that approximately 80% of the force is transmitted across the radiocarpal joint, and 20% across the ulnocarpal joint space (14% across the ulnolunate articulation and 6% across the ulnotriquetral articulation). One study reported that 78% of the longitudinal force across the wrist in the neutral position is transmitted through the radiocarpal articulation, with 46% transmitted by the radioscaphoid fossa and 32% by the lunate fossa. Forces across the midcarpal joint in neutral position have been estimated to be 31% through the STT joint, 19% through the scaphocapitate joint, 29% through the lunocapitate joint, and 21% through the triquetrohamate joint. Forearm pronation increases ulnocarpal force transmission (up to 37% of total forces transmitted), with a corresponding decrease in radiocarpal force transmission. This has been theoretically linked to the relative distal prominence of the ulna that occurs as the forearm is pronated. Ulnocarpal force transmission increases to 28% of the total in ulnar deviation of the wrist, while radiocarpal forces increase to 87% of the total in radial deviation. Wrist flexion and extension have only a modest effect on the relative forces transmitted through the radiocarpal and ulnocarpal joints.

Using pressure-sensitive film placed in the radiocarpal joint space, 3 distinct areas of contact through the radiocarpal joint have been identified—radioscaphoid, radiolunate, and ulnolunate. The actual area of contact of the scaphoid and lunate against the distal radius and TFCC is quite limited regardless of joint position, averaging 20% of the entire available articular surface. The scaphoid contact area is greater than that of the lunate by an average factor of 1.5. Centroids of the contact areas shift with varying positions of the wrist, as do the actual areas of contact. Flexion of the scaphoid, for example, results in a dorsal and radial shift of the radioscaphoid contact centroid, and a progressive diminution of contact area. With externally applied loads, the peak articular pressures are quite low, ranging from 1.4 N/mm^2 to 31.4 N/mm^2. The midcarpal joint has been difficult to evaluate with pressure-sensitive film because of its complex shape. It has been estimated that less than 40% of the available articular surface of the midcarpal joint is in actual contact at any one time. The STT joint has been estimated to contribute 23% of the total contact; the scaphocapitate joint, 28%; the lunatocapitate joint, 29%; and the triquetrohamate joint, 20%. Thus, it may be surmised that more than 50% of the midcarpal load is transmitted through the capitate across the scaphocapitate and lunatocapitate joints.

Using the rigid body spring model, simulated limited intercarpal arthrodeses involving the STT, scaphocapitate (SC), and capitohamate (CH) joints have shown no more than 15% reduction of load transmission through the radiolunate joint; however, the combination of CH arthrodesis and capitate shortening has a dramatic effect of radiolunate load reduction and concomitantly increased radioscaphoid, ulnotriquetral, triquetrohamate, and scaphotrapezial joint forces. This effect is probably due primarily to the capitate shortening. Nearly all joint contact shifts to the radioscaphoid joint with STT and SC arthrodeses. Scapholunate, scapholunocapitate, and lunatocapitate arthrodeses tend to distribute loads more proportionately through the radioscaphoid and radiolunate joint spaces, but do not duplicate normal joint contact areas.

Joint Force Alteration with Changes in Radius and Ulna Length Studies of change in load transmission related to the relative length of the radius and ulna have shown that simulation of a positive ulnar variance of 2.5 mm (either by ulnar lengthening or radial shortening) shifts the majority of the transmitted load from the radiocarpal joint (58%) toward the ulnocarpal joint (42%). The reverse trend occurs with a 2.5-mm negative ulnar variance, with a reduction in ulnocarpal load transmission to only 4%. Excision of the TFCC has been shown to reduce ulnocarpal force transmission

from 20% to 16%. Additional studies have been carried out to determine the effect of changing the ulnar inclination of the distal radius, a treatment advocated by some for Kienböck's disease in patients with neutral ulnar variance. Lateral closing, lateral opening, and medial closing radial osteotomies have been simulated in cadaver wrists and compared to normal values for joint loading characteristics. The lateral opening and medial closing osteotomies increased force transmission across the ulna and nearly eliminated radiolunate forces. In contrast, the lateral closing osteotomy decreased ulnar loading while increasing the loads transmitted through the radiolunate joint. In all 3 situations, the degree of load shift was proportionately related to the osteotomy angle.

Material Properties of Carpal Ligaments The material properties of the carpal ligaments have been evaluated to define parameters such as yield strength, stress, strain, and histeresis in isolated bone-ligament-bone cadaveric preparations. The ligaments of the wrist have not been found to be substantially different in material properties from other mammalian ligament systems. The extrinsic ligaments of the wrist, such as the palmar capsular radiocarpal ligaments, are viscoelastic structures, exhibiting stiffness behavior proportional to strain rate with failure at approximately 100 N. The scapholunate and lunatotriquetral interosseous ligaments have been identified as the strongest ligaments in the wrist, requiring force applications greater than 300 N to fail. The strain at deformation for the scapholunate and lunatotriquetral interosseous ligaments is substantially greater (over 50%) than that of the other carpal ligaments (10% to 35%). Distraction testing of the RSL ligament has shown it to be extremely weak, failing at less than 50 N of applied tensile load. A recent series of experiments evaluated the material properties of the anatomic subregions of the scapholunate interosseous ligaments. In these experiments, the dorsal, palmar, and proximal (membranous) regions were subjected to deformation testing in isolated torsion, translation, and distraction to failure. The dorsal region was found the strongest of the 3, requiring greater than 250 N of applied tensile load. The dorsal region is the principal stabilizer of the scapholunate complex in dorsal and palmar translation, as well as flexion and extension. The palmar region also contributes to joint stability, but to a smaller degree. The proximal region, composed of fibrocartilage, has little measurable influence on joint stability. The proximal region is also the weakest in distraction testing, generally failing with application of less than 25 N of tension.

The ligamentous stabilizers of the transverse carpal arch have also been recently evaluated; posteroanterior compressive loads were applied after sectioning the flexor retinaculum

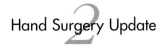
and the distal row palmar and dorsal interosseous ligaments. The transversely oriented interosseous ligaments had a significant effect on transverse carpal instability. The flexor retinaculum did not have a significant effect on transverse carpal stability, reducing stiffness to compressive load by less than 8% when divided; however, the width of the carpal tunnel increased significantly (up to 10%) with division of the flexor retinaculum. Division of the flexor retinaculum has not been associated with measurable changes in carpal kinematics.

Pathomechanical Simulations

Pathologic conditions of the wrist have been simulated in the laboratory to add to our understanding of wrist pathomechanics and the mechanics of treatment options.

Distal Radius Fracture   As ulnar inclination of the distal radius articular surface decreases (a situation often encountered in a malreduced distal radius fracture), ulnar column force increases proportionally. Additionally, changes occur within the radiocarpal joint, with a palmar shift of the radiolunate centroid and a dorsoradial shift of the radioscaphoid centroid. These trends are seen with malposition increments of as little as 10°. Dorsal inclination of the distal radius also affects the load characteristics of the wrist, by progressively increasing the radioscaphoid and radiolunate load pressures. These changes are noted consistently with dorsal angulation greater than 30°. Dorsal angulation of the distal radius beyond 20° leads to significant load shifts across the midcarpal joint, due to the relative DISI posture of the proximal carpal row. Shortening of the radius also affects the load patterns, with gross ulnar impingement and disruption of the TFCC noted with radial shortening more than 5 mm. Thus, it has been suggested that relatively normal mechanical loading of the wrist is a reasonable expectation if less than 2 mm of radial shortening, less than 10° loss of ulnar inclination, and less than 20° loss of palmar inclination can be achieved and maintained.

Scaphoid Nonunion/Malunion   Recent radiographic studies have determined that the normal intraosseous scaphoid angle measures ± 32° in the sagittal plane (the angle between tangents drawn on the palmar cortex of the proximal scaphoid and the dorsal cortex of the distal scaphoid) and ± 40° in the coronal plane (the angle between tangents drawn on the midcarpal cortex of the proximal half of the scaphoid and the flattened subchondral surface of the distal scaphoid). Just as ligamentous dissociation between the scaphoid and lunate can lead to instability patterns, so can nonunion or malunion of the scaphoid after fracture. In an evaluation of carpal kinematics in cadaver specimens with scaphoid osteotomies placed to simulate scaphoid waist

fractures, proximal and distal fragments were found to move independently, with an increase in motion of the proximal fragment and a decrease in motion of the distal fragment. This led to a typical humpback deformity of the scaphoid, as the proximal pole fragment extended with the lunate in a DISI pattern. Contact area and pressure studies of simulated scaphoid fractures have revealed that there is no change in the contact area through the scaphoid fossa between intact specimens, specimens with a proximal pole fracture, or specimens with excised proximal poles. There is, however, a redistribution of contact, tending to increase contact of the scaphoid fossa with the distal fragment, and an increase in the contact pressure in this region. No changes through the radiolunate joint were noted. These studies do not, however, address loading trends encountered with cyclic loading following scaphoid osteotomy.

Annotated Bibliography

Vascular Anatomy

Sheetz KK, Bishop AT, Berger RA: The arterial blood supply of the distal radius and ulna and its potential use in vascularized pedicled bone grafts. *J Hand Surg* 1995;20A:902–914.

The arterial anatomy of the distal radius and ulna is defined in a practical manner, with emphasis on potential corticocancellous grafts from the distal radius with a pedicled blood supply. These grafts have potential use in the treatment of conditions such as scaphoid nonunion and osteonecrosis of the carpal bones.

Ligament Anatomy

Berger RA: The ligaments of the wrist: A current overview of anatomy with considerations of their potential functions. *Hand Clin* 1997;13:63–82.

This is a comprehensive overview of the known carpal and distal radioulnar ligaments with a synopsis of functional attributes of the ligaments.

Ischii S, Palmer AK, Werner FW, Short WH, Fortino MD: An anatomic study of the ligamentous structure of the triangular fibrocartilage complex. *J Hand Surg* 1998;23A:977–985.

The TFCC can be artificially divided into a proximal and distal complex, with stabilizing responsibilities for the DRUJ and ulnocarpal joint, respectively. The details provided in this study help clarify this often confusing and complex anatomy.

General Biomechanics

An K-N, Berger RA, Cooney WP III (eds): *Biomechanics of the Wrist Joint.* New York, NY, Springer-Verlag, 1991.

This comprehensive reference of anatomy and current biomechanics of the wrist compiles the research experience of 13 investigators into

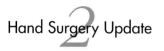

one volume. Heavily referenced, topics of discussion include anatomy, individual carpal bone and global wrist motion, force analysis, joint contact area and pressure, osseous strain, material properties, and muscle function.

Individual Carpal Bone Kinematics

Kobayashi M, Berger RA, Linscheid RL, An KN: Intercarpal kinematics during wrist motion. *Hand Clin* 1997;13:143–149.

The largest collection of kinematic data from cadaveric specimens is published to optimize the statistical significance of measurements. The authors confirmed that the distal row bones move largely as a fixed unit, while the scaphoid, lunate, and triquetrum exhibit significant out-of-plane motion.

Kobayashi M, Berger RA, Nagy L, et al: Normal kinematics of carpal bones: A three-dimensional analysis of carpal bone motion relative to the radius. *J Biomech* 1997;30:787–793.

This is a continuation of the *Hand Clinics* article above, with concentration on radiocarpal displacement.

Kinetics

Viegas SF, Patterson R, Peterson P, Roefs J, Tencer A, Choi S: The effects of various load paths and different loads on the load transfer characteristics of the wrist. *J Hand Surg* 1989;14A:458–465.

Using pressure-sensitive film in cadaver radiocarpal joints, the authors studied contact areas and pressures within the radiocarpal joint with varying loading pathways (loading proximally through the tendons versus loading distally through various metacarpal pathways). A consistent finding was a 3:2 ratio of scaphoid fossa to lunate fossa contact area. Loads greater than 46 lbs do not change the contact areas; however, joint contact pressures correlate positively with load applications. The overall joint contact area does not exceed 40% of the available joint surface area.

Material Properties of Ligaments

de Lange A, Huiskes R, Kauer JM: Wrist-joint ligament length changes in flexion and deviation of the hand: An experimental study. *J Orthop Res* 1990;8:722–730.

Using roentgenstereophotogrammetric analysis, the length changes of 7 carpal ligaments were measured in cadaver wrists. Short ligaments, such as the short radiolunate ligament, experienced length changes up to 30%, whereas other longer ligaments did not lengthen more than 20%. The longer ligaments also displayed a greater tendency to curve than did the shorter ligaments. The authors concluded that the radioscaphocapitate ligament plays an important role in stabilizing the capitate in extension and deviation, just as the lunate is stabilized by the long radiolunate ligament. The dorsal radiocarpal and palmar triquetrocapitate ligaments stabilize the carpus in the neutral position.

Nowak MD, Logan SE: Strain rate dependent permanent deformation of human wrist ligaments. *Biomed Sci Instrum* 1988;24:61–65.

These authors have published several articles providing comprehensive evaluations of the material properties of the major carpal ligaments.

Schuind F, An K-N, Berglund L, et al: The distal radioulnar ligaments: A biomechanical study. *J Hand Surg* 1991;16A: 1106–1114.

In this stereophotogrammetric analysis of the palmar and dorsal radioulnar ligaments, cadaveric forearms were positioned in varying degrees of pronation and supination. Qualitative analysis indicated that the dorsal ligament becomes taut in pronation, and the palmar ligament taut in supination. Quantitative confirmation was obtained with consistent length changes in the respective ligaments. Mechanical testing applying axial loads to the triangular fibrocartilage revealed significant laxity that decreased with forearm pronation. Transverse loading revealed diminished stiffness of the triangular fibrocartilage in neutral forearm rotation.

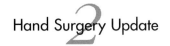
Chapter 7
Imaging and Evaluation of the Carpus and Distal Radius

Thomas J. Graham, MD

Introduction

To confirm a suspected diagnosis, the hand surgeon can supplement physical examination findings with appropriate imaging. The scope and level of sophistication of the available modalities has evolved considerably. The surgeon must understand the appropriateness of each imaging study and recognize the importance of cost-effective test selection. The right choice of imaging technique can optimize patient treatment.

Cooperation between the musculoskeletal radiologist and the hand surgeon will enhance the ultimate diagnostic capability. The surgeon's ability to extract from plain radiography critical information that may impact the immediate care of the patient will likely exceed that of the radiologist; however, the performance and interpretation of ultrasound, arthrography, bone scintigraphy, and advanced cross-sectional imaging modalities remain the purview of the radiologist. The hand surgeon must increase his or her level of comfort in interpreting these sophisticated studies while maintaining a dialogue with the radiologist.

Enhanced imaging capabilities now offer the clinician totally new depictions of normal and abnormal anatomy. Integrating and comparing this information with the patient's history, physical examination, and surgical findings will be the mechanism by which the sensitivity and specificity of the imaging modalities will be increased.

This chapter is organized using an algorithm-building approach for specific pathologies about the wrist. This approach, focused on surgical decision making, provides a foundation on which a systematic battery of tests can be built to accompany the surgeon's clinical evaluation. Special consideration is given to comparison of differential effectiveness of imaging modalities for work-up of the same pathologic entity, cost comparisons of radiographic work-ups, and difficult diagnoses of pathologic conditions of the wrist.

Advances in Imaging of Normal Anatomy

No hand surgeon would dispute the value of biplanar posteroanterior (PA) and true lateral radiographs in the initial evaluation of wrist pathology. In addition, many treatment centers have developed a standard wrist series, consisting of PA, true lateral, 45° semisupinated oblique, and ulnar deviation PA views. Debate on positioning of the entire upper extremity has been largely resolved with recent recommendations for standardized circumstances under which studies are obtained. Shoulder abduction to 90° and elbow flexion to 90° places the hand-forearm unit at the same height as the shoulder; the PA film should be obtained in this position, with the forearm in neutral rotation. To obtain the true lateral image, the technician can reposition the cassette for the lateral view, or adduct the patient's shoulder while maintaining the same elbow position. Standardizing the methods by which films are obtained enhances the ability of the surgeon to compare and contrast the individual patient's anatomy in a longitudinal survey, improve comparisons between patient populations, and facilitate communication among physicians.

One of the most cost-effective mechanisms by which the surgeon can improve the clinical value of diagnostic studies is to extract more information from a routine evaluation. The importance of imaging the contralateral wrist in unilateral pathology has been corroborated. Normal contralateral wrist radiographs provide a superior reference for measurement of radiocarpal and intercarpal angles, as well as carpal height indices. Radiographic parameters of the radius platform (radial inclination and palmar tilt) and ulnar variance should be compared to established standards and to the contralateral wrist.

To assist the surgeon in determination of fragment size and position in fractures about the distal radius, anatomic studies with radiographic correlates have recently been published. Determination of the relative contact area of the radiocarpal relationships in recent radiographic studies has recapitulated

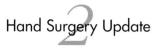
earlier anatomic investigations; the lunate facet exceeds the scaphoid facet in articular surface area. Performance of antero-posterior radiographs with the beam directed 30° cephalic results in a more precise characterization of the posteromedial aspect of the distal end of the radius, both by orientation and magnification of this critical portion of the bone.

Variations in intercarpal relationships exist without pathologic consequences; this fact may diminish reliance on adjunctive radiographic studies. Normal disruption in the carpal arcs (Gilula's lines) can occur in certain wrist positions. On PA films taken in radial deviation, carpal arcs I and II are predictably disrupted at the lunatotriquetral (LT) joint. In ulnar deviation, arc II becomes malaligned at the scapholunate (SL) joint in roughly a third of normal wrists; type II lunate morphology accentuates these findings. Arc III is nearly immutable in any wrist position due to the stability that exists between the bones of the distal carpal row.

Interpretation of the external geometry of each of the carpal bones can be challenging in both the injured and uninjured states. In a recent study conducted to better delineate specific anatomic features of the scaphoid and to direct the radiographic examination toward specific scaphoid injuries, particular landmarks were identified with wire, and then a series of radiographs were taken. The authors suggested that up to 5 individual views would be needed to completely characterize the scaphoid, and they recommended specific views to reduce radiation and cost.

The waist of the scaphoid, the most frequent site of fracture, is best visualized in an ulnar-deviated PA view, with a 20° beam angle relative to the elbow; the semipronated 45° PA and a lateral projection with the wrist in extension are also good views. These 3 images all show the scaphoid perpendicular to its longitudinal axis (the distal half of the scaphoid is best visualized on the 45° semipronated oblique). The ulnar-deviated PA view, often called the scaphoid view, was found to distort the bone's anatomy consistently; however, it remains the best study for visualizing the proximal scaphoid pole.

The anatomy and articular relationships of the lunate were also studied to determine if plain radiographs were effective in characterizing that bone. Lateral lunate morphology was scrutinized with plain radiographs to see if the volar aspect of the lunate was thicker than the dorsal pole. The authors found that two thirds of studied lunates were indeed thinner dorsally, while a quarter had the opposite finding of a thinner volar pole. The remainder were roughly symmetric when bisected on the lateral projection. This may have implications with regard to intercalated segment postures associated with specific ligament injuries.

Another recent study of the lunate emphasized the poor predictive value of routine radiographs in identifying the type of lunate morphology. A third of the lunates found to have a separate medial facet for hamate articulation (type 2) upon anatomic study were incorrectly identified as having a single midcarpal facet (type 1) on routine radiographs. Conversely, 26% of the type 1 bones were incorrectly labeled as type 2 by the radiograph reviewers. In over 60% of the wrists with a medial lunate facet, the proximal pole of the hamate had significant cartilage erosion; this may be an underappreciated source of wrist pain.

Interpretation of plain radiographs of the distal radioulnar joint (DRUJ) has traditionally been limited to measurement of ulnar variance. An appreciation for the angles of inclination of the sigmoid notch and ulnar seat has been fostered by recent work in which this relationship was studied. Relative to the longitudinal axis of the ulna, the sigmoid notch is inclined approximately 8° toward the ulna, while the ulnar seat has an articular inclination that exceeds 20°. There is relative correlation between the 2 inclination angles, and even a relationship with the ulnar variance; however, the degree of variability not only has implications for normal function of the DRUJ but may also explain why symptomatic articular incongruity can follow ulnar shortening osteotomy.

Fractures of the Distal Radius

Imaging about the distal radius plays an integral role in identifying and classifying patterns of fracture, assessing the adequacy of closed or open reduction, and cataloging the long-term outcome with regard to well-established radiographic parameters. Objective data continue to emerge concerning the use and reliability of classification systems based solely on plain radiography; however, all schema have limitations. Consistent findings of low intra- and interobserver agreement for popular classifications discourage the use of any single classification as the sole method for determining treatment or even comparing reported series. One study even demonstrated that the same experienced clinician can be internally inconsistent to a high degree when repeatedly assessing a particular image.

Computed tomography (CT) is considered a superior imaging modality for discerning bony detail in the wrist. Because of cost considerations, criteria should be developed for selection of patients in whom CT scanning might have the greatest impact on treatment. The surgeon should use CT scans for assessing fractures with intra-articular extension into the radiocarpal joint, fracture propagation into the metadiaphysis, and ulnar styloid fractures. Cross-sectional imaging offers the advantages of detailing DRUJ involvement, the amount of fracture comminution, and articular surface depression (Fig. 1).

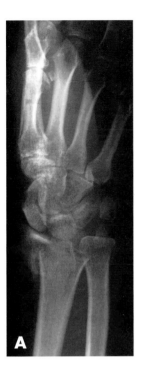
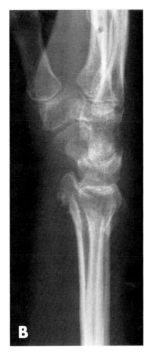
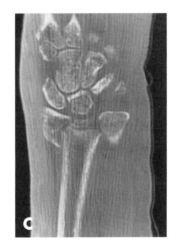
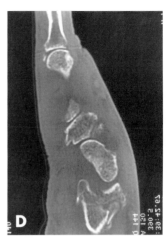
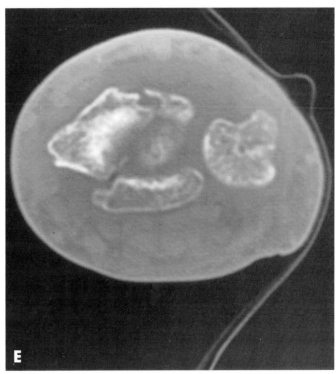

Figure 1

A and **B**, Posteroanterior and lateral images of a comminuted, intra-articular fracture of the distal radius. A prior attempt at external fixation was performed before referral. **C**, **D** and **E**, Three useful computed tomography cuts, detailing the articular depression and fragment position. Additional information about the status of the carpal bones can be gleaned simultaneously with this modality.

In comparisons of plain radiographs and CT scans, CT scans consistently demonstrated a greater ability to detect and quantify articular incongruities after fracture of the distal radius. Authors of a recent article detailed 2 innovative methods for gleaning objective data from plain radiographs and CT scans. The Longitudinal Axis Method was used to measure "step and gap" parameters from lateral radiographs of the fractured radius, and the Arc Method was used to quantify these values from CT scans (Fig. 2). More reproducible measurements were obtained for the Arc Method. Furthermore, plain radiographs were found to either significantly underestimate or overestimate displacement when compared to CT scans.

Cineradiographs, or "real-time fluoroscopy," have the advantage of studying radiocarpal and intercarpal motion. The technique has been used to study the effect of dorsal distal radius tilt on wrist motion. Findings indicate that motion decreased and intercarpal alignment was altered as loss of normal palmar tilting escalated. When dorsal tilt was less than 10°, however, the effects on wrist motion and dynamic carpal alignment were negligible.

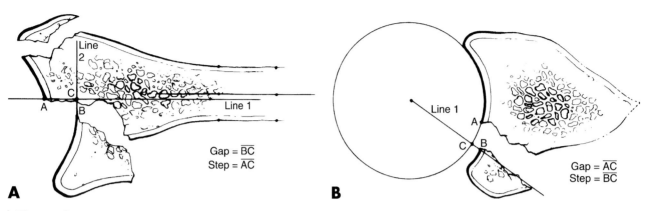

Figure 2

A, Description of the Longitudinal Axis Method measured on plain radiographs. **B,** Description of the Arc Method measured on computed tomography scans. (Reproduced with permission from Cole RJ, Bindra RP, Evanoff BA, Gilula LA, Yamaguchi K, Gelberman RH: Radiographic evaluation of osseous displacement following intra-articular fractures of the distal radius: Reliability of plain radiography versus computed tomography. *J Hand Surg* 1997;22A:792–800.)

The role of magnetic resonance imaging (MRI) in evaluating the wrist continues to evolve. Although the technique has limited application in the typical assessment of distal radius fractures, MRI is appropriate for some situations. Periphyseal injuries, especially those due to chronic repetitive stress, may be best evaluated with MRI. In populations of young gymnasts, MRI has proved useful in identifying abnormalities about the growth plate. The role of MRI may be to detect subtle stress injuries when other more specific modalities fail to demonstrate a source of pain.

Fractures of the Carpal Bones

Although new techniques for the plain radiographic assessment of scaphoid morphology have been described and referenced, defining the optimum method for precise identification of occult fractures of the scaphoid remains a challenge. Much of the interest in this field of study has surrounded the emerging role of MRI in detection and follow-up assessment of the fractured scaphoid. MRI has been shown to have a high degree of sensitivity, specificity, and interobserver agreement for identification of scaphoid fractures, even in a setting of "negative" plain radiographs. The technical aspects of the study included performance of T1-weighted spin-echo, T2-weighted gradient echo, and short inversion time-inversion recovery (STIR) sequences; fractures are typically detected from a combination of the T1 and STIR images. Similar success was achieved when MRI was used to detect suspected scaphoid fractures in adults and

in skeletally immature patients. Associated injuries to other carpal bones and the distal radius that went unrecognized in conventional imaging were also detected on MRI.

The ultimate value of any imaging technique is determined by capability and cost comparisons. When MRI was compared to bone scintigraphy in one uncontrolled study, both had less than optimal performance yet were roughly comparable in their ability to detect carpal pathology (Fig. 3). Another investigation contrasted routine radiography, high-definition macroradiology, and MRI. The findings support early use of MRI in detection of occult scaphoid fractures, citing the benefits of early identification of fractures and determination of patients who will not need lengthy immobilization and repeat follow-up if the MRI scan is negative. Compelling cost data showed nearly equivalent charges for an initial MRI versus repeated plain radiographs and clinic visits. The study also supported MRI use with "time off work" data. Macroradiography, essentially a 4 × magnification view that minimizes blurring, was unsuitable for detection of occult scaphoid fractures.

A short-sequence wrist MRI series was developed at one institution for detection of suspected scaphoid fractures not demonstrated on plain radiographs. Dedicated wrist coils and careful positioning have enabled clinicians to increase the information yield and make this evaluation cost-competitive with other modalities, such as bone scan and computed axial tomography.

Another new technology is 3-dimensional reconstruction of CT images about the wrist. This technology is evolving from an investigation tool into a modality with broader clinical applications that will soon have implications in

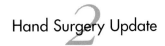

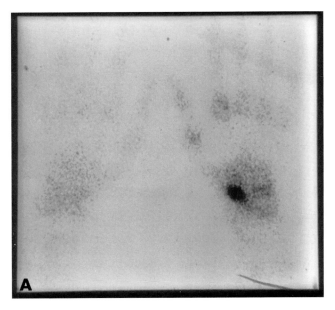

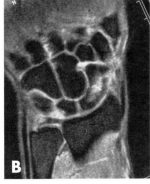

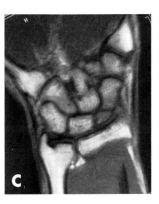

Figure 3

A, A patient in whom a scaphoid fracture was suspected. Plain radiographs fail to reveal bony pathology. Collimated bone scintigraphy can be a very useful diagnostic examination. **B,** A T2-weighted magnetic resonance imaging scan demonstrates edema within the scaphoid. **C,** A fracture line in the scaphoid is better demonstrated on the T1-weighted magnetic resonance image.

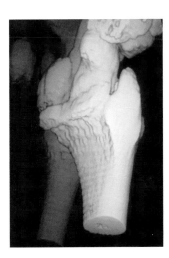

Figure 4

This 3-dimensional computed tomography reconstruction of a malunited volar margin fracture and the adjacent carpal bones details the pertinent anatomy and can assist in preoperative planning.

assessment of the fine anatomy of the carpus. It is particularly well-suited for characterizing the malunited distal radius (Fig. 4).

Interosseous Ligament Injuries

The diagnosis of a tear or rupture of an intrinsic ligament of the wrist can be difficult, especially in the acute period after injury. Whether presenting as an isolated injury or in combination with fractures of the carpal bones and radius, interosseous ligament failure is often suspected but can rarely be proven by physical examination and routine imaging alone. Some of the suboptimal results experienced by patients with wrist trauma may be due to neglected or inadequately treated intercarpal ligament disruptions.

A static wrist instability pattern is rarely present immediately after acute wrist trauma. Provocative maneuvers can be used to obtain "stress" views, which can result in incremental improvement in diagnostic specificity. These views should be compared to the contralateral, presumably uninjured, wrist in order to establish a definitive diagnosis.

Posteroanterior plain radiographs imaged under longitudinal distraction can be helpful in identifying certain intercarpal ligament injuries. In a laboratory setting, division of the LT ligament has a high correlation with significant disruption of carpal arc II and the LT joint in specimens subjected to distraction of 15 lbs through the index and long rays. Scapholunate ligament division has a similar effect on the relationship at the SL junction but the magnitude of the displacement is less, due to a slight amount of scaphoid rotation. The SL and LT intervals also show statistically significant widening when their respective ligaments are sectioned. Normalized carpal height ratios are poor predictors of intercarpal injury under the influence of distraction. These distraction findings are consistently seen in a clinical setting (Fig. 5). Knowledge of the behavior of the normal and injured carpus under distraction may enhance recognition of intrinsic and extrinsic ligament injuries, thereby reducing the need for expensive and invasive testing.

If an unequivocal diagnosis cannot be made with plain radiographs, economical and judicious use of advanced

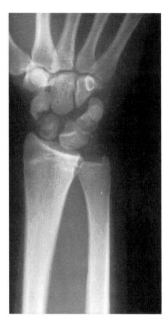

Figure 5

In this patient with an obvious fracture of the scaphoid, a rupture of the lunatotriquetral (LT) ligament was also suspected because of a small bone fragment in the region. Based on laboratory studies, a significant disruption of carpal arc II at the LT interval (under distraction) denotes a rupture of this ligament.

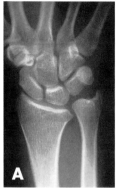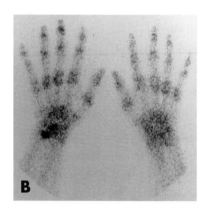

Figure 6

A and **B,** Zero-rotation posteroanterior radiographs characterize the relationship at the distal radioulnar joint. When ulnocarpal abutment is suspected, bone scintigraphy can support this diagnosis when increased uptake in both the lunate and ulnar pole is seen.

imaging should be considered. The most reasonable imaging choices available to the surgeon and radiologist are arthrography and MRI. Other modalities, such as bone scan and CT scan, have little application in this diagnostic arena. These imaging choices must be weighed against wrist arthroscopy as the evolving gold standard; there is little argument that direct visualization offers certain advantages over potentially fallible imaging techniques.

While wrist arthrography is an invasive procedure, it is a safe and relatively inexpensive technique for wrist evaluation. Triple injection (radiocarpal, followed by DRUJ and midcarpal) is now the technically established standard, but radiocarpal injection alone can yield important information about the SL and LT ligaments, as well as the triangular fibrocartilage complex (TFCC). One drawback to arthrography is its lack of specificity. Leaks, often interpreted as tears, are prevalent, even in asymptomatic individuals. One series related that over 25% of young volunteers without wrist complaints or antecedent trauma had an abnormal communication on radiocarpal arthrography.

MRI avoids the invasiveness of arthrography, but is in a nascent stage of development with respect to wrist ligament imaging. The technique is subject to the vicissitudes of anatomic inaccuracy due to sectioning and the lack of experience in interpreting its images. Several recent studies have added greatly to our knowledge of how normal extrinsic and intrinsic wrist ligaments should appear on MRI. Identification

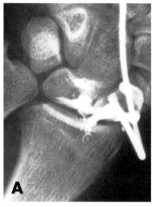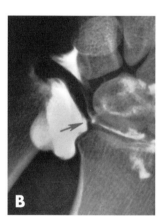

Figure 7

A, Radiocarpal dye injection in a patient with significant positive ulnar variance and ulnar-sided wrist pain. **B,** Dye passage through a tear in the radial aspect of the articular disk (arrow) fills the distal radioulnar joint capsule.

of the SL ligament in normal and pathologic states is now accomplished with more confidence, but definitive characterization of the status of the LT ligament is slower in development. Addition of an arthrogram component to the MRI study, however, significantly enhances the diagnostic capabilities of the technique. Cinemagnetic resonance arthrography, in which images are collected at intervals during injection, is a promising technique that may prove definitive in the diagnosis of subtle SL and LT tears.

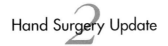

The Ulnar Wrist

Defining the source of pathology at the ulnar aspect of the wrist is particularly challenging. Although the physical examination is critical, it may establish only a working diagnosis, not a definitive one. Certain pathology can be ruled out by a focused and well-performed physical examination. Provocative maneuvers and injection of the extensor carpi ulnaris tendon sheath with local anesthetic, for example, can differentiate tendinitis or a subsheath rupture from an intra-articular problem. Fracture of the ulnar styloid can usually be detected on plain radiographs. Extreme ulnar length resulting in ulnocarpal abutment can typically be appreciated on routine zero-rotation radiographs or can be exposed by imaging the wrist in pronation and ulnar deviation, as well as during grip maneuvers. Carefully columnated bone scans may offer certain critical information, but are plagued by a lack of specificity (Fig. 6).

When the differential diagnosis of ulnocarpal pathology includes TFCC tear, ulnocarpal abutment, subtle destabilizing injury of the DRUJ, and LT ligament tear, the complexity of the work-up increases and imaging choices become more critical. Arthrography can be a valuable entry level test. Injection of the radiocarpal joint can identify ligament communications in both the LT ligament and TFCC (Fig. 7). Performance of a DRUJ injection is technically more difficult, yet can yield additional information (Fig. 8). The potential for false positive findings exists; asymptomatic communications at either site can distract the surgeon's attention from the true pathology causing the patient's symptoms and signs.

The role of MRI in imaging presents the greatest promise as a noninvasive examination of the ulnar wrist, but it remains in a nascent stage of development. The LT ligament is poorly visualized, and only recently have the ulnolunate and ulnotriquetral ligaments been appreciated with MRI. High signal intensity of the triangular fibrocartilage has been seen in the wrists of many asymptomatic individuals, with a prevalence approaching 50% in some studies. Although this is an unacceptably high rate of false positive studies, MRI appears capable of detecting intrasubstance tears of the articular disk, and may be even better suited to demonstrating avulsions from the radial or ulnar insertions (Fig. 9).

Ulnocarpal abutment is nicely demonstrated by MRI on STIR or fat suppression techniques. The findings of low signal intensity on T1 images, and increased signal intensity on T2, can be confused with osteonecrosis of the

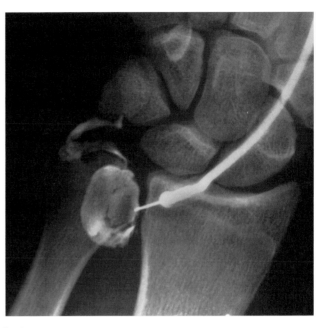

Figure 8
Injection of dye into the distal radioulnar joint capsule demonstrates an avulsion injury of the triangular fibrocartilage complex from the basilar region of the ulnar styloid.

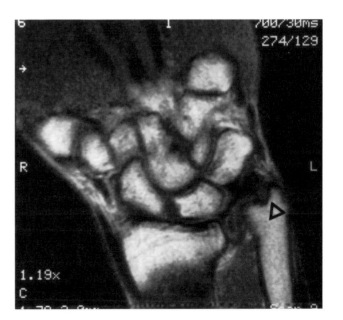

Figure 9
Magnetic resonance imaging of a patient with ulnar-sided wrist pain and intermittent mechanical symptoms related to forearm pronosupination. Avulsion of the triangular fibrocartilage complex with invagination of the articular disk into the distal radioulnar joint was seen on the image and corroborated at surgery.

lunate, but similar findings on the pole of the ulna mitigate against Kienböck's disease in favor of ulnocarpal impaction syndrome.

With improvements in magnets and coils, newer techniques of imaging (gradient-recalled-echo sequences, dynamic MRI, MRI arthrography), and higher levels of sophistication on the part of radiologists, MRI will likely become preeminent in imaging of the ulnar aspect of the wrist. Cost-effectiveness will need to be addressed in the future, and clinical efficacy will have to be enhanced relative to the effectiveness of arthroscopy or arthrotomy.

Osteonecrosis

Identifying idiopathic or posttraumatic osteonecrosis of the carpal bones can be a challenging diagnosis; often the diagnosis is made by exclusion. Radiographic imaging may accelerate the identification of the pathology and/or the initiation of treatment. When Kienböck's disease is suspected, for example, plain radiographs may reveal sclerosis and fragmentation of the lunate and a potentially pathologic relationship between the radius, ulna, and carpus (Fig. 10). Images of the contralateral films of the wrist will provide an internal control for comparison of lunate density and ulnar variance.

The sophisticated imaging techniques used in the diagnosis and staging of avascular necrosis include transpiral tomography, CT absorptiometry, and MRI. Transpiral tomography provides advantages over routine PA and true lateral radiographs, which are the present standard for staging of lunatomalacia (including anatomic definition of both the sagittal and coronal planes). In a large series of patients with Kienböck's disease imaged with tomography, the most common fracture patterns were the transverse shear fracture and the midcoronal fracture. Nondissociative intercalated segment palmarflexion was the predominant instability pattern seen in stage III disease. While not ubiquitous, tomography is available at most hospitals. The technique is cost-competitive.

MRI provides the potential to detect osteonecrosis at an early stage, before it can be identified on plain radiographs (Fig. 11). As the disease process responds to treatment, correlating clinical parameters with MRI will advance our understanding of the pathology as well as the role of MRI in its management.

Carpal Tunnel Syndrome

Carpal tunnel syndrome is a clinical diagnosis that in many cases is corroborated by an electrodiagnostic work-up. To date, imaging modalities have had little role in the evaluation of carpal tunnel syndrome with the possible exception of posttraumatic deformity of the radius as a potential etiologic factor. One study estimated that radiology charges per significant finding in carpal tunnel syndrome ranged from

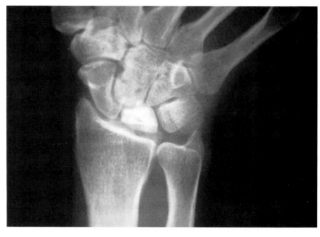

Figure 10

Advanced sclerosis of the lunate, pathognomonic of Kienböck's disease, is demonstrated on a posteroanterior radiograph.

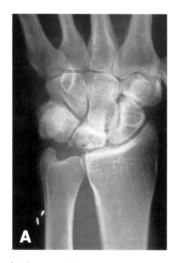
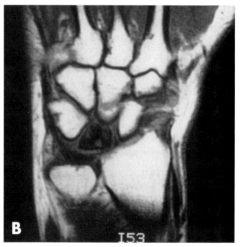

Figure 11

A, Sclerosis, mild cystic change, and early fragmentation of the lunate is seen on plain radiographs. **B,** Findings on magnetic resonance imaging are consistent with osteonecrosis of the lunate.

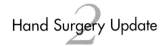

$5,000 to $20,000; thus, radiographs are not recommended routinely in the work-up of compression median neuropathy at the wrist.

Recent reports outline the use of MRI and ultrasonography in the diagnosis of carpal tunnel syndrome. While it is premature to support any of these modalities as a primary diagnostic tool, there may be an adjunct for determining the adequacy of release of the transverse carpal ligament in recurrent carpal tunnel syndrome. MRI may be a valuable investigational tool for characterizing the volumetric and morphologic characteristics of the carpal canal.

Neoplasms

Imaging plays a central role in the diagnostic evaluation of occult and overt neoplastic conditions. Whether single modalities are selected, or a combination of techniques employed, the surgeon must understand the potential yield of each test and how to conduct a global tumor work-up, including evaluation of possible metastases.

Ultrasound plays a role in the evaluation of suspected occult ganglia of the wrist, especially in clinically inconclusive situations. Masses can be characterized by their cystic or cellular nature and their anatomic location can be better defined, with accuracy rates in the 90% range. Studies have found less-costly ultrasound to be as effective as MRI in diagnosing occult ganglia. The lower cost, equivalent diagnostic accuracy, and usefulness in dynamic evaluations support ultrasound as a viable first-line imaging technique for nonpalpable and equivocal lesions.

There has been great interest in the role of MRI in the imaging of bone and soft-tissue tumors about the hand and wrist. The pathologies for which it has been employed include interosseous and periarticular ganglia, peripheral nerve tumors, lipomas, and a variety of benign and malignant cellular tumors. Increased experience and improved technology have enhanced the diagnostic accuracy of MRI considerably. One study demonstrated that the ability of MRI to correctly identify the specific pathology of a hand/wrist mass exceeded the surgeon's preoperative clinical impression.

Inflammatory Conditions

Ultrasound and MRI may play a supplemental role in the diagnosis of inflammatory arthropathy and crystal deposition diseases. Plain radiographic findings that are characteristic of certain diseases are well documented, but the appearance of inflammatory entities on more sophisticated imaging studies is only recently being defined.

MRI has been used for the early diagnosis of both tophaceous gout and rheumatoid arthritis. Urate deposits have been detected along fascial planes and compartmental boundaries, giving insight into the mode of early spread of disease. Radiographs and clinical examination may underestimate the extent of soft-tissue disease in gout. With respect to rheumatoid arthritis, symmetric periarticular contrast enhancement at the wrist and metacarpophalangeal joints was found to have a high correlation with early disease. The integrity of extensor tendons and the degree of pannus or synovial effusion can also be assessed by MRI in the rheumatoid patient.

Reflex Sympathetic Dystrophy

The hand surgeon is occasionally called on to evaluate a patient with a symptom complex consistent with autonomic dysfunction. When the clinical features associated with reflex sympathetic dystrophy (RSD) are present, bone scintigraphy has been suggested to provide objective evidence of the organic manifestations of pain-dysfunction syndromes. Three-phase studies correlate best with the clinical diagnosis of RSD in the first 6 months after onset, but sensitivity is in the neighborhood of 50%. The accuracy of the test declines as the longevity of the process extends. Consequently, bone scintigraphy is not recommended as a confirmatory examination for the diagnosis of RSD.

Summary

The hand surgeon should develop and maintain a systematic approach to the diagnosis of wrist pain and dysfunction. When evaluating an acute or chronic presentation of wrist pathology, appropriate integration of physical examination findings with radiographic imaging results is critical. Although algorithms have been published to assist with the assessment of wrist trauma, the surgeon's experience and individual patient factors will be the deciding influence in what tests are chosen, and at what stage of the diagnostic work-up they are employed (Fig. 12). The expense of performing these diagnostic tests is under greater scrutiny now than ever before. The efficacy of each modality must be demonstrated by clinical and surgical corroboration to yield the most meaningful outcomes data.

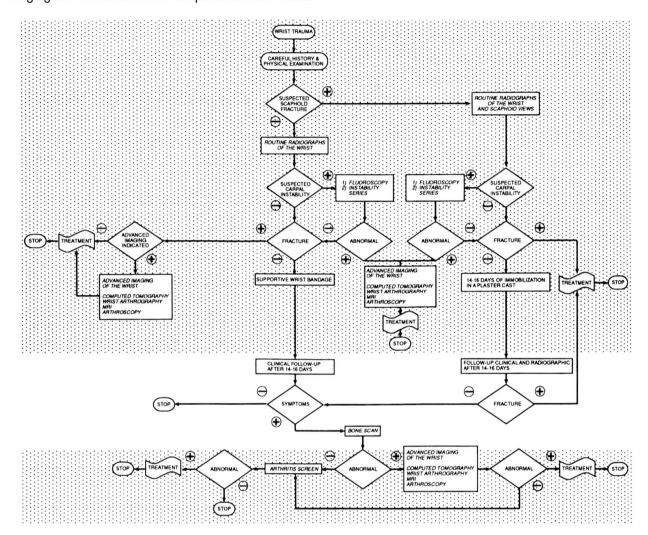

Figure 12

A well-designed algorithm for systematic evaluation of acute wrist injuries derived from a prospective study. (Reproduced with permission from Larsen CF, Brndum V, Wienholtz G, Abrahamsen J, Beyer J: An algorithm for acute wrist trauma: A systematic approach to diagnosis. *J Hand Surg* 1993;18B:207–212.)

Annotated Bibliography

Advances in Imaging of Normal Anatomy

Compson JP, Waterman JK, Heatley FW: The radiological anatomy of the scaphoid: Part 2. Radiology. *J Hand Surg* 1997;22B:8–15.

Because the scaphoid is complex in shape, it is difficult to characterize radiographically. It is even more challenging when the dynamics of scaphoid motion are taken into account. This investigation is extremely thorough, and does yield clinically applicable information about scaphoid imaging. Before the clinician chooses a secondary study, one of the special views described could assist in the diagnosis of an occult scaphoid fracture.

Mekhail AO, Ebraheim NA, McCreath WA, Jackson WT, Yeasting RA: Anatomic and X-ray film studies of the distal articular surface of the radius. *J Hand Surg* 1996;21A:567–573.

This is a combination study of the osteology of the distal radius and its radiographic appearance. Each facet of the study has important intellectual implications for the student of the wrist. A clinically applicable recommendation for characterizing the dorsomedial radius fracture fragment was described.

Peh WC, Gilula LA: Normal disruption of carpal arcs. *J Hand Surg* 1996;21A:561–566.

There is increasing recognition of the importance of the carpal arcs in identification of pathology; knowledge of their normal variation is critical. Study of arc variations may yield additional information about the integrity of the intercarpal ligaments.

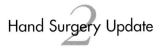
Sagerman SD, Hauck RM, Palmer AK: Lunate morphology: Can it be predicted with routine x-ray films? *J Hand Surg* 1995;20A:38–41.

This study updates information on the anatomy and radiographic appearance of the lunate. Understanding the morphology and projection of the lunate is central to the diagnosis of carpal instability, carpal arthrosis, and Kienböck's disease.

Sagerman SD, Zogby RG, Palmer AK, Werner FW, Fortino MD: Relative articular inclination of the distal radioulnar joint: A radiographic study. *J Hand Surg* 1995;20A:597–601.

This study focuses on one of the fine osteology elements of the distal radioulnar joint that has received little attention. Although these authors emphasize the possibility that a mismatch may cause problems after ulnar shortening, there is very little articular contact between the sigmoid notch and the ulna seat.

Schuind F, Alemzadeh S, Stallenberg B, Burny F: Does the normal contralateral wrist provide the best reference for X-ray film measurements of the pathologic wrist? *J Hand Surg* 1996;21A:24–30.

This study supports the common clinical practice of using the contralateral wrist as the control for assessing more subtle pathologies. The correlation was best for intercarpal relationships imaged on the lateral projection, and for the carpal height index. Many of the radius platform parameters are best compared to the accepted normals, rather than to the contralateral wrist of the same patient. Some differences between the sexes and age-specific findings were also reported.

Watson HK, Yasuda M, Guidera PM: Lateral lunate morphology: An x-ray study. *J Hand Surg* 1996;21A:759–763.

This study updates information on the anatomy and radiographic appearance of the lunate. Understanding the morphology and projection of the lunate is central to the diagnosis of carpal instability, carpal arthrosis, and Kienböck's disease.

Fractures of the Distal Radius

Andersen DJ, Blair WF, Steyers CM Jr, Adams BD, el-Khouri GY, Brandser EA: Classification of distal radius fractures: An analysis of interobserver reliability and intraobserver reproducibility. *J Hand Surg* 1996;21A:574–582.

This is one of the most complete and current studies analyzing inter- and intraobserver agreement in determining the classification of distal radius fractures. It adds more credence to the concept that all classifications have limitations, and no single method should be prime in guiding treatment of these common fractures.

Cole RJ, Bindra RR, Evanoff BA, Gilula LA, Yamaguchi K, Gelberman RH: Radiographic evaluation of osseous displacement following intra-articular fractures of the distal radius: Reliability of plain radiography versus computed tomography. *J Hand Surg* 1997;22A:792–800.

This study forwards two mechanisms by which intra-articular displacement of distal radius fractures can be quantified. The Longitudinal Axis Measurement is used to analyze plain radiographs, while the Arc Method is employed for CT scans. Both methods are reasonably simple to use. Computed tomography better characterizes the intra-articular incongruities; the Arc Method could occupy a valid clinical and scientific place.

Kazuki K, Kusunoki M, Yamada J, Yasuda M, Shimazu A: Cineradiographic study of wrist motion after fracture of the distal radius. *J Hand Surg* 1993;18A:41–46.

This study correlated radiographic parameters of the radius platform (particularly dorsal tilt) with intercarpal angles and wrist motion. Perhaps the most important element of this study is its promotion of cineradiography as an evaluation tool for wrist pathoanatomy. The advantages of evaluating the wrist in real time deserve emphasis.

Kreder HJ, Hanel DP, McKee M, Jupiter J, McGillivary G, Swiontkowski MF: X-ray film measurements for healed distal radius fractures. *J Hand Surg* 1996;21A:31–39.

This article is a more comprehensive, objective treatment of radius fracture X-ray reading. Eight parameters measured from radiographs of healed fractures were established and interobserver responses were compared. This study takes an important step toward relating radiographic appearance of the radius platform and functional outcomes.

Pruitt DL, Gilula LA, Manske PR, Vannier MW: Computed tomography scanning with image reconstruction in evaluation of distal radius fractures. *J Hand Surg* 1994;19A:720–727.

This study strengthens the position of computed tomography scanning in the evaluation of complex distal radius fractures and emphasizes its role in a cost-effective evaluation scheme. Computed tomography is recommended only for those patients who are candidates for surgical intervention.

Shih C, Chang CY, Penn IW, Tiu CM, Chang T, Wu JJ: Chronically stressed wrists in adolescent gymnasts: MR imaging appearance. *Radiology* 1995;195:855–859.

This is one of several reports that mark the growing recognition of stress injuries to the physis of the radius. This injury is chronic and cumulative. This article supports a modification of the Heuter-Volkmann principle, that intermittent high-compressive load at the physis can retard growth. The number of radii without plain radiographic abnormalities was equivalent to those with changes (positive ulnar variance, altered styloid anatomy, physeal widening).

Fractures of the Carpal Bones

Breitenseher MJ, Metz VM, Gilula LA, et al: Radiographically occult scaphoid fractures: Value of MR imaging in detection. *Radiology* 1997;203:245–250.

Hunter JC, Escobedo EM, Wilson AJ, Hanel DP, Zink-Brody GC, Mann FA. MR imaging of clinically suspected scaphoid fractures. *Am J Roentgenol* 1997;168:1287–1293.

These two recent reports detail the use of MRI for detection of the occult yet clinically suspected scaphoid fracture. Not only did MRI reveal many scaphoid fractures that were undetectable by plain radiography, but additional fractures of the radius were likewise identified. The sensitivity and specificity of MRI may supplant the bone scan, but cost-effectiveness must be established. Incomplete follow-up and de-emphasized reporting of the image appearance through the healing phases hampers these works, but together with thorough cost analyses

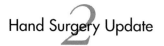

these studies may promote MRI to first-line in cases of diagnostic dilemmas about the distal radius and carpus.

Kukla C, Gaebler C, Breitenseher MJ, Trattnig S, Vécsei V: Occult fractures of the scaphoid: The diagnostic usefulness and indirect economic repercussions of radiography versus magnetic resonance scanning. *J Hand Surg* 1997;22B:810–813.

The true value of this study is that it considers the entire patient encounter and the impact of our recommendations on the patients' livelihood. Magnified radiography is dismissed as a viable technique for scaphoid imaging, and early MRI for detection of occult scaphoid fractures and other wrist injuries is supported. This study then presents data that globally assess the economic differences between a rapid diagnosis of scaphoid fracture, and presumptive treatment when plain radiographs are used as the diagnostic modality.

Tiel-van Buul MMC, Roolker W, Verbeeten BWB Jr, Broekhuizen AH: Magnetic resonance imaging versus bone scintigraphy in suspected scaphoid fracture. *Eur J Nucl Med* 1996;23:971–975.

Although this investigation has a small sample size (19 patients), it is nonetheless thorough in comparing modalities. Their finding that MRI's utility is promising, but not necessarily superior to that of bone scan, may have greater economic implications if these findings are recapitulated with larger cohorts.

Interosseous Ligament Injuries

Berger RA, Linscheid RL, Berquist TH: Magnetic resonance imaging of the anterior radiocarpal ligaments. *J Hand Surg* 1994;19A:295–303.

This report is one of many articles in the radiology and hand surgery literature concerning the use of MRI in the detection of interosseous ligament pathologies. Other reports focus on techniques of demonstrating tears, radiological anatomy papers, and the use of MRI in clinical studies. The radiology and surgical communities are clearly gaining greater experience and comfort with this technique of wrist imaging, but there is still a long way to go before there can be strong reliance on the technique.

Kirschenbaum D, Sieler S, Solonik D, Loeb DM, Cody RP: Arthrography of the wrist: Assessment of the integrity of the ligaments in young asymptomatic adults. *J Bone Joint Surg* 1995;77A:1207–1209.

This is a good example of the false positive potential of the arthrogram. Over 25% of the normal adults studied had positive arthrographic findings. A positive ulnar variance seemed to correlate with the occurrence of false arthrographic positivity. Guarded interpretation of leaks or tears is recommended, and clinical correlation is emphasized.

Smith DK: MR imaging of normal and injured wrist ligaments. *Magn Reson Imaging Clin N Am* 1995;3:229–248.

This is another of the numerous articles focusing on MRI to detect ligament pathologies.

The Ulnar Wrist

Escobedo EM, Bergman AG, Hunter JC: MR imaging of ulnar impaction. *Skeletal Radiol* 1995;24:85–90.

This article and others forwarded the concept that MRI was sensitive and specific for the purpose of detecting ulnocarpal abutment or impingement. By utilizing STIR or fat suppression sequences, the subchondral bone abnormalities characteristic of ulnocarpal abutment can be detected with greater certainty than that offered by other techniques (specifically bone scan). Furthermore, greater anatomic detail throughout the wrist can be imaged with MRI.

Sugimoto H, Shinozaki T, Ohsawa T: Triangular fibrocartilage in asymptomatic subjects: Investigation of abnormal MR signal intensity. *Radiology* 1994;191:193–197.

Totterman SM, Miller RJ: MR imaging of the triangular fibrocartilage complex. *Magn Reson Imaging Clin N Am* 1995;3:213–228.

MRI of the triangular fibrocartilage has received considerable attention in the literature, with articles on such topics as definition of its normal anatomy, interpretation of abnormal signal intensity, and establishment of the appearance of pathologic entities. Assessment of early degenerative change or partial tearing and avulsion of the articular disk and radioulnar ligaments from the basistyloid area are the pathologies for which MRI holds particular promise.

Osteonecrosis

Quenzer DE, Linscheid RL, Vidal MA, Dobyns JH, Beckenbaugh RD, Cooney WP: Trispiral tomographic staging of Kienböck's disease. *J Hand Surg* 1997;22A:396–403.

Rettig ME, Raskin KB, Melone CP Jr: Clinical applications of MR imaging in hand and wrist surgery. *Magn Reson Imaging Clin N Am* 1995;3:361–368.

Kienböck's disease is a rare entity, yet there continues to be a great interest in its diagnosis and treatment. The modalities of MRI and specialized tomography have been shown to be useful in the early diagnosis and staging of Kienböck's disease. These specialized imaging techniques play a role when plain radiographs are equivocal.

Carpal Tunnel Syndrome

Bindra RR, Evanoff BA, Chough LY, Cole RJ, Chow JC, Gelberman RH: The use of routine wrist radiography in the evaluation of patients with carpal tunnel syndrome. *J Hand Surg* 1997;22A:115–119.

There has been a proliferation of recent literature describing imaging modalities used for the evaluation of carpal tunnel syndrome. This study discusses the associated costs, and prudently concludes that carpal tunnel syndrome is a clinical diagnosis for which routine imaging need not be performed.

Neoplasms

Cardinal E, Buckwalter KA, Braunstein EM, Mih AD: Occult dorsal carpal ganglion: Comparison of US and MR imaging. *Radiology* 1994;193:259–262.

This study focuses on the diagnosis of occult dorsal carpal ganglia, but is chosen mainly to applaud a study design that should be followed for future investigations into the utility of imaging. Two modalities, ultrasound and MRI, are compared on many parameters, including cost. Ultrasound, the less expensive option, compares

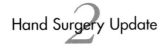
favorably to the diagnostic capability of MRI, and is thus supported as the initial procedure for diagnostic work-up of suspected ganglia. For imaging of other neoplasms, these two modalities will likely be among the primary choices.

Read JW, Conolly WB, Lanzetta M, Spielman S, Snodgrass D, Korber JS: Diagnostic ultrasound of the hand and wrist. *J Hand Surg* 1996;21A:1004–1010.

Although the imaging of cystic and cellular neoplasms is only one facet of this article, it is recommended as a good general overview of the role of ultrasound in upper extremity surgery. The operator-dependent nature of the modality is stressed.

Inflammatory Conditions

Rubens DJ, Blebea JS, Totterman SM, Hooper MM: Rheumatoid arthritis: Evaluation of wrist extensor tendons with clinical examination versus MR imaging: A preliminary report. *Radiology* 1993;187:831–838.

Sugimoto H, Takeda A, Masuyama J, Furuse M: Early-stage rheumatoid arthritis: Diagnostic accuracy of MR imaging. *Radiology* 1996;198:185–192.

These two studies represent excellent work that is being done to diagnose and stage rheumatoid arthritis with a combination of clinical examination and advanced imaging modalities. Characteristic findings on MRI may assist in the early diagnosis of the disease, accurately differentiating it from other pathologic entities. The technique may be useful in assessing the integrity of tendons; this capability would have particular value in surgical planning.

Reflex Sympathetic Dystrophy

Lee GW, Weeks PM: The role of bone scintigraphy in diagnosing reflex sympathetic dystrophy. *J Hand Surg* 1995;20A:458–463.

Most hand surgeons encounter patients with symptom constellations reminiscent of autonomic dysfunction. The role of bone scintigraphy in their work-up has been supported in the past. The article demonstrated that bone scan was not highly correlative, with sensitivity approximating 50% in the early stages (less than 26 weeks after onset). Furthermore, the longer the symptoms persisted, the poorer the correlation became. The study concluded that the diagnosis of RSD should be made by an experienced clinician on the basis of examination, not by findings on bone scintigraphy.

Algorithm

Larsen CF, Brondum V, Wienholtz G, Abrahamsen J, Beyer J: An algorithm for acute wrist trauma: A systematic approach to diagnosis. *J Hand Surg* 1993;18B:207–212.

This is an excellent algorithm-based patient analysis. The diagnostic algorithm, replete with suggestions for the judicious use of imaging modalities, is reprinted in the text.

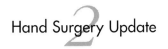
Chapter 8
Distal Radius Fractures

William H. Seitz, Jr, MD

Introduction

The distal radius is probably the most commonly fractured long bone in adults. Although the highest incidence is in adults aged 60 to 70 years, distal radius fractures can occur in all age groups. Injuries occurring later in life are usually the result of low-velocity mechanisms through more osteopenic bone, while injuries to younger patients frequently reflect a higher level of energy dissipation. Fracture patterns vary depending on the mechanism of injury, with a combination of axial load through an extended (or sometimes flexed) wrist and varying degrees of shear, rotational, and angular forces. Based on the quality of the bone, the line of force application, and magnitude of the force, a distinct fracture pattern occurs. This fracture pattern, placed in the framework of surrounding soft-tissue and/or associated injuries, should be the determining factor in treatment choice.

Classification

A number of classification systems have been developed to describe fractures of the distal radius. The Frykman classification system has been widely used, and includes the presence or absence of an ulnar styloid fracture. It has not, however, been helpful in designing an appropriate treatment rationale. The Melone classification system describes major articular fragments and provides valuable focus on location and displacement of major articular fragments. The AO classification is quite complex, with over 25 subtypes that become more confusing than helpful in trying to determine an appropriate plan of treatment.

The more recent treatment-based universal classification system has 4 major categories, based on the appearance of plain radiographs (Table 1). These 4 fracture types can be divided into intra- and extra-articular fractures. Type I is a nonarticular, nondisplaced fracture; type II, nonarticular, displaced; type III, articular, nondisplaced; and type IV,

articular, displaced. Based on the degree of displacement, comminution, angulation, and associated injuries, types II and IV can be further categorized as reducible and stable, reducible and unstable, irreducible, or complex.

Well-detailed plain radiographs can be quite helpful in sorting these fractures into major subtypes, as a basis for outlining a treatment plan. It has been suggested by some that multiplane computed tomography (with and without 3-dimensional reconstruction) can be helpful in defining distal radius fractures; however, these additional studies are of benefit only in the more comminuted, complex intra-articular fractures. Although these studies have not altered the treatment plan, they have provided greater definition of the extent of articular injury, thereby improving the ability to predict outcomes (Fig. 1).

Principles of Treatment

The goal of treating distal radius fractures should be to restore anatomy as closely as possible, while reconciling the cost of doing so with the patient's needs and demands. Not every fracture about the distal radius can or should be anatomically restored. The degree of treatment must reflect the needs of the patient, as well as an understanding of the anatomy, interrelationships, and kinematics of the distal radius, ulna, and carpus. To determine the relationship of the distal radius and ulna, radiographs should be obtained in 2 views: (1) a posteroanterior view of the wrist, with the shoulder abducted to 90°, the elbow flexed to 90°, and the wrist and palm flat on the X-ray cassette (zero rotation view); and (2) a true lateral view, with the shoulder in neutral position, the elbow flexed to 90° with the ulnar side of the hand on the plate, and the thumb pointing up. These should be compared to comparable views of the contralateral wrist. Ulnar variance should be recorded and compared. The typical uninjured wrist has a neutral ulnar variance with an angle of inclination of the radial articular surface of approximately 23° and a palmar tilt of 11° to 12° on the lateral view.

Articulations of the distal radius include the scaphoid fossa, the lunate fossa, and the sigmoid notch of the radius. These articulate with the scaphoid, lunate, and head of the distal ulna, respectively. Alterations and articular incongruence at any of

The author or the department with which he is affiliated has received something of value from a commercial or other party related directly or indirectly to the subject of this chapter.

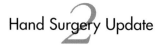
78   Distal Radius Fractures

Table 1

Treatment guide based on an adaptation of Cooney's universal classification system and patient activity level

Extra-articular Distal Radius Fractures	High Demand Patient	Moderate Demand Patient	Low Demand Patient
Nondisplaced	LAC	SAC	Splint
Displaced/stable	Cast/KIF	SAC	SAC
Displaced/unstable	KIF/ORIF	LAC	SAC
Irreducible	ORIF	ORIF	ORIF
Intra-articular Distal Radius Fractures			
Nondisplaced	LAC/pins/EF	LAC	SAC
Displaced/stable	EF/pins	LAC/EF	SAC
Displaced/unstable	EF/IF/BG	EF/IF/BG	LAC
Irreducible	ORIF/EF/BG	ORIF/EF/BG	Splint/Fusion

LAC = long-arm cast, SAC = short-arm cast, EF = external fixation, IF = internal fixation, ORIF = open reduction and internal fixation, BG = bone graft, KIF = Kapandji intrafocal

these facets can alter the normal mechanics of flexion/extension, radial and ulnar deviation, and pronosupination. Malalignment after trauma can have a profound effect on the patient's ability to transfer load from hand to the forearm, and may result in a significantly painful outcome.

Nonsurgical fixation techniques vary from immobilization in situ with a short-arm cast or splint, to closed reduction and long-arm cast fixation. More invasive techniques include percutaneous Kirschner wire (K-wire) fixation in the transstyloid, transulnar, or intrafocal mode. Internal fixation with plates and screws, and interfragmentary screws with and without bone grafting have also been widely used. External fixation alone affords a self-limited traction apparatus, which provides reduction of the major fracture fragments through ligamentotaxis. Combinations of external fixation, internal fixation, and subarticular bone grafting have become more widely used with increased understanding of the biomechanics of fracture fixation. Newer techniques include an injectable bone grout substitute and use of arthroscopically guided articular surface reconstruction.

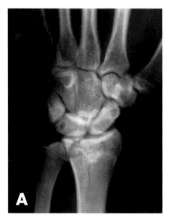
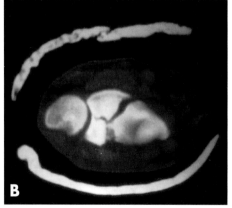
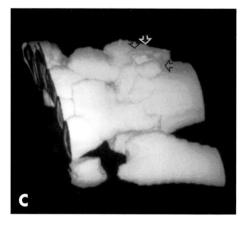

Figure 1

A, Plain radiograph of an intra-articular distal radius fracture in a 26-year-old man who fell 10 feet from a ladder demonstrates impaction, loss of radial tilt, and intra-articular extension. **B,** Computed tomography scan shows the degree of articular comminution. **C,** 3-dimensional reconstruction demonstrates the degree of displacement and cortical comminution (arrows), and can be helpful in surgical planning. The additional information from these special studies must be weighed against their cost.

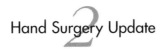
A Classification-Based Treatment Rationale

The universal classification system is helpful in selecting the appropriate treatment modality for the various patterns of distal radius fracture (Table 1). This contemporary system is a guide for considering the spectrum of treatment options; exact treatment will vary based on individual fracture characteristics, surgeon capability, and preference.

Nonarticular, Nondisplaced Fractures (Type I)

Frequently the result of a fall on an outstretched hand, resulting in a bending moment through the metaphysis, this fracture type is characterized by minimal dorsal radius comminution, minimal or no shortening, and little significant displacement or angulation (less than 5° change in the normal palmar tilt or angle of inclination). Fractures resulting from an extension injury should be held in a well-padded sugar-tongs splint with the wrist gently flexed. Those resulting from a flexion injury should be held in slight extension and full supination, using the pronator quadratus to prevent palmar displacement of the metaphyseal fragment. The sugar-tongs splint allows maintenance of the fracture in a reduced position, while preventing pronation and supination. The sugar-tongs splint allows the expected degree of postinjury swelling to occur. Seven to 10 days after injury, the temporary splint may be replaced by a long-arm cast or Muenster-type cast, which allows some elbow flexion/extension but restricts pronosupination. In lower-demand, older patients, a short-arm cast or splint can be used.

Nonarticular, Displaced Fractures (Type II)

Reducible, Stable Fractures   Although these fractures do not involve injury of the radiocarpal articulation, they may involve the distal radioulnar joint (DRUJ). Enough impact is absorbed, usually the result of a bending moment, to cause displacement through the metaphyseal region. Reducible and stable fractures generally demonstrate displacement less than 2 mm, shortening under 5 mm, angulation less than 15°, and only mild comminution. These fractures usually have an ulnar-sided injury as well, either an ulnar styloid avulsion or an injury to the triangular fibrocartilage complex (TFCC). To achieve satisfactory reduction in such cases, adequate anesthesia must be administered to

both the radial and ulnar sides of the wrist; this can be achieved by an axillary block, intravenous Bier block, or local anesthesia with a hematoma block. Cooperation and relaxation of the patient is critical to a gentle satisfactory reduction; consequently, some additional intravenous sedation may be beneficial.

The fracture should be gently manipulated with modest longitudinal traction. Forceful maneuvers and overreduction should be avoided to prevent further comminution and fracture instability. Once the fracture is reduced, a sugar-tongs splint should be applied and radiographs obtained. When satisfactory reduction has been confirmed, follow-up radiographs should be obtained within 1 week. The extremity can be placed in a long-arm cast in 7 to 10 days.

Reducible, Unstable Fractures   Failure to maintain satisfactory reduction indicates a need for supplementary internal fixation. K-wires can be helpful in maintaining the reduced bony alignment. Intrafocal pinning can also be very effective, especially in younger patients with normal bone stock (there is a tendency in more osteoporotic bone for some collapse around these pins). Combining intrafocal pinning with an oblique radial styloid pin can be very effective (Fig. 2). The addition of multiple K-wires can reduce the need for long-arm casting; in some cases, this technique may be preferential to closed reduction alone.

Irreducible Fractures   Irreducible fractures usually result from a high level of energy dissipation with significant injury in the metaphyseal area, without extension into the radiocarpal joint. These fractures are characterized by significant metaphyseal compression and bone loss, wide

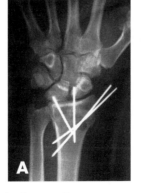 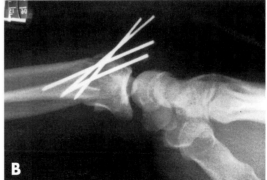

Figure 2

Intrafocal pinning can be helpful in stabilizing the nonarticular, displaced unstable fracture. In more osteopenic bone, additional radial styloid pins can be useful in preventing collapse around the pins, as remodeling occurs during fracture healing.

displacement and angulation, and potential interposition of soft tissues (eg, the pronator quadratus), all of which may prevent satisfactory fracture fragment realignment. Because of the high level of energy associated with these injuries, patients should be carefully observed for evidence of median nerve injury as well as possible compartment syndrome. Irreducible fractures may require open reduction with either external or internal fixation and/or bone grafting. Internal fixation with a buttress plate is the most commonly used technique in treating these fractures. Dorsally displaced fractures should be approached through a dorsal incision with the plate applied along the extensor surface of the distal radius, while palmarly displaced fractures should be approached through a palmar incision, with concomitant decompression of the carpal canal. Distal radius T-plates have been developed to stabilize these fractures. When applied dorsally, these plates may require some contouring; removal of Lister's tubercle may be helpful in achieving a smooth application. When the palmar approach is used, the plate should be contoured to the curve of the palmar distal radius. Distal screws must be angled proximally to avoid violation of the distal radius articular surface. Specialized low-profile, limited distal radius plates have been designed and used successfully (Fig. 3).

Articular Nondisplaced Fractures (Type III)

These relatively rare fractures may result from a low-energy fall onto the outstretched hand in osteopenic bone, creating a T-type pattern in the older patient. The injury mechanism could also be a direct blow, such as in a chauffeur's fracture. Articular nondisplaced fractures are frequently treatable with a sugar-tongs splint, followed by a long-arm cast. If follow-up radiographs show any suggestion of displacement, however, additional fixation with K-wires or interfragmentary screws may be applied (Fig. 4).

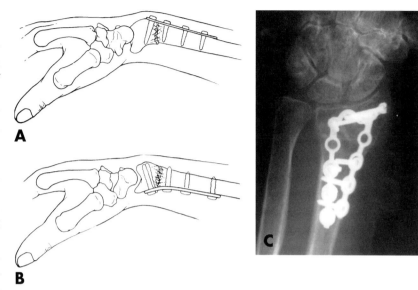

Figure 3

Buttress plate fixation. **A,** Dorsal application for dorsally-displaced fracture. **B,** Palmar application for palmarly-displaced fractures. (**A** and **B** are reproduced with permission from Seitz WH Jr: Fractures of the distal radius, in Peimer C (ed): *Surgery of the Hand and Upper Extremity.* New York, NY, McGraw-Hill Health Professions Division, 1996, pp 637–666.) **C,** A new low-profile design provides both buttress and interfragmentary fixation capabilities.

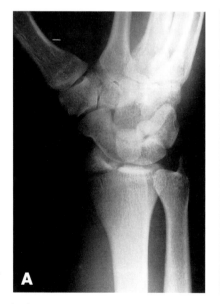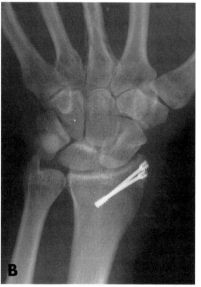

Figure 4

A, Displaced distal radius styloid fracture. **B,** Fixation with interfragmentary buried Herbert screws.

Articular Displaced Fractures (Type IV)

Reducible, Stable Fractures These fractures represent a combination of axial compression and shear, resulting in displacement of larger articular fragments that can be well-fit back into their original bed. The degree of comminution is relatively minor, with minimal subarticular bone loss. These fractures can be treated with K-wires, interfragmentary screws, plates, external fixation, or a combination of methods (Fig. 5).

Reducible, Unstable Fractures These fractures are characterized by more extensive comminution, wide displacement or step-off of articular fragments (more than 2 mm), impaction (shortening greater than 5 mm), and loss of supportive bone stock. Treatment will usually require a combination of external fixation, augmented by K-wire fixation for fine articular restoration, and subarticular supportive bone grafting performed through a limited extra-articular approach.

External fixation employs the principles of ligamentotaxis; traction is applied through the soft tissue to help realign major bone fragments. Although restoration of anatomic length and general alignment can certainly be obtained through ligamentotaxis, fine articular restoration requires percutaneous joystick manipulation of the smaller fragments. The smaller fragments can then be held with a combination of K-wires

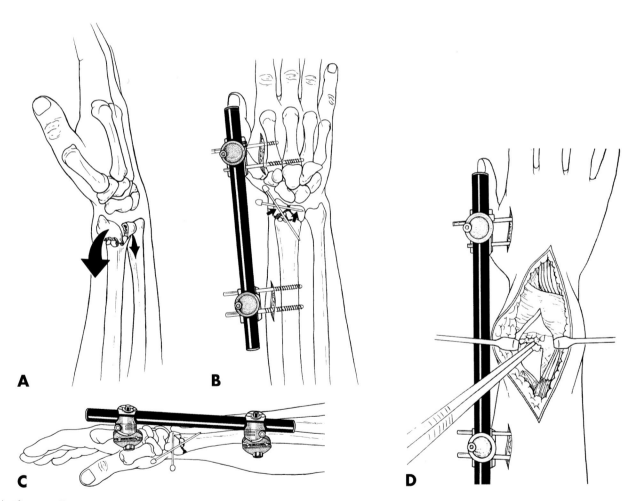

Figure 5

External fixation is performed through a limited open approach. This exposes the radial shaft and index metacarpal to direct vision, reducing the risk of the drill skiving off center and causing bone damage or injury to soft-tissue structures. A lightweight, carbon-fiber, radiolucent design is shown here. This design allows X-ray fracture visualization in all planes, while aiding in activities of daily living. Interfragmentary augmentation with K-wires restores articular congruity, while extra-articular subchondral bone grafting helps resist late collapse. (Reproduced with permission from Seitz WH Jr: Fractures of the distal radius, in Peimer C (ed): *Surgery of the Hand and Upper Extremity.* New York, NY, McGraw-Hill Health Professions Division, 1996, pp 637–666.)

placed through the radial styloid under the subchondral bone of the lunate facet. In some cases dorsal intrafocal insertion is necessary to restore appropriate palmar tilt. A small dorsal incision can be used just proximal to Lister's tubercle to insert supportive subarticular bone graft into the fracture site itself (Fig. 5).

External fixation is best achieved through a limited open approach. Important soft-tissue structures can be seen and protected while directly visualizing the radius and index metacarpal for insertion of fixator pins. Predrilling minimizes the potential for microfractures or loosening at the pin–bone interface. Three- and 4-mm self-tapping, threaded half-pins are most frequently used for external fixation of distal radius fractures. Four-mm pins should be considered for younger, muscular patients to avoid pin-bending or breakage, and for older patients with osteopenic bone to afford better pin purchase.

The fixator choice should allow pin insertion and frame application prior to fracture fragment reduction. The device should facilitate gentle fracture reduction, and provide the ability to rereduce the fracture if necessary. Radiolucent devices are now available that are lightweight, easy to use, and provide complete X-ray visibility of the fracture in all planes (Fig. 5). Overdistraction could lead to stiffness and/or reflex sympathetic dystrophy. One-mm distraction through the radiocarpal joint will provide enough soft-tissue tension to achieve the desired degree of ligamentotaxis. The physiologic elongation of the radiocarpal ligaments is sufficient to allow early radiocarpal range of motion fairly easily after removal of the device. One-mm radiocarpal distraction will also avoid the degree of overdistraction associated with reflex sympathetic dystrophy. The device is usually left in place for a minimum of 6 weeks.

Irreducible Fractures These fractures, usually characterized by an extreme amount of comminution, cannot be restored to an anatomic configuration by closed means. They have fragments so widely displaced that soft-tissue structures become interposed, or the articular fragments are so severely rotated that manual derotation maneuvers must be performed. These fractures frequently require a combination of open reduction, external fixation, internal fixation, and bone grafting (Fig. 6).

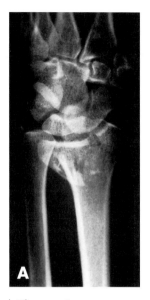
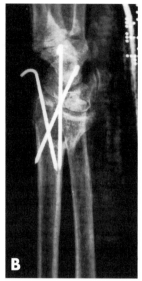
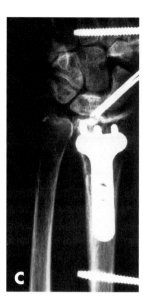

Figure 6

A and **B,** Irreducible distal radius fracture that has been inadequately treated with attempted closed reduction and percutaneous pinning. **C,** A combined approach of external fixation, open reduction and internal fixation, and bone grafting is required to adequately restore anatomy.

Complex Fractures Complex fractures may be associated with significant other skeletal or soft-tissue injuries. These high-energy injuries include open fractures; fractures with significant nerve or vascular injury with or without compartment syndrome; concomitant carpal fractures; intercarpal ligamentous disruption; and significant fractures of the head or neck of the distal ulna.

For open fractures, external fixation is quite useful for maintaining fracture alignment, while providing ready access for wound care. Acute median or ulnar neuropathy associated with distal radius fracture should be managed by exploration and decompression. Concomitant fractures of the scaphoid should be treated by internal fixation, using a compression screw if possible. If K-wires are used, caution should be exercised to avoid distraction via the external fixator. Intercarpal ligamentous injuries can be treated by percutaneous pinning, with or without open ligamentous repair, depending on the degree of ligament disruption. Comminuted ulnar head or neck fractures, in association with fractures of the distal radius, are very difficult to treat, and prevent early resumption of forearm pronosupination. When these fractures occur, excision of the fragments with reconstruction of the soft-tissue sling of the TFCC and ulnar collateral ligament complex has proven successful in allowing early motion, while avoiding DRUJ problems (Fig. 7).

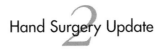

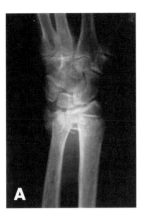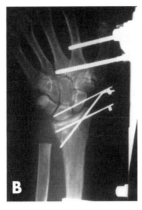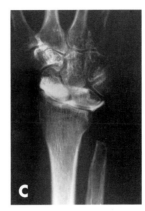

Figure 7

A and **B,** A complex distal radius fracture with comminuted ulna head/neck fracture and scapholunate dissociation is managed by stabilization with external and internal fixation, and excision of the ulna head fragments with ulnar-sided soft-tissue reconstruction. The excised bony fragments have been morcellized and used as subchondral bone graft. **C,** Follow-up arthrogram at 2 years shows ulnar remodeling within its periosteal/ligamentous sling and a water-tight radiocarpal joint.

Complications

Complications from distal radius fractures include infection, tendon dysfunction and rupture, posttraumatic arthritis, neuropathy, reflex sympathetic dystrophy, malunion, nonunion, stiffness, and contracture. Many of these complications can be avoided with careful attention to detail and appropriate recognition and treatment of the various fracture patterns.

Infection can be minimized with judicious use of perioperative antibiotics, thorough patient education, and meticulous pin-site care when external fixation or percutaneous K-wires are used. Pin-site care includes twice-daily cleansing of the pins with hydrogen peroxide for the first week after insertion, followed by twice-daily alcohol swab-cleansing for the duration of fixation. When pin tract infections do occur, prompt administration of oral antibiotics will usually cure the problem. Deep-seated infection, although rare, must be treated more aggressively.

Tendon rupture over the site of fracture can occur after even the most simple fracture; however, when any form of open procedure is performed, especially through a dorsal approach, removal of Lister's tubercle and transposition of the extensor pollicis longus can prevent tendon rupture. The extensor retinaculum may also be step-cut to allow adequate coverage of the extensor tendons. Half the retinaculum can be used deep to the tendons to cover exposed hardware (eg, plates and screws), avoiding deep tendon irritation.

Extensor tendon bowstringing following iatrogenic retinaculum disruption can be avoided by careful reconstruc-

tion. Posttraumatic arthritis may result from severe articular damage, but this can be minimized if careful reconstruction of the articular surface is provided by open reduction and internal fixation.

Damage to the peripheral nerves may be a direct result of trauma, or may be iatrogenic. Recognition of median or ulnar nerve dysfunction should provide a very low threshold for surgical decompression and repair. The arborization of the superficial branch of the radial nerve and the terminal branches of the lateral antebrachial cutaneous nerve are at risk for injury during fixator pin insertion. Retraction of these nerves in a careful, limited open approach minimizes the potential for injury.

Although malunion is usually the result of too-conservative treatment, even with external or internal fixation the surgeon must be careful to restore not only normal length and radiocarpal alignment but rotational alignment as well. This restoration will avoid alternation in the mechanics of the DRUJ.

Nonunion is rare in the distal radius, but can certainly result from overdistraction with an external fixator. Reflex sympathetic dystrophy is probably the most vexing complication following a distal radius fracture. As with stiffness and contracture, the best prevention is afforded by early intervention, aggressive hand therapy, and careful observation and surveillance. At the first sign of reflex sympathetic dystrophy, more aggressive sensory bombardment with or without adjunctive stellate ganglion blocks should be instituted.

New Developments

Several new forms of plates have been designed specifically for management of distal radius fractures and are FDA class III devices. An injectable bone grout has also been developed to fill fracture voids and to maintain internal fixation in stable fractures and in displaced fractures that are reducible and stable. This bone grout has chemical, crystalline, and has structural characteristics very similar to bone; the substance is gradually replaced by host bone after the fracture has healed (Fig. 8).

Although some authors have reported increased success using arthroscopic techniques to achieve anatomic reduction, arthroscopy adds significant cost, raises the potential for

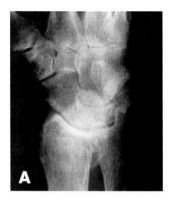

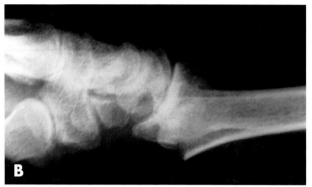

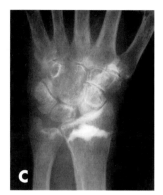

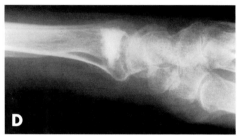

Figure 8

An injectable tricalcium phosphate bone grout, used to fill the fracture void and resist compressive forces, has been shown to be effective by itself in managing simpler fractures, and has great promise for more complex fracture management when combined with other forms of fixation.

fluid extravasation through the fracture site, and creates a potential hazard for nerve compression and increased intra-compartmental pressures.

Annotated Bibliography

General

Altissimi M, Antenucci R, Fiacca C, Mancini GB: Long-term results of conservative treatment of fractures of the distal radius. *Clin Orthop* 1986;206:202–210.

The authors reviewed subjective and objective clinical parameters and X-ray features of 297 cases involving conservative treatment of wrist fractures. Radial deviation, palmar tilt, and radioulnar index were often out of normal range. Postreduction problems with grip strength, clinical deformity, pain, and numerous compressive neuropathies were noted. Conservative management of distal radius fractures may not produce acceptable results.

Aro HT, Koivunen T: Minor axial shortening of the radius affects outcome of Colles' fracture treatment. *J Hand Surg* 1991; 16A:392–398.

Results suggest that minor axial shortening of the radius increases the risk of permanent disability, even in the absence of malalignment of the articular surfaces.

Dias JJ, Wray CC, Jones JM: Osteoporosis and Colles' fractures in the elderly. *J Hand Surg* 1987;12B:57–59.

A group of 127 patients older than 50 years with unilateral Colles' fractures were studied to determine the incidence of osteoporosis and investigate its influence on bony deformity. Seventy- eight percent were found to be osteoporotic. The final deformity was significantly greater in patients with osteoporosis.

Larsen CF, Lauritsen J: Epidemiology of acute wrist trauma. *Int J Epidemiol* 1993;22:911–916.

This report details the relatively high frequency of Colles' type fractures.

Short WH, Palmer AK, Werner FW, Murphy DJ: A biomechanical study of distal radial fractures. *J Hand Surg* 1987; 12A:529–534.

An experiment using fresh cadaver arms was designed to study the distribution of forces and change in pressure across the distal radial and ulnocarpal joints after a distal radius fracture. As dorsal angulation increases, the changes in the pressure distribution of the ulnar and radial articular surfaces become more concentrated.

Classification

Cooney WP: Fractures of the distal radius: A modern treatment-based classification. *Orthop Clin North Am* 1993;24:211–216.

This is an excellent review of the evolving classification systems for fractures of the distal radius. The modern treatment-based universal classification system is discussed in detail.

Melone CP Jr: Articular fractures of the distal radius. *Orthop Clin North Am* 1984;15:217–236.

Based on a review of 330 articular fractures of the distal radius, the author defines patterns of injury and proposes a classification system to

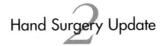
guide optimal treatment. Consistently successful techniques for more complex injuries are also described.

Principles of Treatment

Johnston GH, Friedman L, Kriegler JC: Computerized tomographic evaluation of acute distal radial fractures. *J Hand Surg* 1992;17A:738–744.

Use of computed tomography increases the recognition of fracture comminution and instability.

Melone CP Jr: Distal radius fractures: Patterns of articular fragmentation. *Orthop Clin North Am* 1993;24:239–253.

This study describes the patterns of articular fragmentation of distal radius fractures and the subsequent treatment based on radiographic recognition of fracture patterns.

Rayhack JM: The history and evolution of percutaneous pinning of displaced distal radius fractures. *Orthop Clin North Am* 1993;24:287–300.

The author provides a review of the history of percutaneous pinning of displaced distal radius fractures and the clinical application of this technique.

Seitz WH Jr: External fixation for fractures of the distal radius, in Blair WF, Steyers CM (eds): *Techniques in Hand Surgery*. Baltimore, MD, Williams & Wilkins, 1996, pp 309–321.

This chapter provides a detailed description of the principles of external fixation of distal radius fractures, including surgical techniques and avoidance of complications.

Seitz WH Jr, Putnam MD, Dick HM: Limited open surgical approach for external fixation of distal radius fractures. *J Hand Surg* 1990;15A:288–293.

A safe, reliable technique for application of external fixation in the management of unstable fractures of the distal radius is presented. The technique allows central pin placement, while avoiding injury to important soft-tissue structures. Clinical results in 66 cases document the efficacy and safety of this technique.

Warwick D, Prothero D, Field J, Bannister G: Radiological measurements of radial shortening in Colles' fracture. *J Hand Surg* 1993;18B:50–52.

Three different methods of assessing radial shortening were evaluated in a group of 100 patients. Techniques that used the radial or ulnar styloid as a landmark were found to correlate poorly with outcome due to involvement of the styloid in the fracture pattern. Axial shortening as measured from the radial articular surface to the ulna articular surface did correlate with outcome.

Treatment Rationale

Dowdy PA, Patterson SD, King GJ, Roth JH, Chess D: Intrafocal (Kapandji) pinning of unstable distal radius fractures: A preliminary report. *J Trauma* 1996;40:194–198.

This article presents a detailed discussion of the Kapandji procedure and its application to fractures of the distal radius.

Hastings H II, Leibovic SJ: Indications and techniques of open reduction: Internal fixation of distal radius fractures. *Orthop Clin North Am* 1993;24:309–326.

The authors provide an excellent review of distal radius fracture types and their management. They cover closed reduction techniques, surgical methods and approaches, and problems encountered in each of the specific fracture types. Their own experience demonstrates that better reductions produce better overall results.

Kaempffe FA, Wheeler DR, Peimer CA, Hvisdak KS, Ceravolo J, Senall J: Severe fractures of the distal radius: Effect of amount and duration of external fixator distraction on outcome. *J Hand Surg* 1993;18A:33–41.

Twenty-six patients were retrospectively reviewed, and carpal height index used to quantitate distraction. Increasing the amount or time of distraction was found to diminish the final outcome. The variable most significantly affected was final range of motion.

Knirk JL, Jupiter JB: Intra-articular fractures of the distal end of the radius in young adults. *J Bone Joint Surg* 1986;68A:647–659.

This classic article defines the importance of restoring articular congruity in the young, active patient. Fractures with a depressed articular surface component (even when initially reduced anatomically) were found to be responsible for residual incongruity. This was noted in 75% of the incongruous joints at late follow-up, suggesting redisplacement from lack of subarticular support.

Kongsholm J, Olerud C: Plaster cast versus external fixation for unstable intraarticular Colles' fractures. *Clin Orthop* 1989; 241:57–65.

The authors compare 75 consecutive patients with Frykman type 8 fractures of the distal forearm treated by primary external fixation to a historic control of 32 patients with similar injuries who were treated with closed reduction and cast immobilization. All fractures treated with external fixation remained well-reduced and aligned, while 88% of the historic controls treated with cast immobilization alone had an unsatisfactory alignment, despite a second reduction in 30% of that population. Treatment with external fixators also demonstrated superior results in functional outcome, range of motion, and grip strength.

Seitz WH Jr: Fractures of the distal radius, in Peimer C (ed): *Surgery of the Hand and Upper Extremity*. New York, NY, McGraw-Hill Health Profession Division, 1996, pp 637–666.

This chapter presents an in-depth analysis of distal radius fractures, including clinical and radiographic diagnosis, classification, treatment options, and details of surgical techniques.

Extra-articular Fractures

Greatting MD, Bishop AT: Intrafocal (Kapandji) pinning of unstable fractures of the distal radius. *Orthop Clin North Am* 1993;24:301–307.

A careful review of the literature on the Kapandji technique is presented, as well as the authors' own clinical experience. Excellent X-ray results were achieved in 79% of the patients under 65 years of age, and 60% of patients over age 65. Clinical and X-ray results demonstrated that this technique provides acceptable clinical results, but some loss of reduction after pinning in the elderly population may be expected due to osteopenic bone.

Kopylov P, Johnell O, Redlund-Johnell I, Bengner U: Fractures of the distal end of the radius in young adults: A 30-year follow-up. *J Hand Surg* 1993;18B:45–49.

In this long-term follow-up of extra-articular and intra-articular fractures, the best predictors of long-term degenerative changes were found to be shortening with ulnar positive variance greater than 2 mm or an intra-articular step-off greater than 1 mm.

Szabo RM: Extra-articular fractures of the distal radius. *Orthop Clin North Am* 1993;24:229–237.

The author suggests that extra-articular distal radius fractures are frequently undertreated with the use of immobilization in plaster. He recommends that if failure to maintain reduction with plaster is noted, closed reduction of the displaced fracture should be accompanied by external fixation. This method preserves radial length and palmar tilt.

Intra-articular Fractures

Bartosh RA, Saldana MJ: Intraarticular fractures of the distal radius: A cadaveric study to determine if ligamentotaxis restores radiopalmar tilt. *J Hand Surg* 1990;15A:18–21.

Nineteen fresh cadaver wrists were divested of all dorsal and palmar tissues and intrinsic and extrinsic ligaments. A Frykman type 7 fracture was introduced across radiocarpal and radioulnar joints and attempts were made to reestablish radiopalmar tilt by ligamentotaxis. The authors concluded that ligamentotaxis is limited as the sole method for restoring radiopalmar tilt.

Bradway JK, Amadio PC, Cooney WP: Open reduction and internal fixation of displaced, comminuted intra-articular fractures of the distal end of the radius. *J Bone Joint Surg* 1989;71A:839–847.

A step-off of 2 mm or more in the distal radius articular surface at the time of healing is shown to be significant. All patients with this amount of incongruity developed posttraumatic arthritis.

Jupiter JB, Lipton H: The operative treatment of intraarticular fractures of the distal radius. *Clin Orthop* 1993;292:48–61.

The authors provide an excellent discussion of preoperative planning, fracture classification, and surgical tactics used in the management of complex intra-articular fractures of the distal radius.

Melone CP Jr: Open treatment for displaced articular fractures of the distal radius. *Clin Orthop* 1986;202:103–111.

Maximum recovery of wrist function following articular distal radius fractures depends on acceptable and stable reduction of the radial articular surfaces. In injuries with major disruption, the fracture site may need to be opened in order to preserve the distal radius articulation. The author describes open treatment techniques and analyzes results of treatment in cases of complex articular fractures.

Porter ML, Tillman RM: Pilon fractures of the wrist: Displaced intra-articular fractures of the distal radius. *J Hand Surg* 1992;17B:63–68.

The authors compare these comminuted intra-articular fractures to pilon fractures of the distal tibia, as the mechanisms of injury are similar. They report a high incidence of associated injuries. Scapholunate dissociation was present in 18%, and 23% had disruption of the DRUJ.

Seitz WH Jr, Froimson AI, Leb R, Shapiro JD: Augmented external fixation of unstable distal radius fractures. *J Hand Surg* 1991;16A:1010–1016.

The principles of additional internal fixation for precise articular reconstruction and subchondral bone graft for metaphyseal support are detailed, and clinical results presented.

Complications

Geissler WB, Fernandez DL, Lamey DM: Distal radioulnar joint injuries associated with fractures of the distal radius. *Clin Orthop* 1996;327:135–146.

These authors review distal radioulnar joint injuries associated with distal radius fracture, their management, and effect on outcome.

Kozin SH, Wood MB: Early soft-tissue complications after fractures of the distal part of the radius. *J Bone Joint Surg* 1993;75A:144–153.

In this review of soft-tissue complications (skin, tendon, and nerve injuries, as well as compartment syndrome), special emphasis is placed on nerve injuries; early anatomic reduction is advocated to minimize trauma to the nerve. In cases with a persistent deficit, early surgical decompression is advocated.

Roysam GS: The distal radio-ulnar joint in Colles' fractures. *J Bone Joint Surg* 1993;75B:58–60.

This review of 170 patients without radiocarpal extension of their fractures shows a poorer outcome in those with DRUJ involvement. Grip strength was decreased, supination was decreased, and pain increased when the fracture involved the DRUJ.

Seitz WH Jr, Froimson AI, Leb R: Reduction of treatment-related complications in the external fixation of complex distal radius fractures. *Orthop Rev* 1991;20:169–177.

The authors present methods for avoiding problems in the management of distal radius fractures, highlighting surgical approach, technique, choice of pins and devices, and after-care.

Seitz WH Jr: Complications and problems in the management of distal radius fractures. *Hand Clin* 1994;10:117–123.

Problems associated with various treatment modalities are discussed, and strategies designed to minimize them are offered.

New Developments

Levy HJ, Glickel SZ: Arthroscopic assisted internal fixation of volar intraarticular wrist fractures. *Arthroscopy* 1993;9:122–124.

A description of the technique used and some of its difficulties are outlined.

Whipple TL: The role of arthroscopy in the treatment of wrist injuries in the athlete. *Clin Sports Med* 1992;11:227–238.

The article reviews the application of arthroscopy to acute wrist injuries. Management of both soft-tissue and osseous injuries is described.

Chapter 9
Triangular Fibrocartilage and Ulnar Wrist Problems

Jeffrey A. Greenberg, MD

Introduction

Interest in anatomy, biomechanics, afflictions, and treatment of the ulnar side of the wrist has grown substantially since the first edition of this book was published. No longer do hand and upper extremity surgeons consider the ulnar wrist to be a "black box," or the "low back pain" of the wrist. This chapter highlights the significant recent advances in diagnostic and treatment modalities that have contributed to our further understanding of the ulnar side of the wrist.

Nomenclature and Anatomy

Standardized nomenclature facilitates communication. The cartilage-covered surface of the ulnar head has 2 parts. The convex portion of the head, which articulates with the sigmoid notch of the radius, is the seat, the cartilage-covered distal surface, nonarticular and deep to the articular disk, is the pole. These two components combine to form the articular cartilage-covered surface of the lateral distal ulna (Fig. 1).

The triangular fibrocartilage complex (TFCC) has multiple components, well-documented in the literature. Central to this complex is the articular disk, centrum, or triangular fibrocartilage (TFC) proper, located distal to the pole of the ulnar head, immediately between the carpus and the ulnar pole. The richly vascularized dorsal and palmar radioulnar ligaments (DRUL and PRUL, respectively) are comprised of thickened, longitudinally-oriented collagen fiber bundles that blend in with the central avascular fibrocartilaginous centrum (Fig. 2).

The ulnocarpal portion of the TFCC includes the disk-lunate and disk-triquetral ligaments, critical to the carpal-suspensory function of the TFCC. These ligaments originate from the palmar margin of the TFC itself (Figs. 1 and 2). This contrasts with the prior terminology of ulnotriquetral and ulnolunate ligaments, which connotate a bony origin. It has been shown embryologically that these ligaments take

their origin from dense ligamentous condensations on the dorsal and palmar aspects of the articular disk, and not from bone. The ulnocarpal volar ligament includes the disk-carpal ligaments as well as the more superficial ulnocapitate ligament (Fig. 3). The ulnar collateral ligament, which also attaches to the fovea, thickens distally to form the vestigial meniscal homolog. This structure is one component of the floor of the extensor carpi ulnaris subsheath, the final component of the TFCC.

There are 2 distinct insertions of the TFC into the ulna. The deep portion, or ligamentum subcruetum, inserts into the fovea near the axis of forearm rotation; the superficial components of the DRUL and PRUL insert into the base of the ulnar styloid (Fig. 4).

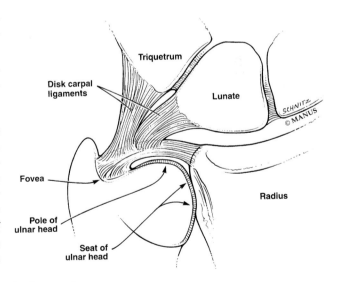

Figure 1

Diagrammatic representation of the head of the ulna, demonstrating the weightbearing seat and the articular cartilage-covered pole, proximal to the centrum of the triangular fibrocartilage complex. (Reproduced with permission from Kleinman WB, Graham TJ: Distal ulnar injury and dysfunction, in Peimer CA (ed): *Surgery of the Hand and Upper Extremity.* New York, NY, McGraw-Hill, 1996, pp 667–709. Illustrated by Gary Schnitz, © MANUS 1996.)

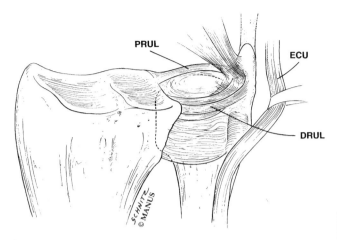

Figure 2

Soft-tissue relationships about the distal ulna. The vascularized dorsal radioulnar ligaments (DRUL) and palmar radioulnar ligaments (PRUL) blend in with the avascular fibrocartilagenous articular disk. (Adapted with permission from Kleinman WB, Graham TJ: Distal ulnar injury and dysfunction, in Peimer CA (ed): *Surgery of the Hand and Upper Extremity.* New York, NY, McGraw-Hill, 1996, pp 667–709. Illustrated by Gary Schnitz, © MANUS 1996.)

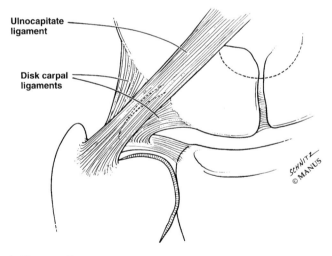

Figure 3

Relationship of the superficial ulnocapitate ligament to the disk-carpal ligaments. These comprise the ulnocarpal volar ligament portion of the triangular fibrocartilage complex. (Reproduced with permission from Kleinman WB, Graham TJ: Distal ulnar injury and dysfunction, in Peimer CA (ed): *Surgery of the Hand and Upper Extremity.* New York, NY, McGraw-Hill, 1996, pp 667–709. Illustrated by Gary Schnitz, © MANUS 1996.)

Biomechanics

One cannot think in isolated terms when discussing, diagnosing, or treating pathology about the distal radioulnar joint (DRUJ), TFC, or supporting soft-tissue elements. The

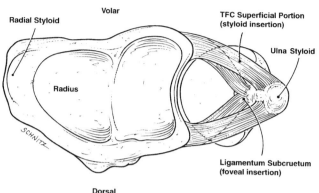

Figure 4

Diagrammatic view of the triangular fibrocatrtilage (TFC) from a distal perspective, illustrating Hagert's description of deep and superficial components of the ligamentous support about the distal ulna. The arrangement of the crossing fibers of the ligamentum subcrueteum and the fibers of the superficial components supports the disparate theories of ligament tension changes during forearm rotation. (Illustrated by Gary Schnitz, © MANUS 1996.)

DRUJ itself can be considered the distal half of a bicondylar forearm joint; the proximal half is the proximal radioulnar joint. Most daily activities involving the upper limb are performed with the elbow flexed and the forearm in neutral rotation. This places the seat of the ulna in a weightbearing position, and in a perfect position to provide a stable fulcrum around which the radius and carpus can rotate. Because of differences between the articulating surface of the ulnar seat and the concave articular surface of the sigmoid notch, there are both rotational and translational movements at this distal articulation. At the end range of pronation, due to this combination of movements, the palmar border of the ulnar seat rests against the dorsal rim of the sigmoid notch; conversely, at the end range of supination, the dorsal border rests against the palmar rim of the sigmoid notch.

One of the central controversies in the area of kinematics is the issue of ligament tension in the radioulnar ligaments during forearm rotation. The initial controversy resulted from conflicting data and theory regarding ligament tension and kinematics. Schuind supported his theory that PRUL tension increased with supination and DRUL tension increased with pronation using a stereophotogrammetric method. There has been great recent interest in settling this debate. One group confirmed Schuind's hypothesis in cadaveric experiments, using measurements of displacement in the PRUL and DRUL. Studying surface strains in the articular disk, other investigators also supported Schuind's hypothesis, demonstrating decreased strain along the dorsal margin during supination. They also noted changes in TFC

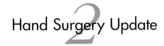
configuration during forearm rotation, and presented biomechanical evidence that supported the development of the most common Palmer class 1A TFC tear. Another author used measurements of the stabilizing structures of the DRUJ to create a mathematical model and 3-dimensional computed tomography reconstructions to lend further support to Schuind's hypothesis. In analyzing factors that contribute to DRUJ stability, one group not only emphasized the importance of the interosseous membrane, but also supported the hypothesis that the DRUL is an important stabilizer in pronation, while the PRUL is more important in supination.

The majority of the laboratory and cadaveric data support the theory that tension increases in the DRUL and decreases in the PRUL as the forearm pronates from full supination to full pronation; however, one of the initial proponents of the opposite theory now proposes anatomical support for both theories. Hagert suggests that ligament tension is directly dependent upon which section of the TFC is studied, supporting both theories; tension develops differentially in each of the 2 different portions (Fig. 4) of the TFC ligaments. The deep portion, or ligamentum subcruetum, inserts into the fovea at the junction of the ulnar styloid and pole, whereas the superficial portion of the ligament inserts at the proximal portion of the ulnar styloid itself. Hagert feels that the majority of biomechanical studies are indeed correct, as they relate directly to the superficial ligaments; opposite tensions develop in the deep DRUL and deep PRUL. Functional anatomic studies, as well as detailed magnetic resonance imaging (MRI) studies of the TFC, support Hagert's description of separate functional components of the TFC, as well as different TFC anatomic insertions.

Diagnosis

The key to an accurate diagnosis of ulnar-sided wrist pain is detailed knowledge of anatomy, surface landmarks, and provocative maneuvers. Although great advances in imaging technology have been made, the fundamentals of history and physical examination remain critical to making an appropriate diagnosis. The ulnar side of the wrist is comprised of a large number of structures. These different structures can be examined individually simply by altering the position of the clinician's examining fingers only a few millimeters. Provocative maneuvers are specific tests designed to apply load to potentially injured structures in a specific, focused fashion. Patient reaction to provocative testing is paramount to formulating a diagnosis and treatment plan.

Great controversy has been generated over the most appropriate imaging techniques for evaluation of the ulnar wrist,

DRUJ, and associated ligament structures. The accuracy and diagnostic capability of the triple injection wrist arthrogram has been challenged, adding skepticism to the interpretation of arthrographic results. One investigator showed only an 86% correlation between arthrography and arthroscopy in 20 patients with wrist injuries. Another group demonstrated 15 TFC tears in 39 patients with wrist pain; only 7 of these tears could be documented arthrographically. In one study of 52 asymptomatic adults, only 27% had positive arthrograms. Investigators have also demonstrated symmetrical defects in the symptomatic and asymptomatic wrists of patients. Other studies have emphasized a poor correlation between wrist pain and arthrographically-demonstrated noncommunicating defects. This work has provided significant insight to ligament anatomy, but has tempered enthusiasm for the routine use of the arthrogram in the diagnosis of wrist pain.

Although MRI techniques continue to be widely applied for a variety of conditions that affect the wrist, arthroscopy currently holds the lead position as both a diagnostic and therapeutic tool for evaluation of the ulnar side of the wrist. Arthroscopy has been shown to be highly accurate in the detection of ligament, soft-tissue, and cartilage lesions; in addition, therapeutic intervention is possible at the time of diagnosis. The interface of imaging techniques with arthroscopy was nicely demonstrated in a 1997 series of 43 patients who underwent clinical examination, plain radiography, wrist MRI, and arthroscopy. In 20 patients with a preoperative MRI diagnosis, 8 diagnoses were changed following arthroscopy. The sensitivity and specificity of MRI compared to arthroscopy was highest for TFC lesions; false positives, however, have prompted these investigators to view MRI results regarding the TFC with skepticism. MRI was not useful in the diagnosis of instability or other intercarpal ligament lesions. This clinical study is consistent with cadaveric and other clinical studies in which MRI was useful for TFC pathology, but not as accurate as arthroscopy. MRI proved to be useful in another study, correlating a nonspecific ulnocarpal stress test with arthroscopy. Signal changes within the proximal ulnar portion of the lunate correlated with abutment; however, the correct diagnosis was established by arthroscopy in all 45 patients on whom this nonspecific provocative test was performed. The interpretation of findings on MRI studies can be further complicated by false positive results. Signal intensity changes in the wrists of 50% of asymptomatic volunteers and overstaging of TFC lesions near the PRUL, DRUL, and the ulnar origin of the TFC have all been reported. Although MRI remains a useful tool for the detection of avascular necrosis, occult fractures, and space-occupying lesions, it is less sensitive and specific than arthroscopy as a diagnostic tool for ulnar-sided wrist pain.

Triangular Fibrocartilage

Significant advances have been made in the arthroscopic and limited open management of symptomatic and potentially destabilizing tears of the TFCC. The classification of traumatic and degenerative lesions of the triangular fibrocartilage recommended by Palmer and Werner continues to be a useful system, and facilitates communication regarding TFC pathology. Many authors have reported good results using totally arthroscopic techniques for repair of Palmer class 1B peripheral lesions. Commercial meniscal repair instrumentation can facilitate these repairs (Fig. 5).

Elegant studies have demonstrated the rich vascularity of the TFC at its palmar, dorsal, and ulnar peripheral margins, and shown that the fibrocartilaginous radius border origin of the TFC is essentially avascular. Despite the paucity of blood supply along the radius border of the TFCC, direct repair of Palmer class 1D lesions—previously not recommended—is now being advocated by some; good results have been obtained with both open and transradial arthroscopic techniques. One group demonstrated 18 good or excellent results in 23 patients who underwent repair of Palmer class 1D lesions with an open trans-DRUL approach, and another group had good results in 12 patients using a totally arthroscopic technique. Other studies have corroborated good results with arthroscopic repair techniques. Two groups also yielded good results combining TFC repairs with ulnar shortening osteotomies in patients with positive ulnar variance.

Ulnar Impaction

Impaction or ulnocarpal abutment must be distinguished from distal ulnar impingement on the radius secondary to instability after distal ulna resection (Fig. 6). Ulnocarpal abutment is usually associated with positive ulnar variance. Positive ulnar variance can be congenital, developmental, or acquired. Common causes of acquired ulnar positive variance are distal radius fractures with shortening, severe Essex-Lopresti injuries with progressive ulnar shortening after radial head resection, and premature medial radius physeal closure with the acquired variation of Madelung's deformity. Although impaction is usually seen in patients with positive ulnar variance, some patients with ulnar impaction have static zero-rotation view radiographs that are ulna-neutral or slightly ulna-minus. The clinician must order a dynamic grip zero-rotation view, as dynamic ulnar positivity has been demonstrated and reported.

The surgical treatment of ulnar impaction should be individualized. The importance of the position of the ulnar head against the sigmoid notch as a fulcrum for forearm rotation—the keystone of forearm stability—is well-known. The ulnar head must be ablated with caution, and a healthy respect for potential loss of the distal load-bearing fulcrum of forearm rotation. The Darrach resection of the distal ulna is successful only in patients with low upper-extremity demands. Surgery for patients who have failed conservative management and manifest early stages of ulnar impaction (Palmar class 2A and 2B) should focus

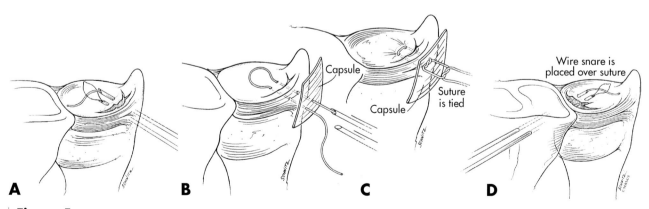

Figure 5

Arthroscopic techniques used for peripheral and radial-sided triangular fibrocartilage (TFC) tears. The technique incorporates cannulated needles (which can be passed through the TFC, allowing passage of suture) and instruments that facilitate tying of mattress sutures to anchor the tear. **A,** Two parallel cannulated needles are passed through the tear. The snare passed through one cannulated needle extracts one limb of the suture, forming a mattress configuration (**B**). **C,** The suture can then be tied over the joint capsule. **D,** A similar technique can be used for radial-sided tears, passing the cannulated needles through the dorsal distal radius. (Illustrated by Gary Schnitz, © MANUS 1996.)

only on decompression of the ulnocarpal joint. Although the distal ulna hemisection procedure can be used for impaction, it is more appropriate for arthrosis or instability, as both ulnar seat and pole are sacrificed. One team studied the results of hemiresection in 49 wrists with derangement of the DRUJ, including ulnar impaction. Similar to earlier studies, 72% achieved pain relief, with an 84% overall satisfaction rate. A partial resection of the distal ulna head can be performed in patients with less than 4 mm of positive ulnar variance and an intact and stable DRUJ. Another study yielded good long-term (36 months) follow-up in 7 wrists treated with an open wafer procedure.

In more advanced cases of ulnar impaction (Palmer class 2C and 2D), the ulnar head is accessible through the worn TFC. Arthroscopic techniques can be applied through the TFC lesion for treatment of the ulnar head. Many authors have reported successful results with a variation of the Feldon open wafer procedure, using arthroscopic techniques. The advantage of the arthroscopic wafer resection technique is that the TFC, as well as frayed synovium and associated radiocarpal and ulnocarpal pathology, can be addressed directly. Nevertheless, good results after arthroscopic TFC debridement have been reported by many authors. Arthroscopic debridement must be limited only to the pole, so that the intra-articular, load-bearing seat is not disturbed. One report proposed that as long as the peripheral 2 mm of the TFC remain intact, then DRUJ stability will not be compromised, lending further justification to arthroscopic debridement.

For advanced cases of ulnar impaction, or in patients with either static or dynamic positive ulnar variance, formal ulnar shortening osteotomy is still a viable option. This is the recommended treatment for advanced cases with associated partial lunatotriquetral lesions, based on laboratory evidence that suggests ulnar-sided wrist ligaments tighten after ulnar shortening. Ulnar shortening osteotomies can be performed in association with arthroscopic debridement. Formal ulnar shortening osteotomy has the advantage of being performed proximal to the articular surface of the DRUJ, but is a technically demanding procedure. Prior to performing ulnar shortening, attention must be paid to sigmoid notch morphology. One cadaveric study reported a 12% incidence of type III (reverse obliquity) inclination of the sigmoid notch as classified by Tolat and associates. In these situations, ulnar shortening osteotomy would be contraindicated; shortening would likely increase joint reaction forces on the seat of the ulna. In cases of reverse obliquity of the DRUJ, ulnar impaction is more appropriately treated by hemiresection or Sauvé-Kapandji procedure.

The Sauvé-Kapandji procedure has recently received renewed interest. The technique, first described in 1936, creates a distal radioulnar fusion and an ulnar pseudarthrosis proximal to the fusion site through which forearm rotation can occur. Many authors have reported successful results using the Sauvé-Kapandji procedure for DRUJ arthrosis, ulnar impaction, DRUJ instability, and acquired disorders such as Madelung's or impaction secondary to malunited distal radius fractures. The advantage of the Sauvé-Kapandji technique, unlike other ablative procedures, is that ulnocarpal support is not sacrificed. Some remain critical of the Sauvé-Kapandji procedure, commenting that instability of the proximal ulna may result, leading to impingement. The success of the Sauvé-Kapandji procedure is related to the effectiveness of the DRUJ fusion, and to technical factors that help support the distal end of the proximal ulna through the arc of pronosupination (periosteal stabilization and pronator quadratus interposition).

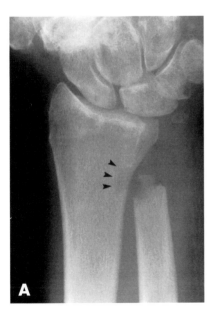

Figure 6

Comparison radiographs demonstrating radioulnar impingement (**A**) and ulnocarpal impaction or abutment (**B**). Cortical scalloping is associated with chronic mechanical impingement of the unstable distal stump of the ulna against the medial radius. Most cases of impaction are associated with positive ulnar variance; radiolucent lesions can also be seen on the proximal lunate. In this case, a large chondral lesion was diagnosed and treated with arthroscopic debridement at the time of ulnar shortening.

Radioulnar Impingement

Distal radioulnar impingement usually involves a mechanical irritation of an unstable shortened ulna against the distal medial radius cortex (Fig. 6). Most commonly, impingement is associated with resection of the entire distal ulna. A variety of soft-tissue and bony reconstructive procedures have been described for treatment of this challenging and often debilitating condition; no single treatment has been proven superior. Published reports on these procedures involve small samples; no randomized prospective studies comparing treatments have been presented. A soft-tissue reconstruction for relief of post-Darrach impingement was designed by Kleinman and Greenberg. They described a unique multicomponent soft-tissue reconstruction incorporating 2 tendon transfers, coupled with temporary pinning of the radioulnar relationship. They achieved satisfactory results in their small group of patients with severe post-Darrach distal ulna instability.

Creation of a one-bone forearm has been traditionally recommended for salvage of the upper extremity with radioulnar impingement symptoms that failed to respond to conservative management. Although pain relief can be achieved, fusion of the forearm has devastating functional consequences. Investigators continue to search for alternatives to this procedure.

Based on the clinical outcomes of patients who have undergone extensive and radical ulnar resections for malignancy, surgeons are investigating the use of an extensive resection of the distal ulna as an alternative to creation of a one-bone forearm. One group reported a group of patients with minimal functional deficits after extensive resection of the ulna. A recent multicenter study demonstrated favorable functional outcome after extensive distal ulnar resections for a number of conditions. Biomechanical testing is currently underway to justify use of this technique as an alternative to the creation of a one-bone forearm.

DRUJ Capsular Contracture

Loss of forearm rotation is a frequent occurrence after trauma, and can be severely disabling to function. Intra-articular fractures that involve the DRUJ, malunions, and shortening of the distal radius, as well as local trauma to the joint capsule itself, are all factors in posttraumatic loss of forearm rotation. The importance of the DRUJ capsule has only recently been recognized. In those patients in whom bony and extra-articular factors have been ruled out, contracture of the DRUJ capsule is most frequently the cause of loss of forearm rotation. The authors of a laboratory and clinical study on the subject emphasized the functional benefits that can be derived from DRUJ capsular release. The technique and indications for the "silhouette" capsulectomy have been further elucidated. Palmar DRUJ capsulectomy is indicated when functional supination has been lost; dorsal capsulectomy is indicated for loss of functional pronation. Both palmar and dorsal releases can be performed for concomitant supination and pronation losses. In one cadaveric study on rotational losses after distal radius fracture, capsular contracture was cited as a factor in rotational loss following uniplanar malalignment; bony restriction of motion was not noted in these cases.

DRUJ Instability

Instability of the DRUJ can be acute or chronic. Chronic conditions are usually the sequelae of unrecognized or untreated acute pathology. Injury to the restraining radioulnar ligaments is necessary to produce instability; injury to these ligaments and the DRUJ capsule itself is necessary to produce frank dislocation. Galeazzi fracture-dislocations, Essex-Lopresti injuries, both-bone forearm fractures, and high-energy distal radius fractures are all conditions in which the stability of the distal radioulnar joint should be considered in concert with other bony injuries. Simple DRUJ dislocations can frequently be reduced by treating associated bony pathology of the radius, or by performing simple closed reduction and long-arm cast immobilization in a stable position. Complex dislocations are characterized by profound pathology of the TFC, ulnar styloid, or sigmoid notch, any or all of which must to be addressed in order to restore long-term stability of the distal radioulnar joint.

A simple dislocation is fairly easy to reduce congruently. Simple DRUJ dislocation may occur in an isolated fashion, or may be associated with other trauma, such as fracture of the distal radius. If associated with other injuries, the simple dislocation is usually congruently relocated with treatment of the associated pathology. Stress testing of the DRUJ is important in assessing instability. Slight translational instability at the DRUJ in neutral rotation of the forearm is normal, as palmar and dorsal fibers of the TFC are most lax in this position. Translation of the ulna a few millimeters both dorsally and palmarly in the midrange of forearm rotation is not pathologic; however, at the end-arc of forearm pronosupination, minimal "shuck" should be present. End-range instability is indicative of an injury to one or more of the stabilizing elements of the DRUJ. Simple dislocations can be treated closed, with appropriate immobilization in either supination (for dorsal ulna dislocations) or pronation (for the less common palmar ulna dislocation). If the joint can be reduced congruently, but remains unstable, stabilization of the DRUJ relationship can be maintained by temporary percutaneous Kirschner wire fixation for 6 weeks, in addition to a long-arm cast.

Complex dislocations are those in which the DRUJ either cannot be reduced congruently, or is grossly unstable following reduction. Instability is usually attributed either to an avulsion fracture of the ulnar styloid through its base, or to soft-tissue TFCC pathology. DRUJ instability after stabilization of the distal radius may be seen in association with a large ulnar styloid fragment. Internal fixation of the ulnar styloid fracture is indicated for correction of DRUJ instability. Occasionally, a patient will present with chronic instability if a large radius fragment has been neglected or fixation of the ulnar styloid fragment has been neglected. Instability without bony pathology usually indicates a destabilizing tear of the TFC, which must be carefully repaired and immobilized until healed. Triangular fibrocartilage tears can also occur in association with small bony ulnar styloid avulsions. Stability of the DRUJ must be tested after bony stabilization of the associated radius fracture. If instability of the DRUJ is detected, repair of the TFC must be addressed.

A variety of soft-tissue reconstructions have been recommended for the treatment of chronic DRUJ instability. Because most clinical series are small, it is difficult to compare the results of different treatments. In one study of a variety of soft-tissue reconstructions used to correct both instability and impingement, the authors determined that reconstructions that created a radioulnar sling were most effective. Using previously published data on the important stabilizing function of the DRUL, another group devised a DRUL reconstruction using a free tendon graft. They reported good results in 15 patients with chronic instability. In another series of 23 patients, good to excellent results were reported in 17 patients. The hemiresection procedure was recommended as a salvage for instability in patients with neutral or negative ulnar variance. The authors also recommended combining the procedure with an ulnar shortening osteotomy to avoid ulnocarpal abutment in those patients with neutral or negative ulnar variance.

The ideal management of DRUJ instability is to recognize the problem and address the pathology acutely. Studies on chronic DRUJ instability suggest that the best results occur when anatomic correction can be achieved (eg, late repairs of destabilizing TFC tears). Surgical options for instability in the face of arthrosis include partial resections, with and without ulnar stabilization; complete ulnar resections, which sacrifice the entire distal ulna, and the Sauvé-Kapandji procedure.

Annotated Bibliography

Nomenclature and Anatomy

Hagert CG: Distal radius fracture and the distal radioulnar joint: Anatomical considerations. *Handchir Mikrochir Plast Chir* 1994;26:22–26.

Although this article deals with justifying reconstruction of the distal radioulnar joint after fracture, the majority of the content summarizes the anatomy and biomechanics of the DRUJ and surrounding soft-tissue elements. Hagert summarizes his theory regarding ligament tension during forearm rotation.

Tolat AR, Stanley JK, Trail IA: A cadaveric study of the anatomy and stability of the distal radioulnar joint in the coronal and transverse planes. *J Hand Surg* 1996;21B:587–594.

This excellent cadaveric review details the morphology of the distal radioulnar joint complex, including the sigmoid notch, distal radioulnar joint, and surrounding soft-tissue structures. A classification of sigmoid notch inclination, an important consideration in ulnar shortening osteotomy, is also presented.

Biomechanics

Acosta R, Hnat W, Scheker LR: Distal radio-ulnar ligament motion during supination and pronation. *J Hand Surg* 1993;18B:502–505.

Displacement transducers, used to measure relative tension changes, were placed along the radioulnar ligaments to determine relative ligament displacements during forearm rotation. This cadaver study supports Schuind's hypothesis.

Adams BD, Holley KA: Strains in the articular disk of the triangular fibrocartilage complex: A biomechanical study. *J Hand Surg* 1993;18A:919–925.

The authors used cadavers and a video-imaging system to determine changes in disk configuration and strain in different portions of the centrum and disk margins. Their findings support a mechanism that explains the development of the most common traumatic TFC tear. Findings related to strain changes are consistent with Schuind's hypothesis.

De Smet L, Fabry G: The controversy of the biomechanics of the triangular fibrocartilage complex: A mathematical model to clarify the problem. *Acta Orthop Belg* 1995;61:305–307.

The authors constructed a mathematical model of the distal radioulnar joint in order to elucidate changes in the radioulnar ligaments during forearm rotation. Their model takes into account both rotational and translational motions at the distal radioulnar joint.

Kihara H, Short WH, Werner FW, Fortino MD, Palmer AK: The stabilizing mechanism of the distal radioulnar joint during pronation and supination. *J Hand Surg* 1995;20A:930–936.

The wrist simulator is used in a sequential ligament sectioning study to determine the roles of the radioulnar ligaments, TFC, and interosseous membrane in stabilizing the distal radioulnar joint.

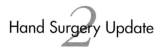

Totterman SM, Miller RJ: Triangular fibrocartilage complex: Normal appearance on coronal three-dimensional gradient-recalled-echo MR images. *Radiology* 1995;195:521–527.

An MRI study of the anatomy of the TFC using cadavers, patients without a history of trauma, and normal volunteers is described. The multiple components and varied insertion sites are demonstrated. Variations in the ulnar attachment of the TFC are also noted and described.

Van der Heijden EP, Hillen B: A two-dimensional kinematic analysis of the distal radioulnar joint. *J Hand Surg* 1996;21B:824–829.

Using 3-dimensional reconstructions and mathematical modeling from computed tomography scans obtained from 11 cadavers, the authors draw conclusions regarding ligament tension and TFC function during forearm rotation.

Diagnosis

Cantor RM, Stern PJ, Wyrick JD, Michaels SE: The relevance of ligament tears or perforations in the diagnosis of wrist pain: An arthrographic study. *J Hand Surg* 1994;19A:945–953.

Bilateral arthrograms were conducted in 56 patients with unilateral wrist pain. The authors found an extraordinarily high incidence of bilaterally symmetric defects—radial lesions of the TFC (88%), lunatotriquetral lesions (59%), and scapholunate lesions (57%). They found poor correlation of tear location noted on arthrograms with findings on physical examination.

Cooney WP: Evaluation of chronic wrist pain by arthrography, arthroscopy, and arthrotomy. *J Hand Surg* 1993; 18A:815–822.

Twenty consecutive patients with chronic wrist pain were evaluated using double contrast arthrography, followed by multiportal arthroscopy and an arthrotomy to confirm arthroscopic findings. The significance of interosseous ligament tears, as well as the extent and location of TFC tears, was most readily diagnosed with the arthroscopic technique. Diagnostic agreement was noted in 50% of the patients. In 2 of the 10 patients with diagnostic agreement, loose bodies not identified on arthrography were also noted.

Johnstone DJ, Thorogood S, Smith WH, Scott TD: A comparison of magnetic resonance imaging and arthroscopy in the investigation of chronic wrist pain. *J Hand Surg* 1997; 22B:714–718.

In this clinical study using preoperative MRI followed by arthroscopy in 43 patients with chronic wrist pain, TFC lesions could be predicted with a 0.8 sensitivity and 0.7 specificity. Lower rates were noted for intercarpal ligament lesions.

Kirschenbaum D, Sieler S, Solonick D, Loeb DM, Cody RP: Arthrography of the wrist: Assessment of the integrity of the ligaments in young asymptomatic adults. *J Bone Joint Surg* 1995;77A:1207–1209.

Fifty-two asymptomatic adults volunteered to have a wrist arthrogram using a single radiocarpal injection. Twenty-seven percent of the arthrograms demonstrated abnormal dye communications. Six of the 14 abnormal communications were through the TFC.

Schers TJ, van Heusden HA: Evaluation of chronic wrist pain: Arthroscopy superior to arthrography. Comparison in 39 patients. *Acta Orthop Scand* 1995;66:540–542.

In this study designed to correlate arthrographic findings with arthroscopy in 39 patients, arthrographic findings were found to be erroneous in 31 of the patients. False positive and false negative preoperative diagnoses were made. The authors advise against using a single injection arthrographic technique, but justify arthrography as a comparative diagnostic tool.

Triangular Fibrocartilage

Adams BD: Partial excision of the triangular fibrocartilage complex articular disk: A biomechanical study. *J Hand Surg* 1993; 18A:334–340.

This cadaveric study supports the clinical use of arthroscopic debridement of TFC tears. Maintenance of a 2-mm rim and preservation of at least 66% of the centrum's surface area produced no kinematic or structural changes.

Cooney WP, Linscheid RL, Dobyns JH: Triangular fibrocartilage tears. *J Hand Surg* 1994;19A:143–154.

The authors describe extensive experience of 56 patients with TFC injuries. Treatment was individualized to the patient and tear morphology. Their open repair technique, useful for radial and anterior tears, is outlined.

Jantea CL, Baltzer A, Ruther W: Arthroscopic repair of radial-sided lesions of the triangular fibrocartilage complex. *Hand Clin* 1995;11:31–36.

The authors present their justification for arthroscopic treatment of radial-sided TFC lesions, and describe a technique using a cannulated guide device. The clinical results in 12 patients with long-term follow-up are presented.

Kalainov D, Culp R: Arthroscopic treatment of TFCC tears. *Techniques in Hand and Upper Extremity Surgery* 1997; 1:175–182.

Lucey S, Poehling G: Arthroscopic treatment of triangular fibrocartilage complex tears. *Techniques in Hand and Upper Extremity Surgery* 1997;1:228–236.

In these technically-oriented articles, the authors provide an excellent perspective on the biological and biomechanical justification for treatment of TFC lesions. Arthroscopic techniques for both traumatic and degenerative TFC tears are also presented.

Trumble TE, Gilbert M, Vedder N: Ulnar shortening combined with arthroscopic repairs in the delayed management of triangular fibrocartilage complex tears. *J Hand Surg* 1997; 22A:807–813.

The authors report an average 29-month follow-up in 21 patients who underwent TFC repair in conjunction with an ulnar shortening osteotomy. Significant pain relief was achieved in 90% of patients. Preoperative arthrograms did not predict any peripheral tears. Follow-up diagnostic studies revealed that 8 of 9 radial and 4 of 5 peripheral lesions studied postoperatively were intact.

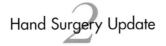
Hand Surgery Update

Ulnar Impaction

Angelini LC, Leite VM, Faloppa F: Surgical treatment of Madelung disease by the Sauvé-Kapandji technique. *Ann Chir Main Memb Super* 1996;15:257–264.

Along with 3 other articles cited below, this article presents clinical experience with patients in whom the Sauvé-Kapandji technique was applied for DRUJ derangements. Clinical diagnoses included posttraumatic impaction and osteoarthritis, primary ulnar impaction, instability, and Madelung's deformity. All 4 articles describe similar operative techniques and present favorable clinical results.

Bain GI, Pugh DM, MacDermid JC, Roth JH: Matched hemiresection interposition arthroplasty of the distal radioulnar joint. *J Hand Surg* 1995;20A:944–950.

Forty-nine wrists were evaluated following matched ulna hemiresection. Patients in this clinical retrospective study had a variety of conditions affecting the DRUJ, including ulnocarpal abutment. Patient satisfaction was high; 35 of 49 reported pain relief. Little correlation was noted, however, between measurable parameters and clinical results. Pain relief was the primary determinant of patient satisfaction.

Köppel M, Hargreaves IC, Herbert TJ: Ulnar shortening osteotomy for ulnar carpal instability and ulnar carpal impaction. *J Hand Surg* 1997;22B:451–456.

In this retrospective review of 47 ulnar shortening osteotomies, undertaken for both impaction and instability, the authors conclude that formal ulnar shortening osteotomy is an acceptable procedure for reducing pain and improving function. The oblique osteotomy was noted to have a reduced nonunion rate and faster healing time compared to the transverse osteotomy.

Minami A, Suzuki K, Suenaga N, Ishikawa J: The Sauvé-Kapandji procedure for osteoarthritis of the distal radioulnar joint. *J Hand Surg* 1995;20A:602–608.

This is one of many good articles about clinical experience with the Sauvé-Kapandji technique.

Schuurman AH, Bos KE: The ulno-carpal abutment syndrome: Follow-up of the wafer procedure. *J Hand Surg* 1995;20B:171–177.

In this retrospective review of a small number of wrists undergoing open wafer distal ulnar resections, good to excellent results were achieved in 5 of the 7 patients. The authors present an excellent discussion justifying the use of this procedure; the results support their continued use of this technique for symptomatic ulnocarpal abutment.

Waizenegger M, Schranz P, Barton NJ: The Kapandji procedure for post-traumatic problems. *Injury* 1993;24:662–666.

This is one of many good articles about clinical experience with the Sauvé-Kapandji technique.

Zachee B, De Smet L, Roosen P, Fabry G: The Sauvé-Kapandji procedure for nonrheumatic disorders of the distal radioulnar joint. *Acta Orthop Belg* 1994;60:225–230.

This is one of many good articles about clinical experience with the Sauvé-Kapandji technique.

Radioulnar Impingement

Cooney WP, Damron TA, Sim FH, Linscheid RL: En bloc resection of tumors of the distal end of the ulna. *J Bone Joint Surg* 1997;79A:406–412.

Eight patients underwent en bloc resection of the distal ulna, measuring between 3.1 and 9 cm. Functional results were excellent in 6 and good in 2. This small retrospective study justifies the possible use of an extensive distal ulnar resection as a salvage for symptomatic impingement. Routine reconstruction of distal ulna bony defects is not supported by study results.

Kleinman WB, Greenberg JA: Salvage of the failed Darrach procedure. *J Hand Surg* 1995;20A:951–958.

The authors present an alternative soft-tissue reconstruction for symptomatic radioulnar impingement following failed Darrach distal ulna resections. Their technique consists of a pronator quadratus interpositional tendon transfer combined with an extensor carpi ulnaris tenodesis, with temporary pinning of the distal radioulnar relationship. Good results were achieved in this small group of patients with a very challenging clinical problem.

Wolfe SW, Mih AD, Hotchkiss RN, Culp RW, Kiefhaber TR, Nagle DJ: Wide excision of the distal ulna: A multicenter case study. *J Hand Surg* 1998;23A:222–228.

This retrospective review of 12 patients collected from the combined experience of the Kiros Hand Study Group was presented at the 52nd annual meeting of the American Society for Surgery of the Hand. Each patient had at least 6 cm of the distal ulna resected for a variety of afflictions, including failed reconstructions. After a 22-month average follow-up, good to excellent results were achieved in 9 of the 12 patients. The authors recommend this technique as an additional salvage procedure that will not necessarily preclude the ultimate DRUJ salvage—a one-bone forearm.

DRUJ Capsular Contracture

Bronstein AJ, Trumble TE, Tencer AF: The effects of distal radius fracture malalignment on forearm rotation: A cadaveric study. *J Hand Surg* 1997;22A:258–262.

These authors studied the effects of fracture malalignment on forearm rotation. Rotational losses noted with uniplanar deformities are attributed to extra-articular and capsular contracture; these investigators were unable to generate rotational losses secondary to some uniplanar malalignments.

Kleinman WB, Graham TJ: The distal radioulnar joint capsule: Clinical anatomy and role in posttraumatic limitation of forearm rotation. *J Hand Surg* 1998;23A:588–599.

The authors describe a laboratory assessment of the components of the DRUJ capsule, and demonstrate how posttrauma fibrosis can lead to limitation of forearm rotation. They also present their clinical experience with palmar DRUJ capsulectomy for posttraumatic limitation of supination and dorsal DRUJ capsulectomy for limitation of pronation. The authors encourage anatomic restoration of bony relationships before considering DRUJ capsulectomy as a motion-enhancing procedure.

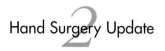
DRUJ Instability

Bruckner JD, Alexander AH, Lichtman DM: Acute dislocations of the distal radioulnar joint, in Pritchard DJ (ed): *Instructional Course Lectures 45.* Rosemont, IL, American Academy of Orthopaedic Surgeons, 1996, pp 27–36.

Acute treatment options for simple and complex DRUJ dislocations are summarized. A very good review of anatomy and biomechanics is also included.

Cheng SL, Axelrod TS: Management of complex dislocations of the distal radiounlar joint. *Clin Orthop* 1997;341:183–191.

The authors describe their experience with complex dislocations treated over a 3-year period. Although the number of clinical cases presented is small, this is an excellent review paper that includes a useful algorithm applicable to the treatment of complex DRUJ dislocations.

Geissler WB, Fernandez DL, Lamey DM: Distal radioulnar joint injuries associated with fractures of the distal radius. *Clin Orthop* 1996;327:135–146.

In this excellent review of both acute and chronic conditions affecting the DRUJ, and associated with fractures of the distal radius, the authors incorporate their combined clinical experience to justify treatment recommendations.

Imbriglia JE, Matthews D: Treatment of chronic post-traumatic dorsal subluxation of the distal ulna by hemiresection-interposition arthroplasty. *J Hand Surg* 1993;18A:899–907.

Average follow-up of 36 months was conducted in a series of 23 patients who had a partial distal ulnar resection for painful subluxation. The technique is recommended as a salvage procedure in patients with painful instability. The authors advocate the addition of a formal ulnar shortening osteotomy in patients with positive ulnar variance.

Peterson MS, Adams BD: Biomechanical evaluation of distal radioulnar reconstructions. *J Hand Surg* 1993;18A:328–334.

A variety of soft-tissue reconstructions are biomechanically analyzed and compared to the intact DRUJ. The authors conclude that a radioulnar tether is most effective, but suggest further investigation of the potential for a more anatomic reconstruction.

Scheker LR, Belliappa PP, Acosta R, German DS: Reconstruction of the dorsal ligament of the triangular fibrocartilage complex. *J Hand Surg* 1994;19B:310–318.

The authors present a reconstruction technique for chronic dorsal ulnar instability. They attempt to recreate the function of the DRUL in a more anatomic fashion using a free tendon graft. Clinical results in 14 of the 15 patients undergoing surgery revealed high satisfaction rates, with 12 of the 14 rendered pain free.

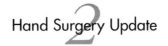

Chapter 10
Ligamentous Injuries and Instability Patterns

Mark S. Cohen, MD

Stability of the wrist is provided by the tight-fitting anatomic design of the individual carpal bones and by the ligamentous interconnections that control movement of one bone on another. A stable wrist has been defined as a wrist that does not deviate from a stable state of equilibrium while being loaded within a physiologic range of stress. Wrist instability results from a disruption of either the intrinsic ligamentous support between the individual carpal bones, the extrinsic carpal ligaments connecting the forearm to the carpus, or both.

Once the normal soft-tissue constraints are lost, the carpal bones may assume a pathologic orientation based on the bony and ligamentous restraints that remain. If the ligamentous injury is incomplete, the bones will maintain normal alignment at rest, but will collapse under applied load. This is termed "dynamic" instability. "Static" carpal instability occurs when enough restraints are lost that the bones assume an abnormal alignment on standard radiographic projections of the wrist. Instability has been further classified as carpal instability dissociative (CID) to denote independent, dissociative rather than normal associative motion between the bones of the proximal carpal row. In a carpal instability nondissociative (CIND) lesion, normal physiologic motion among the 3 bones of the proximal carpal row remains intact. The dissociation occurs between the proximal and distal carpal rows, or between the proximal carpal row and the radius.

Although the term wrist instability is used to describe a pathologic state, the wrist is actually in a more mechanically stable configuration when ligamentous support is lost. Under normal physiologic conditions, the wrist ligaments are under tension, resulting in stored potential energy. As the bones lose their alignment, they assume a collapsed position with kinetic dissipation of this energy. The pathologic resting position is more stable, but less physiologic and less functional. In the collapsed state, wrist motion and load-bearing capacity are compromised. Pain occurs secondary to abnormal shear forces on surface cartilage, synovitis, and abnormal ligamentous tension within the wrist.

Scapholunate Injuries

The most common form of carpal instability occurs between the scaphoid and the lunate. Three anatomic regions of the scapholunate interosseous ligament—a thick dorsal region consisting of short collagen fibers, a thin fibrocartilaginous central membranous portion, and a palmar region composed of thin collagen fascicles—have been described. It has been demonstrated in a cadaveric study that disruption of this ligament complex results from excessive wrist extension, ulnar deviation, and intracarpal supination, such as occurs with a fall onto the outstretched hand with a pronating forearm.

When load-bearing potential of the scapholunate interosseous ligament is rendered completely incompetent by rupture, the scaphoid collapses into a flexed posture, and the triquetrum and lunate extend. The term DISI (dorsiflexion intercalated segment instability) was coined to refer to the extended posture of the lunate following scapholunate ligament disruption as seen on a lateral radiograph of the wrist (Fig. 1).

Scapholunate dissociation significantly alters articular contact areas and stress patterns within the carpus. One investigator showed a 45% reduction in the radioscaphoid contact area with only a 5° subluxation (flexion) of the scaphoid. Arthritic changes begin at the radial styloid articulation with the scaphoid and progress to the proximal radioscaphoid joint, and then to the midcarpal capitolunate joint. This progressive arthritic pattern has been called scapholunate advanced collapse, or the SLAC wrist. The extended lunate is actually unloaded in this setting as a result of its concentric design; the radiolunate joint does not undergo progressive degeneration following scapholunate dissociation (Fig. 2).

The diagnosis of scapholunate ligament disruption may be confirmed clinically by the scaphoid shift test. Palmar pressure is applied at the distal scaphoid pole as the wrist is brought from ulnar deviation to radial deviation (Fig. 3). This maneuver is positive if scaphoid subluxation reproduces the patient's complaints of wrist discomfort and "giving away." Standard plain radiographs will often reveal

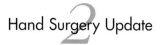
a flexion attitude of the scaphoid and an extended lunate. On the lateral film, the scaphoid assumes a more perpendicular orientation (with respect to the plane of the palm) and the extended position of the lunate can be seen more clearly.

Stress radiographs are very helpful in accentuating scapholunate diastasis. An axial-loading "grip" view in full supination will tend to drive the capitate proximally, wedging apart the scaphoid and lunate. An anteroposterior view in maximum ulnar deviation will distract the scaphoid

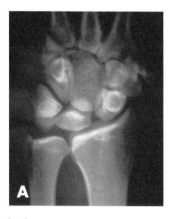
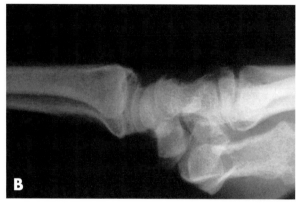
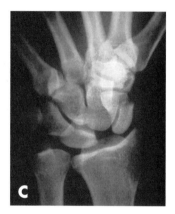

Figure 1

Posteroanterior (**A**) and lateral (**B**) radiographs of a patient with scapholunate dissociation. The frontal projection reveals a foreshortened, flexed scaphoid, resulting in a cortical ring sign. A scapholunate gap is not readily apparent. The lateral view reveals the flexed scaphoid, now more perpendicular with respect to the plane of the palm, and an extended lunate (dorsiflexion intercalated segment instability). **C,** Anteroposterior view in maximum ulnar deviation clearly demonstrates the pathologic scapholunate diastasis. Stress radiographs can be helpful in establishing the diagnosis of scapholunate dissociation.

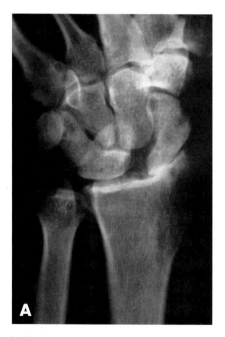
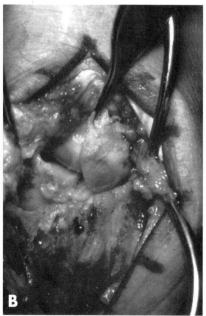
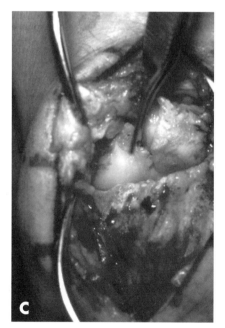

Figure 2

Anteroposterior radiograph (**A**) and intraoperative photograph (**B**) of a patient with the scapholunate advanced collapse (SLAC) pattern of degenerative arthritis secondary to a chronic scapholunate dissociation. Note the advanced degeneration at the radioscaphoid joint and proximal capitate. **C,** The radiolunate articulation (at tip of forceps) is preserved in SLAC arthritis.

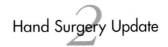

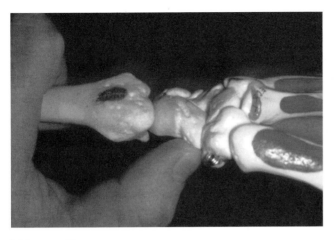

Figure 3

The scaphoid shift test is used to evaluate scapholunate ligament integrity. The wrist is taken from ulnar to radial deviation with the examiner's thumb applying palmar pressure to the distal pole of the scaphoid. This pressure opposes normal scaphoid flexion that occurs in radial deviation. When devoid of ligamentous attachment to the lunate, the proximal pole of the scaphoid loses its carpal shift influence on the lunate and can be subluxated out of the elliptical fossa of the distal radius. Reproduction of pain in the context of pathologic scaphoid motion is diagnostic of scapholunate ligament incompetence.

from the lunate, thereby widening the scapholunate gap by loss of carpal shift influence of the proximal pole of the scaphoid on the lunate (Fig. 1). These views should be compared to identical views of the contralateral uninjured wrist.

Additional studies can be used to confirm the diagnosis of a scapholunate ligament tear if required. Unfortunately, both wrist arthrography and magnetic resonance scanning have variable degrees of sensitivity and specificity for intracarpal ligament tears. Whereas the diagnosis of scapholunate insufficiency can usually be made by the history, physical examination, and plain radiographs, wrist arthroscopy appears to now be the "gold standard" when additional studies are required to make a definitive diagnosis.

Acute complete scapholunate dissociations should be treated by open reduction and internal fixation. Although there are advocates of arthroscopically assisted reduction and percutaneous pin fixation, long-term results of this technique are lacking. A dorsal capsulodesis may be used to augment a direct ligamentous repair, providing a secondary restraint to maintain the scaphoid in a physiologically extended posture (Fig. 4). Although it originally was reserved for acute injuries,

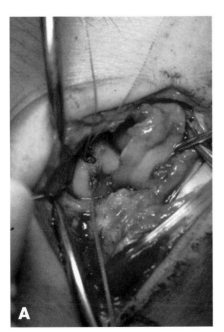 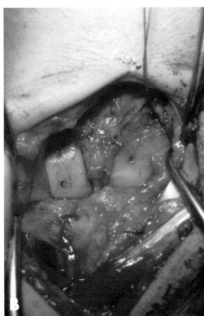 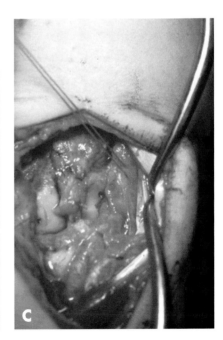

Figure 4

A, Intraoperative photograph depicting an acute scapholunate ligament disruption in which the scapholunate ligament has been avulsed from the lunate. Note the "joy-stick" Kirschner wires (K-wires) that have been placed into the scaphoid and lunate to manipulate these carpal bones. Bone anchors have been placed at the site of detachment to aid in repair. **B,** Following K-wire stabilization of the reduced scapholunate relationship, the ligament has been repaired. Note the additional anchor placed in the distal aspect of the scaphoid. **C,** The dorsal wrist capsule is secured under tension to the distal scaphoid, completing a capsulodesis augmentation. This provides a dorsal tether helping to limit pathologic flexion of the scaphoid.

it has been shown that in the absence of degenerative changes and with an adequate ligament as determined at surgery, soft-tissue reconstruction can successfully stabilize the carpus long after the acute disruption.

The dorsal capsulodesis procedure has also been shown to be effective in cases of dynamic scapholunate instability resistant to conservative treatment. This group of patients will have normal plain radiographs. The unstable scaphoid is demonstrable clinically only with a scaphoid shift test, by video radiography, or by arthroscopy. Subjective and functional improvement has been reported following dorsal capsulodesis in these patients.

If scapholunate dissociation is treated late, when there is no longer adequate ligament remaining for direct suture (before arthritic changes develop at the radioscaphoid joint), a partial wrist arthrodesis can be performed to stabilize the scaphoid, either fusing it distally to the trapezium and trapezoid (termed an STT fusion), or to the capitate (termed an SC fusion). These 2 procedures are essentially equivalent from a biomechanical standpoint, as long as care is taken to anatomically reduce the scaphoid at the time of surgery. Both procedures aid in keeping the scaphoid in a physiologically extended posture. They each result in approximately a 35% loss of wrist motion in the flexion-extension plane. The procedures are associated with significant reported complications.

Once degenerative arthritis is present, the wrist can be treated only by salvage-type procedures. The 2 most common options consist of excision of the scaphoid with fusion of the midcarpal joint (ulnar 4-bone fusion) or proximal row carpectomy. These procedures result in approximately a 50% loss of wrist motion in the flexion-extension plane and a 20% loss of grip strength. Two retrospective and nonrandomized reviews comparing these procedures showed few subjective or objective differences. Both provided satisfactory pain relief, restored adequate grip strength, and preserved a functional arc of motion in short-term follow-up. Advanced midcarpal arthritis at the capitolunate joint is a contraindication to proximal row carpectomy because this would place unhealthy cartilage of the head of the capitate into the lunate fossa of the radius.

Lunatotriquetral Injuries

Ligament tears between the lunate and triquetrum are approximately one sixth as common as those between the scaphoid and lunate. The lunatotriquetral ligament is thinner than its scapholunate counterpart; these 2 bones are also much more tightly coupled during wrist motion. In a kinematic analysis, one group reported only approximately 15°

of average lunatotriquetral rotation in the normal wrist versus approximately 25° between the scaphoid and lunate.

Experimentally, lunatotriquetral tears are produced by wrist extension and radial deviation (with associated intracarpal pronation). Energy of injury enters the proximal carpal row from the ulnar side of the wrist (a mechanism directly opposite of that causing scapholunate injuries). These injuries are associated with the presence of ulna-plus variance. Complete lunatotriquetral tears only rarely lead to volarflexion intercalated segment instability (VISI) (to describe the flexed lunate). The dorsal and palmar extrinsic ligaments have been shown to act as secondary joint stabilizers. The majority of lunatotriquetral injuries are thus dynamic in nature, causing pathologic symptoms only under load or with motion.

Patients with lunatotriquetral injuries typically complain of ulnar-sided wrist pain, weakness, and giving away; patients often report a "click" during wrist loading. The most sensitive provocative clinical test for instability is the lunatotriquetral "shear" test. This maneuver involves palmarly directed pressure against the dorsal body of the lunate, with a dorsally directed force applied to the pisiform (Fig. 5). This provocative maneuver produces a shearing vector across the lunatotriquetral joint and results in crepitation, clicking, and/or symptoms of pain in these patients.

Plain radiographs are normal in the vast majority of lunatotriquetral injuries. Occasionally a slight step-off can be seen along the proximal carpal row at the lunatotriquetral junction in maximum deviation of the wrist (disruption of

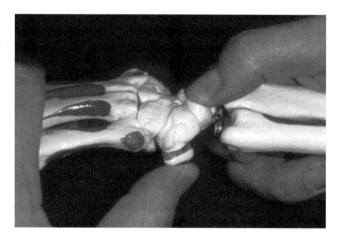

Figure 5

The provocative lunatotriquetral shear test to detect lunatotriquetral insufficiency. Dorsal pressure is applied to the lunate body, with simultaneous palmar pressure applied to the triquetrum (through the pisiform). This creates shearing force at the lunatotriquetral joint. A painful instability is diagnostic of a lunatotriquetral ligament sprain.

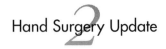

Gilula's line). When secondary joint restraints are also disrupted, a VISI collapse deformity results. Frontal radiographic views may then reveal a step-off at the lunatotriquetral joint, as the lunate and scaphoid flex away from an extending triquetrum (Fig. 6).

Wrist arthrography has variable specificity and sensitivity for lunatotriquetral disruptions; positive findings must be interpreted with caution. A positive arthrogram demonstrates neither the location nor the severity of the ligament disruption. Furthermore, age-related perforations in the lunatotriquetral ligament are not uncommon. A 20% incidence of lunatotriquetral contrast media leaks has been reported in the arthrograms of asymptomatic individuals between the ages of 20 and 60 years. Finally, it has been shown that normal arthrographic findings do not rule out the possibility of an internal derangement of the wrist. Magnetic resonance scanning lacks sensitivity for diagnosing lunatotriquetral disruptions, because the small interosseous signal is difficult to interpret. When ulnar-sided wrist pain persists following appropriate immobilization, wrist arthroscopy remains the most effective way of establishing a definitive diagnosis.

Lunatotriquetral joint tears (without static VISI) do not lead to progressive degenerative arthritis of the wrist. Furthermore, the ligament has an inherent healing capacity. This is a tightly coupled joint that will allow ligament healing in most cases, simply by prolonged immobilization. If conservative measures fail, one group reported an 80% success rate after arthroscopic debridement followed by temporary pin

fixation for isolated dynamic lunatotriquetral ligament tears. It is unclear if pin fixation is really necessary in this setting. Two other groups recently reported symptomatic improvement in most patients undergoing arthroscopic lunatotriquetral ligament debridement alone. It appears, however, that complete tears may not respond as well as incomplete tears to simple arthroscopic debridement.

Arthrodesis of the unstable lunatotriquetral joint is not entirely predictable. The authors of a meta-analysis of the literature reported a 27% nonunion rate. The lunatotriquetral joint has a very small surface area with high rotational torque, making union difficult. Furthermore, even successful lunatotriquetral fusion can lead to between 20% and 30% loss of wrist motion in all planes; pain relief is not uniform. Ligament reconstructions using a supplementary free-tendon graft are being performed at some centers, although long-term results are presently not available.

Ulnar shortening osteotomy is currently a commonly performed procedure for dynamic lunatotriquetral tears without VISI, especially in ulna-positive individuals. By shortening the ulna approximately 2.5 mm, one group showed that the ulnocarpal joint force could be reduced from 20% to 4%. Load across the lunatotriquetral joint is correspondingly reduced as the load across the triangular fibrocartilage is reduced. Ulnar shortening also theoretically tightens the disk-carpal palmar ligament complex, further increasing the stability of the lunatotriquetral relationship.

Lunatotriquetral injuries resulting in static VISI collapse patterns are rare. They require a clear understanding that

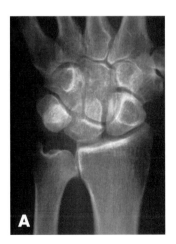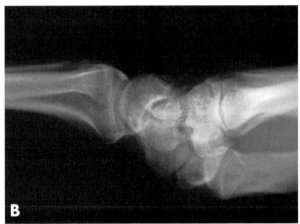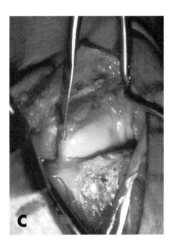

Figure 6

Posteroanterior (**A**) and lateral (**B**) radiographs of a patient with complete lunatotriquetral instability and volarflexion intercalated segment instability (VISI) collapse deformity. The frontal view depicts a flexed scaphoid and lunate, with a step-off disruption of the normal smooth contour between the lunate and triquetrum. The lateral radiograph better depicts flexed posture of the lunate. **C,** An intraoperative photograph documenting complete lunatotriquetral disruption (at tip of elevator). Note the intact scapholunate interosseous ligament (right). Most lunatotriquetral tears do not result in a VISI collapse deformity, because of the integrity of secondary extrinsic ligamentous stabilizers.

simply addressing the lunatotriquetral joint is not sufficient treatment. A component of the injury in addition to the complete lunatotriquetral disruption is a loss of secondary extrinsic ligamentous support. Stabilization of the lunatotriquetral relationship alone will convert a CID pattern to a CIND pattern; midcarpal collapse will persist unless treated. Partial wrist arthrodesis of the midcarpal joint, or proximal row carpectomy are 2 options for this rare condition.

Midcarpal Instability

All injuries discussed thus far result in loss of ligamentous support and integrity within the proximal carpal row. Ulnar midcarpal instability is a form of CIND. It is seen less frequently than lunatotriquetral ligament disruption.

Patients with midcarpal instability commonly complain of a painful and spontaneous wrist "clunk" occurring with ulnar deviation of the pronated wrist. The clunk represents a pathologic carpal shift of the proximal row from a flexed to an extended posture. In ulnar midcarpal instability, normal ligamentous support between the carpal rows is lost; the entire proximal row sags into flexion in the neutral position of the hand-forearm unit. A smooth transition during ulnar deviation does not occur until late in ulnar deviation, when the proximal row suddenly clunks into a reduced extended posture, termed a "catch-up clunk".

The diagnosis of ulnar midcarpal instability is often difficult to make. On physical examination, the physician can often see an indentation or sulcus over the dorsoulnar border of the wrist. This indentation may create the illusion of a prominent ulnar head. However, it actually represents a pathologic sag of the midcarpal joint, with flexion of the proximal carpal row relative to the forearm and the distal row.

Radiographs often reveal a mild to moderate VISI collapse pattern. The frontal projection reveals a foreshortened scaphoid resulting from the flexed attitude of the entire proximal row; however, there is no disruption or step-off at the lunatotriquetral articulation, as is seen with VISI collapse from severe lunatotriquetral dissociation. Midcarpal instability is associated with ligamentous laxity and a hypermobile wrist. The provocative maneuver used to confirm the diagnosis is performed by applying an axial load to a pronated and slightly flexed wrist, which is then brought into ulnar deviation. This commonly reproduces the painful and characteristic clunk of this midcarpal (CIND) instability pattern.

The treatment of ulnar midcarpal instability is still evolving. The pathologic lesion is believed to be attenua-

tion or incompetency of the ulnar limb of the palmar arcuate (triquetrohamate-capitate) ligament of the wrist, although radial-sided deficiency has been described. Initially, surgical efforts were directed at stabilizing or reinforcing the medial ligament complex. More recently, 2 groups reported a high rate of failure following soft-tissue reconstructions for this condition. Current recommendations include midcarpal fusion, or simple splinting and activity modification for these individuals.

Triangular Fibrocartilage Complex

The triangular fibrocartilage complex (TFCC) is the major stabilizer of the distal radioulnar joint and helps support the ulnar carpus in a load-bearing capacity. On a gross level, the TFCC consists of a central articular disk and dorsal and palmar radioulnar ligaments, spanning from the radius to the base of the ulnar styloid. The articular disk is the load-bearing component of the complex. The dorsal and palmar ligaments principally stabilize the distal radioulnar joint. In the past, controversy existed regarding which radioulnar ligament (palmar or dorsal) was the primary stabilizer of the distal radioulnar joint in terminal pronation and supination. However, deep and superficial components to these radioulnar ligaments have been identified. The deep portion, referred to as the ligamentum subcruetum, inserts into the fovea, just ulnar to the articular surface of the pole of the distal ulna. The superficial portion of the dorsal and palmar ligaments inserts more distally, onto the base of the ulnar styloid. It is now recognized that the palmar fibers of the deep portion tighten in pronation, and the dorsal fibers tighten in supination; the opposite occurs in the superficial portion (Fig. 7).

TFCC tears are associated with individuals who have positive ulna variance and frequently are seen in conjunction with lunatotriquetral ligament disruptions (eg, the end stages of ulnocarpal abutment syndrome). The diagnosis can be confirmed by arthrography, magnetic resonance scanning, or arthroscopy in those individuals who fail conservative measures. Arthrography lacks sensitivity and specificity. Magnetic resonance scanning is more useful in the evaluation of the TFCC than evaluation of other internal wrist derangements. Recently, investigators reported a 100% sensitivity, 90% specificity, and 97% accuracy when using high-resolution magnetic resonance scanning with a wrist surface coil to evaluate the triangular fibrocartilage. Arthroscopy, however, allows determination of the location and extent of TFCC tears in addition to associated ligamentous and cartilaginous lesions. Unfortunately, isolated injuries to the ligamentum subcruetum (in the face of a normal superficial component) may appear normal on arthroscopic evaluation. In these cases, the physical examination findings are critical.

TFCC tears can be posttraumatic or attritional (degenerative). TFCC lesions have been classified based on the anatomic location of the tear and whether the lesion is more consistent with acute trauma or a degenerative process. Treatment is based on the class and type of the tear. Central tears, for the most part, can be treated with arthroscopic debridement. One group reported excellent results following arthroscopic debridement of posttraumatic tears alone in individuals without positive ulnar variance or associated lunatotriquetral disruptions. Another group showed ulnar shortening to be effective if debridement alone fails to adequately relieve symptoms in individuals with central or nondetached peripheral TFCC disruptions. Thus, strong consideration must be given to ulnar shortening in individuals with TFCC tears who have positive ulnar variance, or when there are associated lunatotriquetral tears or articular cartilage injury as defined by arthroscopy (Fig. 8).

Peripheral or marginal tears of the TFCC, associated with either gross or slight instability, can heal with conservative measures or surgical repair. The peripheral 20% of the TFCC in the adult is well-vascularized and possesses inherent healing capacity. Investigators reported excellent results in ulnar-sided TFCC tears treated by arthrotomy and direct open repair after failure of conservative measures. More recently, in a multicenter study, 93% satisfactory results were reported with arthroscopic repair of peripheral TFCC lesions. This appears to now be possible, in part, because of newer arthroscopic instrumentation. Excellent functional results were also recently reported in peripheral TFCC tears treated with combined arthroscopic repair and ulnar shortening osteotomy.

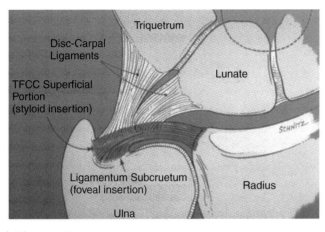

Figure 7

Diagram depicting the deep and superficial portions of the triangular fibrocartilage. The deep portion, referred to as the ligamentum subcruetum, inserts onto the fovea just ulnar to the articular surface of the distal ulna. The palmar fibers of this portion tighten in forearm pronation, and dorsal fibers tighten in supination. The superficial portion of the triangular fibrocartilage complex inserts directly onto the base of the ulnar styloid. The dorsal fibers of this portion tighten in pronation; the palmar fibers tighten in supination. (Reproduced with permission from Kleinman WB, Graham TJ: Distal ulnar injury and dysfunction, in Peimer CA (ed): *Surgery of the Hand and Upper Extremity.* New York, NY, McGraw-Hill, 1996, pp 667–709.)

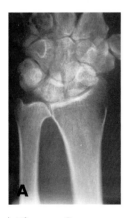 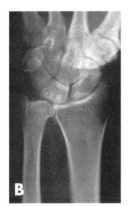 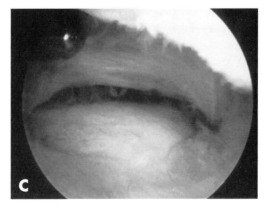 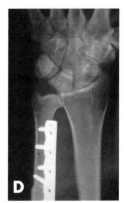

Figure 8

A, Neutral rotation posteroanterior (PA) radiograph of a patient with positive ulnar variance, a triangular fibrocartilage complex (TFCC) tear, and a lunatotriquetral disruption. **B,** Pronated grip view reveals dynamic impaction at the ulnocarpal joint, with associated degenerative changes (ulnocarpal abutment syndrome). **C,** Arthroscopic photograph following debridement of central TFCC attritional tear, the lunatotriquetral ligament, and chondromalacia of the lunate. **D,** Neutral rotation PA view following ulnar shortening osteotomy with compression plate fixation. This procedure significantly unloads the ulnocarpal joint.

Annotated Bibliography

Scapholunate Instability

Ashmead D IV, Watson HK, Damon C, Herber S, Paly W: Scapholunate advanced collapse wrist salvage. *J Hand Surg* 1994;19A:741–750.

The authors report the results of 100 cases of SLAC wrist salvage with scaphoid excision and limited wrist midcarpal arthrodesis. Pain relief was good to excellent in most cases. Flexion-extension averaged 53% and grip strength 80% of the opposite side. Technical details are discussed.

Berger RA: The gross and histologic anatomy of the scapholunate interosseous ligament. *J Hand Surg* 1996;21A:170–178.

The scapholunate interosseous ligament was evaluated histologically revealing 3 anatomic regions: a thick dorsal region composed of short collagen fibers, a proximal region consisting principally of fibrocartilage, and a palmar region composed of thin collagen fascicles. Clinical implications are discussed.

Burgess RC: The effect of rotatory subluxation of the scaphoid on radio-scaphoid contact. *J Hand Surg* 1987;12A:771–774.

The effect of progressive rotary subluxation of the scaphoid on radio-scaphoid contact area was examined in a cadaveric model. Only 5° of pathologic scaphoid flexion reduced the contact area of the proximal pole by 44%. A 20% subluxation of the scaphoid reduced contact area by 77%. These findings explain the progression of arthritis following scapholunate ligament disruption.

Kirschenbaum D, Sieler S, Solonick D, Loeb DM, Cody RP: Arthrography of the wrist: Assessment of the integrity of the ligaments in young asymptomatic adults. *J Bone Joint Surg* 1995;77A:1207–1209.

Fifty-two asymptomatic adults between 20 and 35 years old were studied with the use of single injection arthrography. Abnormal arthrograms were found in 27% of patients. Four of 14 had multiple areas of communication. The authors concluded that perforation of a ligament of the wrist is common in young asymptomatic adults.

Lavernia CJ, Cohen MS, Taleisnik J: Treatment of scapholunate dissociation by ligamentous repair and capsulodesis. *J Hand Surg* 1992;17A:354–359.

Twenty-one patients with scapholunate dissociation were treated with direct ligamentous repair supported by a dorsal radioscaphoid capsulodesis. At an average follow-up of 33 months, grip strength, pain, and radiographic appearance improved in all cases. A loss of motion was only seen in palmar flexion (average 12°). The results were not dependent on the age of the ligament disruption.

Mayfield JK, Johnson RP, Kilcoyne RK: Carpal dislocations: Pathomechanics and progressive perilunar instability. *J Hand Surg* 1980;5A:226–241.

The pathomechanics of progressive carpal instability were studied experimentally in a cadaver wrist. The mechanism of injury was extension,

ulnar deviation, and intercarpal supination. Stage I perilunar instability resulted in scapholunate ligament disruption. Stage IV perilunar instability resulted in volar lunate dislocation.

Tomaino MM, Miller RJ, Cole I, Burton RI: Scapholunate advanced collapse wrist: Proximal row carpectomy or limited wrist arthrodesis with scaphoid excision? *J Hand Surg* 1994;19A:134–142.

Twenty-four wrists were retrospectively reviewed at an average of 5.5 years postoperatively to compare proximal row carpectomy with scaphoid excision to ulnar midcarpal fusion for the SLAC wrist disorder. There were no differences in subjective or objective results between groups with the exception of slight increased residual motion following proximal row carpectomy. A stage-dependent surgical approach for this condition is presented.

Watson HK, Ashmead D IV, Makhlouf MV: Examination of the scaphoid. *J Hand Surg* 1988;13A:657–660.

The anatomic basis and technique of performing the "scaphoid shift" test is described. Clinical interpretation is discussed.

Weiss AP, Akelman E, Lambiase R: Comparison of the findings of triple-injection cinearthrography of the wrist with those of arthroscopy. *J Bone Joint Surg* 1996;78A:348–356.

Fifty consecutive patients were prospectively studied to compare the findings of triple-injection arthrography with those of wrist arthroscopy. When compared with arthroscopy, the sensitivity, specificity, and accuracy of triple-injection cinearthrography were 56%, 83%, and 60%, respectively. This study suggests that normal arthrographic findings do not rule out the possibility of an internal derangement of the wrist.

Wintman BI, Gelberman RH, Katz JN: Dynamic scapholunate instability: Results of operative treatment with dorsal capsulodesis. *J Hand Surg* 1995;20A:971–979.

Twenty dorsal radioscaphoid capsulodesis procedures were performed for dynamic scapholunate instability. At a mean postoperative follow-up of 34 months, objective and functional status improved in most patients. An average loss of 12° of wrist flexion was noted.

Wyrick JD, Stern PJ, Kiefhaber TR: Motion-preserving procedures in the treatment of scapholunate advanced collapse wrist: Proximal row carpectomy versus four-corner arthrodesis. *J Hand Surg* 1995;20A:965–970.

Seventeen patients were retrospectively reviewed at 27 to 37 months postoperatively to compare proximal row carpectomy to 4-corner arthrodesis for the SLAC wrist. Proximal row carpectomy led to a slightly improved final flexion-extension arc and grip strength. Because the study was retrospective and not randomized, the authors were unable to prove the superiority of either procedure over the other.

Zdravkovic V, Jacob HA, Sennwald GR: Physical equilibrium of the normal wrist and its relation to clinically defined "instability". *J Hand Surg* 1995;20B:159–164.

The rotational stability of the wrist was experimentally tested under load. A truly stable state of equilibrium could be found in the normal wrist only under axial load. A unidirectional coupling was observed

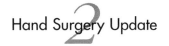
through the scapholunate ligament as a counteraction to a tendency for the lunate to extend and the scaphoid to flex. The triquetrum and lunate were closely coupled.

Lunatotriquetral Instability

Brown JA, Janzen DL, Adler BD, et al: Arthrography of the contralateral, asymptomatic wrist in patients with unilateral wrist pain. *Can Assoc Radiol J* 1994;45:292–296.

The authors compared the prevalence and site of wrist ligament perforation bilaterally in individuals with unilateral wrist pain. The authors concluded that asymptomatic perforation was common, even in young individuals.

Kirschenbaum D, Coyle MP, Leddy JP: Chronic lunotriquetral instability: Diagnosis and treatment. *J Hand Surg* 1993; 18A:1107–1112.

Fourteen patients with lunotriquetral instability were evaluated. Injury mechanism and clinical findings are discussed. Lunotriquetral arthrodesis resulted in approximately a 20% loss of wrist motion.

Larsen CF, Jacoby RA, McCabe SJ: Nonunion rates of limited carpal arthrodesis: A meta-analysis of the literature. *J Hand Surg* 1997;22A:66–73.

The results and union rates for limited intracarpal arthrodesis reported in the literature between 1946 and 1993 were reviewed. Ninety-five percent confidence intervals were calculated, and the studies were combined. Nonunion rates were highest for lunotriquetral and scapholunate arthrodesis.

Nelson DL, Manske PR, Pruitt DL, Gilula LA, Martin RA: Lunotriquetral arthrodesis. *J Hand Surg* 1993;18A:1113–1120.

Lunotriquetral arthrodesis was retrospectively studied in 22 patients. Fixation with a Herbert screw supplemented with a Kirshner wire was superior to fixation with wires alone. Postoperatively, 12 patients had minor pain, 10 patients had moderate pain, and none had severe pain. Technical details are discussed.

Osterman AL, Seidman GD: The role of arthroscopy in the treatment of lunatotriquetral ligament injuries. *Hand Clin* 1995; 11:41–50.

A group of 20 patients with intractable ulnar wrist pain from lunatotriquetral disruption were treated with arthroscopic debridement and percutaneous pin fixation. Eighty percent of patients reported good to excellent relief of pain and preoperative symptoms. Patients lost an average of 20% of wrist motion in a flexion-extension arc.

Ruby LK, Cooney WP III, An KN, Linscheid RL, Chao EY: Relative motion of selected carpal bones: A kinematic analysis of the normal wrist. *J Hand Surg* 1988;13A:1–10.

The relative motion of individual carpal bones was studied using cadaveric specimens and a combination of orthoradiography, sonic digitization, and computer analysis. The wrist was found to function as 2 carpal rows with the proximal row functioning as a variable geometry intercalated segment between the distal row and the radius-triangular fibrocartilage. The lunate and triquetrum were more tightly coupled than the scaphoid and lunate.

Ruch DS, Poehling GG: Arthroscopic management of partial scapholunate and lunotriquetral injuries of the wrist. *J Hand Surg* 1996;21A:412–417.

Fourteen patients with partial scapholunate and lunotriquetral ligament tears were treated with arthroscopic debridement alone. Thirteen were highly satisfied and 11 had complete relief of symptoms. No further instability of the wrist was noted at a minimum 2-year follow-up.

Sennwald GR, Fischer M, Mondi P: Lunotriquetral arthrodesis: A controversial procedure. *J Hand Surg* 1995;20B:755–760.

Twenty-three patients underwent lunotriquetral arthrodesis for painful lunotriquetral instability. The authors report a 57% rate of pseudarthrosis even with compression screw techniques. Results were found to be unpredictable.

Viegas SF, Patterson RM, Peterson PD, et al: Ulnar sided perilunate instability: An anatomic and biomechanic study. *J Hand Surg* 1990;15A:268–278.

A staging system for ulnar-sided perilunate instability is presented based on cadaveric dissections and load studies. A pattern of increasing ulnar-sided instability was defined starting with lunotriquetral interosseous ligament disruption and progressing to a static VISI (CID) pattern. The importance of the dorsal ligamentocapsular structures was demonstrated.

Weiss AP, Sachar K, Glowacki KA: Arthroscopic debridement alone for intercarpal ligament tears. *J Hand Surg* 1997; 22A:344–349.

Arthroscopic debridement alone was evaluated for complete and incomplete intercarpal ligament tears in 43 wrists at an average follow-up of 27 months. Between 80% and 100% of patients with partial or complete lunotriquetral tears or partial scapholunate tears had complete symptom resolution or improvement. The data suggest that complete intercarpal ligament tears may not respond as well as incomplete ones to arthroscopic debridement alone.

Wright TW, Del Charco M, Wheeler D: Incidence of ligament lesions and associated degenerative changes in the elderly wrist. *J Hand Surg* 1994;19A:313–318.

Sixty-two cadaveric wrists were studied to determine the incidence of pathologic changes in asymptomatic elderly wrists. Defects involving the scapholunate, lunotriquetral, and triangular fibrocartilage were very common. These ligament defects appear to occur as a process of aging and behave in a manner quite differently from traumatic lesions in younger individuals.

Midcarpal Instability

Brown DE, Lichtman DM: Midcarpal instability. *Hand Clin* 1987;3:135–140.

The anatomy, pathomechanics, and clinical treatment of midcarpal instability are reviewed. The evolution of various treatment strategies are discussed, and current recommendations are presented.

Lichtman DM, Bruckner JD, Culp RW, Alexander CE: Palmar midcarpal instability: Results of surgical reconstruction. *J Hand Surg* 1993;18A:307–315.

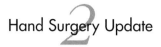
Thirteen patients who underwent 15 surgical procedures for mid-carpal instability are reviewed. Six of 9 soft-tissue reconstructions failed. All 6 patients treated with limited midcarpal arthrodesis were successful. The authors suggest that nonsurgical management of mid-carpal instability, including splinting can be effective in many cases.

Wright TW, Dobyns JH, Linscheid RL, Macksoud W, Siegert J: Carpal instability non-dissociative. *J Hand Surg* 1994; 19B:763–773.

Forty-five patients with nondissociative carpal instability are presented. Patients had a high incidence of hypermobility syndrome. Unpredictable results were found using a variety of soft-tissue procedures. Joint leveling procedures in the patients with ulnar negative variance had the best results. The authors discuss the current understanding and treatment options for this subset of patients.

Triangular Fibrocartilage Complex

Corso SJ, Savoie FH, Geissler WB, Whipple TL, Jiminez W, Jenkins N: Arthroscopic repair of peripheral avulsions of the triangular fibrocartilage complex of the wrist: A multicenter study. *Arthroscopy* 1997;13:78–84.

A multicenter study was performed to assess the results of arthroscopic repair of peripheral TFCC tears in 45 wrists using a zone-specific repair kit. Twenty-seven wrists had associated injuries. Patients were evaluated 1 to 3 years postoperatively. Twenty-nine of 45 wrists were rated excellent, 12 good, 1 fair, and 3 poor.

Hagert CG: Distal radius fracture and the distal radioulnar joint: Anatomical considerations. *Handchir Mikrochir Plast Chir* 1994;26:22–26.

The author reviews the anatomy and pathologic conditions affecting the distal radioulnar joint and TFCC. Effects of distal radius fractures on distal radioulnar joint mechanics are discussed. The role of the deep and superficial portions of the TFCC with respect to stability during forearm rotation is discussed.

Hermansdorfer JD, Kleinman WB: Management of chronic peripheral tears of the triangular fibrocartilage complex. *J Hand Surg* 1991;16A:340–346.

The authors report on the management of chronic peripheral TFCC tears treated with open repair and stabilization. Thirteen patients are reviewed at follow-up of more than 1 year. Eight of 11 patients were able to return to normal painless activities. Indications and details of the surgical technique are discussed.

Hulsizer D, Weiss AP, Akelman E: Ulna-shortening osteotomy after failed arthroscopic debridement of the triangular fibrocartilage complex. *J Hand Surg* 1997;22A:694–698.

The authors report on 13 patients who underwent ulnar shortening osteotomy after failing debridement alone for central or nondetached peripheral tears of the TFCC. At an average of 2.3 years' follow-up, 12 of 13 had complete relief of ulnar-sided wrist pain. Nonunion or loss of fixation occurred in 2 patients. The authors recommend a 2-mm ulnar shortening osteotomy in those patients with central or stable peripheral TFCC tears that fail debridement alone.

Kleinman WB, Graham TJ: Distal ulnar injury and dysfunction, in Peimer CA (ed): *Surgery of the Hand and Upper Extremity.* New York, NY, McGraw-Hill, 1996, pp 667–709.

This comprehensive chapter reviews the normal and pathologic conditions affecting the ulnar side of the wrist. Included are relevant anatomic descriptions of the distal radioulnar joint and triangular fibrocartilage. Physical examination methods, the use of diagnostic imaging, and pathology-specific management procedures are reviewed for bony and soft-tissue ulnar-sided wrist pathology.

Minami A, Ishikawa J, Suenaga N, Kasashima T: Clinical results of treatment of triangular fibrocartilage complex tears by arthroscopic debridement. *J Hand Surg* 1996;21A:406–411.

The results of arthroscopic debridement of the TFCC were reviewed in 16 patients with either posttraumatic or degenerative tears. Patients with positive ulnar variance and lunotriquetral interosseous ligament tears had a poor clinical outcome. Patients with degenerative tears also did poorly. All patients with posttraumatic tears had a good clinical outcome.

Palmer AK: The distal radioulnar joint: Anatomy, biomechanics, and triangular fibro-cartilage complex abnormalities. *Hand Clin* 1987;3:31–40.

This article reviews the basic anatomy and biomechanics of the distal radioulnar joint. The different types of TFCC injuries are reviewed and treatment options are discussed in terms of traumatic and degenerative lesions.

Potter HG, Asnis-Ernberg L, Weiland AJ, Hotchkiss RN, Peterson MG, McCormack RR Jr: The utility of high-resolution magnetic resonance imaging in the evaluation of the triangular fibrocartilage complex of the wrist. *J Bone Joint Surg* 1997;79A:1675–1684.

The authors review the use of high-resolution magnetic resonance imaging (MRI) with a dedicated wrist surface coil for evaluation of the TFCC. With the use of arthroscopy as the standard, MRI had a sensitivity of 100%, a specificity of 90%, and an accuracy of 97% for the detection of a tear. The authors concluded that high-resolution MRI permits accurate description and localization of tears of the TFCC.

Trumble TE, Gilbert M, Vedder N: Ulnar shortening combined with arthroscopic repairs in the delayed management of triangular fibrocartilage complex tears. *J Hand Surg* 1997; 22A:807–813.

Twenty-one patients were reviewed following a combined arthroscopic repair of the TFCC with ulnar shortening for traumatic lesions deemed repairable at arthroscopy. Pain relief was significant and 12 of 13 returned to their original job or sports activities. Indications and surgical techniques are discussed.

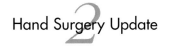

Chapter 11
Carpal Fractures

Gary M. Lourie, MD

Introduction

Less than 10% of carpal injuries are isolated fractures, but the potential for disabling sequelae from these injuries is significant. Nearly 70% of carpal fractures involve the scaphoid; the remaining 30% are distributed among the other bones. Although recent advances have focused on the scaphoid, the potential for morbidity in the other carpal bones should not be overlooked. This chapter addresses recent advances in anatomy and vascularity, mechanism of injury, diagnosis, treatment, and complications.

Scaphoid Fractures

Over 90% of scaphoid fractures heal, leaving nearly 35,000 nonunions in the US every year. Nearly every published theory on carpal kinematics—most notably Navarro's columnar concept, Fisk's mechanical tie-rod linkage, and Lichtman's ring theory—emphasizes the importance of the scaphoid as a major contributor to carpal stability. Loss of bony integrity and collapse will predispose the wrist to patterns of instability. Two precarious arterial systems have been noted—the dorsal ridge vessels, which supply the proximal 70% to 80% of the bones, and the volar branches of the radial artery, supplying the remaining 20% to 30%, including the tuberosity. Although no vessels enter the proximal pole through the scapholunate interosseous ligament, recent studies have shown that the radioscapholunate ligament (ligament of Testut) is primarily a neurovascular structure containing terminal branches of the anterior interosseous artery and nerve. Unfortunately, little of this blood supply reaches the proximal scaphoid pole. Results of a study undertaken over 50 years ago, in which vascular foramina were painstakingly counted to determine vascularity, closely parallel conclusions from recent latex injection studies. Clinical studies document an approximate 30% incidence of osteonecrosis with waist fractures, and even higher incidence with proximal pole fractures (100%).

Mechanism of Injury

Loading the radial aspect of the palm with the wrist extended more than 95° to 100° consistently reveals that scaphoid waist fractures result from forces applied to the distal pole as the proximal pole remains strongly stabilized by the radius, and the volar aspect of the scaphoid is stabilized by the radioscaphocapitate ligament. A unique mechanism of injury termed the "puncher's" scaphoid fracture has been described recently. This injury is caused by the clenched fist punching an object so that the concentration of force is directed along the second metacarpal, then dispersed to the trapezium and trapezoid and finally through the scaphoid, resulting in fracture (Fig. 1).

The simultaneous occurrence of fracture of the distal radius and scaphoid has been reported with incidence up to 5%. In a recent study of over 2,000 fractures of the distal radius, and approximately 400 fractures of the scaphoid, this pattern was observed 12 times. Considering that the angle between the wrist and ground at impact will determine the subsequent fracture pattern (angle between 45° and 90°, radius fracture; greater than 90°, scaphoid fracture), it was postulated that the same mechanism would produce fracture of each bone. The fact that fracture of one bone will dissipate energy and protect adjacent bones from fracture serves to underscore that this simultaneous fracture pattern can only result from high-energy impact.

Another unique fracture pattern recently described involves concomitant scapholunate dissociation with fracture of the scaphoid. Thought previously to be mutually exclusive injuries, this pattern has been reported with increasing frequency. One author hypothesized that the same mechanism of injury could actually cause this double injury, by initial hyperextension resulting in scapholunate dissociation, then further injury to the intact scaphoid tubercle, resulting in its fracture. The resultant severe instability of this injury mandates treatment of both injury patterns, to decrease the possibility of nonunion and/or intercalated carpal instability.

Another new fracture pattern of the scaphoid involves a dorsal avulsion component. The isolated dorsal avulsion fracture arises from the dorsal ridge of the scaphoid, and can

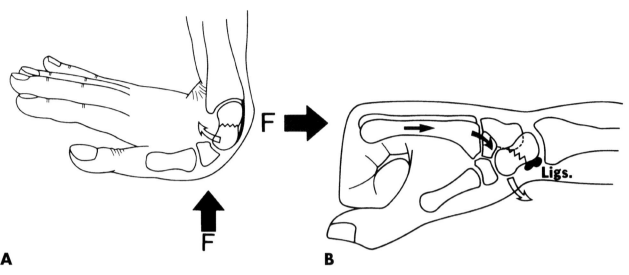

Figure 1

The "puncher's" scaphoid fracture. **A,** The bending force at the distal pole of the scaphoid (white arrow) is the main factor producing fracture, which has been stated to occur in extension. **B,** In neutral or slight palmarflexed position, the external force (F) transmitted through the second metacarpal disperses to the trapezoid and trapezium (shown by black arrows), resulting in flexion moment on the distal pole of the scaphoid (white arrow). The palmar ligaments (Ligs), which hold the proximal pole of the scaphoid, are the fulcrum. Because of the obliquity of the scaphoid, the external force creates shear stress at the waist. (Reproduced with permission from Horii E, Nakamura R, Watanabe K, Tsunoda K: Scaphoid fractures as a "puncher's" fracture. *J Orthop Trauma* 1994;8:107–110.)

only be visualized on a supinated oblique radiograph of the wrist. This fracture may mimic a more complete lesion through the scaphoid waist. Misdiagnosis may result in prolonged immobilization. This fracture is thought to occur from avulsion by the dorsal intercarpal ligament. If properly diagnosed, it should respond to a short period of casting with satisfactory outcome.

Diagnosis

A careful history and physical examination, coupled with a high index of suspicion, will suggest to the clinician the possibility of a scaphoid fracture. Routine radiographs should include posteroanterior, true lateral, and pronated oblique views. The supinated oblique view may reveal a dorsal avulsion fracture. Although minimal ulnar deviation will extend the scaphoid, increasing the likelihood of fracture exposure, this can be a painful experience for the patient. A proximal tilt view, in which the beam is 30° off the vertical, toward the elbow, can eliminate the need to move the injured wrist.

Trispiral tomography and/or computed tomography (CT) scans can also be helpful in visualizing scaphoid fractures. A longitudinal axis CT scan of the scaphoid is useful in detecting fresh fractures as well as chronic nonunions, or malunions with a humpback deformity.

The high sensitivity of bone scans in detecting occult scaphoid fractures remains of some value. One study indicates that occult scaphoid fractures can be ruled out if the bone scan is negative (0% false negative) at 72 hours. Specificity, however, remains low because of the relatively high incidence of false positives. False positive bone scans are most likely secondary to injuries such as scapholunate ligament disruption and capsular tears. Bone scans are still useful, though, particularly for the high performance athlete; a negative bone scan will allow return to sport activity.

Ultrasound (or a variation termed intrasound) has been used in an attempt to improve early diagnosis while avoiding radiation. The test is considered positive when an application of ultrasound over the scaphoid produces pain, burning, or a tingling sensation. Unfortunately, early enthusiasm has been tempered by more recent studies showing low specificity and poor reproducibility. One investigator recently reported on the use of intrasound vibration as a simple, low-cost method to diagnose occult scaphoid fractures. Of 50 patients who presented with a significant clinical history, palpable anatomic snuffbox tenderness, and negative plain radiographs, the intrasound vibration demonstrated 100% sensitivity and nearly 95% specificity. Although the false positive rate was much lower than with conventional bone scanning, the use of intrasound vibration still depends primarily on the patient's subjective positive response, determined by retracting the extremity with application of the noxious

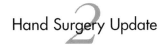

Hand Surgery Update

stimulus. Vibratory testing, however, is inexpensive, non-invasive, and easy to perform. It involves no ionizing radiation and may prove useful as an adjunct to accurate diagnosis.

Classification

Various classifications have been described for the scaphoid based on fracture location, pattern, and intrinsic stability. Waist fractures are the most common, with an incidence of up to 65%. Up to 30% involve the proximal pole, and the remaining fractures involve the distal pole.

Russe classified scaphoid fractures over 30 years ago based on orientation—transverse, vertical oblique, or horizontal oblique. The vertical oblique pattern was considered the most unstable (Fig. 2). Herbert's classification described 4 basic types—acute stable, acute unstable, delayed union, and nonunion. Within each type, he further classified the location—waist, proximal pole, distal pole, and tubercle—and noted sclerotic or fibrous nonunions (Fig. 3).

Classifications based on inherent fracture stability remain well accepted. Instability is determined by displacement more than 1 mm in any projection, or scapholunate angulation greater than 60°, and/or radiolunate angulation greater than 15°, and a lateral intrascaphoid angulation exceeding 20°. The importance of this classification is that uncorrected instability is associated with an increased incidence of fracture nonunion. One series of conservatively treated fractures displaced more than 1 mm had a nonunion rate of nearly 92%.

Treatment

Closed cast treatment remains the undisputed recommendation for nondisplaced scaphoid fractures, with the union rate approaching nearly 95%; fracture location should determine the duration of casting required. Distal pole fractures usually require up to 8 weeks of immobilization, waist fractures up to 12 weeks, and more proximally situated fractures sometimes require as much as 5 to 6 months. Short-arm versus long-arm cast, thumb interphalangeal joint immobilization, and even index/middle finger immobilization

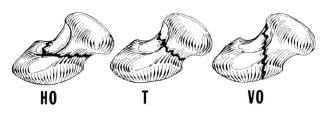

Figure 2

Russe's classification of scaphoid fractures (HO = horizontal oblique, T = transverse, VO = vertical oblique). (Reproduced with permission from Taleisnik J: *The Wrist*. New York, NY, Churchill Livingstone, 1985. © 1985 Elizabeth Roselius.)

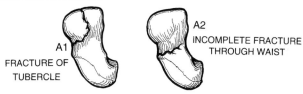
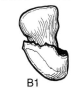
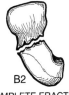
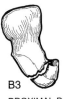
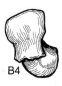
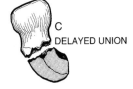
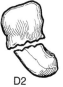
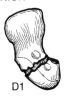

TYPE A:
STABLE ACUTE FRACTURES

A1 FRACTURE OF TUBERCLE

A2 INCOMPLETE FRACTURE THROUGH WAIST

TYPE B:
UNSTABLE ACUTE FRACTURES

B1 DISTAL OBLIQUE FRACTURE

B2 COMPLETE FRACTURE OF WAIST

B3 PROXIMAL POLE FRACTURE

B4 TRANS-SCAPHOID-PERILUNATE FRACTURE DISLOCATION OF CARPUS

TYPE C:
DELAYED UNION

C DELAYED UNION

TYPE D:
ESTABLISHED NONUNION

D1 FIBROUS UNION

D2 PSEUDARTHROSIS

Figure 3

Herbert's classification of scaphoid fractures. (Reproduced with permission from Amadio PC, Taleisnik J: Fractures of the carpal bones, in Green DP (ed): *Operative Hand Surgery*, ed 3. New York, NY, Churchill Livingstone, 1993, pp 799–860.)

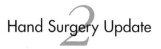
have all been argued extensively in the literature. Support can be found for nearly every type of cast and position. Biomechanical studies seem to support slight wrist flexion and radial deviation, to relax the radioscaphocapitate ligament and allow closer approximation of the fragments. One study showed that a long-arm thumb spica cast applied for 6 weeks will accelerate the time to union in middle and proximal pole scaphoid fractures. There were no reported nonunions and only 2 delayed unions in the long-arm cast group, compared to 2 nonunions and 6 delayed unions in the short-arm group.

There has been some recent support in sports medicine literature for immediate internal fixation of acute stable scaphoid fractures in the high performance athlete. In one report on 12 athletes treated with Herbert screw fixation for acute waist scaphoid fractures, the average union rate was greater than 90% by 9.8 weeks, and the athletes returned to sports in less than 6 weeks. The authors advise longer follow-up before internal fixation can be more widely recommended.

The acute unstable fracture, however, requires surgical reduction and internal fixation. Closed reduction of an unstable fracture by manipulation alone has proved unsuccessful in obtaining and maintaining anatomic alignment, crucial for a satisfactory outcome. The best surgical approach and type of internal fixation remain controversial. The palmar approach through the floor of the flexor carpi radialis sheath avoids injury to the precarious dorsal blood supply, but causes injury to the extrinsic radiocarpal ligaments. While the potential for iatrogenic carpal instability exists, this has not occurred with meticulous repair of the capsule. In addition, obtaining reduction in cases of acute displaced fracture and late humpback malunions is easier through the palmar approach. Proponents of the dorsal approach, however, believe that the dorsal approach will not impair the blood supply, and will avoid the morbidity of operative trauma to the palmar extrinsic radiocarpal ligaments. These advocates report a union rate of approximately 90%. They do not, however, mention the incidence of osteonecrosis (ON), nor the potential for correction of a humpback deformity through the dorsal approach. Fractures of the proximal pole can be easily approached dorsally.

Recent studies have compared different fixation devices to improve selection of the most appropriate type. In one investigation of 5 available commercial screws, the authors found no statistical difference in compression, but significant differences in resistance to cantilever bending. In a cadaveric study of different screws, another investigator found the AO screw, the Acutrak screw, and the Herbert-Whipple screw superior to the Herbert screw under cyclical bending loads; clinical relevance is undetermined, however. Even earlier reports demonstrating the use of multiple Kirschner wires have reported excellent union rates. Because of prominent hardware and the potential for persistent fragment distraction, use of an Ender's plate or staples is probably not indicated.

Delayed Union

For the nondisplaced stable scaphoid fracture seen late (4 to 6 months), casting is still successful in up to 90% of cases, although prolonged immobilization may be needed. Initial enthusiasm for the use of pulsed electromagnetic field stimulation has been tempered by further long-term follow-up; one report indicated a decline in the success rate from 80% in the initial study to 69% on follow-up. There is general agreement that this treatment should be recommended only as an alternative to bone grafting. Scaphoid nonunion usually involves fractures of the waist and proximal pole, and remains challenging. Nonunion of fractures of the scaphoid tuberosity have been described, but much less frequently because of the rich vascularity of the distal portion of this bone (Fig. 4). Mody and associates presented 4 cases of persistent nonunion of the tuberosity, all intra-articular, which required open reduction and internal fixation.

Nearly 100% of patients with untreated scaphoid fracture nonunion will go on to develop degenerative arthritis. In a younger, high-demand population, surgical treatment cannot be criticized; however, the occasional incidence of asymptomatic scaphoid nonunion advanced collapse in the general population suggests that conservative treatment may be the more prudent choice in the low-demand wrist.

Scaphoid fracture nonunions have also been classified as stable versus unstable, with or without associated degenerative changes. The stable nonunion can be effectively treated with a Russe graft, using corticocancellous bone graft (Fig. 5). Current literature supports adjunctive internal fixation. Another significant problem involves treatment of the patient with a second nonunion after undergoing internal fixation and bone grafting. Comparing cannulated screws to Herbert screws in scaphoid nonunion, one study found no difference in union rates but did find that the proximal position of the screw affected time to union. Placement of the screw in the central third of the scaphoid was associated with a significant shorter time to union, and increased chance of nonunion.

Three recent articles have addressed repeat bone grafting for a second nonunion. One article reported results on

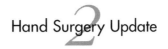

25 patients, 19 of whom had a second bone grafting procedure. Using a modification of the Mayo Wrist Score, they report somewhat poor subjective results, but still recommend repeat treatment. They provide a useful treatment algorithm to help the hand surgeon (Fig. 6). Another

researcher reported on 8 patients with persistent nonunions after primary failure of Herbert screw fixation, documenting union on 6 patients following repeat bone grafting and Herbert screw fixation. Both studies concluded that the initial procedure usually failed because of inadequate placement of the Herbert screw. The third article reported on the outcome of repeat Russe bone grafting after failure of a previous Russe graft in 15 patients; 53% achieved union with a second procedure, and an additional 25% united after a third procedure. The authors recommended supplementary internal fixation if repeat Russe bone grafting is undertaken.

Treatment for patients with scaphoid nonunion and early degenerative radioscaphoid arthritis at the distal pole has also received recent attention. One author proposed limited arthrodesis for the scaphoid nonunion, in which the distal pole is excised and the proximal pole fused to the lunate and capitate. Biomechanically, this procedure is warranted, because initial degenerative changes usually occur between the malpositioned distal pole and the radius. Pain relief was excellent in this patient group; range of

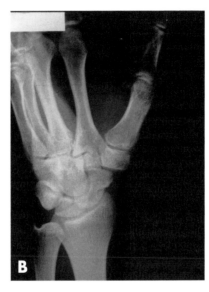

Figure 4

A, This patient had chronic nonunion of the scaphoid tuberosity. Exploration revealed a small fragment, which was treated with simple excision and ligament repair. **B,** Postoperative radiograph.

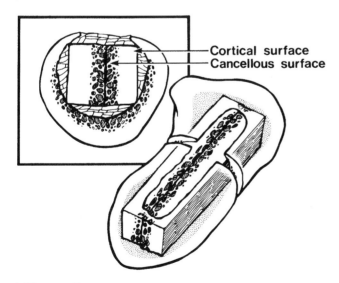

Figure 5

Russe graft performed for a stable nonunion. (Reproduced with permission from Green DP: The effect of avascular necrosis on Russe bone grafting for scaphoid nonunion. *J Hand Surg* 1985;10A:597–605.)

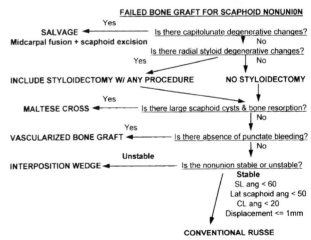

Figure 6

Treatment algorithm for failed bone grafting in scaphoid nonunion. SL ang = scapholunate angle; CL = capitolunate angle; Lat = lateral. (Reproduced with permission from Smith BS, Cooney WP: Revision of failed bone grafting for nonunion of the scaphoid. *Clin Orthop* 1996;327:98–109.)

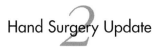

motion averaged 50% of the contralateral side. Incorporating a similar rationale, another study reported on simple excision of the distal scaphoid fragment, retaining the proximal pole. The 12 patients were able to return to work; 9 were pain-free. This procedure offers an excellent alternative to partial wrist fusion, and does not preclude further surgical reconstruction, if needed.

Osteonecrosis

Osteonecrosis (ON) of the proximal pole, and its influence on healing of scaphoid fracture nonunion, are topics of continuing debate. The majority feel that in the presence of ON, scaphoid healing can still occur, but with difficulty. With an absence of punctate bleeding from the proximal pole, the success rate of the Russe bone grafting procedure approaches zero. One researcher found that in 5 patients with presumed ON who underwent histologic scaphoid examination, the pattern of necrosis was patchy at best; random biopsy alone cannot accurately predict the histologic status of the entire specimen. Another report found MRI to be 100% accurate in both sensitivity and specificity, compared to only 80% for surgical visualization, 86% for tomography, and 40% for plain radiography.

Treatment of ON of the scaphoid without degenerative changes has received extensive attention. One study describes a pedicled vascularized bone graft off the ascending branch of the radial artery, and reports an approximate 90% union rate (Fig. 7). Using a modified Spalteholtz technique in a cadaveric study of 41 upper limbs, the arterial blood supply of the distal radius and ulna and their potential use in vascularized pedicled bone grafts were documented. One article described a pedicled bone graft off the first dorsal metacarpal artery in 4 patients, with a 100% union rate; another report was of 11 patients treated with a combination of bone grafting from the iliac crest and implantation of the second dorsal intermetacarpal artery, with union in all but one patient. These articles suggest a potential for pedicled vascularized grafts to revascularize necrotic bone and accelerate healing. Nonetheless, conventional techniques have convincing advocates. In one study of 26 nonunions with an avascular proximal pole treated with iliac crest bone grafting and Herbert screw fixation, 9 healed and 7 patients had an incomplete union or fibrous union. All patients had high subjective scores, suggesting that a fibrous union may impart enough stability to be relatively painless. The authors emphasized the importance of iliac crest bone grafting, rigid fixation, and appropriate postoperative immobilization (thumb spica cast for 3 months).

Malunion

Amadio and associates provided clinical evidence that malunion of the scaphoid directly affected outcome. In their series of 45 patients, 83% had satisfactory clinical outcomes, and degenerative arthritis occurred in only 22% of patients with healed normal scaphoid configuration; however, patients with greater than 45° of lateral intrascaphoid angulation had only 27% satisfactory clinical outcomes and 54% occurrence of degenerative arthritis. Their conclusion was that healing alone was not sufficient to indicate success. Another report provided experimental evidence that for 5° of experimental humpback deformity, there was a 24° loss of wrist extension.

The challenge of osteotomizing a healed scaphoid with a malunion to establish anatomic alignment continues to cause trepidation for most hand surgeons. In one study, patients with healed malunions returned to work with significant relief of discomfort. Of 25 patients treated for nonunion with Russe bone-grafting, 12 of 13 who healed with intrascaphoid angles greater than 45° reported success. Longer-term follow-up is needed to determine if this success is lasting. In a series of patients who underwent corrective osteotomy for symptomatic scaphoid malunion, 5 patients underwent osteotomy; all had symptomatic improvement. Union was achieved in less than 6 months, and there were no cases of ON. The authors proposed that reconstructive osteotomy for scaphoid malu-

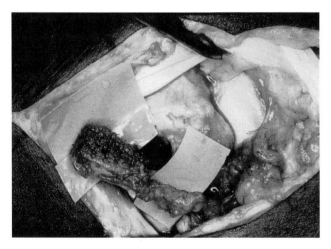

Figure 7

Intraoperative view of the pedicled vascularized bone graft described by Zaidemberg. (Reproduced with permission from Alex Mih, MD, Indiana Hand Center, Indianapolis, IN.)

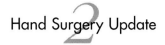

nion may be indicated to reduce the incidence of degenerative arthritis in young patients with high-demand wrists and symptomatic malunion.

Lunate Fractures

The literature on acute fractures of the lunate is sparse. Incidence has been reported as low as 1.3% and as high as 6.5%; the high incidence, however, included cases of Kienböck's disease. The mechanism of injury includes hyperextension of the wrist. Half of the patients manifest concomitant fractures of the radius, capitate, and even the proximal ends of the metacarpals. Diagnosis requires a high index of suspicion. Plain radiographs may fail to reveal the fracture; CT scanning and/or tomography will usually demonstrate the fracture. In one classification scheme, group I involves the palmar pole; group II, chip fractures; group III, fractures of the dorsal pole; group IV, sagittal fractures through the body; and group V, transverse fractures through the body of the lunate. The majority of fractures described have involved groups I and II. Treatment of acute nondisplaced fractures should be by cast immobilization. Displaced fractures, especially those involving the palmar pole, are best treated by open reduction and internal fixation. In the majority of cases, the lunate is fed by a rich vascular supply involving both the palmar and dorsal surfaces, with a variety of branching patterns; 20% of lunates, however, are fed by a single palmar blood supply, which courses retrograde in the lunate. As in the scaphoid, this vascular anatomy places certain patients at risk for ON.

Magnetic resonance imaging remains a fairly accurate way of diagnosing ON. Lunates at risk, those with a tenuous blood supply, may have a relationship to Kienböck's disease; a direct cause and effect theory, however, has not been definitely established at this point. Repeated trauma with compression fracture in a lunate that relies on a limited palmar blood supply may lead to segmental interruption, placing the lunate at a greater risk for Kienböck's disease.

Triquetral Fractures

Fractures of the triquetrum range from the innocuous dorsal chip fracture to the unstable body fracture associated with the greater arc perilunate dislocation. Triquetral fractures are the second most frequent carpal fracture type, with an incidence of approximately 14%. The dorsal chip fracture results from an impact hyperextension injury in ulnar deviation. The ulnar styloid may be driven into the triquetrum. One group proposed that the same fracture can result from the chisel action of the dorso-proximal edge of the hamate striking against the fully extended and ulnar-deviated wrist. Although there is some controversy over the etiology of the chip fracture, it is not believed to be a destabilizing injury. The bony pathology is best seen on a lateral or slightly pronated radiograph. Three weeks of immobilization in a short-arm cast is usually all that is required; most patients heal uneventfully. Because of a rich triquetral blood supply (dorsal and palmar), ON is not usually observed following triquetral fracture. If a patient has pain from a triquetral nonunion, simple excision of the ununited fragment is usually successful.

Most body fractures of the triquetrum result from forced hyperextension, ulnar deviation, and intercarpal supination, and are associated with progressive perilunar dislocations. Left untreated, carpal instability may result. A volar intercalated segment instability (VISI) pattern can result if progressive treatment is not performed. This requires appropriate reduction and internal fixation of the fracture, and repair of damaged ligaments.

A new fracture of the triquetrum involving an avulsion of the palmar radial aspect of the bone has recently been reported. The authors described 5 palmar radial triquetral avulsion fractures resulting from falls onto the hyperextended wrist during sport activity. Initial standard radiographs (posteroanterior, true lateral, and 45° supinate views) failed to reveal the fracture; only an 8-view instability series succeeded in visualizing the fracture. The best view was the posteroanterior view with the wrist radially deviated. In this view, the avulsed fragment was displaced from the adjacent triquetral and hamate bones. The authors felt that these injuries represented a significant ulnar-sided perilunate instability pattern, similar to the stage II or stage III progressive ulnar-sided instability created by serial section of the lunotriquetral ligament complex. The patients all eventually developed a VISI collapse deformity, underscoring the importance of recognition of this injury. Once the diagnosis is made, the lunotriquetral complex can be repaired or reconstructed.

Pisiform Fractures

Fractures of the pisiform are rare, comprising only 1% of carpal fractures. They usually result from direct trauma to the palmar ulnar aspect of the wrist. Fractures have been classified as transverse (usually involving a chip off the distal end of the bone), longitudinal, or comminuted. Fractures are best visualized on a 30° supinated or carpal tunnel view, or may require a CT scan or conventional tomography. Local tenderness over the pisiform is usually present. Because of the proximity to Guyon's canal, ulnar nerve symptoms may be present. Multiple ossification regions present in the pisiform in adolescents can make the diagnosis of pisiform fracture difficult.

Most fractures of the pisiform are nondisplaced, and respond well to 3 to 4 weeks of short-arm cast immobilization. Nonunions, malunions, fractures healing with degenerative arthritis, and acute fractures involving the articular surface of the pisotriquetral joint are best treated by pisiform excision. In a recent report of 8 patients seen with pisotriquetral loose bodies, 50% gave a history of trauma, in which the loose body was thought to be a fracture resulting from a shearing injury. The loose body required simple excision; however, excision of the entire pisiform was recommended for patients manifesting concomitant degenerative changes. When treated conservatively, fractures of the pisiform may go on to develop symptomatic loose bodies, emphasizing the need for longer follow-up in these seemingly benign injuries.

Trapezial Fractures

Fractures of the trapezium comprise 2% to 5% of all carpal bone fractures. Two types of trapezial fractures have been identified: the trapezial ridge, which usually occurs from a direct blow; and trapezial body fractures, which result from more severe trauma. The trapezial body fracture is usually intra-articular and can be associated with ligament injuries involving the thumb. Fractures of the ridge are commonly missed by conventional radiographs, and may require a carpal tunnel view or even CT scan. Fractures of the body can best be seen with an oblique radiograph, with the ulnar border of the hand resting on the cassette and the forearm placed in 20° pronation from a perpendicular attitude.

Ridge fractures involving the tip (type II) are usually treated successfully by simple cast immobilization for 4 to 6 weeks. Fractures at the base of the ridge (type I) may go on to painful nonunion, requiring excision of the ununited fragment.

Body fractures are usually intra-articular and may be combined with fractures at the base of the first metacarpal. If displaced, body fractures require open reduction and internal fixation, and occasionally concomitant external fixation (Fig. 8).

Trapezoid Fractures

Because of the trapezoid's well-protected location, fractures of this bone are extremely rare, comprising only 0.2% of carpal fractures. ON can occur with dislocation; the blood supply of this bone lacks a dorsopalmar intraosseous connection, making it prone to vascular compromise. Fractures usually respond to simple cast immobilization for 4 to 6 weeks. If incongruity results, limited intercarpal fusion may be necessary to control pain.

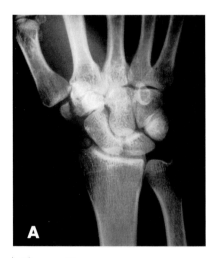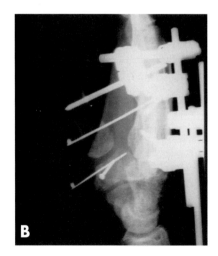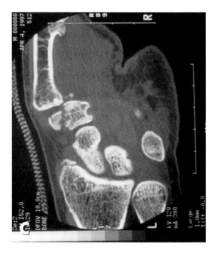

Figure 8

A and **B,** Plain radiographs of a concomitant trapezium fracture, subluxation of the first metacarpal, and radial styloid fracture. **C,** Computed tomography scanning with 3-dimensional reconstruction further defines the fracture, which was fixed with K-wire, AO minicortical screw, and supplemental external fixation.

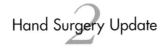
Capitate Fractures

Fractures of the capitate are also rare, comprising approximately 1% of all carpal fractures. Because the blood supply of the capitate is similar to that of the scaphoid (retrograde flow), ON and nonunion of the proximal pole can occur in displaced fractures. Isolated fractures are rare. A capitate fracture can occur with a scaphoid fracture—the naviculocapitate syndrome. The proximal fragment of the capitate may rotate 180°, dictating careful radiographic imaging.

The mechanism of injury is believed to be from direct trauma to the dorsal wrist, hyperextension, or trauma delivered to the heads of the second and third metacarpals with the wrist flexed. A useful imaging technique involves angling the tube 30° off the vertical, toward the fingertips, which elongates the capitate and makes the fracture more identifiable.

Nondisplaced capitate fractures are best treated by cast immobilization for up to 6 weeks. Displaced fractures require open reduction and internal fixation, achieved with K-wires or a headless screw. The tenuous blood supply can result in ON in displaced fractures. One group reported on 5 cases in which curettage and bone grafting was successful in patients without degenerative changes, while midcarpal fusion succeeded in patients with pericapitate arthritis.

Hamate Fractures

Hamate fractures are another rare type, comprising 1.5% of carpal fractures. These fractures can involve either the uncinate process (hook) or the body. Fractures of the hook usually result from direct palmar trauma. Conventional radiographs do not always demonstrate the fracture; suspicion should lead to either a 20° supinate oblique or carpal tunnel view, or a CT scan in the prayer position. Pain in the area of the proximal ulnar palm is usually present, with tenderness over the hook of the hamate. Sometimes the patient may be more tender over the dorsoulnar aspect of the proximal hand. Manipulative maneuvers such as resisted distal interphalangeal flexion of the ring and small fingers with a flexed and ulnar-deviated wrist may be helpful in eliciting hamate pain. Treatment for the acute nondisplaced hamate hook fracture has historically been excision; however, one group recommends a trial of short-arm cast immobilization for 6 to 8 weeks to determine if healing will take place. Open reduction and internal fixation has also been recommended; this is actually unnecessary, because nonunion of the hamate hook responds so well to simple excision. An established nonunion should be excised; complications such as flexor tendon rupture, ulnar nerve compression, and chronic pain have been reported. In a recent study of the pattern and size of the hamate hook vascular foramina, the author found 2 entry sites—one at the radial base (always present) and one at the ulnar tip (absent in 30% of specimens). In these at-risk hamate hooks, fracture at the base could impair vascular supply and result in nonunion.

Body fractures of the hamate are usually in the coronal plane, and associated with fourth or fifth carpometacarpal fracture–dislocation. Conventional radiography must often be supplemented with CT scan to clearly define fracture anatomy. Nondisplaced, stable fractures of the hamate body may heal with simple cast immobilization. Unstable body fractures, particularly those accompanied by carpometacarpal dislocation, require open reduction and internal fixation. Chronic, overlooked fracture–dislocations of the fourth and fifth carpometacarpal joints associated with hamate body fracture may require open reduction and fusion (Fig. 9).

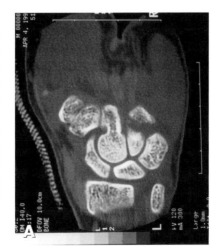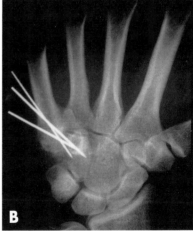

Figure 9

A, Computed tomography scan of a hamate body fracture. Three-dimensional reconstruction further defined a base of the hook fracture, which was associated with concomitant fourth and fifth carpometacarpal joint dislocation. **B,** Fracture healed with subluxation and degenerative arthritis requiring reduction and fusion.

Annotated Bibliography

Scaphoid Fractures

Adams BD, Frykman GK, Taleisnik J: Treatment of scaphoid nonunion with casting and pulsed electromagnetic fields: A study continuation. *J Hand Surg* 1992;17A:910–914.

In a follow-up to their earlier study on electrical stimulation for scaphoid nonunion, the authors found that the initial success rate of 80% had decreased to 69%. They recommend the treatment only as an alternative to bone grafting.

Amadio PC, Berquist TH, Smith DK, Ilstrup DM, Cooney WP III, Linscheid RL: Scaphoid malunion. *J Hand Surg* 1989; 14A:679–687.

This classic article is one of the first to discuss scaphoid malunion and its deleterious effects, showing that malunion can result in an unsatisfactory clinical outcome. The authors concluded that healing alone was not sufficient for a successful outcome.

Braithwaite IJ, Jones WA: Scapho-lunate dissociation occurring with scaphoid fracture. *J Hand Surg* 1992;17B:286–288.

The incidence of concomitant scapholunate injury with scaphoid fracture is rare. The authors document the etiology and treatment of 4 cases. The concomitant occurrence must be identified so that proper treatment can be directed toward both injuries.

Bynum EB, Culp RW, Bonatus TJ, Alexander CE, McCarroll HR: Repeat Russe bone grafting after failed bone graft surgery for scaphoid non-union. *J Hand Surg* 1995;20B:373–378.

A long-term outcome of repeat Russe bone grafting after unsuccessful previous Russe grafting is presented. The authors recommend supplementary internal fixation when repeat bone grafting is performed.

Compson JP, Waterman JK, Spencer JD: Dorsal avulsion fractures of the scaphoid: Diagnostic implications and applied anatomy. *J Hand Surg* 1993;18B:58–61.

The authors present a new fracture pattern of the scaphoid involving a dorsal avulsion. A 45° supinated oblique is required to reveal this fracture. The injury should not be confused with a complete fracture through the waist. Treatment requires only short-term immobilization.

Eddeland A, Eiken O, Hellgren E, Ohlsson NM: Fractures of the scaphoid. *Scand J Plast Reconstr Surg Hand Surg* 1975; 9:234–239.

Despite its age, this study remains a landmark. The authors report a nonunion rate of almost 92% in scaphoids which were displaced more than 1 mm, when treated conservatively, highlighting the need for surgical stabilization in displaced scaphoid fractures.

Fernandez DL, Eggli S: Non-union of the scaphoid: Revascularization of the proximal pole with implantation of a vascular bundle and bone-grafting. *J Bone Joint Surg* 1995;77A:883–893.

Revascularization of the scaphoid proximal pole, with implantation of a vascular bundle and bone grafting using the second dorsal intermetacarpal artery, is discussed. The union rate was over 90%. Patients presenting with scaphoid nonunions and avascular proximal poles remain a challenge; a surgical alternative is provided.

Finkenberg JG, Hoffer E, Kelly C, Zinar DM: Diagnosis of occult scaphoid fractures by intrasound vibration. *J Hand Surg* 1993; 18A:4–7.

Vibratory testing is inexpensive, noninvasive, and easy to perform. It involves no ionizing radiation and may prove useful as an adjunct to diagnosis. With a sensitivity approaching 100%, the specificity still is lower. The technique does depend on the patient's subjective response to the stimulus, which can be variable, and will certainly affect the interpretation.

Ganel A, Engel J, Oster Z, Farine I: Bone scanning in the assessment of fractures of the scaphoid. *J Hand Surg* 1979; 4A:540–543.

The authors describe the use of the bone scan in detecting acute scaphoid fractures, discussing its high sensitivity and low specificity. A negative bone scan at 72 hours is useful in determining a high performance athlete's return to sport.

Horii E, Nakamura R, Watanabe K, Tsunoda K: Scaphoid fracture as a "puncher's fracture." *J Orthop Trauma* 1994;8:107–110.

The authors review 18 cases of scaphoid fracture due to a mechanism of injury not discussed previously. Each scaphoid fracture occurred when the clenched fist punched an object. This was felt to direct the longitudinal force through the second metacarpal into the trapezium and trapezoid, finally resulting in injury to the scaphoid. Most clenched fist injuries result in open metacarpal head fractures. This study should alert the clinician to the possibility of a scaphoid injury.

Hove LM: Simultaneous scaphoid and distal radial fractures. *J Hand Surg* 1994;19B:384–388.

The rare simultaneous occurrence of distal radius and scaphoid fracture, along with its proposed etiology and treatment, is discussed. This high-energy injury may become more common.

Inoue G, Kuwahata Y: Repeat screw stabilization with bone grafting after a failed Herbert screw fixation for acute scaphoid fractures and nonunions. *J Hand Surg* 1997;22A:413–418.

Reviewing a series of failed Herbert screw fixation, the authors found that failure was caused by inadequate screw placement in the majority of cases. Repeat stabilization with bone grafting and a second Herbert screw can be successful.

Jiranek WA, Ruby LK, Millender LB, Bankoff MS, Newberg AH: Long-term results after Russe bone-grafting: The effect of malunion of the scaphoid. *J Bone Joint Surg* 1992;74A:1217–1228.

The simple presence of malunion of the scaphoid after bone grafting for nonunion was not predictive of a poor long-term subjective outcome in this series of patients. This report clearly shows objective evidence that a malunion can result in decreased range of motion and strength even though healing of the nonunion is satisfactory.

Kerluke L, McCabe SJ: Nonunion of the scaphoid: A critical analysis of recent natural history studies. *J Hand Surg* 1993;18A:1–3.

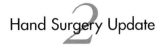

In a critical analysis of recent natural history studies, the authors assert that the initial studies were flawed, in that they did not involve an inception cohort. They conclude that the natural history of this presentation is not as severe. Nearly 100% of patients with scaphoid nonunions will go on to develop degenerative arthritis, however; the hand surgeon must clearly recognize the pathophysiology in our intense medicolegal climate.

Lynch NM, Linscheid RL: Corrective osteotomy for scaphoid malunion: Technique and long-term follow-up evaluation. *J Hand Surg* 1997;22A:35–43.

This is the first published series of patients undergoing corrective osteotomy for symptomatic scaphoid malunion. The authors feel that reconstructive osteotomy may be indicated in diminishing degenerative arthritis in young patients with high-demand wrists.

Malerich M, Clifford J, Eaton R, Littler JW: Distal scaphoid resection arthroplasty for the treatment of degenerative arthritis secondary to scaphoid nonunion. *Orthop Trans* 1995; 19:833.

Simple excision of the distal scaphoid fragment, retaining the proximal pole, was successful in 12 patients. The authors feel that this procedure offers an excellent alternative to partial wrist fusion and does not preclude further surgical reconstruction.

Mody BS, Belliappa PP, Dias JJ, Barton NJ: Nonunion of fractures of the scaphoid tuberosity. *J Bone Joint Surg* 1993; 75B:423–425.

Fracture of the scaphoid tuberosity, because of its rich vascularity, usually does not go on to nonunion. The authors report a small series, alerting the clinician to the unusual possibility of nonunion so that it can be recognized and treated effectively.

Newport ML, Williams CD, Bradley WD: Mechanical strength of scaphoid fixation. *J Hand Surg* 1996;21B:99–102.

Five commercially available screws for scaphoid fixation were tested and found to have no statistically significant difference in compression. Resistance to cantilever bending, however, did show differences that could have clinical implications.

Perlik PC, Guilford WB: Magnetic resonance imaging to assess vascularity of scaphoid nonunions. *J Hand Surg* 1991; 16A:479–484.

Magnetic resonance imaging was found to be 100% accurate in both sensitivity and specificity, compared to visualization, tomography, and plain radiography. This modality has been proven useful in assessing vascularity of the proximal pole.

Rettig AC, Kollias SC: Internal fixation of acute stable scaphoid fractures in the athlete. *Am J Sports Med* 1996; 24:182–186.

The authors report that internal fixation for acute stable scaphoid fractures in the athlete has a union rate greater than 90% at an average duration of 9.8 weeks, with a return to sports in less than 6 weeks. They do, however, recommend longer-term follow-up. Although applicable to professional athletes, the technique remains questionable for recreational athletes.

Robbins RR, Ridge O, Carter PR: Iliac crest bone grafting and Herbert screw fixation of nonunions of the scaphoid with avascular proximal poles. *J Hand Surg* 1995;20A:818–831.

Conventional bone grafting and rigid fixation with a Herbert screw remains useful in treating patients with nonunions and avascular proximal poles. This is an excellent report on the attributes of conventional bone grafting. The authors introduce the concept that a persistent fibrous union can be successful in providing pain relief, range of motion, and strength.

Sanders WE: Evaluation of the humpback scaphoid by computed tomography in the longitudinal axial plane of the scaphoid. *J Hand Surg* 1988;13A:182–187.

This article remains highly useful for its description of an accurate method for viewing the anatomic axis of the scaphoid, so difficult to evaluate with conventional radiographs. The method is helpful not only in acute fracture detection, but also in monitoring healing of delayed unions. The author also describes an excellent method for assessing the degree of humpback deformity.

Sheetz KK, Bishop AT, Berger RA: The arterial blood supply of the distal radius and ulna and its potential use in vascularized pedicled bone grafts. *J Hand Surg* 1995;20A:902–914.

This article presents an elegant description of the extra- and intraosseous blood supply of the distal radius and ulna, and defines potential vascularized pedicle bone grafts that can be used in surgical reconstruction. A clear description of Zaidemberg's pedicle vascularized graft is also provided.

Smith BS, Cooney WP: Revision of failed bone grafting for nonunion of the scaphoid: Treatment options and results. *Clin Orthop* 1996;327:98–109.

A useful algorithm is provided for patients who have had a failed bone graft for nonunion of the scaphoid, providing the hand surgeon a useful outline for addressing this difficult problem.

Toby EB, Butler TE, McCormack TJ, Jayaraman G: A comparison of fixation screws for the scaphoid during application of cyclical bending loads. *J Bone Joint Surg* 1997;79A:1190–1197.

In an investigation of different screws used for fixation, the authors found the AO screw, the Acutrak screw, and the Herbert-Whipple screw superior under cyclical bending load to the Herbert screw. Proponents of the Herbert screw feel that with the use of the jig, significant compression can be exerted to the fracture. Because of its headless design and universal appeal, the Herbert screw remains a popular physiologic screw.

Trumble TE, Clarke T, Kreder HJ: Non-union of the scaphoid: Treatment with cannulated screws compared with treatment with Herbert screws. *J Bone Joint Surg* 1996;78A: 1829–1837.

In this retrospective review comparing Herbert screws with AO-cannulated screws, the authors found no clinical or radiographic difference. Regardless of the screw type, the time to union was significantly shorter when the screw was placed in the central third of the proximal scaphoid. The technical aspects of screw placement are emphasized.

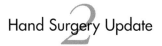

118   Carpal Fractures

Urban MA, Green DP, Aufdemorte TB: The patchy configuration of scaphoid avascular necrosis. *J Hand Surg* 1993;18A: 669–674.

In a follow-up report to an earlier study, these authors conclude that random biopsy alone cannot accurately predict the histologic status of the proximal scaphoid pole. Visualization for punctate bleeding at time of surgery or preoperative use of magnetic resonance imaging may be helpful.

Viegas SF: Limited arthrodesis for scaphoid nonunion. *J Hand Surg* 1994;19A:127–133.

Limited fusion for the scaphoid nonunion, in which the distal pole is excised and the proximal pole is fused to the lunate and capitate, is described in this article; biomechanical usefulness is also presented. Pain relief and preservation of range of motion marked this series.

Watson HK, Pitts EC, Ashmead D IV, Makhlouf MV, Kauer J: Dorsal approach to scaphoid nonunion. *J Hand Surg* 1993; 18A:359–365.

The dorsal approach to the scaphoid eliminates surgical trauma to the palmar radiocarpal ligaments, theoretically avoiding iatrogenic carpal instability. The dorsal approach remains useful for nondisplaced waist scaphoid fractures and proximal pole fractures, but the palmar approach is still superior for distal pole fractures and long-standing nonunion of the waist, when humpback deformity is present. Iatrogenic carpal instability was not borne out if meticulous repair of the radiocarpal ligaments is performed.

Yuceturk A, Isiklar ZU, Tuncay C, Tandogan R: Treatment of scaphoid nonunions with a vascularized bone graft based on the first dorsal metacarpal artery. *J Hand Surg* 1997; 2B:425–427.

Four patients with chronic nonunion of the scaphoid were treated with a vascularized bone graft based on the first dorsal metacarpal artery, with a 100% union rate. The technique provides an alternative vascularized pedicle bone graft for the hand surgeon in treating scaphoid nonunion.

Lunate Fractures

Teisen H, Hjarbaek J: Classification of fresh fractures of the lunate. *J Hand Surg* 1988;13B:458–462.

These authors provide a useful classification of lunate fractures, along with a discussion on mechanism of injury and treatment.

Triquetral Fractures

Hocker K, Menschik A: Chip fractures of the triquetrum: Mechanism, classification and results. *J Hand Surg* 1994;19B: 584–588.

This article is a review of chip fractures of the triquetrum, along with mechanism, classification, and treatment. The hand surgeon is alerted to the different types that can directly affect treatment.

Smith DK, Murray PM: Avulsion fractures of the volar aspect of triquetral bone of the wrist: A subtle sign of carpal ligament injury. *Am J Roentgenol* 1996;166:609–614.

This article presents a new injury type and its clinical implications. Recommendations for radiographic visualization needed to detect this previously unreported type fracture are provided.

Pisiform Fractures

Steinmann SP, Linscheid RL: Pisotriquetral loose bodies. *J Hand Surg* 1997;22A:918–921.

Fractures of the pisiform may result in the development of loose bodies in the pisotriquetral joint. The authors provide a way to detect and treat the lesion.

Trapezial Fractures

Palmer AK: Trapezial ridge fractures. *J Hand Surg* 1981;6A: 561–564.

In this discussion of trapezial ridge fractures, the author provides recommendations for treatment and radiographic assessments for detection.

Trapezoid Fractures

Yasuwaki Y, Nagata Y, Yamamoto T, Nakano A, Kikuchi H, Tanaka S: Fracture of the trapezoid bone: A case report. *J Hand Surg* 1994;19A:457–459.

Although a case report, this article is useful in its description of the mechanism of injury and the treatment of this rare fracture.

Capitate Fractures

Vander Grend R, Dell PC, Glowczewskie F, Leslie B, Ruby LK: Intraosseous blood supply of the capitate and its correlation with aseptic necrosis. *J Hand Surg* 1984;9A:677–683.

This classic article clearly emphasizes the susceptibility of the capitate to avascular necrosis, and provides a useful discussion of its presentation and treatment.

Hamate Fractures

Bishop AT, Beckenbaugh RD: Fracture of the hamate hook. *J Hand Surg* 1988;13A:135–139.

This is a thorough discussion of fractures involving the hamate hook. Treatment for the acute nondisplaced fracture by immobilization is supported. Although open reduction and internal fixation of an acute nondisplaced fracture is discussed, simple excision is advanced as the treatment choice.

Failla JM: Hook of hamate vascularity: vulnerability to osteonecrosis and nonunion. *J Hand Surg* 1993;18A:1075–1079.

The blood supply to the hook of the hamate is described, noting its vulnerability to avascular necrosis and nonunion.

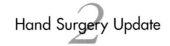
Chapter 12
Osteonecrosis of the Carpus

Arnold-Peter C. Weiss, MD

Introduction

Osteonecrosis (ON) of the carpal bones is an uncommon event with several possible etiologic mechanisms, none of which has been definitively demonstrated. Different theories have attributed avascularity to a primary ischemic event, possibly involving increased intraosseous pressure and subsequent vascular stasis, or to pericarpal or intercarpal trauma involving vascular disruption and resultant necrosis. Fracture of the subchondral structure of the carpal bones has also been implicated in patients with ON; however, there is uncertainty as to whether this is a secondary phenomenon resulting from the ON itself (with subsequent revascularization), or the primary phenomenon responsible for disruption of the vascular supply and causing fragmentation. Repetitive microtrauma may also produce a higher degree of vascular compromise in specific carpal bones where only 1 or 2 nutrient vessels are present.

Recently, magnetic resonance imaging (MRI) has improved our understanding of ON in the clinical setting, and has facilitated earlier detection. Findings sometimes correlate to the histologic osteoid and granulation zones noted in explanted specimens. Improved ability to make an earlier diagnosis has led to earlier treatment, which has proven more successful in long-term clinical studies.

Osteonecrosis of the Lunate

Etiology

Although Kienböck described ON of the lunate almost 90 years ago, the exact cause of the condition remains elusive. There has been support for both primary ischemic and primary traumatic etiologies of this condition. Fragmentation of the lunate in the later stages of the disease is fairly uniform; however, recent reports have noted a higher incidence of lunate fractures with tomograms, even in earlier stages. Osteonecrosis of the lunate has also been reported in diseases characterized by periods of ischemia, such as sickle cell anemia, and with the use of large-dose steroids. Dislocation of the lunate, with its concomitant disruption of all

major vascular supply, leads to an increased radiodensity of bone similar to stage 2 of Kienböck's disease; however, this increased radiodensity is usually transient and resolves, unlike that seen in Kienböck's.

A generalized decrease in mineralization in the lunates of patients with Kienböck's disease has been reported in recent literature. One clinical study measuring intraosseous pressure in 12 normal and 12 necrotic lunates found increased intraosseous pressure in the necrotic lunates, especially in wrist extension. Increased intraosseous pressure was also demonstrated in the normal lunates, when compared to normal capitates. Impairment of venous drainage and potential arterial disruption may also be factors in the development of this disorder.

The role of ulnar length in the etiology of Kienböck's disease has been debated for decades. Hulten demonstrated the association between ulna-negative variance and Kienböck's disease, and theorized that increased load transfer to the lunate via the lunate fossa of the distal radius resulted in the development of ON. Nevertheless, Kienböck's disease can be seen in patients who are ulna-neutral or even ulna-positive. This observation requires questioning whether ulnar length itself is an etiologic agent, rather than merely an advancing component to the disease process already started. No statistically significant association of negative ulnar variance with Kienböck's disease has been demonstrated.

Subchondral bone formation in the lunate fossa of the radius has been demonstrated in long-term studies of patients treated conservatively for Kienböck's disease. This accumulation of subchondral bone leads to the development of a "pseudo" ulna-negative wrist in patients who may have originally had an ulna-neutral variance. However, most patients are seen relatively soon after onset of their condition; there would be insufficient time to develop subchondral bone formation affecting ulnar variance.

The type of vascular supply to the lunate influences its propensity to develop ON. Experimental studies have demonstrated that 20% of lunates are supplied by only one nutrient vessel, and are thus at high risk for ON via any mechanism that disrupts this tenuous vascular supply. Both bony microfractures and soft-tissue pericapsular and ligamentous disruption could result in a cutoff of the blood supply to this subgroup of lunates. The remaining 80% of lunates receive

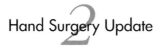

blood from 2 or more nutrient arteries at nonadjacent, nonarticular surfaces. They also have intraosseous anastomoses, decreasing the overall risk of ON.

Development of Kienböck's disease likely requires interaction of a number of variables. The varied factors known to be associated with Kienböck's disease can arise in different scenarios, providing for a multifactorial etiology. In assessing these patients, awareness of each of the variables that might increase suspicion of the disorder is critical in the early stages.

Diagnosis

Kienböck's disease is most commonly seen in young, active adults in their 20s and 30s. The condition is characterized by pain and stiffness at the wrist, frequently without a history of specific trauma. Physical examination demonstrates tenderness over the dorsal aspect of the lunate, a decrease in grip strength, and pain with hyperextension. Standard posteroanterior (PA) and lateral radiographs should be used for the initial evaluation. Because of the change in ulnar variance associated with different techniques, the radiographs should be taken with the shoulder abducted to 90°, the elbow flexed to 90°, the forearm in neutral rotation, and the wrist in neutral extension/flexion. Ulnar variance should be determined from the zero-rotation PA radiograph. On the lateral view, a change in the shape of the lunate, decreasing height with increasing PA width, is a common finding (decreasing Stahl index). Increase in osseous density of the lunate, or obvious fragmentation and carpal collapse, are both associated with the diagnosis of Kienböck's disease. The classification of Kienböck's disease, initially described by Stahl in 1947 and later modified by Lichtman and Weiss (Fig. 1), is a descriptive representation of the lunate on the PA radiograph. In the modified classification, stage 1 has no evidence of radiographic change. Stage 2 demonstrates sclerosis of the lunate without alteration in shape of the lunate itself, or carpal collapse. Stage 3A is characterized by collapse of the lunate with fragmentation, while stage 3B combines stage 3A with associated fixed rotation of the scaphoid (Fig. 2). Stage 4 demonstrates degenerative changes in the perilunate region and intercarpal articulations, frequently accompanied by subchondral cyst formation in advanced cases.

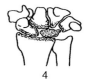
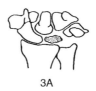

Figure 1

Radiographic classification of Kienböck's disease according to the methods of Lichtman and associates, and Weiss and associates. Stage 1, No visible change in the lunate. Stage 2, Sclerosis of the lunate. Stage 3A, Sclerosis with fragmentation or collapse of the lunate, or both. Stage 3B, stage 3A changes combined with fixed rotation of the scaphoid. Stage 4, stage 3A or 3B changes combined with degenerative changes in adjacent intercarpal joints. (Reproduced with permission from Weiss APC, Weiland AJ, Moore JR, Wilgis EF: Radial shortening for Kienböck's disease. *J Bone Joint Surg* 1991;73A:384–391.)

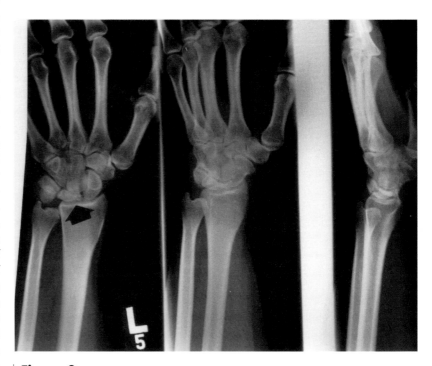

Figure 2

Posteroanterior, oblique, and lateral radiographs of a patient with stage 3B Kienböck's disease. Note flattening and fragmentation of the lunate (arrow), negative ulnar variance, and loss of carpal height.

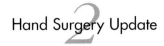
Bone scans have been helpful in the establishment of the diagnosis in both stage 1 and stage 2 disease. Focal-increased uptake of tracer in the location of the lunate is diagnostic. Although the sophistication and accuracy of MRI has essentially replaced bone scans for the early diagnosis of all stages, its primary role is establishment of the stage 1 and 2 diagnoses. Regardless of whether or not standard radiographs are normal, ON is noted by a decrease in signal intensity on both T1- and T2-weighted images. Recent studies have demonstrated that MRI has greater accuracy than both plain radiographs and bone scans in establishing a diagnosis. The addition of contrast enhancement in MRI has provided even greater sensitivity and specificity in the very early stages of the disease. Loss of signal on T1-weighted images is diagnostic for ON. A normal or increased signal intensity on T2-weighted images indicates less damage and improved prognosis. Computed tomography and trispiral tomograms have been proven effective in assessing the overall skeletal morphology of the lunate, both in the early and late stages of the disease. A recent histopathologic study of extracted lunate bones correlated with MRI, computed tomography, and tomography demonstrated that fractures of the articular cartilage and subchondral bone occurred secondary to overloading; however, the findings of the 3 techniques were not definitively predictive of the degree of bone necrosis and the revascularization zone.

Treatment

Treatment of Kienböck's disease varies widely, but is generally correlated to the stage of disease. Authors have advocated immobilization, ulnar lengthening, radial shortening, limited intercarpal fusion, lunate resection with or without soft-tissue interposition, revascularization with or without external fixation, radiocarpal fusion, and total wrist arthrodesis. Recently, vascularized bone grafting, capitate shortening, radial wedge osteotomy, and proximal row carpectomy have also been supported.

Patients with stage 1 disease are almost always treated by cast immobilization, occasionally combined with nonsteroidal anti-inflammatory medication. Immobilization is generally maintained for 1 to 3 months, producing a relative osteopenia of the carpus and making lunate sclerosis more prominent on subsequent radiographs. If any evidence of a fracture is present, immobilization may facilitate healing during the initial stages. Although long-term results of nonsurgical treatment for Kienböck's disease have been poor, with symptom progression as well as radiographic deterioration, surgical treatment should be considered only if immobilization does not alleviate symptoms early and completely. Unfortunately, patients with stage 1 Kienböck's disease rarely present to physicians.

In patients with stage 2 disease, immobilization can be attempted for a trial period; however, surgical intervention is more frequent due to the visible changes already present in the lunate. Patients most often present stage 3A or 3B disease to physicians; for these cases, surgery is invariably the primary treatment option. Immobilization alone has been uniformly unsuccessful. Theoretically, revascularization of the necrotic lunate would be an attractive option; it directly reconstitutes intraosseous blood flow, and does not preclude other treatment options. Procedures involving the use of vascularized distal radius bone attached to the pronator quadratus, second dorsal metacarpal artery and venae comitantes, and vascularized pisiform; and, more recently, vascularized distal radius bone grafts on branches of the posterior division of the anterior interosseous artery system have been described by advocates. Revascularization in stages 3A and 3B has also been accompanied by hand-forearm external fixation across the lunate, to decrease compressive forces present during healing. Long-term follow-up studies on these techniques are not available; however, some preliminary evidence suggests good to excellent results in the majority of patients. Because experimental studies have indicated an association of lunate collapse with revascularization, some form of external support for carpal height appears prudent, regardless of the technique performed.

The mainstays of surgical treatment for Kienböck's disease are those procedures directed towards either joint leveling, or unloading compressive forces via limited intercarpal arthrodesis. Radial shortening or ulnar lengthening of approximately 2 mm and scapho-trapezio-trapezoid (STT) fusions have been shown to reduce lunate load via experimental strain gauge measurement; other intercarpal arthrodeses, such as capitohamate fusion, are less effective in this regard. A mathematical model of the wrist demonstrated a 30% contribution of the radiolunate articulation to the total radioulnar-carpal load. Joint leveling procedures reduce the contribution of the radiolunate articulation by 45%; limited intercarpal fusions decrease this force only 15%. Capitate shortening demonstrates similar radiolunate joint unloading; however, the procedure transfers load with increased force at the scaphotrapezial and triquetrohamate joints.

Joint leveling procedures attempt to decrease compressive forces at the radiolunate joint by load-sharing from the distal ulna-triangular fibrocartilage complex. Joint leveling has been very popular for patients with negative ulnar variance and an absence of degenerative changes at the radiolunate articulation. Although ulnar-lengthening procedures were used to accomplish joint leveling in the past, radial-shortening osteotomy is now a more popular alternative because there is no need for bone grafting. Significant improvement in patient symptoms following joint leveling procedures has been demonstrated in several published studies. Radiographic appearance of the lunate does not change in the majority of patients, but the progression of fragmentation appears to stabilize. Joint leveling procedures have been advocated for stages 1 to 3A and possibly stage 3B of Kienböck's disease. These procedures have provided pain relief in 70% to 80% of patients, improved grip strength 30% to 50%, and increased postoperative range of motion. Carpal collapse and disease progression appear to stabilize in the majority of patients. Younger patients treated by radial shortening have also exhibited significantly improved results (Fig. 3). Joint leveling procedures are undertaken to effect a 2- to 3-mm change in the preoperative ulnar variance; they are not usually performed to obtain an ulna-neutral wrist. The danger of excessive

radial shortening must be recognized, as ulnar-sided wrist pain due to secondary ulnar impaction is a known complication of overshortening the radius. Radial wedge osteotomy, reducing wrist radial inclination to unload joint forces around the lunate, has been advocated recently as an alternative to formal radial shortening osteotomy. Curiously, other authors have advocated increasing the radial inclination as a treatment option. The initial clinical results of these procedures are encouraging, although short term, and are similar to large series of radial shortening osteotomies.

Decreasing load across the lunate by intercarpal fusion is also popular. Reports of STT, scaphocapitate, capitohamate, and other intercarpal fusions have indicated improvement of symptoms comparable to joint leveling. There is generally no significant improvement in range of motion, however. The long-term success of intercarpal fusion is still unknown, both from the perspective of the lunate itself, and whether the alteration of joint forces will prevent eventual secondary degenerative arthrosis. Joint leveling procedures have the advantage of being an extra-articular treatment option, leaving intra-articular procedures for possible later salvage. Lunate excision, with or without soft-tissue interposition using the palmaris longus, has had isolated reports of success; however, a significant incidence of overall carpal collapse has been reported recently. Replacement of the lunate by silicone arthroplasty is currently contraindicated, due to the incidence of silicone synovitis, microfragmentation, and prosthesis failure. The use of other types of materials to replace the carpus should be considered with caution; no long-term results are available. Proximal row carpectomy has also been advocated, most commonly for the older patient who has some early evidence of adjacent joint arthrosis. Any evidence of capitate head or radiolunate degenerative changes should be considered a contraindication for this procedure.

Patients with stage 4 disease who have substantial evidence of pancarpal arthritis are best treated by either radiocarpal or total wrist arthrodesis. With radiocarpal arthrodesis, arthroscopic evaluation of the distal lunate articular surface should be

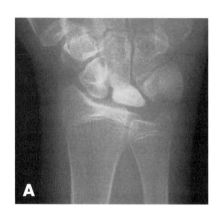
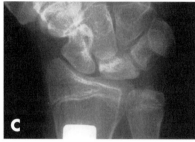
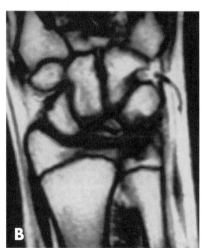
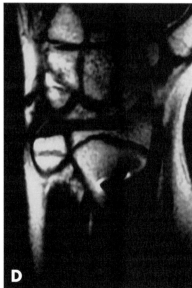

Figure 3

A, A 14-year-old female presented with stage 3A Kienböck's disease and a 2-mm negative ulnar variance. B, MRI demonstrated fragmentation and loss of signal at the lunate. C, Radiographs revealed improvement in lunate density and contour 1 year after radial shortening osteotomy (neutralizing the ulnar variance). D, Follow-up MRI demonstrated normal signal intensity of the lunate, indicating revascularization.

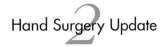
considered to ensure that no substantial fragmentation has occurred. If evidence of midcarpal and radiocarpal disease is present, total wrist arthrodesis should be performed.

Osteonecrosis of the Scaphoid and Capitate

In 1910, Preiser described 5 cases of ON of the scaphoid that had no radiographic evidence of fracture. The incidence is low, documented primarily by scattered case reports. Isolated cases associated with oral steroid use have been described in the literature. The risk of ON is enhanced by the fact that the large proximal portion of the scaphoid is frequently supplied by a single dorsal blood vessel with a limited intraosseous anastomotic supply. The diagnosis is made from evidence of increased radiographic density of the scaphoid, or obvious sclerosis. On occasion, fragmentation of the proximal pole of the scaphoid can be identified without evidence of distal fracture. A large number of authors discuss ON in light of nonunion or scaphoid fracture, but limited data is available on patients who develop ON with no evidence of previous trauma. Patients frequently present with dorsal wrist pain over the scaphoid area that is worsened by activity. Tenderness is noted on palpation of the scaphoid and range of motion is decreased, especially in extension. Soft-tissue swelling can also be seen, although this symptom is frequently absent. PA and lateral radiographs demonstrate sclerosis of the scaphoid, most frequently involving the proximal pole. In advanced cases, subchondral cyst formation and radioscaphoid arthritis may be found.

Initial treatment consists of cast immobilization, which is generally unsuccessful. The majority of patients eventually require some form of surgical intervention. Procedures advocated for this condition include arthroscopic subchondral drilling of the scaphoid, revascularization procedures, scaphoid excision and four-corner fusion, proximal row carpectomy, and total wrist arthrodesis. Data on any of these techniques is scant; evidence of success is anecdotal.

Osteonecrosis of the capitate is extremely rare, documented only in case reports. Patients complain of pain and stiffness of the wrist; radiographs demonstrate sclerosis of the head of the capitate. Initial treatment by prolonged cast immobilization yields some success; surgical intervention is required only in patients with persistent symptoms. Partial capitate excision with tendon interposition arthroplasty, and scapholunate-capitate fusion have both been described with good early results.

Annotated Bibliography

Etiology and Diagnosis

Aspenberg P, Wang JS, Jonsson K, Hagert CG: Experimental osteonecrosis of the lunate: Revascularization may cause collapse. *J Hand Surg* 1994;19B:565–569.

A literature review was conducted to determine if lunates were avascular at the time of collapse; no evidence was found. One small experimental study using excised lunates that were replanted in 2 monkeys demonstrated spontaneous revascularization leading to increased osteoblastic activity. The authors argue that revascularization may be a cause of lunate collapse.

Chen WS, Shih CH: Ulnar variance and Kienböck's disease: An investigation in Taiwan. *Clin Orthop* 1990;255:124–127.

In this study of 1,000 normal subjects in Taiwan, a significant association between negative ulnar variance and Kienböck's disease was demonstrated, in a population with a relatively high incidence of the disease.

D'Hoore K, De Smet L, Verellen K, Vral J, Fabry G: Negative ulnar variance is not a risk factor for Kienböck's disease. *J Hand Surg* 1994;19A:229–231.

No statistical difference between patients with Kienböck's disease and normal wrists was demonstrated with respect to overall ulnar variance, although an association between these 2 factors was present in the data.

Gelberman RH, Gross MS: The vascularity of the wrist: Identification of arterial patterns at risk. *Clin Orthop* 1986;202:40–49.

In this experimental study, injection techniques were used to examine 75 cadaver limbs. Ninety-two percent of lunates had excellent intraosseous anastomotic vascularity, while 8% had only one surface-supplying vessel or large at-risk areas of bone in the lunate due to single-vessel supply.

Giunta R, Lower N, Wilhelm K, Keirse R, Rock C, Muller-Gerbl M: Altered patterns of subchondral bone mineralization in Kienböck's disease. *J Hand Surg* 1997;22B:16–20.

Computed tomographic osteoabsorptiometry was used to compare normal subjects with Kienböck's patients. Overall mineralization was less in the lunates of the Kienböck's patients.

Hashizume H, Asahara H, Nishida K, Inoue H, Konishiike T: Histopathology of Kienböck's disease: Correlation with magnetic resonance and other imaging techniques. *J Hand Surg* 1996;21B:89–93.

Ten patients with stage 3 Kienböck's disease underwent histopathologic studies of their excised lunates. This study revealed inability of MRI to specifically distinguish bone necrosis, histologic reactive interface between new bone and granulation tissue, and surrounding hyperemia with respect to the histologic localization of each of these findings.

Quenzer DE, Linscheid RL, Vidal MA, Dobyns JH, Beckenbaugh RD, Cooney WP: Trispiral tomographic staging of Kienböck's disease. *J Hand Surg* 1997;22A:396–403.

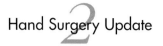

124   Osteonecrosis of the Carpus

One hundred five patients with Kienböck's underwent trispiral tomograms, which caused an upward revision in the stage classification in a majority of patients with stage 1 or 2 disease. Tomograms revealed that 91% of patients with Kienböck's disease had some evidence of lunate fracture, either primary or secondary.

Schiltenwolf M, Martini AK, Mau HC, Eversheim S, Brocai DR, Jensen CH: Further investigations of the intraosseous pressure characteristics in necrotic lunates (Kienböck's disease). *J Hand Surg* 1996;21A:754–758.

Intraosseous pressures were measured in 12 normal and 12 necrotic lunates in various degrees of flexion and extension. Intraosseous pressure was significantly higher in necrotic lunates than normals in wrist extension. Impairment of venous drainage may play a role in lunate necrosis.

Schmitt R, Heinze A, Fellner F, Obletter N, Struhn R, Bautz, W: Imaging and staging of avascular osteonecroses at the wrist and hand. *Eur J Radiol* 1997;25:92–103.

This article describes the changes in ON noted on MRI. The initial stage is bone marrow edema, followed by trabecular sclerosis, cystic formation, and bone fragmentation. The authors advocate contrast-enhanced MRI to evaluate the initial stages of Kienböck's.

Trumble T, Glisson RR, Seaber AV, Urbaniak JR: A biomechanical comparison of the methods for treating Kienböck's disease. *J Hand Surg* 1986;11A:88–93.

This experimental biomechanical evaluation used strain gauges to evaluate joint leveling and intercarpal arthrodesis and their effect on lunate forces. Scapho-trapezio-trapezoid fusions and joint leveling procedures were equally effective in relieving lunate loads, while capitohamate fusions did not significantly alter lunate mechanics. Intercarpal fusions significantly decreased overall wrist range of motion.

Watanabe K, Nakamura R, Horii E, Miura T: Biomechanical analysis of radial wedge osteotomy for the treatment of Kienböck's disease. *J Hand Surg* 1993;18A:686–690.

A 2-dimensional mathematical model was used to simulate force transmission through the lunate after theoretical radial wedge osteotomy. In 29 patients who had radial wedge osteotomy, force transmission through the lunocapitate joint decreased 23%, with similar changes at the radiolunate and ulnolunate joints.

Treatment

Begley BW, Engber WD: Proximal row carpectomy in advanced Kienböck's disease. *J Hand Surg* 1994;19A:1016–1018.

Sixteen patients with stage 3 Kienböck's disease underwent proximal row carpectomy. At average 3-year follow-up, all patients experienced improvement in pain, slight improvement in wrist motion, and grip strength to 72% of the unaffected side. All patients resumed normal activity.

Bochud RC, Buchler U: Kienböck's disease, early stage 3: Height reconstruction and core revascularization of the lunate. *J Hand Surg* 1994;19B:466–478.

In this study, 28 cases of internal debridement of the lunate, recontouring, height reconstruction with bone grafting, and core revascu-

larization in stage 3 Kienböck's were reviewed with average follow-up of 6.5 years. Pain lessened in the vast majority of patients, with slight motion gain and improved grip strength. One third of the patients demonstrated revascularization on radiographs. The results were graded as excellent or good in 86%.

Carroll RE: Long-term review of fascial replacement after excision of the carpal lunate bone. *Clin Orthop* 1997;342:59–63.

Ten patients who had lunate excision and fascial interposition were reviewed at a minimum 10-year follow-up. Most of these patients had pain relief without evidence of carpal collapse; however, only 25% of the entire group of patients receiving the procedure were available for this study.

Condit DP, Idler RS, Fischer TJ, Hastings H II: Preoperative factors and outcome after lunate decompression for Kienböck's disease. *J Hand Surg* 1993;18A:691–696.

Twenty-three patients treated with either radial shortening or STT fusion were evaluated 5 years after surgery. Although outcomes in the radial shortening group were superior to the STT group, lunate collapse was not improved by either method and radiographs remained static in the postoperative follow-up period.

De Smet L, Verellen K, D'Hoore K, Buellens C, Lysens R, Fabry G: Long-term results of radial shortening for Kienböck's disease. *Acta Orthop Belg* 1995;61:212–217.

Seventeen patients who had radial shortening osteotomy were followed an average of 4.5 years. The authors reported that no patients were completely pain-free, and that mobility and strength were approximately 70% of the unaffected side.

Miura H, Sugioka Y: Radial closing wedge osteotomy for Kienböck's disease. *J Hand Surg* 1996;21A:1029–1034.

Twenty-six patients were treated with a radial closing wedge osteotomy, with an average follow-up of 4.5 years. Seventy-three percent of patients had good or excellent results. Poor results were correlated to a poor postoperative lunate height index and abnormal radiolunate angle.

Quenzer DE, Dobyns JH, Linscheid RL, Trail IA, Vidal MA: Radial recession osteotomy for Kienböck's disease. *J Hand Surg* 1997;22A:386–395.

Sixty-eight patients were followed after radial shortening osteotomy, although a large number had additional concurrent procedures. Pain decreased in 93% of patients; grip strength and motion improved. Seventy-five percent of patients resumed normal activity and work. One third of the patients demonstrated some evidence of lunate healing on radiographs.

Sennwald GR, Ufenast H: Scaphocapitate arthrodesis for the treatment of Kienböck's disease. *J Hand Surg* 1995;20A:506–510.

Eleven patients treated with scaphocapitate arthrodesis for Kienböck's stages 2 and 3 were followed for an average of 3 years. All but one patient had excellent pain relief, and no complications were reported.

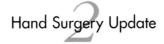
Shin AY, Bishop AT, Berger RA: Vascularized pedicle bone grafts for disorders of the carpus. *Tech Hand and Upper Extremity Surg* 1998;2:94–109.

In this review article, the authors demonstrate the vascular anatomy to the dorsal aspect of the carpus, including the numerous branches that can be taken as vascularized distal radius bone grafts in the treatment of Kienböck's disease.

Watanabe K, Nakamura R, Imaeda T: Arthroscopic assessment of Kienböck's disease. *Arthroscopy* 1995;11:257–262.

Thirty-two patients underwent arthroscopic evaluation of the wrist for Kienböck's disease. Arthroscopy was able to identify osteoarthritic changes in the articular surface that were not present on some preoperative radiographs. Interosseous ligament tears correlated with the radiographically determined stage. The authors feel that arthroscopy is a useful tool in staging the disease and planning further treatment.

Watson HK, Monacelli DM, Milford RS, Ashmead D IV: Treatment of Kienböck's disease with scaphotrapezio-trapezoid arthrodesis. *J Hand Surg* 1996;21A:9–15.

Twenty-eight patients treated with scapho-trapezio-trapezoid arthrodesis were followed for an average of 4.5 years. Excellent or good results were obtained in 77%. Range of motion averaged 48° of extension and 52° of flexion.

Weiss AP, Weiland AJ, Moore JR, Wilgis EF: Radial shortening for Kienböck disease. *J Bone Joint Surg* 1991;73A:384–391.

In this study, 30 consecutive wrists underwent radial shortening osteotomy for stages 1 to 3B of Kienböck's disease. Seventy percent of wrists had no pain at 3.8-year average follow-up; 17% of patients had decreased symptomatology. No significant change in radiographs was noted on final follow-up.

Zelouf DS, Ruby LK: External fixation and cancellous bone grafting for Kienböck's disease: A preliminary report. *J Hand Surg* 1996;21A:746–753.

Seventeen patients with stages 1 to 3 Kienböck's disease underwent external wrist fixation and cancellous bone autografting of the lunate. Good or excellent results were achieved in 71%; approximately one third demonstrated some postoperative improvement in signal intensity of the lunate.

Osteonecrosis of the Scaphoid and Capitate

Arcalis Arce A, Pedemonte Jansana JP, Massons Albareda JM: Idiopathic necrosis of the capitate. *Acta Orthop Belg* 1996; 62:46–48.

In this case report of ON of the capitate, the patient was treated successfully by scapholunate-capitate fusion; excellent pain relief was achieved.

De Smet L, Aerts P, Walraevens M, Fabry G: Avascular necrosis of the carpal scaphoid: Preiser's disease: Report of 6 cases and review of the literature. *Acta Orthop Belg* 1993;59: 139–142.

Six cases of nontraumatic osteonecrosis of the scaphoid were reported; 2 had taken oral steroids. Three were treated successfully with proximal row carpectomy.

Herbert TJ, Lanzetta M: Idiopathic avascular necrosis of the scaphoid. *J Hand Surg* 1994;19B:174–182.

This report of 8 patients with idiopathic osteonecrosis of the scaphoid involving the proximal pole noted a positive ulnar variance in 88%. Treatment was by cast immobilization and partial silastic replacement of the scaphoid.

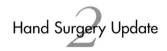

Section III
Tendons

American Society for Surgery of the Hand

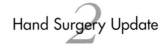
Chapter 13
Experimental Studies of the Structure and Function of Flexor Tendons

Thomas E. Trumble, MD

Introduction

"If flexor tendons are severed in the finger, the usual place opposite the proximal phalanx, one cannot join them together by sutures with success, as the junction will become adherent in the narrow fixed channel and will not slip. It is better to remove the tendons entirely from the finger and graft in new tendons smooth throughout its length."—Sterling Bunnell, MD, 1928

Nearly 4 decades passed before reports of successful repairs in zone 2 were published. In the last 5 years, clinicians and scientists have published well over 1,000 reports regarding tendon injury and repair. Based on epidemiologic data from Norway, it appears that the incidence of flexor tendon injury is approximately 1 in 7,000 in industrialized countries. The injuries occur predominately in males aged 15 to 30 years.

Tendon Injury and Repair

Key Information for Surgeons Performing Tendon Repair

In order to properly perform tendon repairs and prescribe appropriate rehabilitation, the surgeon needs information regarding the loads, friction, and excursion that the flexor tendons experience during digital flexion with active and passive motion. Surgeons must also know the strength of a particular tendon repair, and how the repair strength changes as the flexor tendon heals and remodels.

Few injuries are as critically dependent on postoperative rehabilitation as flexor tendon lacerations. To develop an appropriate rehabilitation program, surgeons and hand therapists must strike a balance. The therapy must be aggressive enough to provide some form of digit motion that produces tendon gliding to minimize tendon adhesions, and safe enough to avoid tendon rupture. Flexor tendon lacerations are infrequent injuries, but they consume a great deal of physician time and institutional resources; consequently, flexor tendon repair and rehabilitation methods should not be developed using clinical studies alone.

Research Models for Studying Flexor Tendon Injuries

Although many animals have digital flexor tendons resembling those of humans, primate, canine, avian, and rabbit models (in that order) most closely approximate the healing of human flexor tendons. Although one of the major problems with animal models of flexor tendon injury has been the difficulty of simulating active range of motion after tendon repair, electrical stimulation of the flexor tendon muscles has been employed with limited success. Theoretically, primates would seem to be the best animal model; however, monkeys are extremely difficult to immobilize in a manner that allows protective motion.

Determination of Tendon Repair Strength

Because tendon gapping is the hallmark of tendon failure, the cyclic load required to produce gapping is the standard by which the strength of flexor tendon repair is measured. The ultimate tensile strength (UTS) is the load that is required for failure of the tendon repair. Failure of the tendon repair can be defined as gapping of 2 mm or more rather than by the UTS. The loads to tendon failure by gapping or disruption are reported in newtons (N) or as kilogram force (kgf). A newton is the force required to move a mass of 1 kg a distance of 1 meter; however, this is not a measurement that most surgeons use in clinical practice. A kgf is the weight of a kilogram assuming the earth's gravity; 1.0 kgf equals 9.8 N. Most grip and pinch meters provide measurements in kgf, and most force measurements in this chapter will be expressed as kgf. As a reference point, most tendon repairs can withstand a single load of 2.0 to 4.0 kgf.

Using a special buckle transducer, one group measured the forces on flexor tendons during active and passive motion as well as during pinch under local anesthetic in patients undergoing open carpal tunnel release (Fig. 1). They noted that up to 3.5 kgf were required for active flexion of the proximal interphalangeal (PIP) joint. Tendon forces up to 12.0 kgf were recorded during pinch, which produced a pinch force of 3.5 kgf. Passive range of motion required only 0.9 kgf for digit motion. Passive mobilization of the wrist produced load in the flexor tendons of up to 0.6 kgf. Using electrical stimulation of canine flexor tendon muscles to stimulate active motion after flexor tendon repair, the force required for digit flexion varied with wrist motion. With full wrist extension, a force of 3.4 kgf was required to produce digital flexion; only 0.5 kgf was required when the wrist was in full flexion.

Tendon Friction During Digital Flexion

Because many tendon repairs increase the size or volume of the tendon, it seems intuitive that the friction during digit flexion is increased after tendon repair. The increased friction of tendon gliding can be measured by subtracting the force required to flex a digit after tendon repair. In cadaver studies, investigators determined that the work of flexion is directly proportional to the amount of suture material at the repair site. (The work of flexion is the measurement of the total amount of energy required to flex the digit; mathematically, the work of flexion is determined by the integral of the force applied and the resulting tendon excursion reported in joules.) In one report, the additional friction produced by the suture material increased the work of flexion by 12.2% for 4-strand repair with a 4-0 core suture placed dorsally, and by 92.7% for a tendon repair with a volar Dacron splint used to reinforce the repair.

Flexor Tendon Repair Strength

Using a special pneumatic loading device to produce 1,000 cycles of flexor tendon loading in a laboratory setting, one group found that the strength of the flexor tendon repair (and the ability of the repair to resist gapping) appear to be directly proportional to the number of sutures crossing in the repair site. Because no published research compared 2-, 4-, and 6-strand repairs in an animal model during the critical phases of tendon healing, the investigators extrapolated data from various reports to provide a graphic representation of the strength of tendon repair over time (Fig. 2). The graph in

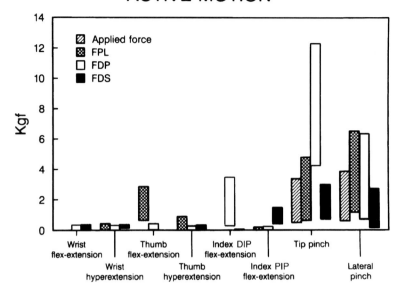

Figure 1

Flexor tendon load was measured during passive and active digit motion and pinch activities with a special buckle strain gauge. (Reproduced with permission from Schuind F, Garcia Elias M, Cooney WPD, et al: Flexor tendon forces: In vivo measurements. *J Hand Surg* 1992;17A:291–298.)

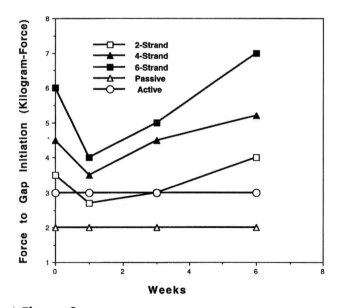

Figure 2

Assuming that active motion requires a tendon repair strength of at least 3.0 kgf, the 2-strand repair in this model has insufficient strength during the first week of healing to prevent tendon rupture.

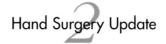
Figure 2 shows that most reports demonstrate a 20% to 40% decrease in tendon strength during the first 3 to 7 days after tendon repair. If the repair strength dips below the threshold of the loads produced by active or passive motion, the tendon will rupture. Nearly all models were based on a passive range of motion program because of the difficulty of producing an active range of motion program in an animal model. In a chicken model, controlled active motion was approximated by splinting the adjacent digits in hyperextension following repair of the profundus tendon. The tendons subjected to early active motion did not experience a drop in repair strength in the early phase of tendon healing (Fig. 3). The concept that early active motion produces stronger tendon repairs without an increased rate of tendon rupture is a very attractive theory; however, there are no other reports of active motion in an animal model to confirm these results.

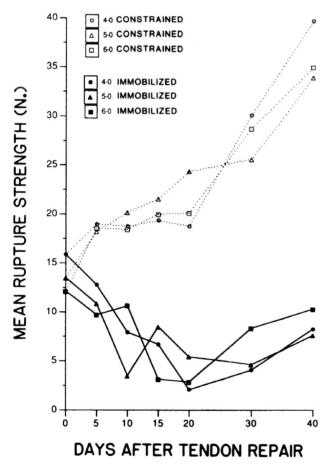

Figure 3

In a chicken model, early active motion caused no decrease in tendon strength after repair. (Reproduced with permission from Hitchcock TF, Light TR, Bunch WH, et al: The effect of immediate constrained digital motion on the strength of flexor tendon repairs in chickens. *J Hand Surg* 1987;12A:590–595.)

Suture Locking and Tendon Repair Strength

Early data with wire sutures suggested that locking loops result in collapse of the loop and failure of the repair as the wires cut through the tendon. More recent evidence indicates that suture locking with nonmetallic sutures increases the strength of the tendon repair, and locking only 1 side of each tendon end produces the optimal effect.

Effect of Knot Location of Core Sutures on Tendon Strength and Healing

In one report, the knots-outside technique was initially 1.14 kgf stronger than the knots-inside technique; however, at 6 weeks there was no significant difference between the 2 techniques. The knots-inside technique may not be strong enough for the initial phases of an active range of motion program. When the knots-outside technique was employed after a running epitenon repair, the amount of suture material at the repair site was significantly less than the modified Kessler technique. Suture material occupied only 2.6% of the surface area of the tendon coaptation site with the epitenon first technique, compared to 22% for the knots-inside technique after core suture placement.

Placement of Core Sutures

Using conventional logic, sutures should be placed in the palmar aspect of the tendon because the blood supply to part of the tendons is via the vinculae that are attached to the dorsal surface of the tendon. Theoretically, sutures placed in the dorsal aspect of the tendon would obstruct the blood supply and cause tendon ischemia. However, more recent studies indicate that imbibition of synovial fluid may be the key to tendon nutrition following tendon injury. During digit flexion, the dorsal aspect of the tendon is under the greatest tension; accordingly, dorsal placement of core sutures is the best mechanical location for tendon repair. The failure load of a modified Kessler suture placed dorsally was 26.5% greater than that of a palmar-side modified Kessler suture. Even when combined with an epitenon suture, dorsally placed sutures were consistently stronger with a variety of core suture types, and dorsal core sutures resulted in less work of flexion.

Effect of Epitenon Suture on Tendon Repair Strength and Quality

Although epitenon repairs were initially recommended to improve the contour of the repair, subsequent research has shown that the epitenon suture significantly increases the resistance of the tendon repair to gap formation and adds to the UTS of the repair. The running Halsted epitenon suture added substantial strength to the repair, especially with a running, locking suture procedure. Because of the growing body of evidence that the epitenon suture substantially increases the mechanical strength of the tendon repair, the option of placing the epitenon sutures deeper into the tendon has also been investigated with positive results on tendon repair strength. By placing the "back wall" or dorsal edge of the epitenon suture after the core sutures were placed (but not yet tied), or by placing the entire epitenon suture before the core suture, bunching and overlapping at the tendon repair site were dramatically reduced. Consequently, it appears that the alignment and strength of the tendon repair will be augmented by placing all or part of the epitenon suture before the core sutures are tied and by using deep epitenon suture as grasping or locking sutures.

Repair of One Versus Two Tendons in Zone 2
Most reports favor repair of both flexor tendons in zone 2. In one retrospective study, 74% of digits with both tendons repaired had good or excellent results, compared to 47% of digits with repair of only the profundus tendon. Dividing zone 2 into 3 separate areas (A = A4 pulley, B = C1 pulley, and C = A2 pulley), a higher rate of reoperation for the tenolysis of adhesions was noted when 2 tendons were repaired in the region under the A2 pulley (zone 2C), compared to the region under the C1 pulley (zone 2B) or under the A4 pulley (zone 2A). Although no other reports confirm this finding, studies investigating tendon excursion in the different segments of the tendon sheath suggest that separate data analysis for the different portions of zone 2 is warranted.

Impact of Surface Area on Repair Strength
Two different methods of increasing surface contact at the tendon repair site have been described—a beveled cut (Becker method), and a step-cut technique. A step-cut repair was 65% stronger in resisting gap formation and yielded 84% more UTS than the Kessler-Tajima repair. The Becker method employs a technique of beveling the tendons to accomplish the same increase in surface area, allowing the epitenon sutures to be placed perpendicular to the long axis of the tendon. Both these techniques carry the risk of tendon shortening and producing an extension deficit.

Influence of Tendon Repair Timing on Functional Results
Several reports suggest that results following tendon repair that is delayed 3 to 4 weeks will still be equivalent to results of immediate repair. In one model using animals that were not allowed to have controlled mobilization after surgery, the best results were achieved when repairs were performed within hours of the injury. The next best result was with repair any time after the tenth day; the worst results

occurred when repairs were performed between the fourth and seventh days. Histologic evidence indicates that tendons lose 40% of their dry weight, as well as substantial portions of the proteoglycans and collagen, within 12 weeks of tendon division. Changes occur in flexor tendons after laceration, but the ideal time for tendon repair with a passive or active rehabilitation program is not defined.

Other New Developments in Tendon Repair
In one study, addition of a separate tendon suture looping around both transverse components of the core suture increased the load to cause gap initiation 100% greater than that in tendons repaired with the modified Kessler epitenon suture. Tendon splints made out of a Dacron mesh yielded a dramatic increase in tendon repair strength in animal models. These splints were stronger when used on the dorsal surface of the tendon (4.89 kgf), but work of flexion increased 25.1% when the splint was placed dorsally and 92.7% with the splint placed on the palmar surface of the tendon.

Repair of Partial Tendon Lacerations
Using a canine model of partial tendon lacerations, unrepaired tendons treated with early mobilization resulted in better tendon excursion as well as increased tendon strength compared to tendons that were repaired or immobilized. Lacerations of less than 60% of the cross-sectional area of the tendon should be treated with early mobilization but without repair. Partial lacerations on both the dorsal and volar surface produced increased vascular ingrowth. Both dorsal and palmar lacerations healed promptly without need of repair.

Tendon Sheath Repair
The ideal research model for tendon sheath repair would include complete laceration of the tendon and repair, because partial tendon lacerations perform differently than complete tendon lacerations. The model would also employ a rehabilitation program encompassing either passive or active motion, but not immobilization. Although some studies support the use of patch grafts or primary sheath repair, these models fail to include mobilization of the digits, complete tendon laceration, and an evaluation of total tendon excursion following tendon healing. A smooth gliding surface was established in both monkeys and chickens regardless of whether the sheath was repaired or excised. Another study compared tendon sheath repair, tendon sheath excision, and tendon sheath grafting in a canine model following flexor tendon repair. No significant difference was observed between the sheath repair and excision groups in terms of ultimate strength of the tendon repair and histologic evidence of adhesion formation (Fig. 4). In

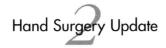
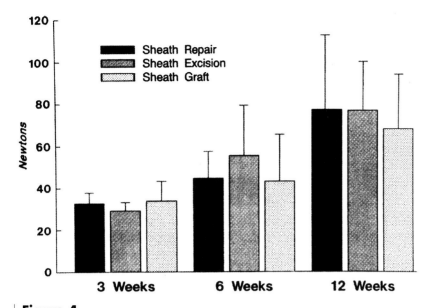

Figure 4

No significant differences were noted in a comparison of canine tendon sheath excision and tendon sheath repair groups at 3, 6, and 12 weeks. (Reproduced with permission from Gelberman RH, Woo SL, Amierl D, et al: Influences of flexor sheath continuity and early motion on tendon healing in dogs. *J Hand Surg* 1990;15A:69–77.)

the tendon sheath. When autologous synovial grafts have been used to restore the function of the tendon sheath, hyaluronic acid is present in the tendon sheath at normal levels if only a portion of the tendon sheath has been grafted. When a substantial portion of the tendon sheath has been replaced with grafted material, there is a dramatic decrease in the hyaluronic acid concentration indicating poor nutrition and lubrication of the tendon. Because of the poor clinical results with tendon injuries that involve bone, the use of interposition grafts between the proximal phalanx and the tendon sheath has been proposed in animal models; however, this concept has not yet been tested in clinical studies. Accumulated evidence suggests that only the essential portions of the tendon sheath should be replaced with autogenous grafts when required; autogenous tissue with a synovial lining is recommended.

the group with the patch graft, the strength of the tendon did not increase over time; furthermore, a high degree of disorganization of the collagen fibers was present. These findings demonstrate that reconstruction of the tendon sheath, either by suture or autogenous graft, does not significantly improve the biochemical or morphologic characteristics of repaired tendons treated with early motion rehabilitation. Although clinical reports indicate that repair of the tendon sheath appears to be safe, a clinical comparison of patients treated with sheath repair showed no significant improvement over patients treated without sheath repair.

Reports investigating the use of artificial materials for reconstruction of the tendon sheath have focused on biomaterials such as polytetrafluoroethylene (PTFE). This material is strong enough to prevent tendon bowstringing; however, the strength of the reconstructed pulley was generally less than that of an intact A3 pulley. Although the PTFE grafts permitted cellular migration and proliferation with minimal inflammation in animal models, protein synthesis within the sheath was slightly depressed in repaired tendons after use of PTFE grafts. Given the limited success of autogenous grafts, the role of artificial tendon sheath grafts is uncertain at this time. When a large portion of the tendon sheath has been destroyed or excised due to excessive scar tissue during 2-stage reconstruction, autogenous tendon sheath graphs are required for reconstruction of

Minimizing Tendon Adhesions

Intrinsic Versus Extrinsic Tendon Healing

The understanding of tendon repair and rehabilitation has been significantly advanced by a series of investigations that have established the mechanisms by which tendons can heal based on nutrition from imbibition by capillary action from the synovial fluid. Early reports suggested that adhesions were necessary in order to bring in the required blood supply for tendon healing. However, a rabbit model using tendons transplanted to the knee joint clearly demonstrated that tendons could heal without formation of adhesions, even when the tendons were wrapped in a membrane that prevented migration of the cells from the knee joint to the tendon. Irradiation of the tendon in order to kill the cells within the tendon demonstrated that cells could migrate from the joint fluid, providing the means for tendon healing without a contribution from the cells within a tendon. These experiments could be repeated with the tendons in tissue culture, an environment free of other cells, growth factors, and cytokines. These studies were later expanded to confirm that the same phenomenon could occur in a variety of animal species and in humans (using tendon segment placed in tissue culture). The epitenon was the most active portion of the tendon in the early phases of tendon repair.

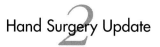

Using electron microscopy, the epitenon cells can be shown to migrate across the site of tendon laceration.

Rehabilitation to Optimize Functional Results

Earlier clinical reports of tendon repair with passive motion demonstrated 75% good results when there was no injury to the underlying bone, but the results dropped to 23% with injury to the proximal or middle phalanx. To prevent patients from moving their digits against resistance and maintain the digits in a protective position, the Kleinert technique maintains injured digits in flexion by using an elastic band attached to the level of the wrist (Fig. 5). The Durran technique uses a protective splint, but no elastic bands. Passive flexion is achieved by the therapist, with the patients using their uninjured hand. The Durran technique reportedly decreased the incidence of flexion contractures at the PIP joint. By combining these 2 techniques, 2 different teams of investigators reported an increase in the number of good and excellent results; one report demonstrated 98% good and excellent results.

Clinical studies preceded many of the laboratory investigations of the safety and efficacy of passive motion in rehabilitation of flexor tendon lacerations. Using passive digit motion in a canine model, the repair site revascularized faster in the early motion group than in the group with delayed motion or immobilization. Animals treated with immediate passive motion demonstrated fewer adhesions and a better gliding surface than animals treated by immobilization for the first 3 weeks after surgery before initiation of passive exercises. Passive mobilization generated 3.8 ± 0.1 mm of tendon excursion, which is correlated with decreased adhesion formation. Immediate passive motion demonstrated enhanced functional results not only in animal models but also in clinical studies. In one prospective randomized trial, patients using a continuous passive motion device an average of 75 hours per week with 12,000 cycles per week of digital flexion fared significantly better than patients treated with the conventional passive motion programs described by Kleinert and Durran. Besides the amount of passive motion, increased frequency of passive motion (from 1 cycle/min to 12 cycles/min) also improved the functional results in an animal model.

Impact of Splint Design on Tendon Excursion During Rehabilitation

In order to enhance flexion at the PIP and distal interphalangeal (DIP) joints, splint designs have been altered to include a pulley at midpalm level (Fig. 5). The palmar pulley for the dorsal splint produces greater tendon excursion and improved clinical results. In one prospective study with all 4 fingers in dynamic flexion regardless of the number of

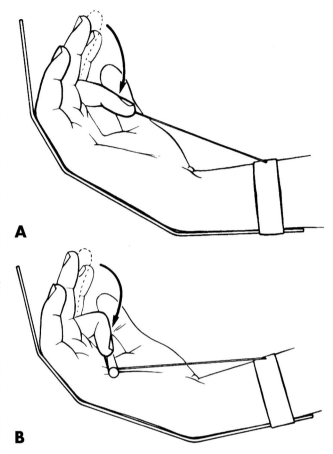

Figure 5

A, The conventional Kleinert splint uses a pulley at the wrist level. **B,** By moving the pulley to midpalm, proximal and distal interphalangeal flexion increases. (Reproduced with permission from Horii E, Lin GT, Cooney WP, et al: Comparative flexor tendon excursion after passive mobilization: An in vitro study. *J Hand Surg* 1992;17A:559–566.)

injured digits, the patients regained better motion than historic controls. The advantage of splinting all 4 fingers may be predominately psychological, as other studies have shown that splinting all 4 digits did not decrease forces on the tendon regardless of wrist position. In order to further enhance tendon excursion, a hinge or S-splint was developed that takes advantage of the tenodesis effect of wrist extension upon finger flexion as well as the facilitation of finger extension by wrist flexion (Fig. 6). The synergistic or S-splint significantly increases tendon excursion (Figs. 6 and 7). Wrist extension dramatically increases the fo'rce required for both active and passive digit flexion. The force of active finger flexion decreased from 3.4 kgf in wrist extension to 0.4 kgf with the wrist in flexion. Passive motion decreased from 0.9 kgf to 0.1 kgf as the wrist moved from extension to flexion. Flexion of the metacarpophalangeal joints with the wrist

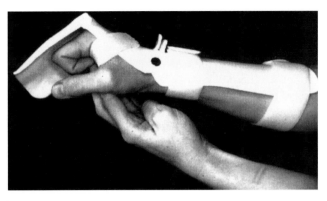

Figure 6

The tenodesis action produces finger extension during wrist flexion and finger flexion during wrist extension.

ZONE 2

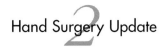

Figure 7

The synergistic splint (S-splint) provides greater tendon excursion than the Kleinert splint (K-splint) or the splint with the pulley in the palm (P-splint). (Reproduced with permission from Horii E, Lin GT, Cooney WP, et al: Comparative flexor tendon excursion after passive mobilizatrion: An in vitro study. *J Hand Surg* 1992;17:559–566.)

produces 1.3 mm of excursion between the 2 tendons for every 10° of joint flexion.

Active Digit Motion in Rehabilitation of Zone 2 Flexor Tendon Injuries

Active motion places much higher loads on the flexor tendons. Will the tendon load exceed the strength of the tendon repair? Several clinical studies have demonstrated a tendon rupture rate of approximately 6% to 8% using active motion, but these studies lack a comparison group of patients treated with passive motion. In one report using biplanar radiographs to accurately track tendon motion after implanting metal markers during flexor tendon repairs in zone 2, patients treated with active motion were compared to patients treated with passive flexion and active hold to maintain the position of flexion. The patients with active motion had increased tendon excursion at the level of the A3 and A4 pulleys, but less benefit at the A2 pulley. In another report comparing patients treated with active motion to those with historic controlled passive motion, there was a slight increase in tendon rupture rate; however, the comparison was not a controlled prospective trial, and therefore a statistical analysis was not possible. The active program does appear to increase tendon excursion, with 2.3 mm along the middle phalanx and 11.7 mm along the proximal phalanx. In order to resolve the issue of early active motion versus passive motion, a prospective randomized trial was initiated in 1996 as a joint effort of the Division of Hand and Microvascular Surgery at the University of Washington and the Indiana Hand Center. Patients were randomized to either an active range of motion program using the synergistic splint or a combined program of dynamic splinting plus passive Durran splinting as described by Chow.

Impact of Drugs or Electrical Stimulation on Tendon Healing and Adhesions

Although many reports have addressed the effect of drugs or electrical stimulation on tendon healing, to date few have clinical applications. The only drug or treatment that has been subjected to a clinical trial has been hyaluronic acid. After using a rabbit model to determine the correct molecular weight and concentration to use, hyaluronic acid was applied in a randomized prospective

extended helped decrease the force on finger flexor tendons. Passive joint motion not only enhances motion of the tendons with respect to the phalanges but also with respect to one another. DIP joint flexion produces excursion of the flexor digitorum profundus (FDP) on the flexor digitorum superficialis (FDS) of 1 mm for every 10°; PIP joint flexion

clinical trial; however, no improvement was noted in the group treated with hyaluronic acid injected into the flexor tendon sheath.

Two-Stage Tendon Reconstruction Using Tendon Grafts

Vascularity of Tendon Grafts

Despite Dr. Bunnell's warnings, recent studies have indicated that functional results with primary tendon repair are superior to results with tendon grafts. In one early study, 60% of the patients had good to excellent results with primary tendon suture compared to only 42% with tendon grafts. Using an animal model of 2-stage reconstruction, revascularization of the graft was observed with vessels penetrating the proximal and distal stumps of the grafted tendon within 1 week after surgery. Two weeks after surgery, additional vessels penetrated the tendon from areas of contact with the pseudosheath. By the fifth and sixth weeks after tendon grafting, vascular anastomoses appeared between the vessels in the tendon and the pseudosheath. At 10 weeks, the vascular anastomosis of the graft tendon was more abundant than that of the normal tendon; this phenomenon corrected by week 15. This revascularization of tendon grafts was at least 2 to 3 weeks behind that of primary tendon repairs.

To prevent the development of adhesions during this relative ischemia, vascularized free tendon grafts have been proposed using FDS tendons or the extensor indicis proprius (EIP). The vascular pedicle for the FDS tendons was based on branches from the ulnar artery, and the EIP tendon graft was based on the second dorsal metacarpal artery. Two clinical cases of vascularized extensor tendon transfer to replace the FDP have been reported with good results.

Tendon grafts frequently fail at the distal bone-tendon junction. One author demonstrated the use of prefabricated bone-tendon grafts by inserting a flexor tendon into the bone several weeks prior to the final harvest for tendon grafting. Although allografts and transplantation have been performed successfully, concerns about rejections of tendon allografts, delayed revascularization, and failure have discouraged the widespread use of tendon allografts.

At the site of proximal tendon attachment to the recipient muscle, the strength of the proximal tendon weave increases directly with the number of weaves. A cross-stitch provides greater strength than horizontal sutures.

Intrasynovial Versus Extrasynovial Tendons

One very exciting avenue of research is the study of intrasynovial tendon grafts (eg, digital flexor tendons) com-pared to extrasynovial tendons (eg, palmaris longus). Intrasynovial grafts demonstrate more rapid incorporation, decreased vascular response, and less tendon degradation than extrasynovial tendons. In a canine model using a digital flexor tendon as intrasynovial graft and the peroneus longus tendon as an extrasynovial graft, the intrasynovial grafts showed minimal adhesion formation with rapid proliferation and migration of cells from the epitenon to provide improved collagen production. The extrasynovial tendons went through a process of neovascularization, with vessels penetrating from the synovial sheath; intrasynovial tendon grafts did not form vascular adhesions. The intrasynovial grafts produced greater joint rotation at the interphalangeal joint at 3 and 6 weeks than the extrasynovial grafts. However, the source of intrasynovial grafts is quite limited. Harvesting an adjacent FDS tendon for use as a tendon graft will result in strength loss in the donor digit. The flexor digitorum longus in the foot averages only 12 cm, compared to the 22-cm tendons in the hand. At this time, no clinical studies have confirmed the results of using intrasynovial tendon grafts.

Functional Results

The 6 commonly used rating schemes for digit function following flexor tendon repair are the Buck-Gramcko classification system, Grossman system II, the Louisville classification system, Strickland's original and adjusted classifications, and the rating system of the American Society for Surgery of the Hand (ASSH). The ASSH rates results as excellent if full motion is achieved, good if greater than 75% of normal motion is achieved, fair if over 50%, and poor if less than 50%. Jansen and Watsen determined that Strickland's original system and the Louisville system provided the most critical ratings, and found only fair agreement among the different rating systems. They recommended Strickland's original classification system because it conformed most closely to measurement principles. Another group conducted a similar comparison and recommended that the Buck-Gramcko classification be used. They noted that the ASSH classification system proved to be the most stringent. All of these rating systems that involve excellent, good, fair, and poor classifications have much less statistical power than simply reporting the total active motion. Validated standardized questionnaires, such as the Disabilities of the Arm, Shoulder, and Hand (DASH) or the Carpal Tunnel Syndrome questionnaire, provide the most reliable means of assessing patient satisfaction after treatment. Although it is not possible to obtain measurements before and after injury, these are still

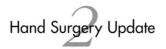

very useful tools for evaluating patient satisfaction. Key factors associated with decreased active motion at follow-up evaluation were increased patient age, increased digit swelling and an increased number of tendons and digits that were injured. However, these 3 predictive factors only explained 19% of the total variance in the result; a large percentage of the variance was unexplained and may be due to biologic or psychologic factors.

Published reports indicate that patients with flexor tendon injuries regain 75% of their grip strength, 77% of finger pressure, and 75% of their pinch strength. Because many of the reports on results of flexor tendon repair use a variety of classification systems that have nonordinal rankings (excellent, good, fair, or poor), it is difficult to determine the actual degrees of motion obtained. The preliminary results of the prospective randomized multicenter study by the University of Washington and the Indiana Hand Center suggest that the average motion of the PIP joint obtained is 80° (76% of the uninjured contralateral digit), and 45° at the DIP joint (75% of the uninjured contralateral digit).

Cellular and Biochemical Factors in Tendon Healing

Passive Physiology of Tendon Injury and Repair
The tendon injury stimulates a potent chemotactic response resulting in migration of cells into the zone of injury from either the epitenon or the synovial sheath. These cells histologically resemble myofibroblasts and synthesize collagen with an increased ratio of type III to type I, a general characteristic of scar tissue formation. The epitenon is clearly the most active segment of the tendon, for collagen synthesis with initiation of α-procollagen as well as for phagocytosis of collagen debris resulting from the injury. Evidence suggests that metalloproteinases are an important component in regulating collagen synthesis. Metalloproteinases have been implicated as one of the factors regulating the synthesis of collagen proteins. Metalloproteinases are identified early in the repair process (day 4 to 9), before the increase in sulfated and nonsulfated glycosaminoglycans (GAGs). GAGs appear 2 weeks after tendon repair. At 6 to 9 weeks, there is a significant increase in net collagen formation. As a characteristic component of the repair process, fibronectin has been identified in both the tendon and the sheath synovium. The epitenon contains 3.8 times more fibronectin than the endotenon; the sheath synovium contains 21 times more fibronectin than the fibro-osseous portion of the tendon sheath. The larger the gap between the tendon ends, the greater the contribution from the epitenon. The more closely the tendon ends are coapted,

the greater the contribution from the endotenon. The endotenon can contribute to wound healing, and the cells in the endotenon appear to form a more mature form of collagen than the cells in the epitenon.

Cytokines and Growth Factors
Platelet-derived growth factor and epidermal growth factor were identified in healing flexor tendons from 3 to 17 days after repair. Notably absent from the repair process was fibroblastic growth factor.

Hyaluronic acid, which is a normal component of tendon synovial fluid, did not increase collagen synthesis and actually depressed cellular proliferation. Ascorbic acid was essential at a concentration of at least 50 μg/ml for tendon healing. Transforming growth factor beta (TGF-β) was also noted in healing tendons as well as in the tendon sheath. Increased levels of TGF-β were noted in experimental models in regions of the tendon that were under increased loads; TGF-β has been associated with proteoglycan synthesis. Proteoglycans appear to be present in increased concentrations in regions of the tendon and tendon sheath that are subjected to tendon load.

Tendon Nutrition and Blood Supply
Tendon nutrition is provided by a combination of blood vessels entering through the vinculae and vessels penetrating from the musculotendinous junction, as well as by direct diffusion of nutrients from the synovial fluid. The region of the tendon between the musculotendinous junction and the vinculae is the area most dependent on synovial diffusion. Synovial diffusion is enhanced by the capillary pumping mechanism known as imbibition. This pumping process is enhanced by finger flexion as the tendon glides into the fibrous pulleys; this helps draw fluid into the interstices of the tendon through small ridges or conduits that are oriented at 90° to one another. The extent of tendon dependency on nutrition delivered through the vascular supply as compared to the synovial diffusion has not been determined in a clinical setting. In an animal model with ligation of the vinculae, there was no decrease in collagen or noncollagen protein synthesis, suggesting that the process of diffusion is quite efficient. There did not appear to be any difference between the different digits in the extent of the tendon nutrition supplied by blood vessels from the vinculae versus the blood vessels penetrating from the musculotendinous junction. Tendon lacerations combined with vincular injuries have been associated with a decreased active motion of the digits; this may correspond to a greater dependence on the vincular blood supply in humans than in animal models. However, vincular injuries also correlate with injuries that have a greater degree of trauma of the surrounding tissues.

Tendon Structure and Biomechanics

Flexor tendons are strong when tested in tension; they can resist up to 150 kfg. Ideally, tendon grafts to replace these long structures will average 20 cm in length and be able to expand by up to 26 mm. Tendons are composed of 78% type I collagen and 19% type III collagen; the remaining 3% includes a variety of other collagen types and noncollagen proteins. A unique relationship exists between the FDP and FDS because the FDP travels through the decussation of the superficialis (Champer's chiasm). During digit flexion, the 2 slips of the FDS move toward the midline and compress the FDP tendon. The chiasm moves proximally during tendon flexion in a manner similar to a bat's tendon locking mechanism. Tendon growth corresponds directly with the growth of the phalanges and metacarpals. Much like the long bones in the lower extremity, the stimulus for tendon growth likely stems from tension applied during bone growth. Tendons demonstrate a nonlinear viscoelastic property. Tendon load increases in a linear fashion with tendon grip strength. Excursion increases exponentially with increasing tendon load.

Annotated Bibliography

Tendon Injury and Repair

Biomechanical and Clinical Studies

Aoki M, Manske PR, Pruitt DL, Larson BJ: Work of flexion after tendon repair with various suture methods: A human cadaveric study. *J Hand Surg* 1995;20B:310–313.

After flexor tendon repair there is often increased resistance to tendon gliding at the repair side; this increased friction may be measured as the work of flexion in the laboratory setting. The average increase in work of flexion after zone 2 tendon repair in human cadaver hands was 4.8% for the 2-strand Kessler technique, 6.5% for the lateral Becker, 10.9% for 6-strand Savage, 19.3% for the internal tendon splint, 16.2% for the dorsal tendon splint, and 44.3% for the external mesh sleeve. The work of flexion was found to increase in direct proportion to the amount of suture material at the repair site.

Groth GN, Bechtold LL, Young VL: Early active mobilization for flexor tendons repaired using the double loop locking suture technique. *J Hand Ther* 1995;8:206–211.

The authors describe a double loop locking suture (DOLLS) technique that provides sufficient in vitro strength (average 4,400 g) for early active mobilization of the flexor tendon. Early active mobilization was initiated 3 to 7 days postoperatively. Two patients achieved excellent results, 1 a good result, and 1 fair. With the use of a protective splint, early active mobilization of tendons repaired by the DOLLS technique appears to be an effective method for postoperative management.

Komanduri M, Phillips CS, Mass DP: Tensile strength of flexor tendon repairs in a dynamic cadaver model. *J Hand Surg* 1996;21A:605–611.

Twenty-six fresh-frozen cadaver hands (78 tendons) underwent sharp zone 2 profundus tendon transection and repair with Bunnell, Kessler, Kessler with circumferential epitenon, or epitenon-alone sutures. In all cases, dorsally placed sutures provided significantly more tensile strength than palmarly placed sutures. In light of the previous evidence that tendon viability is dependent on diffusion and not on the vascular supply, a dorsally placed core suture and circumferential epitenon repair for zone 2 profundus repairs should be considered because of the increased strength provided by this technique.

Papandrea R, Seitz WH Jr, Shapiro P, Borden B: Biomechanical and clinical evaluation of the epitenon-first technique of flexor tendon repair. *J Hand Surg* 1995;20A:261–266.

After 13 matched pairs of canine flexor tendons were repaired using both the epitenon-first and the modified Kessler with an epitendinous running suture, they were tested to failure with a longitudinal force. Human cadaver flexor digitorum profundus tendons were used to determine the cross-sectional area of the tendon that is displaced by suture material of the Kessler repair and epitenon-first core suture. The epitenon-first technique was 22% stronger than the modified Kessler technique. Comparison of tendon repair cross-sectional contact areas demonstrated that 20% of the surface area of the repair is occupied by the knot of the modified Kessler technique, while the core suture of the epitenon-first repair consumed only 2.6%.

Pruitt DL, Tanaka H, Aoki M, Manske PR: Cyclic stress testing after in vivo healing of canine flexor tendon lacerations. *J Hand Surg* 1996;21A:974–977.

This study evaluated the effects of cyclic tension applied to lacerated and repaired canine flexor tendons after various periods of in vivo healing for up to 30 days. Final gaps obtained after cyclic stress testing were found to increase from a baseline of 0.75 ± 0.17 mm (zero time controls) to a maximum of 1.14 ± 0.24 mm at 3 days after repair, before returning to baseline at 10 days (0.63 ± 0.27 mm). Gap formation at 30 days after repair (0.65 ± 0.27 mm) was similar to that of control tendons. This canine study suggests that continued protection of flexor tendons from strong repetitive tensile stress should extend at least through 30 days after repair.

Tang JB: Flexor tendon repair in zone 2C. *J Hand Surg* 1994; 19B:72–75.

A randomized prospective clinical study was carried out in 33 patients (37 fingers) with lacerations of both FDS and FDP tendons in the area covered by the A2 pulley (zone 2C). Both lacerated tendons were repaired in 19 fingers and repair of only FDP with regional excision of FDS was performed in 18 fingers. Follow-up of average 12 months revealed that there was no significant different in the end results evaluated according to the total active motion (TAM) system. The average TAM was 204° in the fingers with suture of FDP only, and 187° in those with suture of both tendons. The fingers with suture of both tendons showed a higher rate of reoperation due to adhesions or rupture of repair. This study suggests that it is better to repair only FDP with regional excision of FDS when both tendons are injured in zone 2C.

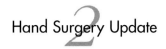

Thurman RT, Trumble TE, Hanel DP, Tencer AF, Kiser PK: The two-, four-, and six-strand zone II flexor tendon repairs: An in situ biomechanical comparison using a cadaver model. *J Hand Surg* 1998;23A:261–265.

A dynamic in vitro model of zone 2 flexor tendon repair was used to compare gliding resistance, gap formation, and ultimate strength of the 2-, 4-, and 6-strand repair techniques. Tendons were sectioned and each was repaired using a different technique so that each specimen acted as its own control. Following repair, each hand was remounted on the loading frame with 3 flexor tendons attached to individual pneumatic cylinders, and cycled 1,000 times. The 2-strand repair had significantly greater gap formation after cyclic loading (mean gap = 2.75 mm) than either 4-strand (0.30 mm) or 6-strand repairs (0.31 mm). The tensile strength of the 6-strand repair (mean = 78.7 N) was significantly greater than either the 4-strand (mean = 43.0 N) or 2-strand repair (mean = 33.9 N).

Williams RJ, Amis AA: A new type of flexor tendon repair: Biomechanical evaluation by cyclic loading, ultimate strength and assessment of pulley friction in vitro. *J Hand Surg* 1995;20B:578–583.

Experiments were performed to evaluate biomechanical aspects of the performance of a deep-biting peripheral suture (DBPS) for flexor tendon repair, either when used alone or with a square or modified Kessler core stitch, and the technique was compared to the Kleinert repair. Tests included progressively increasing cyclic loads, force to pull the repair into the A2 pulley, and ultimate failure strength. Half of the Kleinert repairs failed under 30 N cyclic loading, while 100% of the DBPS plus Kessler core stitch repairs survived. There was no discernable difference in gliding function or repair bulk between these sutures, but ultimate strength increased significantly with the DBPS repairs. The DBPS plus Kessler-type core stitch will survive active mobilization better than the Kleinert method.

Adhesion Formation and Tendon Rehabilitation

Bainbridge LC, Robertson C, Gillies D, Elliot D: A comparison of post-operative mobilization of flexor tendon repairs with "passive flexion-active extension" and "controlled active motion" techniques. *J Hand Surg* 1994;19B:517–521.

This study reports the outcome of flexor tendon repairs mobilized by either a passive flexion-active extension or a controlled active motion regimen. The controlled active motion regimen conferred significant benefits on the final range of motion and extensor lag. The rupture rate was raised with controlled active motion, but no more than levels reported by other authors using passive flexion-active extension regimens.

Horii E, Lin GT, Cooney WP, Linscheid RL, An KN: Comparative flexor tendon excursion after passive mobilization: An in vitro study. *J Hand Surg* 1992;17A:559–566.

In 2 experimental studies conducted to investigate flexor tendon excursions, tendon excursions due to passive joint motion in various loading conditions were evaluated, and the efficacy of a new technique that used synergistic wrist motion (S-splint) was compared with traditional dorsal splinting methods—the Kleinert splint (K-splint) and the Brooke Army Hospital/Walter Reed modified Kleinert splint with a palmar bar (P-splint). The measured tendon excursion under a condition of low tendon tension was almost half that of the-

oretically predicted values. In zone 2, the magnitude of excursion was greatest for the S-splint, then P-splint, and then the K-splint ($p <$ 0.05). Differential tendon excursion between the FDP and FDS had a mean value of 3 mm and was not significantly different among the 3 methods. Passive PIP joint motion was the most effective means of providing increased amplitude of tendon gliding in zone 2. Passive DIP joint motion did not increase excursion in zone 2 as much as had been predicted.

Mass DP, Tuel RJ: Intrinsic healing of the laceration site in human superficialis flexor tendons in vitro. *J Hand Surg* 1991; 16A:24–30.

The intrinsic capability of the human superficialis flexor tendon to heal a reapproximated laceration site in vitro was examined. Segments of lacerated and sutured human superficialis flexor tendons from zone 2 were cultured for 2, 4, or 8 weeks in vitro and analyzed by use of light and electron microscopy. A specific pattern of intrinsic healing at the repair site was noted during the incubation period. After 2 weeks, the cells of the epitenon from both tendon stumps proliferated and appeared to migrate into the repair site. By 8 weeks, a smooth contiguous tendon surface was restored and the internal collagen bundles were brought into intimate contact. The cells in the repair site were active in protein synthesis, and new collagen fibers were present. The results indicate that human superficialis tendons possess an intrinsic capacity to heal with diffusion and without dependence on extratendinous cells or on adhesions.

Silfverskiold KL, May EJ: Flexor tendon repair in zone II with a new suture technique and an early mobilization program combining passive and active flexion. *J Hand Surg* 1994;19A:53–60.

A new epitendinal suture technique (cross-stitch) was used for flexor tendon repair in zone 2 in 46 consecutive patients with 55 injured digits. For the first 4 weeks after the operation, the digits were mobilized with a combination of active extension and passive and active flexion. Postoperative tendon excursions and gap formation were measured with intraoperatively placed metal markers. There were 2 ruptures. In the remaining digits, the mean active range of motion 6 weeks after surgery was 50° (DIP) and 83° (PIP). This increased to 63° (DIP) and 94° (PIP) at 6 months. Three weeks postoperatively the mean tendon excursions per 10° of joint motion varied from 82% (DIP) to 88% (PIP) of the maximum possible. The results indicate that the cross-stitch is a reliable suture technique that, when used in combination with a program incorporating early active and passive flexion, can produce very good results after zone 2 flexor tendon repair.

Wittemann M, Blumenthal K, Hornung RW, Germann G: Washington regime after-care of flexor tendon injuries in zone 2. *Handchir Mikrochir Plast Chir* 1996;28:191–197.

The Washington regimen for the rehabilitation of flexor tendon injuries (Chow and associates) represents a combination of the established Kleinert method and the controlled passive motion of Durran and Houser. This paper presents the results of a study that was carried out in 99 patients with 113 injured fingers. The Washington regimen yielded an improvement of up to 27% of very good and good results in injured fingers compared to the Kleinert method. In cases with additional laceration of digital nerves, the subjective evaluation of two thirds of the patients was significantly worse than the objective functional results.

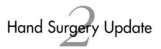

Tendon Grafts

Gabuzda GM, Lovallo JL, Nowak MD: Tensile strength of the end-weave flexor tendon repair: An in vitro biomechanical study. *J Hand Surg* 1994;19B:397–400.

In a study designed to investigate the tensile strength of the end-weave method of tendon repair, flexor tendons were removed from 13 fresh-frozen human cadavers. The tendons were transected and repaired with the end-weave technique varying form 1 to 5 weaves, with 2 suture techniques—the commonly used horizontal mattress suture and a new method termed the cross stitch. Tensile strength increased linearly with the number of weaves for both suture methods. The cross stitch demonstrated significantly greater strength per weave compared to the horizontal mattress suture ($p < 0.05$). The results from this in vitro model suggest that active rehabilitative exercises might safely be performed in the immediate postoperative period after procedures that involve tendon weaving.

Morrison WA, Cleland H: Vascularised flexor tendon grafts. *Ann Acad Med Singapore* 1995;24(suppl 4):26–31.

Tendon grafts can be implanted with their own living sheaths as free or pedicled vascularized transfers from the foot or forearm to either extensor or flexor sites in the hand. These tendon grafts can be inserted into the intact or reconstructed tunnel systems of the digit and repaired proximally and distally to the tendon remnants. Gliding is enhanced, although limitations still potentially exist at the proximal tendon junctions.

Seiler JG III, Gelberman RH, Willams CS, et al: Autogenous flexor-tendon grafts: A biomechanical and morphological study in dogs. *J Bone Joint Surg* 1993;75A:1004–1014.

Intrasynovial and extrasynovial donor autogenous flexor tendon grafts were placed in the synovial sheaths of the medial and lateral digits of the forepaw in 20 dogs (40 tendons). The extrasynovial tendon grafts healed with early ingrowth of peripheral adhesions, which appeared to become larger and more dense over time. These grafts exhibited decreased cellularity and early neovascularization at 10 days, and there was evidence of progressive revascularization and cellular repopulation at 3 and 6 weeks. In contrast, the intrasynovial tendon grafts demonstrated minimum adhesions, and both cellularity and collagen organization were normal at each time interval. The intrasynovial grafts had significantly more angular rotation at the PIP joint at 3 and 6 weeks than did the extrasynovial grafts ($p < 0.05$).

Functional Results of Flexor Tendon Repair

Jansen CW, Watson MG: Measurement of range of motion of the finger after flexor tendon repair in zone II of the hand. *J Hand Surg* 1993;18A:411–417.

This study compared classification systems of active range of motion of the finger after flexor tendon surgery in zone 2 of the hand. Active range of motion of 20 fingers (16 subjects) was classified according to 5 systems. Agreement between the systems was only fair. Strickland's original system and the Louisville system rated the results most strictly, followed by Strickland's adjusted system. Buck-Gramcko's systems rated the results least strictly. Stickland's systems conformed most closely to measurement principles. The authors conclude that Strickland's original classification system is preferable for scientific and clinical purposes.

Silfverskiold KL, May EJ, Oden A: Factors affecting results after flexor tendon repair in zone II: A multivariate prospective analysis. *J Hand Surg* 1993;18A:654–662.

A stepwise multiple regression procedure was used to examine the influence of 12 to 13 independent variables on 5 outcome variables 1 year after flexor tendon repair in zone 2 in a consecutive series of 135 patients treated with early controlled motion. Of the included variables, controlled interphalangeal joint range of motion 3 weeks postoperatively was the singlemost influential factor with regard to final active interphalangeal joint range of motion. A large part of the variance in all the outcome variables was probably related to the psychological and biologic characteristics of the patient.

Cellular and Biomechanical Factors in Tendon Healing

Duffy FJ Jr, Seiler JG, Gelberman RH, Hergrueter CA: Growth factors and canine flexor tendon healing: Initial studies in uninjured and repair models. *J Hand Surg* 1995;20A:645–649.

Although the role of growth factors in a variety of bone and soft-tissue healing processes has been studied extensively, little is known about the specific growth factors that may play a role in flexor tendon healing. Data from this study provide evidence that basic fibroblast growth factor, a potent angiogenic growth factor, is present in normal canine intrasynovial flexor tendons. Repaired canine flexor tendons were studied to further elucidate the role of growth factors in the tendon healing process. Heparin-sepharose elution profiles from 3 repair intervals (3, 10, and 17 days) were graphed and compared to known profiles of isolated growth factors. The 3 repair intervals demonstrated 2 elution profile peaks, consistent with varying amounts of platelet-derived growth factor and epidermal growth factor. These data provide compelling evidence that a variety of growth factors are present in uninjured and healing digital flexor tendons.

Packer DL, Dombi GW, Yu PY, Zidel P, Sullivan WG: An in vitro model of fibroblast activity and adhesion formation during flexor tendon healing. *J Hand Surg* 1994;19A:769–776.

The authors studied fibroblast activity during tendon healing with an in vitro tendon culture model. Tendons were embedded in a translucent collagen gel matrix whose porous nature permitted free nutrient diffusion, fibroblast migration out of the tendon, and microphotographic documentation of fibroblast activity. Experiments were performed using one or more tendons cultured in the same collagen gel. Three zones of fibroblast activity were identified in the gel. The collagen gel used in the culture system may help maintain a chemotactic concentration gradient that allows fibroblasts to locate other distal cut tendon surfaces also embedded in the collagen gel.

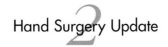

Chapter 14
Flexor Tendon Injuries

John S. Taras, MD

Introduction

Repair of the injured flexor tendon system continues to challenge surgeons, therapists, and patients. Despite efforts to improve the outcome of flexor tendon repairs, restrictive adhesions that form between the injured tendon and the flexor tendon sheath remain the most common problem compromising functional recovery. Joint contracture and repair rupture present additional hazards to primary repair of the flexor tendons. The irreparable tendon and its sheath also remain a troublesome clinical presentation requiring reconstruction.

This chapter presents recent flexor tendon literature that enhances our understanding of the flexor tendon system's response to injury and surgical reconstruction. Evolving techniques focus on promoting tendon gliding and limiting postoperative adhesions. Predictable restoration of normal hand function after flexor tendon injury may soon become an achievable goal.

Acute Injuries

Recent research supports the premise that active mobilization following primary tendon repair can produce greater and more reliable excursion than can passive mobilization. Several studies describe postoperative passive flexion and active extension therapy regimens following flexor tendon repair, documenting a decrease in adhesion formation compared to historically less successful results from immobilization. Variations of the passive flexion-active extension hand therapy regimen have become the treatment standard following primary flexor tendon repair in compliant patients; however, such protocols have not yielded uniformly favorable recovery of motion. One group employed Chow's active extension and rubber band passive flexion regimen in their series of primary flexor tendon repairs, yet their results contrasted sharply with Chow's encouraging report of 82% good and excellent results; a minority (48%) of their patients achieved good or excellent results when evaluated using the Strickland-Glogovac criteria. Typical primary flexor tendon repairs may fall far short of reliable restoration of normal function.

Silfverskiöld evaluated the efficacy of passive flexion and active extension after primary flexor tendon repair, measuring the magnitude of tendon excursion during the early mobilization period by tagging tendon repairs with metallic sutures. He concluded that passive flexion techniques can yield tendon excursions approaching those produced by active flexion, but the variation of excursion among individuals is great. Not all tendons glide to the same degree after primary repair with initiation of passive flexion–active extension. Without gliding, restrictive adhesions are more likely to form. Silfverskiöld believes that early active flexion should elicit more predictable and possibly longer tendon excursions, if combined with a suture technique strong enough to withstand the greater stress on the repair.

Biomechanics of Tendon Repair

Surgeons continue to consider active mobilization a safe modality to optimize excursion after primary repair, constructing suture techniques capable of withstanding the tensile rigors of active mobilization. To bolster this assertion, authors have scrutinized the internal and external elements influencing tendon repairs. Biomechanical models have been constructed to define the tensile requirements of tendon repairs. Factors such as motion and tension, drag after repair, gap formation, and suture placement within the tendon influence tendon gliding, return of repair site strength, and healing. As these variables become better defined, hand surgeons will be better prepared to mitigate the risks that Bunnell set forth in his early work on tendon repair.

A canine study provided evidence that repaired tendons lose nearly half their initial repair strength within 1 week after immobilization. Since publication of that study, researchers have known that the tensile strength of common repair techniques is insufficient to reliably support active tendon mobilization. By devising tendon repair techniques using more suture material, most commonly by increasing the number of suture strands passed across the repair, surgeons have demonstrated an increase in repair strength. One cadaveric "work of flexion" study posits a relationship between the amount of suture and resistance to gliding. The

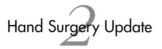

increased resistance to tendon gliding measured 4.8% in the 2-strand modified Kessler repair, 6.5% in the lateral margin Becker repair, and 19.3% in the 6-strand Savage repair. Bulkier experimental repair techniques, including the internal tendon splint, external mesh sleeve, and dorsal tendon splint, interfere with tendon gliding up to 44% more than the simpler constructs. Although the study did not factor in elements such as tissue swelling and edema, work of flexion clearly increases in direct proportion to the amount of suture used to achieve the repair.

Another group elucidated the individual efforts of motion and tension on partially transected and repaired chicken flexor tendons. Histologically, the alliance of motion and tension promotes the greatest increase in cellular activity, while the absence of both components generates the least activity. Motion or tension induce independent intermediate changes in cellular activity, but of a lesser degree than when combined. The collaborative efforts of motion and tension appear to enhance the tendon's response to injury.

One recent report addressed the concern that strong repetitive tensile stress applied too early to repaired tendons may lead to increased gap formation and subsequent adhesions at the repair site. A canine model of cyclic stress testing on tendon repair corroborated prior observations of repair site weakening. Gap formation with cyclic testing in vitro was greatest at 3 days after repair. Following in vivo healing for up to 30 days, gap length and frequency were consistent with that seen after the first week of healing. However, the authors advise protecting healing flexor tendons from strong repetitive tensile stress for 30 days after repair.

In a report on the biomechanical and histologic characteristics of canine flexor tendon repairs subject to early active motion, the weaker Kessler repairs ruptured in 89% of specimens; however, none of the Savage or dorsal tendon splint repairs ruptured. Most significantly, successful tendon repairs stressed during the healing process appear to lose little initial repair strength when tested for gap formation and tensile strength 5 days after repair. In this model, initial repair strength returned within 10 days following repair. Tendons subjected to tensile stress in an active motion postoperative regimen maintained their strength to a far greater extent than did immobilized tendons.

Two separate studies examined core suture placement in cadaveric flexor tendons to determine whether dorsal or volar position influences repair strength. In one report, repaired tendons were harvested before stressing them to longitudinal tensile failure. Dorsally placed suture provided 26.5% greater strength prior to failure than volarly placed suture. The other investigators repaired and tested specimens within their tendon beds, preserving in vivo angula-

tion, loading, and frictional interference. In this curvilinear model, dorsal suture placement proved nearly twice as strong as volar placement.

Following reports that epitendinous suture techniques augment repair strength significantly, another team investigated depth of placement of running epitendinous suture. They found that deep suture placement is nearly 80% stronger than superficial placement, when used to complement a Kessler core suture. This technique, combining deep epitendinous suture and a Kessler core suture, can tolerate loads up to 40 N; however, the authors were concerned that this technique may not provide adequate support for an active mobilization program.

In a comparison of the strengths of Kessler, suture-locking, and Savage techniques in an in vivo immobilized canine model, the Savage method was found to be stronger initially and at 1, 3, and 6 weeks after repair. The authors suggest that it is possible to maintain a significant degree of initial repair strength during the early recuperative period using the Savage technique. During the immediate postoperative phase, however, repair technique has more influence on strength than tendon healing properties.

A study of core suture caliber indicates that greater suture gauge significantly increases repair strength. Kessler, Bunnell, and double-grasping repairs constructed with 4-0 braided polyester failed because of suture rupture. For these 2-strand techniques, the core suture strength is independent of technique. As suture gauge increases, however, the technique's grasping characteristics become more significant. Kessler repairs pull out of the tendon ends more easily than do Bunnell or double-grasping sutures. The combination of a 3-0 double-grasping core suture with the cross-stitch epitendinous repair developed by Silfverskiöld withstood an average ultimate tensile strength of 72 N. Theoretical models indicate that this construct affords sufficient strength to support an active mobilization protocol.

One team developed a theoretical model to determine force application at the repair site. In a posture of 20° wrist extension, 83° metacarpophalangeal (MCP) joint flexion, 75° proximal interphalangeal (PIP) flexion, and 40° distal interphalangeal (DIP) flexion, an external load of 50 g exerts 41 g of tension on the flexor digitorum profundus (FDP) and 605 g of tension on the flexor digitorum superficialis (FDS). Increasing flexion angles by 2° (MCP), 20° (PIP), and 35° (DIP) caused a sharp tension increase—1,650 g on the FDP and 2,050 g on the FDS. Even minimal deviation from the posture associated with the least tension increases the load beyond the repair's tensile capacity. The authors caution against extreme joint positions during active motion rehabilitation exercises when the repair technique might not support these forces.

Clinical Series of Flexor Tendon Repair

Elliot and associates applied a controlled active motion program to 254 digits that underwent primary repair of flexor tendon lacerations. Their repair technique combined a 3-0 or 4-0 Kessler monofilament core suture with a 6-0 running epitendinous nylon suture for FDP and flexor pollicis longus lacerations. For FDS repairs, they used a 4-0 or 5-0 nylon mattress stitch. Using this regimen, 5.8% of the fingers and 16.6% of the thumbs ruptured. During the last year of this study, patient outcomes were appraised using the Strickland and Glogovac criteria. Of the 63 fingers with zone 2 lacerations, 79.4% demonstrated good or excellent results. The study's rupture rate resembles most previous series reporting passive flexion and active extension regimen results (4% to 7% zone 2 repair ruptures).

Silfverskiöld has offered a different epitendinal suture technique—the cross-stitch—used to repair 55 digits with zone 2 flexor tendon lacerations. The cross-stitch creates an external weave resembling a Chinese finger trap. The repair technique combines this cross-stitch epitendinal suture with a 4-0 braided Kessler core stitch. His postoperative regimen consists of active extension with passive and active flexion. Two repairs (3.6%) ruptured. The mean active DIP and PIP joint motion at 6 months after surgery was 157° (71% excellent and 25.5% good). These results represent an improvement of 15° motion over results obtained at the same clinic with a passive flexion and active extension regimen.

Another group applied a program of active and passive flexion to 14 digits with flexor tendon laceration that was repaired using Silfverskiöld's cross-stitch combined with a 3-0 braided polyester core suture incorporating an extra grasping throw at each corner of the stitch (Fig. 1). Recovery of motion was 87%, and no ruptures occurred. The therapy protocol starts with place and hold exercises on the day following surgery and progresses to active tendon gliding exercises at 3 weeks; resistive exercises are initiated by 6 weeks.

Strickland's 4-strand suture technique pairs a modified Kessler core stitch of 3-0 braided synthetic suture with a horizontal mattress stitch and a 6-0 nylon epitendinous suture (Fig. 2). Thirty-four patients with zone 1 and 2 injuries completed an active motion hand therapy program. Nine patients recovered over 150° interphalangeal motion, 17 reclaimed 125° to 149°, 9 recovered 90° to 124° motion, and 2 recovered less than 90° when discharged from therapy. Active interphalangeal motion averaged 130°. Long-term follow-up of 19 digits in this series showed a 19° improvement in interphalangeal joint motion over motion measured at the time of discharge from formal hand therapy. This rep-

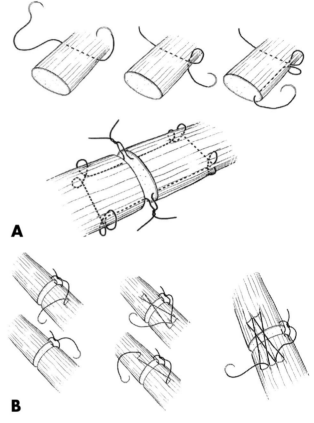

A

B

Figure 1

A, Double-grasping core suture technique using a 3-0 braided polyester suture. **B,** The cross-stitch epitendinous technique developed by Silfverskiöld is added. (Reproduced with permission from Taras JS, Skahen JR III, Raphael JS, Marczyk SC, Bauerle WB: The double-grasping and cross-stitch for acute flexor tendon repair, in Taras JS, Schneider LH (eds): *Atlas of the Hand Clinics.* Philadelphia, PA, WB Saunders, 1996, pp 13–27.)

resents a significant improvement over results from a passive flexion and active extension regimen in patients with comparable repairs.

Two clinical series of 6-strand core suture repair techniques have been presented. One team modified Savage's technique by placing a single cross-grasp for fixation of each suture limb (Fig. 3). They also describe a new tendon-holding device that simplifies this technically demanding suture technique. Twenty-three tendons in 18 patients with zone 2 repairs underwent a program of active mobilization; 78% received an excellent or good rating using the Strickland and Glogovac criteria. Mean active interphalangeal motion measured 135°, and no ruptures were reported.

Another group used a loop suture technique to construct a 6-strand repair. A rehabilitation regimen of controlled active and passive motion was used in 32 digits. One patient

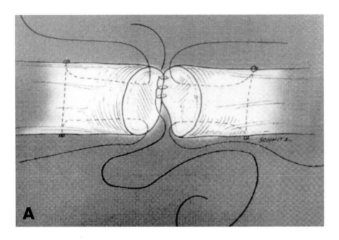

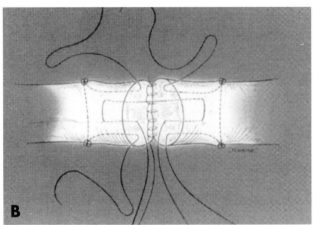

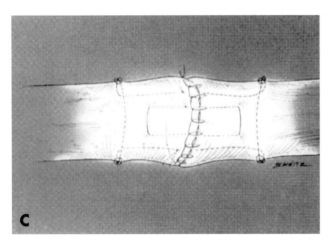

Figure 2

Strickland's Indiana method of flexor tendon repair combines a modified Kessler core stitch with a horizontal stitch and epitendinous suture. **A,** The double-locking suture has been placed, and the back wall epitendinous suture is in place. **B,** The mattress suture has been placed. **C,** The epitendinous suture is completed. (Reproduced with permission from Strickland JS: The Indiana method of flexor tendon repair, in Taras JS, Schneider LH (eds): *Atlas of the Hand Clinics.* Philadelphia, PA, WB Saunders, 1996, pp 77–103.)

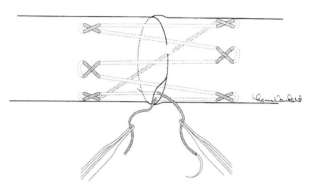

Figure 3

Sandow's modified Savage single cross-grasp 6-strand flexor tenorrhaphy technique, which will be completed by tying the knot. (Reproduced with permission from Sandow MJ, McMahon MM: Single-cross grasp six-strand repair for acute flexor tenorrhaphy: Modified Savage technique, in Taras JS, Schneider LH (eds): *Atlas of the Hand Clinics.* Philadelphia, PA, WB Saunders, 1996, pp 41–64.)

developed a tendon rupture. When graded according to Strickland's revised criteria, 13 (40.5%) achieved more than 132° of active interphalangeal motion, 13 regained 88° to 131°, and 5 (16%) gained 48° to 87°. Excluding the rupture, no patient gained less than 47° active interphalangeal motion.

Partial Tendon Laceration

Most of the current literature espouses surgical repair using a core suture for tendon lacerations through more than 60% of the flexor tendon. Lacerations of less than 30% do not warrant repair. The recommendation for management of tendon lacerations encompassing 30% to 60% of the tendon is less clear. Although the majority of surgeons prefer to repair midrange partial lacerations, some believe that suturing a partially lacerated tendon can be detrimental to tendon strength. One group developed a method to estimate the size of partial tendon laceration in zone 2, using a formula calculating the area of the radial and ulnar bundles of the profundus tendon. This new method factors the cross-sectional area of the profundus tendon and the intratendinous bundles at various levels in zone 2. This formula provides a patient-specific method by which clinicians can assess, accurately and easily, the size of a partial tendon laceration.

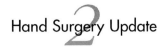

Tendon Reconstruction

Diagnosis

Adhesions are the most common tendon healing complication. The difficulty of distinguishing restrictive adhesions from tendon rupture during the early postoperative period has compelled investigators to seek better methods of visualizing this perplexing clinical situation. In one survey of 16 tendons carrying a clinical diagnosis of rupture less than 8 weeks after repair, clinical examination yielded a 60% accuracy in diagnosis; magnetic resonance imaging (MRI) correctly distinguished adhesions from ruptures in all cases. This study complements earlier work that promoted MRI for evaluation of adhesion formation, tendon ruptures, and gap formation at repair sites.

Bare-handed rock climbing has increased in popularity during recent years. One or 2 fingers may bear the climber's total body weight. Hazards of the sport, including rupture of the pulley system, are more widely encountered today. One group reported 7 cases of pulley rupture confirmed by computed tomography (CT). In each case, CT clearly visualized the rupture and established a correct diagnosis. For pulley ruptures, CT well illustrated the dynamic images of the digits straining against resistance and the resultant bowstringing. Compared to other clinical diagnostic imaging modalities, including standard radiography, ultrasound, and MRI, CT provides an accurate, easy, and cost-effective means to diagnose digital pulley rupture.

The Pulley System

A complex interplay between cams and pulleys employs available excursion and power supplied by the forearm's muscle tendon units. The pulley system enhances the flexors' ability to translate excursion into angular motion across the interphalangeal joints. By preventing bowstringing, the pulleys hold the flexor tendons close to the phalanges. This arrangement enables smooth and efficient digital flexion. One group diverges from historical assertions that the A2 is the most important pulley for optimal flexor tendon function. Although isolated excision of the A2 results in a significant decrease in excursion, absence of the A2 does not alter work ability. Their study demonstrates that a missing A4 pulley dissipates efficiency more than any other pulley. Compared to the intact pulley system, absence of an A4 results in an 85% loss of both work and excursion. The authors also concluded that a 3-pulley system (A2, A3, and A4) maintains work and excursion significantly better than a 2-pulley system (A2 and A4).

A mechanical analysis of the palmar aponeurosis pulley revealed that isolated sectioning of the palmar aponeurosis pulley does not materially change efficiency. Absence of the palmar aponeurosis and loss of either or both proximal annular pulleys (A1 and A2), however, causes a significant decrease in excursion efficiency. This analyst asserts that the palmar aponeurosis pulley is as important as the annular and cruciate flexor tendon pulleys. Another group examined the effects of digital pulley excision and loss of the profundus tendon on superficialis tendon efficiency in a human cadaver model. They concluded that the A2 and A3 are the most important pulleys for superficialis function, and that the profundus is necessary for optimal tendon efficiency.

Grafting

The indications and technique for 1- and 2-stage tendon grafting are well established. Infections, adhesions, concurrent neurovascular and osseous injuries, tendon rupture, and patient noncompliance can compromise the result of a direct flexor tendon repair. Tendon grafting is the standard procedure for digits when direct repair is not feasible or has failed. The common donor tendons—the palmaris, plantaris, and toe extensors—are extrasynovial grafts. Alternative procedures have recently been introduced to ameliorate clinical situations in which standard tendon grafting techniques are not practical. One group described the benefits of intrasynovial autografts including the superficialis tendon in a canine model. The intrasynovial tendon grafts demonstrate superior gliding function compared to extrasynovial grafts after 6 weeks of healing. Although extrasynovial grafts exhibit greater stiffness and ultimate load, adhesions account for much of this biomechanical strength. The extrasynovial graft is still the most practical at this time.

Naam illustrated use of a pedicled FDS tendon as a graft in the second stage of reconstruction. He reported good or excellent results in 64% of patients 3.7 years after surgery. Three of the 33 patients (9.1%) required tenolysis. Patients over 25 years of age with significant soft-tissue injuries and patients who were noncompliant with postoperative therapy achieved poorer results.

Human composite flexor tendon allografts can be used to salvage digits with scarred flexor systems from multiple operations. One group presented 2 cases that were followed for 5 years after human flexor tendon allografting. Both patients achieved real functional improvement without any complications. The authors believe that allografting can restore good function without synovitis, infection, or secondary rupture. Published reports suggest that insoluble collagen is relatively nonantigenic. There has been no significant evidence of antigenicity in grafted patients; however, the issues of antigenicity and transfer of contagious disease with allograft tendon require continued investigation.

Another team investigated the strength of end-weave repair, assessing the impact of the number of weaves on

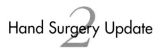

pull-out strength in a human cadaver model. They compared the efficacy of the standard mattress suture to a multiple-pass technique that doubled the amount of suture material used in the mattress technique. A clear relationship was demonstrated between pull-out strength and the number of weaves and suture material used in both methods. They also concluded that the multiple-pass technique grants stronger pull-out resistance per weave than does the mattress suture. The tensile strength of the multiple pass end-weave repairs using 3, 4, or 5 weaves was estimated to be at least 40 N to 50 N. If a moderate contraction produces approximately 15 N of force, the cross-stitch technique using 4 or 5 weaves is likely to support active motion.

When primary repair is unsuccessful, secondary procedures for salvage include tenolysis, in which adhesions are released, and immediate postoperative motion. If the tendon system is not recoverable by lysis (such as in rupture, joint contracture, pulley system disruption, or excessive scarring), salvage can be accomplished by staged tendon reconstruction. A flexible silicone rubber implant is used as a first stage, and is replaced by a tendon graft at a second stage in 3 months. Because of the significant advances in direct repair over the last 15 years, these reconstructive procedures are needed less frequently.

Annotated Bibliography

Acute Injuries

Schenck RR, Lenhart DE: Results of zone II flexor tendon lacerations in civilians treated by the Washington regimen. *J Hand Surg* 1996;21A:984–987.

This review of the results obtained in a civilian application of the Washington regimen of passive flexion—active extension with a palmar pulley is less optimistic than those reported by Chow. Fair or good outcomes were reported by 52% of the patients.

Strickland JW: Flexor tendon injuries: I. Foundations of treatment. *J Am Acad Orthop Surg* 1995;3:44–54.

This is a review of recent and clinically relevant research in flexor tendon surgery, as well as repair techniques and rehabilitation.

Biomechanics of Tendon Repair

Aoki M, Kubota H, Pruitt DL, Manske PR: Biomechanical and histologic characteristics of canine flexor tendon repair using early postoperative mobilization. *J Hand Surg* 1997;22A:107–114.

This in vivo study evaluates the mechanical and histologic healing of flexor tendon repairs using an early active motion protocol. The stronger suture techniques of Savage and the dorsal tendon splint

showed no reduction in ultimate tensile strength when tested during the first 3 weeks of healing, demonstrating the ability to withstand the stress produced by active digital motion protocols. The weaker Kessler repairs ruptured in 8 of 9 specimens.

Aoki M, Manske PR, Pruitt DL, Larson BJ: Work of flexion after tendon repair with various suture methods: A human cadaveric study. *J Hand Surg* 1995;20B:310–313.

This study quantifies the mechanical friction or "work of flexion" before and after tendon repair using the Kessler, Becker, Savage, internal tendon splint, dorsal tendon splint, and external mesh sleeve techniques. Analysis showed that work of flexion increases linearly with the amount of suture material at the repair site. Resistance ranged from 5% for Kessler repairs to 44% for external mesh sleeve repairs.

Diao E, Hariharan JS, Soejima O, Lotz JC: Effect of peripheral suture depth on strength of tendon repairs. *J Hand Surg* 1996;21A:234–239.

Depth of peripheral suture placement was studied to determine its contribution to overall flexor tendon repair strength. Using a modified Kessler core suture, repairs with peripheral sutures placed half the depth to the center of the tendon withstood approximately 80% more distracting force (38.96 N) than those employing superficially placed peripheral sutures (21.68 N).

Evans RB, Thompson DE: The application of force to the healing tendon. *J Hand Ther* 1993;6:266–284.

The authors present a survey of the internal forces applied to a repaired flexor tendon and offer specific guidelines for determining the external load that the repair can withstand. This article presents methods of calculating the stress applied during active mobilization of flexor tendon repairs.

Komanduri M, Phillips CS, Mass DP: Tensile strength of flexor tendon repairs in a dynamic cadaver model. *J Hand Surg* 1996;21A:605–611.

The authors use a dynamic, curvilinear model to more closely approximate the natural forces exerted on a zone 2 flexor tendon repair. Dorsal placement of the core suture demonstrates the ability to withstand significantly more tensile strength than does palmar placement.

Kubota H, Manske PR, Aoki M, Pruitt DL, Larson BJ: Effect of motion and tension on injured flexor tendons in chickens. *J Hand Surg* 1996;21A:456–463.

Isolation of motion and tension components shows that each element exerts a positive effect on flexor profundus repair strength. Histologic evaluation shows the greatest cellular activity from both motion and tension, enhancing the tendon's response to injury with active mobilization protocols.

Pruitt DL, Tanaka H, Aoki M, Manske PR: Cyclic stress testing after in vivo healing of canine flexor tendon lacerations. *J Hand Surg* 1996;21A:974–977.

Flexor tendon repairs underwent in vivo cyclic stress-testing to facilitate observation of gap formation. Strong, repetitive, tensile stress increased gap formation during the 30-day period after repair that was studied.

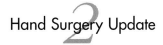
Soejima O, Diao E, Lotz JC, Hariharan JS: Comparative mechanical analysis of dorsal versus palmar placement of core suture for flexor tendon repairs. *J Hand Surg* 1995;20A:801–807.

This in vitro study found a dorsally placed modified Kessler core suture to be 26.5% stronger than a palmarly placed suture, when tested to tensile failure.

Taras JS, Raphael JS, Marczyk SC, et al: Evaluation of suture caliber in flexor tendon repair: Applications for active motion. *Jefferson Orthop J* 1995;24:15–19.

This in vitro study demonstrated that increasing the suture caliber of 2-strand core sutures increased the strength of the repair, while avoiding the technical difficulty encountered in multiple strand repairs.

Wagner WF Jr, Carroll C IV, Strickland JW, Heck DA, Toombs JP: A biomechanical comparison of techniques of flexor tendon repair. *J Hand Surg* 1994;19A:979–983.

The authors presented an in vivo comparison of flexor tendon repairs using the Savage and 2-strand core sutures. The Savage technique is stronger but more technically demanding.

Clinical Series of Flexor Tendon Repair

Elliot D, Moiemen NS, Flemming AF, Harris SB, Foster AJ: The rupture rate of acute flexor tendon repairs mobilized by the controlled active motion regimen. *J Hand Surg* 1994;19B:607–612.

This study tested the safety of controlled active motion after Kessler flexor tendon repair. Small's modified version of the splinting and hand therapy regimen resulted in rupture in 6% of fingers and 17% of thumbs.

Lim BH, Tsai T-M: The six-strand technique for flexor tendon repair, in Taras JS, Schneider LH (eds): *Atlas of the Hand Clinics*. Philadelphia, PA, WB Saunders, 1996, pp 65–77.

The authors present an illustrated description of a 6-strand technique and summarize their postoperative mobilization program for restoring function after zone 2 flexor tendon injuries.

Sandow MJ, McMahon MM: Single-cross grasp six-strand repair for acute flexor tenorrhaphy: Modified Savage Technique, in Taras JS, Schneider LH (eds): *Atlas of the Hand Clinics*. Philadelphia, PA, WB Saunders, 1996, pp 41–64.

The authors present an illustrated description of the single-cross 6-strand (modified Savage) technique for acute flexor tenorrhaphy, and summarize their postoperative mobilization protocol.

Silfverskiöld KL, May EJ: Flexor tendon repair in zone II with a new suture technique and an early mobilization program combining passive and active flexion. *J Hand Surg* 1994;19A:53–60.

This article summarizes a new technique applying an epitendinal circumferential cross-stitch to a modified Kessler core suture. Incorporating this type of repair with a program of early active and passive flexion yielded 90% recovery of motion after zone 2 flexor tendon repair.

Strickland JS: The Indiana method of flexor tendon repair, in Taras JS, Schneider LH (eds): *Atlas of the Hand Clinics*. Philadelphia, PA, WB Saunders, 1996, pp 77–103.

Strickland outlines his preferred method for flexor tendon repair, including scientific rationale, a description of the 2-strand core stitch and running-lock peripheral epitendinous stitch repair technique, and postoperative management.

Taras JS, Skahen JR III, Raphael JS, Marczyk SC, Bauerle WB: The double-grasping and cross-stitch for acute flexor tendon repair, in Taras JS, Schneider LH (eds): *Atlas of the Hand Clinics*. Philadelphia, PA, WB Saunders, 1996, pp 13–27.

The authors describe their technique for zone 2 flexor tendon repair, using a 2-strand core stitch combined with a cross-stitch epitendinous suture. Results are also detailed.

Partial Tendon Laceration

Grewal R, Sotereanos DG, Rao U, Herndon JH, Woo SL: Bundle pattern of the flexor digitorum profundus tendon in zone II of the hand: A quantitative assessment of the size of a laceration. *J Hand Surg* 1996;21A:978–983.

A formula for determining the cross-sectional area of the profundus tendon and the intratendinous bundles at various levels in zone 2 is offered. This formula provides a patient-specific formula by which clinicians can accurately and easily assess the size of a partial tendon laceration.

Tendon Reconstruction—Diagnosis

Le Viet D, Rousselin B, Roulot E, Lantieri L, Godefroy D: Diagnosis of digital pulley rupture by computed tomography. *J Hand Surg* 1996;21A:245–248.

Computed tomography is an adjunct in diagnosing digital pulley rupture. In several cases, hallmark features such as bowstringing or fibrous tissue interposed between the phalanx and the tendon were clearly visible.

Matloub HS, Dzwierzynski WW, Erickson S, Sanger JR, Yousif NJ, Muoneke V: Magnetic resonance imaging scanning in the diagnosis of zone II flexor tendon rupture. *J Hand Surg* 1996;21A:451–455.

MRI differentiated between rupture and adhesion in 11 digits that underwent prior repair with 100% accuracy, compared to 60% accuracy by clinical examination.

Tendon Reconstruction—The Pulley System

Rispler D, Greenwald D, Shumway S, Allan C, Mass D: Efficiency of the flexor tendon pulley system in human cadaver hands. *J Hand Surg* 1996;21A:444–450.

Absence of the A4 produces the largest biomechanically-measured deficit in efficiency of tendon excursion, force generated, and work. The coalition of A2, A3, and A4 preserves both work and excursion efficiency.

Tendon Reconstruction—Grafting

Asencio G, Abihaidar G, Leonardi C: Human composite flexor tendon allografts: A report of two cases. *J Hand Surg* 1996;21B:84–88.

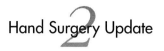

The authors present 2 cases using human composite flexor tendon allografts as an alternative to the more commonly employed 2-stage technique for end-stage flexor tendon reconstruction. Results indicate that composite tendon allografts can restore good function without synovitis, infection, or secondary rupture, and may be considered before amputation in unfavorable cases.

Gabuzda GM, Lovallo JL, Nowak MD: Tensile strength of the end-weave flexor tendon repair: An in vitro biomechanical study. *J Hand Surg* 1994;19B:397–400.

The authors evaluated the tensile strength of the end-weave method of flexor tendon repair, varying the weave technique from 1 to 5 weaves with 2 suture techniques (horizontal mattress suture and cross-stitch). Tensile strength increases linearly with the number of weaves, number of sutures placed to secure the repair, and suture material for each stitch. Results suggest that tendon weaves should be constructed to afford active rehabilitation exercises during the immediate postoperative period.

Naam NH: Staged flexor tendon reconstruction using pedicled tendon graft from the flexor digitorum superficialis. *J Hand Surg* 1997;22A:323–327.

This study details the use of the pedicled flexor digitorum superficialis tendon as a tendon graft in the second stage of flexor tendon reconstruction. Good or excellent results were achieved in 64% of patients.

Noguchi M, Seiler JG III, Boardman ND III, Tramaglini DM, Gelberman RH, Woo L: Tensile properties of canine intrasynovial and extrasynovial flexor tendon autografts. *J Hand Surg* 1997;22A:457–463.

This in vivo study indicates that intrasynovial grafts form fewer adhesions by demonstrating better gliding. Extrasynovial grafts demonstrate greater early strength, perhaps associated with adhesion formation.

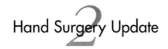
Chapter 15
Extensor Tendon Injuries

Pat L. Aulicino, MD

Introduction

Extension of the digits and wrist is a complex action that is essential for normal hand function. Disruption of the bony architecture, the musculotendinous system, or the integrity of the radial, median, or ulnar nerves will interfere with the delicately balanced mechanism that positions the hand in space and allows it to perform its primary function—prehension. The historic recognition of the importance of the biomechanical systems of grasp has resulted in relegating the treatment of extensor tendon injuries to the least experienced surgeon, who often labors in a less than optimal environment. Emergency rooms often lack adequate assistants, equipment, and sterility to ensure the highest level of care. In addition, these injuries are often composite injuries that have underlying fractures, skin loss, and neurovascular disruption. These complex injuries result in significant scarring between tissue planes, with resultant loss of tendon gliding and associated joint stiffness. The resultant disability usually is not lack of extension, but rather loss of prehension, the primary function of the hand. Secondary procedures, such as tenolysis and capsulotomies to restore flexion, are often necessary in composite injuries.

Recent clinical trials of dynamic extension splinting and early protected motion in selected extensor tendon injuries have been undertaken to decrease the morbidity associated with prolonged immobilization, which has been the traditional postoperative rehabilitation. However, the most important factors in any therapy protocol are a motivated, compliant patient and a capable therapist.

This chapter will deal with isolated acute extensor tendon injuries. Fractures, skin, and nerve injuries will be dealt with in other sections. Wound debridement, rigid internal fixation, bony healing, repair of neurovascular structures, and skin coverage all take precedence over extensor tendon repair.

Anatomy

The extrinsic extensor musculature can be divided into superficial and deep groups. The brachioradialis, extensor carpi radialis longus, extensor carpi radialis brevis, extensor digitorum communis, extensor digiti minimi, extensor carpi ulnaris, and anconeus constitute the superficial group. The supinator, abductor pollicis longus, extensor pollicis brevis, extensor pollicis longus, and extensor indicis proprius are the deep group. Both groups are innervated by the radial nerve. These muscles flex the forearm and extend the wrist, supinate the forearm, and extend the metacarpophalangeal (MCP) joints of the digits.

The lumbricals and the palmar and dorsal interossei abduct and adduct the fingers, flex the MCP joints, and extend the proximal and distal interphalangeal joints. The interossei are innervated by the ulnar nerve. Extension of the digits is accomplished through the synergistic action of both the radial and ulnar innervated musculature. The balance of flexion and extension forces about each joint must be maintained to prevent the collapse of this delicately balanced biomechanical linkage.

The extrinsic extensor muscles become tendinous just proximal to the radiocarpal joint as they enter the hand through 6 discrete fibroosseous compartments. These compartments function as pulleys and prevent bowstringing of the extensor tendons. Loss of a compartment can alter the effective extensor excursion because of vertical displacement of the tendon during attempted extension. This can partially be overcome by wrist flexion, which produces a tenodesis effect.

Because of the minimal clearance in these compartments, degenerative pathologic lesions such as stenosing tenosynovitis may occur. Postoperative or posttraumatic adhesions are frequent in this area.

On the dorsum of the hand, the juncturae tendinum interconnect the extensor tendons proximal to the MCP joints. Although there are usually 3 junctura, they vary in size and shape (Fig. 1). There is also significant variation in the number of extensor tendons themselves. Anomalous muscles such as the extensor digitorum brevis manus are not uncommon.

The anatomy of the extensor tendon on the dorsum of the finger is extremely complex. Although portions of this tendinous system are described as though they were discrete anatomic structures, they are all interconnected and form one complex tendon with multiple insertions. Injuries that affect the function of one portion of the tendon can affect the entire function of the digit (Fig. 2).

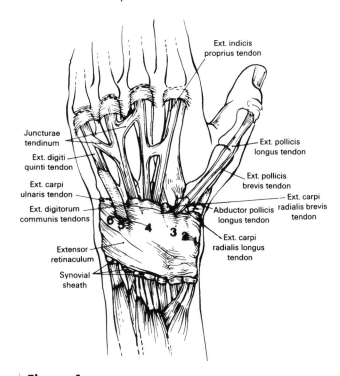

Figure 1

Anatomy of the dorsum of the hand.

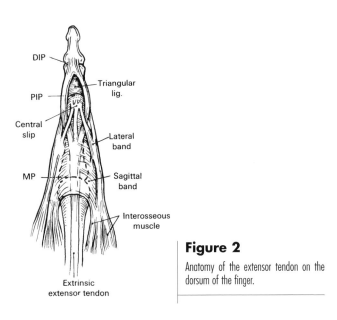

Figure 2

Anatomy of the extensor tendon on the dorsum of the finger.

The extensor tendon is centralized over the MCP joint by the sagittal bands that insert on the volar plate. The sagittal bands provide a support sling for the MCP joint. This support, as well as the attachment of the extensor tendon to the MCP joint capsule, provides MCP joint extension. The lat-

eral bands on each side of the fingers are the tendinous confluence of the termination of the lumbrical and interosseous muscles. The lateral bands join the central tendon at the level of the proximal phalanx, proceed down the digit, and insert on the dorsum of the distal phalanx. The central extensor tendon, which inserts on the dorsum of the midphalanx just distal to the proximal interphalangeal (PIP) joint, is called the central slip. Injuries to the central slip will result in a boutonnière deformity. The lateral bands are stabilized over the PIP joint level by the transverse retinacular ligament, which prevents dorsal subluxation. Dorsal subluxation can result in a swan neck deformity. Distally, the lateral bands are stabilized by the triangular ligament and form the terminal tendon, which inserts on the dorsal aspect of the distal phalanx.

Injuries to the extensor tendons or the stabilizing ligaments will result in loss of motion and deformity. To better categorize these injuries, the extensor tendons have been divided into 8 zones. The odd-numbered zones are located over the joints. Zone I is over the distal interphalangeal (DIP) joint, zone III is over the PIP joint, zone V is over the MCP joint, and zone VII is over the radiocarpal joint. The thumb is numbered differently because of the lesser number of phalanges. TI is over the IP joint; TIII, the MCP joint; and TV, the radiocarpal joint. As with the flexor system, the zone of injury is the level of the tendon injury. The skin wound does not define the zone of injury. The prognosis and treatment of acute extensor tendon injuries will be discussed according to the zone of injury (Fig. 3).

Vascularity of the Extensor Tendons

Extensive studies on the vascular supply of the flexor tendons have greatly influenced surgical technique and placement of sutures. Studies have furthered understanding of the healing process of flexor tendons and influenced postoperative therapy. However, only a few articles have investigated the vascular supply and nutrient pathways of extensor tendons.

Diffusion and perfusion of extensor tendons has been studied in young adult monkeys. It has been found that the synovial diffusion was the major nutrient pathway to the digital and radial wrist extensors beneath the extensor retinaculum. Anatomic studies in human cadavers found 3 distinct zones of vascularization. The first was provided by branches of numerous muscular arteries. In the second zone, under the extensor retinaculum, the vessels reached the tendons through mesotendons. Synovial nutrition and diffusion have greater importance in this region. The third zone is distal to the retinaculum, and the tendons in this area are

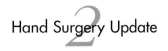

sor tendon reconstruction. Tissue equilibrium and full mobility of joints should also be achieved before tendon transfer or tendon grafting. In severe injuries involving the fourth dorsal compartment tendons, a functional hand occasionally can result without extensor tendon reconstruction. Subdermal scar may result in MCP joint extension that will improve over time.

When there is isolated tendon loss, side-to-side transfer may be adequate to restore finger extension. When 2 tendons are lost, the extensor indicis proprius may be transferred without loss of independent extension of the index finger. If multiple tendons are lost, intercalated grafts or tendon transfers may be necessary.

Suture Technique

The biomechanical characteristics of extensor tendon suture in zone VI have been studied extensively. Mattress, figure-of-8, modified Bunnell, and modified Kessler sutures have all been compared in relationship to the degree of shortening and subsequent loss of PIP joint and MCP joint flexion with each technique. All techniques were considerably weaker than results achieved in repair of flexor tendons, and they all produced significant shortening and loss of motion. The Kleinert modification of the Bunnell technique was the strongest, followed by the modified Kessler. Significantly weaker repairs were obtained using mattress and figure-of-8 techniques.

The excursion of the extensor digitorum communis tendon is approximately 50 mm, whereas the flexor digitorum profundus has an excursion of 70 mm. The extensors of the fingers, therefore, are less tolerant to any degree of shortening. Because of the flattened shape of the tendons, there is a marked propensity for them to bunch during tenorrhaphy. This shortening inevitably results in restriction of MCP joint and PIP joint flexion. This is why the average loss of flexion has been greater than the average loss of extension after extensor tenorrhaphy. It has been reported that the average shortening ranged from 6.8 mm with the Kleinert modification of the Bunnell technique to 5.3 mm with the figure-of-8 technique. The ideal suture technique, which would produce minimal shortening and maximum tensile strength, has not yet been devised. It is extremely important not to shorten the extensor tendons excessively because they have limited excursion to overcome this shortening. The interconnections between the junctura tendini also limit excursion of adjacent tendons in fingers that were not affected by the trauma, as the result of a dorsal "quadriga" effect.

In zones I through VI, suture placement should attempt to produce an anatomic repair. Excessive shortening or scar

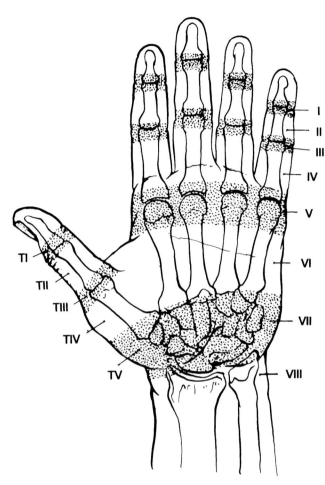

Figure 3
Extensor tendon zones of the digits and thumb.

supplied by arterial branches from the paratenon. The significance and clinical relevance of the blood supply and nutrition of extensor tendons remain to be determined. Because of the flat shape and varying thickness in contour of the extensor tendons, placement of suture material is determined by the tendinous anatomy as opposed to its vascular supply.

Complex Injuries

Injuries that involve substantial loss of bone or overlying skin, such as high-velocity gunshot wounds to the hand, should be treated in the same way as all complex wounds. Irrigation and debridement are paramount. Skeletal stabilization and skin coverage should be obtained. All bone grafts, flaps, or skin grafts should be done before undertaking exten-

elongation should be avoided. Nonabsorbable 4-0 or 5-0 sutures will hold the tendon in an anatomic position; however, it is the postoperative splinting or the transarticular Kirschner wire (K-wire) at the DIP or PIP joint that prevents rupture of the repair.

Nonabsorbable 4-0 sutures usually are sufficient in strength in zones VI and VII. Repair of the fibrous raphe in zone VIII is best accomplished with 3-0 nonabsorbable suture. Epimysial invagination should be performed without strangulation of the muscle, which would cause further necrosis. Small tapered needles in zones VI and VII prevent longitudinal shredding of the tendon, which can occur when cutting needles are used. There is, however, a tendency for the repair to bunch and shorten when a tapered needle is used. Approximation of the tendon ends without gapping and without excessive shortening is the goal. Passive flexion should be tested on completion of the repair. In zone VII, retinacular excision with or without transposition may be performed. In zone VIII injuries, if possible, the forearm fascia should be repaired. If this is not possible, the fascia should be opened proximally and distally to prevent symptomatic muscle herniation.

Rehabilitation

Recent advances using dynamic extension splints and controlled early mobilization have improved the functional outcome of complex injuries. The primary goal of early controlled mobilization is to restore tendon glide and joint motion in the face of an untidy, complex wound. A competent therapist and motivated patient are the primary requirements. Unfortunately, many patients with these types of injuries are not compliant and often are unable to cooperate. Managed care also often limits patients' access to qualified hand surgeons and therapists. In an ideal world, early controlled motion for complex injuries would be the treatment of choice.

Injuries in zones I and II require immobilization of the DIP joint in extension for 6 to 8 weeks. After this period of full-time immobilization, night splinting for another month often is required. The duration of splinting is determined by the nature of the injury and the chronicity of the injury at the time of treatment. Early mobilization of uninvolved joints proximal to the site of injury is very important. Injuries in zones III and IV, which may result in a boutonnière deformity, have been historically treated with prolonged immobilization of the PIP joint in extension, often with a transarticular K-wire. Recent reports of dynamic splinting of these injuries have shown improved results. However, it is very important to follow these protocols vigilantly. Even small (2 to 3 mm) scar elongations of the tendon will result in a residual loss of extension. Under the worst case scenario,

the patient may wind up with a rigid boutonnière deformity, which is an extremely difficult problem to correct. However, anatomic repair of an acute open boutonnière deformity followed by a transarticular K-wire for 6 weeks and then an aggressive range of motion program will usually result in a satisfactory outcome. During the period of immobilization, the DIP joint and the MCP joint should be actively mobilized. The same protocol is followed with closed acute boutonnière deformities.

Acute zone V injuries are characteristically caused by the well-known closed fist injury or "fight bite." These are usually incomplete tendon injuries that do not need immobilization. Irrigation and debridement of the tendon, MCP joint, and articular head of the metacarpal make up the initial treatment. Prophylactic antibiotics must be used to prevent the dreaded sequelae of a septic joint and osteomyelitis of the metacarpal head. Repair of the tendons and wound closure in zone V under these conditions is contraindicated. Early active motion should be encouraged.

Zone I Extensor Tendon Injuries

Injuries to the terminal tendon will result in loss of extension of the DIP joint. If the patient has lax ligaments the combination of proximal migration of the extensor hood with increased extensor force at the PIP joint and laxity of the volar plate may result in a secondary swan neck deformity. The loss of extension at the DIP joint has been termed a "mallet finger" deformity. This injury may be associated with an intra-articular fracture or may be the result of a closed tendon avulsion or open laceration. In skeletally immature individuals, the mallet deformity often represents an open Salter type II fracture.

The treatment of a mallet finger depends on the mechanism of injury, the age of the patient, associated fractures, the presence of preexisting osteoarthritic changes, and the duration of the deformity (Fig. 4). Closed acute mallet fracture deformities are best treated by continuous splinting in extension for at least 6 to 8 weeks. The splint may be placed either dorsally or volarly, as long as the DIP joint is maintained in full extension. It is often better to alternate the placement of the splint to prevent skin maceration and necrosis. Active motion of the PIP joint should be instituted immediately. After 6 to 8 weeks of continuous splint immobilization, the patient may be slowly weaned from the splint. If extensor lag recurs during this period, full-time splinting is reinstituted. The patient should then be night splinted for at least 6 weeks.

If performed properly, closed treatment will yield results that are superior to any open treatment and have less

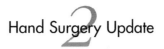

attendant risk. The use of a buried transarticular K-wire has been advocated for certain individuals, such as health-care personnel. A transarticular K-wire, however, is not totally innocuous. Breakage of the wire, pin tract infections with subsequent osteomyelitis, and chondrolysis and joint stiffness are not unusual complications. The patient must be totally compliant to be treated in this fashion. Open repair of the tendon, in a closed injury, usually is indicated only for failure of conservative treatment. Chronic mallet deformities that are up to 12 weeks old, provided they are flexible, may also respond very well to the closed treatment protocol. Failure of a chronic closed mallet deformity to respond to this treatment protocol may be an indication for advancement of the terminal tendon to bone with an associated dermadesis and a transarticular K-wire. In the stiff mallet deformity, or one associated with any degree of osteoarthritis, arthrodesis may be the most viable option.

Chronic mallet deformities associated with significant swan neck deformities, which cause locking or snapping on attempted PIP joint flexion, may be treated by restoring the balance of the DIP joint and PIP joint using a spiral oblique retinacular ligament reconstruction or a superficialis tenodesis. The ligament reconstruction is a complex surgical procedure that is technically challenging and fraught with many potential complications. It should be performed only on young patients with supple, yet significant, deformities of both the DIP and PIP joints. Minor degrees of a swan neck deformity often respond to treatment directed only at the mallet deformity (Fig. 5).

Mallet fractures should be treated in a closed fashion with extension splinting until healed. Some authors suggest that when the DIP joint is subluxed volarly or the fracture involves greater than 30% to 50% of the articular surface, open reduction is indicated. Wehbe and Schneider felt that even in the presence of subluxation, good results could be obtained by closed treatment. Fractures without subluxation of the joint and with less than 30% articular involvement respond well to closed treatment. A small dorsal hump may result with this treatment; however, the articular surface often remodels, and most patients regain nearly full painless range of motion over time (Fig. 6).

Open reduction and internal fixation of a DIP joint intra-articular fracture is technically difficult and rarely indicated. If a surgeon attempts this, the goal should be an anatomic reduction. The type of

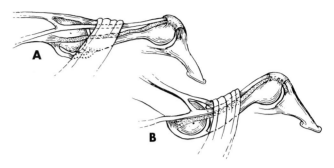

Figure 4

A, Closed ligamentous mallet deformity without secondary swan neck deformity. **B,** Ligamentous mallet deformity associated with laxity of the volar plate and dorsal subluxation of lateral bands resulting in a secondary swan neck deformity.

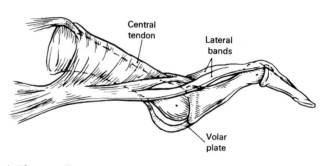

Figure 5

Chronic mallet deformity with significant swan neck deformity, which may cause locking or snapping upon attempted proximal interphalangeal joint flexion. This may be treated by superficialis tenodesis or with a spiral oblique retinacular ligament reconstruction to rebalance the digit.

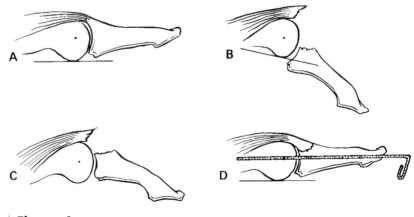

Figure 6

A, Normal distal interphalangeal joint alignment. **B,** Mallet fracture with volar subluxation. **C,** Mallet fracture without subluxation. This injury is best treated with closed splinting. The mallet fracture with volar subluxation can be treated closed (**D**); open treatment is rarely indicated.

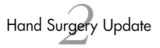
fixation, whether it be K-wire, tension band, screw, or otherwise, is determined by the fracture pattern and the experience of the surgeon. Early motion is not usually possible. Even with anatomic reduction, splinting or a transarticular K-wire often is still necessary.

Zone II Extensor Tendon Injuries

Zone II injuries distal to the insertion of the central slip may result in a mallet deformity if there is a complete transection of the tendon. If this occurs, the treatment protocol is the same as for zone I injuries. This open injury is treated with anatomic repair of the tendon and transarticular fixation of the DIP joint in full extension for 6 to 8 weeks. Partial tendon injuries can be treated with early motion without tendon repair, provided there is no extensor lag at the DIP joint.

Fractures of the middle phalanx are often associated with zone II tendon injuries. In these open crush injuries, the treatment is dictated by the fracture pattern. Concomitant fracture fixation and tendon repair often result in tendon adhesions and DIP joint extension contractures. Tenolysis and capsulotomy may be necessary.

Zone III Extensor Tendon Injuries

The most significant and disabling zone III injury is disruption of the central slip, which can result in volar displacement of the lateral bands. The loss of balance results in a loss of extension at the PIP joint and a secondary hyperextension deformity at the DIP joint. These injuries may be classified as acute or chronic, open or closed, or with associated fractures (Fig. 7).

Open acute lacerations of the central slip should be treated with irrigation and debridement of the joint. Repair of the central slip supplemented with a transarticular K-wire for at least 6 weeks is recommended. Active range of motion of the DIP joint and MCP joint should be instituted early.

A closed acute central slip injury should be treated with extension splinting of the PIP joint with or without a transarticular K-wire followed by early DIP and MCP joint motion. Dynamic splinting of these injuries is advocated by some, but it is not universally accepted at this time.

Acute injuries associated with fractures should be treated in a similar manner. Fracture fixation and/or excision of the fragment with reattachment of the central slip depends on the size of the fracture. The postoperative protocol is the same as with acute tendon injuries.

Chronic boutonnière deformities may be flexible or rigid. If rigid, the flexion contracture should be splinted straight with either a dynamic splint or serial finger casts. This treatment should continue until full passive extension is restored to the PIP joint and full active motion is present at the DIP joint. Then, anatomic reconstruction of the central slip can be done by excising the scar tendon and reattaching the central slip. Usually, only 2 to 3 mm of scar tendon are excised. This procedure should be done under local anesthesia with sedation so that the balance between the lateral bands and the repaired central slip can be evaluated actively at surgery. There must be proper balance of the tendons to allow full extension and flexion at the PIP and DIP joints. Once balance has been restored, the PIP joint is immobilized with a transarticular K-wire. Active DIP and MCP joint motion are instituted immediately (Fig. 8).

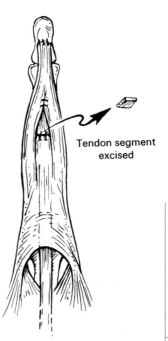

Tendon segment excised

Figure 8

Anatomic reconstruction of the chronic boutonnière deformity is performed by excising a 2- to 3-mm segment from the scarred central tendon. Balance must be maintained between the lateral bands and the central slip. Transarticular Kirschner wire fixation is required for 6 weeks after this procedure.

Figure 7

Central slip disruption results in volar displacement of the lateral bands. The resulting imbalance causes loss of extension at the proximal interphalangeal joint and hyperextension deformity at the distal interphalangeal joint.

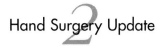

If the flexion contracture of the PIP joint cannot be splinted straight, the prognosis is poor for return of normal function. One option is to perform 2 separate surgical procedures—a volar release to restore passive extension is followed by a subsequent anatomic reconstruction of the central slip after the finger has regained full passive motion.

Salvage procedures, such as tenotomy of the terminal slip to restore DIP joint motion while accepting the PIP joint contracture, is a viable alternative, especially in a patient who does heavy manual labor. This procedure seems to work best on the ulnar aspect of the hand in the fourth and fifth digits because DIP flexion is important in power grip.

Reconstruction of the central slip with free tendon grafts and dorsal suturing of the lateral bands are also salvage procedures that can be used when tendon substance is absent. Results are unpredictable, and joint arthrodesis may be a better alternative in some severe injuries.

Zone IV Extensor Tendon Injuries

Zone IV tendon lacerations may be partial or complete. Partial lacerations of the tendon are repaired, and early protected active motion can be instituted provided the integrity of the tendon repair would not be at risk. Complete lacerations in zone IV are unusual because of the width of the tendon. If there is a complete laceration, then the tendon should be repaired, and the injury may be treated with either static splinting of the PIP joint in full extension or dynamic extension splinting and controlled active flexion. Underlying fractures are often associated with tendon injuries at this level. Because of the large size of the proximal phalanx, rigid internal fixation can usually be done. If possible, early active motion or dynamic extension splinting should be used in these composite injuries.

Zone V Extensor Tendon Injuries

The 2 most common injuries at zone V are the human "fight bite" and the closed rupture of the sagittal band. Closed rupture of the sagittal band may result in recurrent subluxation of the extensor tendon into the ulnar gutter at the MCP joint level.

Fight bite extensor injuries are usually partial injuries and should not be repaired. Cultures, appropriate antibiotic coverage, surgical debridement, and early range of motion are the treatments of choice. Early active motion and/or dynamic extension splinting associated with wound care will allow the skin wound and tendon to heal by secondary intention. Complications of this injury result from articular damage, septic arthritis, and possible osteomyelitis. The extensor injury is usually inconsequential.

Blunt injury to the MCP joints may result in traumatic rupture of the radial sagittal band. This usually occurs in the middle finger. There is a lack of MCP joint extension, and the tendon often can be passively centralized by passively extending the digit and forcing the tendon into a radial direction. Active flexion will produce a painful snap of the tendon into the ulnar gutter. If the diagnosis is made acutely, and the MCP joints are immobilized in extension for 6 weeks with the tendon centralized, this injury may heal nonsurgically. However, the diagnosis is often delayed, and surgical repair is required. Repair of the torn radial sagittal band, augmented with either a free tendon graft or a distal based flap of the ulnar side of the extensor tendon to reinforce the repair, will centralize the tendon and may allow early protected range of motion. This operation should be performed under local anesthesia with sedation to make sure that the tendon is stabilized and full motion is obtained. A posterior splint is used for 3 weeks. Heavy lifting and twisting motions should be avoided for 6 to 8 weeks postoperatively. Buddy strapping of the repaired digit to the index finger will also help stabilize the repair after the splint is removed.

Zone VI Extensor Tendon Injuries

Zone VI, proximal to the MCP joint and distal to the extensor retinaculum, can be subdivided into the area of the junctura tendini and the area proximal to it. Acute lacerations to the extensor tendon proximal to the junctura tendini result in retraction of the proximal stump of the extensor tendon, making repair technically more difficult. Injuries through the junctura tendini are easier to retrieve but may be difficult to diagnose because of the minimal extensor lag at the MCP joints associated with such injuries.

The tendons are very superficial in zone VI and are covered only with paratenon and thin subcutaneous tissue. Full-thickness loss of skin is not uncommon in this area and may require skin grafting or rotational or distant flaps for coverage. In the presence of significant skin injury, tendon adherence may occur, but this usually can be managed with postoperative therapy.

Zone VII Extensor Tendon Injuries

Zone VII has the worst prognosis of the proximal extensor tendon injuries. The extensor retinaculum consists of 2 layers, the supratendinous and the infratendinous. The infratendinous layer is limited to the fourth, fifth, and sixth dorsal compartments. The supratendinous layer inserts by 6 septa into the distal radius. The retinacular tunnels are narrow, and stenosing tenosynovitis is common, even in the absence of significant injury. Injuries of the extensor tendons at this level usually produce mass healing of tendons with adherence to the underlying joint capsule and surrounding retinaculum, resulting in limitation of excursion of the extensor tendons. The resultant limitation of finger flexion with wrist flexion can be very disabling. Limitation of wrist motion, as well as limitation of finger extension with wrist extension also may result.

Retinacular excision or transposition often is required at the time of repair. An attempt should be made to retain some retinaculum, either proximal or distal to this region, especially in the fourth dorsal compartment to prevent subsequent bowstringing and loss of extension. Sometimes, this is not possible.

The dorsal sensory branches of the ulnar and radial nerves often are injured when extensor tendons are injured at this level. Epineural repair can be performed in an attempt to prevent symptomatic neuroma formation. The surgeon may elect to resect the nerve as an alternative technique. The proximal stump of the injured nerve should be resected and allowed to retract or be buried proximal to the radiocarpal joint to prevent a painful contact.

Zone VIII Extensor Injuries

Zone VIII can be divided into the area of musculotendinous origin distal to the point of motor innervation and the proximal third of the forearm at the level of the posterior interosseous nerve. Injuries in zone VIII often are underestimated. The skin laceration may be small and hide multiple tendon injuries. The wound must be enlarged, and the central fibrous raphe that enters the muscle from each tendon must be exposed. Central core sutures of the tendon through this raphe are necessary to provide continuity of the musculotendinous junction. The posterior interosseous nerve branches, if lacerated, should be repaired if possible. The prognosis for reinnervation is good because of the close proximity of the injury to the motor points. At times, repair is not possible, and a decision to proceed with primary tendon transfers is made based on the nature of the wound and the experience of the surgeon.

Extensor Tendon Injuries of the Thumb

The extensor tendon injuries of the thumb are divided into five zones. Zone I is over the interphalangeal joint, zone II is over the proximal phalanx, zone III is over the MCP joint,

and zone IV is proximal to the MCP joint and distal to the third dorsal compartment and extensor retinaculum. Zone V courses around Lister's tubercle to the level of the musculotendinous origin.

Zone TI and TII injuries can result in mallet deformities of the thumb. These are treated in a similar fashion to that of the digits. If open tenorrhaphy is performed, the interphalangeal joint is maintained in extension with a transarticular K-wire. MCP and carpometacarpal motion is encouraged as soon as possible. If an intra-articular fracture is associated with loss of extension, it should be treated with static extension splinting. If the fragment is large and a significant portion of the articular surface, open reduction and internal fixation are required with the proper immobilization time for healing of the fracture fragment.

Zone TIII injuries of the extensor pollicis brevis and extensor pollicis longus are treated with tendon repair and joint immobilization. The thumb and wrist should be splinted in extension, and the thumb should also be placed in adduction. After 6 weeks, aggressive mobilization is instituted. Closed injuries to the extensor pollicis brevis at this level are associated with avulsions of the dorsal capsule and the radial collateral ligamentous complex. If the injury is recognized early, the thumb should be immobilized in a thumb spica cast to permit healing of the dorsal radial ligamentous complex.

The extensor pollicis longus tendon may be injured by laceration or spontaneous rupture in zones TIV and TV. Zone TIV is proximal to the MCP joint and distal to the third dorsal compartment and the extensor retinaculum. The tendon in zone TV courses around Lister's tubercle and is intrasynovial. Just proximal to the retinaculum is the musculotendinous origin of the extensor pollicis longus tendon. The extensor pollicis longus may be injured acutely by laceration or closed rupture. Acute laceration may involve simultaneous injuries to the first and second dorsal compartments as well as the dorsal sensory branches of the radial nerve. Acute repairs in zones TIV and TV should be performed with 3-0 or 4-0 nonabsorbable sutures, using the Kleinert modification of the Bunnell technique with minimal shortening of the tendon. In zone TV, the tendon should be released from the extensor retinaculum to prevent adhesions. Postoperative treatment for simple lacerations involves thumb spica casting for 4 to 6 weeks with MCP and interphalangeal joints in 0° of extension. The thumb should be adducted and extended at the carpometacarpal joint and the wrist extended approximately 30°. If the wound is complex or untidy, controlled early mobilization and dynamic extension splinting may be used.

Lacerations of the abductor pollicis longus and extensor pollicis brevis in the first dorsal compartment are repaired

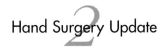
with 3 or 4 nonabsorbable sutures. It is important to release the first dorsal compartment on its dorsal aspect to prevent tendinous adhesions. Immobilization of the wrist and thumb in extension and adduction is also recommended.

Duplay, in 1876, first described closed rupture of the extensor pollicis longus tendon in a patient who fell and sustained a hand injury without fracture. Dums, in 1896, described the rupture of the extensor pollicis longus tendon as a result of chronic tenosynovitis, and coined the term "Drummer Boy's Palsy." Closed rupture of the extensor pollicis longus secondary to a nondisplaced Colles' fracture is a rare, but well recognized, entity. The cause of this injury is still debated. Attritional rupture caused by the fracture site and ischemia secondary to hemorrhage within the intact tendon sheath are the 2 most commonly accepted theories. Regardless of the cause, this tendon rupture can be disabling. It is usually noted 6 to 8 weeks after the fracture and is often anxiety-producing for both the surgeon and the patient.

Loss of interphalangeal extension, adduction, and retropulsion of the thumb are apparent. Direct repair usually is not possible. Intercalated tendon grafting may be performed; however, extensor indicis proprius-to-extensor pollicis longus tendon transfer yields excellent results with no donor site morbidity. The extensor hood at the MCP joint may need repair to maintain independent full extension of the index finger postoperatively.

Postoperative immobilization for 4 weeks with the thumb extended and adducted and the wrist extended to approximately 30° is used. The older patient may be immobilized for a shorter time to prevent joint stiffness. Tenodesis exercises are then performed for approximately 2 weeks after immobilization. At 6 to 8 weeks, the transfer can be used fully. This procedure is simple, and the result usually is gratifying.

Complications of Extensor Tendon Repair

The outcome of extensor tendon injuries on the dorsum of the hand and the forearm varies with the type of injury. Complex injuries with multiple fractures, skin loss, and associated nerve injuries have a much worse prognosis than simple lacerations. The most common complication after extensor tendon repair is adhesion formation, with secondary loss of flexion. Extensor tenolysis and joint capsulotomy can be performed after an adequate trial of hand therapy. Failure to regain motion and associated functional impairment are indications for tenolysis. Tenolysis is best done under local anesthesia with sedation. Dense adhesions often exist between the subcutaneous tissue and extensor tendon, as well as between the extensor tendons and the underlying periosteum and joint

capsule. Immediate active motion is necessary to maintain the motion obtained at the time of tenolysis.

Summary

The results of repair of extensor tendons in the hand and thumb vary with the degree of associated injury. Shortening of the tendon should be minimized at the time of repair. Dynamic extension splinting may help improve results in the compliant patient. The most frequent complication is loss of joint flexion secondary to tendon adhesions. The more complex the wound, the greater the indication for dynamic extension splinting with early controlled active mobilization.

Annotated Bibliography

Anatomy

Wehbe MA: Anatomy of the extensor mechanism of the hand and wrist. *Hand Clin* 1995;11:361–366.

The extensor musculotendinous anatomy from the origin to insertion is described in detail.

Wehbe MA: Junctura anatomy. *J Hand Surg* 1992;17A: 1124–1129.

The author reports 3 types of junctura from detailed dissections of 240 cadaver hands. The 3 types were fascia, ligament and tendon; each hand had 3 juncturae. The most frequent presentation was for the 3 juncturae to be fascia to ligament to tendon, from radial to ulnar.

Boutonnière Deformity

Coons MS, Green SM: Boutonniere deformity. *Hand Clin* 1995; 11:387–402.

The authors present an in-depth review of the treatment of all types of boutonnière deformities. A useful treatment algorithm is presented.

Massengill JB: The boutonniere deformity. *Hand Clin* 1992;8: 787–801.

The author reviews the pathophysiology and treatment of the acute and chronic boutonnière deformity. Various surgical techniques for the late reconstruction of the chronic boutonnière deformity are described. The distinction between the pseudo and the true boutonnière deformities is explained.

Meadows SE, Schneider LH, Sherwyn JH: Treatment of the chronic boutonniere deformity by extensor tenotomy. *Hand Clin* 1995;11:441–447.

The authors present the technique and results of extensor tenotomy of the terminal slip as a salvage procedure for treatment of the chronic

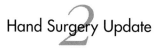

boutonnière deformity. This procedure was originally credited to Fowler and published by Dolphin. The procedure is better indicated in the ulnar digits to restore power grip. The fixed hyperextension deformity may be transformed into a mild mallet deformity.

Extensor Tenolysis

Uhl RL: Salvage of extensor tendon function with tenolysis and joint release. *Hand Clin* 1995;11:461–470.

Extensor tenolysis and joint release under local anesthesia with sedation is described in detail. Postoperative management as well as salvage techniques are discussed.

Mallet Finger

Brzezienski MA, Schneider LH: Extensor tendon injuries at the distal interphalangeal joint. *Hand Clin* 1995;11:373–386.

The authors reviewed the epidemiology, anatomy, and surgical and nonsurgical treatment of the ligamentous mallet injury. Salvage techniques as well as complications of treatment are discussed.

Garberman SF, Diao E, Peimer CA: Mallet finger: Results of early versus delayed closed treatment. *J Hand Surg* 1994; 19A:850–852.

The authors retrospectively compared 2 populations of 40 patients with soft-tissue and bony mallet finger whose treatment was initiated within 2 weeks (early) or more than 2 weeks (delayed) after trauma. The results of both groups were good. The success rate was equivalent to or better than results previously reported for patients surgically treated.

Wehbe MA, Schneider LH: Mallet fractures. *J Bone Joint Surg* 1984;66A:658–669.

Forty-four mallet fractures in 160 mallet injuries, 13 of which had volar subluxation of the distal phalanx, were treated by splinting because the authors believe restoration of joint congruity does not influence the end result. Joint remodeling occurred and led to a near-normal painless joint even in the presence of persistent joint subluxation.

Rehabilitation

Evans RB: Immediate active short arc motion following extensor tendon repair. *Hand Clin* 1995;11:483–512.

The author presents an in-depth review of the immediate short arc motion for repaired zone III and IV injuries. A combined passive and active program for zones V, VI, VII, TIV, and TV is also described. This article is "state of the art" hand therapy for extensor tendon injuries.

Saldana MJ, Choban S, Westerbeck P, Schacherer TG: Results of acute zone III extensor tendon injuries, treated with dynamic extension splinting. *J Hand Surg* 1991;16A:1145–1150.

The authors present their results and technique for the treatment of extensor tendon lacerations in zone III. They describe a rehabilitation technique for micromotion of the repaired central slip.

Review Articles

Newport ML: Extensor tendon injuries in the hand. *J Am Acad Orthop Surg* 1997;5:59–66.

This review article details the evaluation and treatment of extensor tendon injuries. Evaluation, treatment options, surgical technique, and postoperative rehabilitation options are covered in detail.

Swan Neck Deformity

Thompson JS, Littler JW, Upton J: The spiral oblique retinacular ligament (SORL). *J Hand Surg* 1978;3A:482–487.

The authors describe a procedure for reconstruction of the oblique retinacular ligament using a tendon graft in a spiral fashion to act as a dynamic tenodesis to restore DIP joint extension and restrict PIP joint hyperextension. This method is used in the posttraumatic swan neck deformity or mallet deformity. This procedure is a modification of the oblique retinacular ligament reconstruction using the lateral band originally described by Littler.

Suture Technique

Newport ML, Williams CD: Biomechanical characteristics of extensor tendon suture techniques. *J Hand Surg* 1992;17A: 1117–1123.

This study investigated tendon shortening and strength with 4 different repair techniques. Average shortening ranged from 6.8 mm with the Kleinert modification of the Bunnell technique to 5.3 mm with the figure-of-8 technique. The Kleinert modification of the Bunnell technique was the strongest followed by the modified Kessler. Significantly weaker results were obtained with the mattress and figure-of-8 techniques.

Vascularity of the Extensor Tendons

Gajisin S, Zbrodowski A: Vascular anatomy of the digital extensors. *Ann Chir Main* 1986;5:105–112.

This human cadaver study demonstrated 3 distinct zones of vascularization. The first was provided by numerous muscular arteries. The second zone, under the extensor retinaculum, revealed that vessels reached the tendons through mesotendons. Synovial nutrition and diffusion have greater importance in this region. The third zone, distal to the retinaculum, is supplied by arterial branches from the paratenon.

Manske PR, Ogata K, Lesker PA: Nutrient pathways to extensor tendons of primates. *J Hand Surg* 1985;10B:8–10.

The nutrient pathway of primate extensor tendons was investigated using the hydrogen wash-out technique. Synovial diffusion appeared to provide 72% of nutrition to the digital extensor tendon and all nutrition to the wrist extensor tendons.

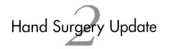

Chapter 16
Tendon Transfers

Waldo E. Floyd III, MD

Introduction

Tendon transfer involves the relocation of functioning muscle and tendon to replace injured or poorly functioning muscle, thereby providing a more equitable distribution of forces in a disabled limb. Tendon transfers may be useful in many conditions, including paralysis due to trauma or disease, cerebral palsy, rheumatoid arthritis, spinal cord injury, or ischemic necrosis. This chapter will review the general principles of tendon transfer and its application in management of peripheral nerve injury and paralytic disease.

Principles of Tendon Transfer

The fundamental principle of tendon transfer is that the recipient musculotendinous unit is more important to limb function than the donor unit. Alternatives to tendon transfer include free muscle transfer, neurorrhaphy, intercalary tendon graft, tenodesis, tendon lengthening, and arthrodesis. Functional restoration using free microneurovascular muscle transfer may be indicated following severe forearm muscle trauma when tendon transfer is not an option. There may be no musculotendinous units available to restore digital flexion or extension following replantation, Volkmann's ischemic contracture, or electrical injuries. The gracilis is the most commonly used muscle for these purposes. The choice between neurorrhaphy and tendon transfer will vary with the clinical circumstances. A younger patient with an uncomplicated radial nerve transection is managed optimally with nerve repair, while an elderly patient with segmental loss of the radial nerve may do better with early tendon transfer. Attritional rupture of the extensor pollicus longus (EPL) tendon associated with a nondisplaced Colle's fracture may be managed with either intercalary palmaris longus tendon graft or tendon transfer of the extensor indicis proprius (EIP) to the EPL. Tenodesis or arthrodesis are alternatives to tendon transfer in relatively simple as well as more complicated settings. Control of the thumb interphalangeal and index distal interphalangeal joints lost consequent to anterior interosseous nerve paralysis may be managed with either arthrodeses,

tenodeses, or tendon transfers. Functions requiring restoration may exceed the number of muscles available for transfer in combined nerve deficits. The reconstructive plan may require selective use of tendon transfer, tenodesis, and arthrodesis. In selected cases, lengthening of the flexor pollicus longus (FPL) at the wrist for reconstruction of distal segmental loss of this tendon may be preferable to transfer of a flexor digitorum superficialis (FDS) or free tendon graft.

The optimal donor tendon is one that is functioning and expendable. The work capacity and the potential amplitude or excursion of the muscle should be appropriate for its new function (Fig. 1). Muscle force is a measure of the pressure exerted by a contracting muscle. Muscle force is directly related to the physiologic or transverse cross-sectional area of a muscle, and is independent of the length or excursion of the muscle. The work capacity of a muscle refers to the ability of the muscle to exert its force over a distance. The work capacity of a muscle is a function of both cross-sectional area and muscle fiber length, and is directly proportional to muscle mass.

The functional purpose of the transfer is the key determinant of donor tendon selection. Tendon transfers for thumb or digital positioning, for example, require less force than those powering grasp. Strength of the selected donor also depends on the force of the antagonist muscle. Recognition of this important relationship can prevent under- or over-correction with resultant deformity.

The amplitude or potential excursion of a transferred tendon must also be appropriate for its new task. The potential excursion of a musculotendinous unit is the sum of the difference between excursion length with applied traction and resting length and the difference between resting length and length at full muscle contraction. Because these distances are usually equal, the total excursion of a muscle from its resting length to its maximum excursion with traction multiplied by 2 determines the muscle amplitude. Among forearm extrinsic muscle, the flexor digitorum profundus (FDP) and FDS have the greatest amplitude—7.0 cm and 6.5 cm. The digital extensors have an amplitude of 5.0 cm; the wrist flexors and extensors, 3 to 4 cm; and the brachioradialis, 3 cm. Wrist motion, through the tenodesis effect, may increase the effective amplitude of a muscle tendon unit by 2.5 cm.

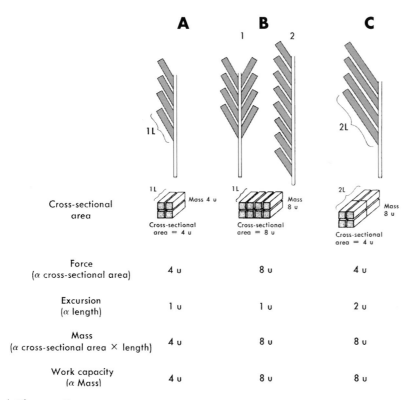

Figure 1

A, A unipennate muscle with a fiber length of 1 and physiologic cross-sectional area of 4. Amplitude is proportional to its fiber length of 1. Potential force of the muscle is proportional to its cross-sectional area of 4. Work capacity is proportional to the mass; the cross-sectional area (4) multiplied by the length (1) equals mass of 4 × 1 = 4. **B,** A bipennate and a unipennate muscle with fiber lengths equal to that of muscle in A, but with twice the cross-sectional area. The potential force of muscle in B is twice that of muscle in A. The amplitude of muscle in B is equal to the one in A. The work capacity of muscle in B is double the muscle in A. **C,** Muscle with the same cross-sectional area as A but twice the fiber length. Potential force of muscle in C is equal to muscle in A, and half of muscle in B. Its work capacity is twice that of muscle in A, and equal to B. (Reproduced with permission from Smith RJ, Hastings H II: Principles of tendon transfers to the hand, in American Academy of Orthopaedic Surgeons *Instructional Course Lectures XXIX.* St. Louis, MO, CV Mosby, 1980, pp 129–152.)

Generally, tendon transfers should follow as straight a route as possible. The functional integrity of a transfer should be redirected so that the transferred musculotendinous unit has but one function. Tendon transfers that are in phase with their new function are synergistic, and the new function is easily learned. Synergistic muscles contract simultaneously to achieve a desired function. The wrist extensors and digital flexors, for example, simultaneously contract when making a fist; therefore, transfer of the extensor carpi radialis longus (ECRL) to the flexor digitorum profundi is an in-phase or synergistic transfer. Transfer of the FDS to extensor digitorum communis would be an out-of-phase transfer; the new function may prove difficult to learn.

Only expendable tendons should be transferred. A wrist flexor and extensor should always be retained to prevent

wrist deformity due to muscle imbalance. Before performing reconstructive tendon transfers, joint contractures should be corrected and edema resolved so that the forearm and hand are in a quiescent state of soft-tissue equilibrium.

Nearly 20 years ago, Smith and Hastings outlined a series of 6 steps for planning tendon transfers; these steps are just as useful today. (1) What works? All regional muscles that are functioning are listed, and the force of contraction graded. (2) What is available? Functioning muscles that are expendable are selected. Unless arthrodesis is to be performed, retain at least 1 wrist flexor, 1 wrist extensor, and 1 flexor and extensor for each digit. (3) What is needed? All functions that require replacement are listed. These functions may include finger and/or thumb flexion and extension, wrist flexion and extension, thumb opposition and adduction, and digital intrinsic muscle function. (4) Available muscles are matched with functional requirements. Selections are made based on force, amplitude, direction, and integrity. (5) If all desired function cannot be obtained by tendon transfer, alternative procedures (eg, arthrodesis, tenodesis, capsulodesis, or pulley releases) are considered. (6) Tendon transfers that pass volarly to the axis of wrist motion are protected during the postoperative phase by wrist palmarflexion; those passing dorsally to the axis of wrist motion are protected by wrist extension. Reconstructive procedures are staged to meet these considerations.

Radial Nerve Paralysis

High (proximal) paralysis of the radial nerve results in significant hand dysfunction. The patient loses the ability to extend the wrist and to extend the thumb and digits. More distal, or low, radial nerve injuries may preserve some radial nerve function. Injuries proximal to the origin of the superficial radial nerve may spare ECRL. A more distal injury may preserve both ECRL and extensor carpi radialis brevis (ECRB). Injuries to the posterior interosseous nerve may preserve the radial wrist extensors as well as EIP and extensor digitorum minimi. Loss of wrist extension substantially weakens grasp strength.

Because the radial nerve is predominantly a motor nerve, with innervation limited to proximal extrinsic musculature, motor return is more often complete following crush injuries or reconstruction than in the case of the median and ulnar nerves, which contain a larger number of sensory fascicles and innervate hand intrinsic as well as forearm extrinsic musculature. Closed injuries of the radial nerve as seen in "Saturday night palsy" and associated with humerus fractures generally recover and do not require tendon transfers. Following uncomplicated radial nerve repair in the distal third of the brachium, clinical or electromyographic evidence of reinnervation in the brachioradialis and radial wrist extensors should be apparent within 4 to 6 months following repair. Tendon transfers are delayed until sufficient time for reinnervation has passed. End to side transfer of the pronator teres to the ECRB can be done at the time of radial nerve repair to provide wrist extension and thereby facilitate grasp during the prolonged period of nerve recovery. In cases of nerve repair performed under less favorable circumstances, early tendon transfers are indicated. In general, patients with radial nerve repair conducted under good circumstances are followed for 6 months before making a decision to proceed with tendon transfer.

Transfers for radial paralysis require a donor tendon for wrist extension, one or more donors for digital extension, and a donor musculotendinous unit for thumb extension. Pronator teres is universally accepted as the optimal donor for wrist extension in uncomplicated radial paralysis. Pronator teres is of appropriate strength and, when transferred into the central wrist extensor—ECRB—effective wrist dorsiflexion and some forearm pronation are produced. A potential limiting factor is the length of the pronator teres. Consequently, the muscle must be prolonged by raising a long strip of radius periosteum in continuity with the pronator teres insertion. The pronator teres is transferred over the brachioradialis and ECRL, and then to the ECRB.

Digital extension in radial paralysis is reconstructed by transfer of either a wrist flexor or FDS muscles. Either flexor carpi ulnaris (FCU) or flexor carpi radialis (FCR) may be transferred to the digital extensors (Fig. 2). The trend has favored using FCR for transfer, and preserving FCU function. The FCU is important for wrist flexion and ulnar deviation, and has twice the force of FCR with less excursion. The digital extensors are positioning tendons and do not require significant force. However, excellent results using FCU continue to be reported. A disadvantage of transferring a wrist flexor for digital extension is that independent digital extension is not possible; furthermore, the amplitude of the wrist flexors limits the ability to extend the digits when the wrist is dorsal to the neutral position. Wrist motion should be preserved to produce the additional 2.5 cm of tendon excursion by a tenodesis action. If independent digital extension is needed, or

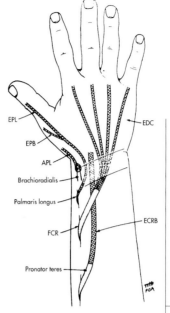

Figure 2

Tendon transfers for high radial paralysis may include pronator teres to extensor carpi radialis brevis (ECRB), flexor carpi radialis (FCR) to extensor digitorum communis (EDC), and extensor digiti minimi and palmaris longus to extensor pollicis longus (EPL) and extensor pollicis brevis (EPB). Abductor pollicis longus (APL) is tenodesed around the brachioradialis. (Reproduced with permission from Smith RJ: *Tendon Transfers of the Hand and Forearm.* Little, Brown and Co, 1987, p 42.)

wrist motion is compromised so that the tenodesis effect is not available to augment the amplitude of a wrist flexor, the FDS transfer developed by Boyes is an option. Through a window in the interosseous membrane, the ring finger FDS is transferred into the EPL and EIP. The middle finger FDS is transferred into the middle and ring finger extensor digitorum communis and the extensor digiti minimi tendons. Because the little finger extensor digitorum communis tendon is frequently ineffective in extending the little finger, all transfers for little finger digital extension should use the extensor digiti minimi as the recipient little finger extensor tendon. Disadvantages of this option are that loss of the FDS in 2 fingers may weaken grip, and deprives the donor digits of independent FDS function. In addition, the new function may be difficult to learn in this out-of-phase transfer.

When palmaris longus is available (80% of the population), it can be used to provide thumb extension. The EPL is released from the third dorsal compartment, and palmaris longus tendon is transferred into the EPL over the first dorsal compartment. Thumb metacarpal extension may be augmented by transferring the extensor pollicis brevis (EPB) into the EPL. If palmaris longus is absent, middle finger FDS is transferred through the interosseous membrane or about the radial aspect of the wrist to rerouted EPL.

Abductor pollicis longus (APL) is the principle extensor of the thumb metacarpal. Restoration of EPL and EPB function will produce first metacarpophalangeal (MCP) joint and interphalangeal (IP) joint extension. However, when the APL is not functioning, flexion-adduction of the thumb metacarpal and compensatory MCP joint hyperextension and IP joint flexion may result. Consequently, in transfers for radial paralysis, restoration of APL function is advisable. This may be produced by tenodesis of the APL about the brachioradialis insertion at the radial styloid. An alternative is transfer of the FCR to EPB and APL for thumb abduction and extension, in combination with FDS transfers to EPL and the digital extensors.

In posterior interosseous paralysis, ECRL function may be preserved. This produces significant radial deviation deformity of the wrist. Transfer of the ECRL to the ECRB based on its third metacarpal insertion, or extensor carpi ulnaris based on its fifth metacarpal insertion proximal to the wrist, can improve the excessive wrist radial deviation (Fig. 3). Thumb and digital extension may be provided with the tendon transfers used for more proximal radial nerve injuries.

Restoring Thumb Opposition

The primary motor loss in distal median nerve injuries is thumb opposition consequent to paralysis of the abductor pollicis brevis (APB), the opponens pollicis, and the superficial head of the flexor pollicis brevis. Thumb opposition requires that the thumb pulp be opposite the middle finger pulp so that the nail of the thumb and digit are in the same plane. Opposition requires the composite motions of thumb abduction, flexion, and pronation at both the carpometacarpal and MCP joints. Prior to opposition transfer, any first web space contracture should be corrected so that this composite motion is passively available. Opposition is required for precision handling of small objects, and places the thumb in position for grasp. Opposition transfers are positioning transfers, which do not require significant force. Opposition transfers generally approach the insertion of the APB at a 45° angle from the pisiform. More radially routed transfers produce better thumb palmar abduction, while more ulnarly routed transfers produce greater thumb flexion. The APB insertion is usually an excellent attachment site for opposition transfers. However, in patients with very mobile MCP joints, the APB insertion site may result in excessive metacarpal joint flexion. In such cases, all or part of

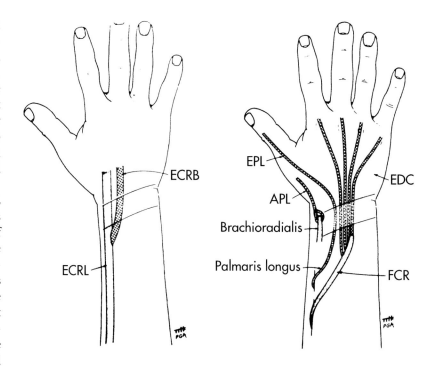

Figure 3

A, Low radial paralysis may spare extensor carpi radialis longus (ECRL) and result in significant wrist radial deviation. Extensor carpi radialis brevis (ECRB) or extensor carpi ulnaris (ECU) may be tenodesed to ECRL. **B,** Transfers for thumb and digital extension may be accomplished at the same location. (Reproduced with permission from Smith RJ: *Tendon Transfers of the Hand and Forearm.* Little, Brown and Co 1987, p 42.)

the transfer can be attached to the EPL or the MCP joint radial collateral ligament. With uncontrollable thumb MCP joint instability, arthrodesis may be required.

The most common opposition transfers are EIP to APB, FDS of ring finger to APB, palmaris longus to APB, and abductor digiti minimi to APB. The EIP transfer avoids use of a potentially injured tendon from a scarred region frequently associated with median nerve injuries at the wrist level. There is no loss of grasp force, as the donor is an extensor tendon and the FDS is retained. Furthermore, no pulley is required. The primary disadvantage of the EIP transfer is that the tendon just reaches its insertion site, with no tendon to spare.

Transfer of uninjured ring finger FDS to APB is an excellent transfer for low median nerve paralysis. A pulley is fashioned at the ulnar aspect of the wrist, using a loop of FCU so that the transferred tendon approaches the APB insertion at the correct angle. This transfer is not an option in patients with high median nerve injuries because the FDS is paralyzed.

The Camitz procedure—the transfer of palmaris longus, prolonged by the distal palmar fascia, to APB—is an excellent technique in the setting of thenar paralysis after longstanding

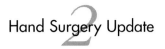
carpal tunnel syndrome. The transfer lies radial to the median nerve, and does not approach the APB insertion at the angle to produce true opposition. Because this transfer provides neither pronation nor flexion, the procedure is an abductorplasty rather than a true opposition transfer.

Transfer of the abductor digiti minimi muscle to APB—the Huber procedure—is primarily used in cases of thumb hypoplasia, as the transferred muscle restores or creates the thenar bulge. The transfer is also useful in patients with combined median and radial nerve paralysis, and for the reconstruction of complex posttraumatic deficits.

Restoring Power Pinch

Low (distal) ulnar nerve injuries result in paralysis of the adductor pollicis and first dorsal interosseous muscles. The adductor pollicis has a large cross-sectional area relative to its volume and thus has a large force potential, second only to the masseter muscle. The dysfunction results from a 33% to 50% loss of grip strength. Therefore, restoration of power pinch is important in patients with intrinsic paralysis. Surgical alternatives include ECRB adductorplasty and flexor superficialis adductorplasty. The ECRB adductorplasty requires prolongation of the ECRB tendon with a tendon graft routed through the second intermetacarpal space and across the volar aspect of the palm into the adductor pollicis insertion. The average preoperative pinch strength is doubled by this operation.

In an alternative procedure, the middle or ring finger FDS is transferred through the palmar fascia to the adductor pollicis insertion. This transfer does not require a tendon graft. In the presence of high ulnar nerve paralysis, the ring finger flexor superficialis should be preserved; this is the only ring finger extrinsic flexor. The middle finger FDS is used for correction of ring and little finger clawing. In patients with high ulnar paralysis or extensive scarring about the digital flexors, the ECRB adductorplasty is preferred. Power pinch may be further improved at the time of adductorplasty by restoration of index finger abduction. Index abductorplasty may be accomplished by prolonging an accessory APL with a tendon graft to the first dorsal interosseous insertion, or by transfer of the EIP from the ulnar aspect of the index MCP joint to the radial aspect of the index MCP joint.

Restoring Intrinsic Muscle Function to the Fingers

Median and ulnar nerve injuries, as well as neurologic disease, may result in paralysis of the digital intrinsic muscles.

Intrinsic muscle paralysis may result in digital deformity, weakened grip, asynchronous motion, and loss of lateral finger mobility. The intrinsic muscles are the primary flexor of the digital MCP joints. In intrinsic paralysis, extensor tendon force is focused on the proximal phalanx. With attempted digital extension, the unbalanced metacarpal joint hyperextends, and the extrinsic muscle force is rendered ineffective in extending the IP joints. The increased flexor tendon tone at the IP joints results in further IP joint flexion. The metacarpal joint hyperextension and IP joint flexion produces the claw deformity characteristic of intrinsic paralysis. Patients with claw deformity can only achieve IP joint extension through extrinsic muscle force if MCP joint hyperextension is prevented or MCP flexion is augmented by tenodesis or tendon transfer. As long as MCP joint hyperextension is prevented, digital IP joint extension may be achieved by the extrinsic digital extensors.

The key to restoring balance to the intrinsic minus hand is achieving MCP flexion; accordingly, all tendon transfers for intrinsic muscle paralysis must pass volar to the axis of the MCP joints. The original Stiles tendon transfer involved transfer of the split FDS into the extensor digitorum communis. This procedure was modified by Bunnell to reroute the FDS tendon along the lumbrical canal, suturing it to the transverse fibers of the dorsal digital aponeurosis. The modified Stiles-Bunnell tendon transfer, using the middle finger FDS, is a good procedure for isolated clawing of the ring and little fingers as seen in low ulnar nerve paralysis. In patients with joint hypermobility, the transfer may produce overcorrection and a swan-neck deformity. In patients with high ulnar nerve paralysis, the ring and little finger intrinsics are absent, and the FDP of ring and little fingers are absent. Clawing may be corrected by transfer of middle finger FDS to the ring and little finger lateral bands. FDP paralysis can be managed by either ring and little finger distal IP joint tenodesis, or side-by-side suture of ring and little finger FDP to middle finger FDP. In patients with hypermobile digits prone to swan-neck deformity, FDS may be transferred directly to the proximal phalanx rather than into the transverse fibers of the dorsal aponeurosis. Transfer to the proximal phalanx should be restricted to patients who can strongly extend the proximal IP joints when the metacarpal joints are blocked in flexion.

Overcorrection at the proximal IP joint and the finding of prior injury or associated paralysis of FDS have prompted development of alternative procedures for intrinsic reconstruction. Extensive experience has been gained using plantaris tendon grafts through the lumbrical canal, motored by ECRL, ECRB, or extensor carpi ulnaris. The transfer can be routed dorsally at the wrist, or volarly through the carpal tunnel. The dorsal route avoids the zone of scar in patients who have sustained extensive injury about the wrist or palm. Use of a wrist motor with a 4-tailed tendon graft for intrinsic reconstruction is appropriate for patients with previous lacerations of the flexor tendons or paralysis of FDS due to high median or ulnar paralysis. Because the FDS remains a proximal IP joint flexor, there is less risk of proximal IP joint hyperextension. This procedure has the significant advantage of increasing grip strength, by adding a wrist motor to provide metacarpal joint flexion. Advocates of the procedure recommend that the tendons be transferred to proximal phalangeal bone.

The Zancolli lasso procedure is another alternative for achieving MCP joint flexion in the claw hand. The FDS of each finger is looped about the A-2 pulley so that contraction of the FDS directly flexes the MCP joints. This transfer does not increase grip strength, nor does it directly contribute to IP joint extension. The procedure is most useful in patients with diffuse muscle paralysis, and in those with a limited number of donor tendons. Metacarpophalangeal joint palmar capsulorrhaphy and pulley advancement are also options in patients with diffuse muscle weakness.

Proximal Median, Ulnar, and Combination Paralyses

Proximal injuries of the median and ulnar nerve may be associated with both intrinsic muscle paralysis and extrinsic flexor paralysis. Deformities due to intrinsic paralysis, such as digital clawing, may not become apparent until the flexor paralysis has been corrected.

Proximal median nerve paralysis is characterized by loss of opposition, FPL paralysis, and loss of index finger flexion. Because the FDP to the middle finger is innervated by both median and ulnar nerves, middle finger flexion is usually retained. Brachioradialis transfer to FPL provides strong thumb flexion. The disadvantage of brachioradialis to FPL transfer is that thumb flexion may weaken with elbow flexion. When the middle finger FDP is functioning, index finger FDP may be sutured side-to-side to the middle finger FDP. If neither the index nor middle FDP is functioning, they can both be sutured to the purely ulnar-innervated ring finger FDP.

For opposition transfer, EIP is usually the best choice in patients with high median paralysis.

Extrinsic musculature reconstruction requirements in high ulnar nerve palsy requires restoration of ring and little finger FDP. The most direct transfer for correction of these deficits is side-to-side suture of the ring and little finger FDP into the FDP of the middle finger. This transfer results in common flexion of the middle, ring, and little fingers. The generally expendable middle finger FDS will allow independent flexion if transferred to ring and little finger FDP.

Following restoration of FDP function in high ulnar paralysis, clawing of the ring and little fingers is produced. Reconstructive options for restoration of digital intrinsic muscle function can then be considered.

In combined high median and ulnar nerve injury, all of the hand intrinsic muscles and the wrist and digital flexors are paralyzed. Digital flexor function may be restored by transfer of the radially innervated brachioradialis to FPL, and transfer of ECRL to FDP. Opposition can be restored by transfer of EIP to APB. Following restoration of digital flexion, clawing is produced and a balancing procedure is necessary. Digital intrinsic function is provided by extensor carpi ulnaris, prolonged by plantaris tendon grafts to the transverse fibers of the dorsal aponeurosis or to the proximal phalanges. As ECRL has been used to motor FDP and extensor carpi ulnaris provides digital intrinsic function, ECRB is not available for adductorplasty. The brachioradialis to FPL transfer may overpower EPL, and produce marked IP flexion with attempts at power pinch. Therefore, at the time of intrinsic reconstruction, thumb IP arthrodesis is frequently necessary.

Combined high median and radial nerve paralysis leaves few muscles available for transfer. The only active wrist motor is FCU. Wrist arthrodesis obviates the requirement for a wrist extensor, and frees FCU for transfer to EPL and the digital extensors in the initial procedure. At the second stage, abductor digiti minimi transfer to APB (the Huber procedure) provides thumb opposition, and index flexion is restored by transfer of index FDP to middle finger FDP if functioning. If middle finger FDP is not functioning through its ulnar innervation, then both index and middle finger FDP are transferred to ring finger FDP. The thumb is stabilized by IP arthrodesis.

Tendon Transfers in Systemic Disease

The majority of upper extremity tendon transfers in the United States are undertaken for posttraumatic reconstruction. However, many techniques for tendon transfer have evolved from the management of paralysis due to disease. Poliomyelitis and Hansen's disease were the impetus for many early tendon transfers.

Hansen's disease (leprosy) is extremely rare in the United States, but remains endemic in developing countries.

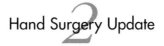
Reconstructive surgery of the contracted and paralyzed lepromatous hand focuses on restoring specific functions. The most common deformity, digital clawing, is due to ulnar or combined ulnar and median nerve palsy. The sensory deficit in Hansen's disease may be more dense than the motor deficit. Resorption of finger or thumb phalanges is common, and the motor deficit may prove progressive. Static procedures such as capsulorrhaphy, pulley advancement, and tenodeses may diminish deformity but will not restore intrinsic power. Because the radial nerve is less frequently involved than the median and ulnar nerves, transfer using the ECRL and a 4-tailed plantaris graft may be useful for intrinsic reconstruction. Principles of procedures for opposition and restoration of power pinch are useful in addressing the problem of intrinsic thumb weakness.

The last severe epidemic of poliomyelitis in the United States was in 1955. Many of the muscles weakened during the early and subacute stages of poliomyelitis will regain function and strength after the acute inflammation has subsided. Tendon transfers for poliomyelitis must not be performed until the condition of the limb has become static.

Charcot-Marie-Tooth (CMT) disease is the most common inherited peripheral neuropathy of the upper extremity. CMT disease is characterized by wide variation in expression, from virtually absent clinical symptoms to severe involvement of the upper and lower extremities. Patients usually first present with lower extremity weakness in the peroneal nerve distribution, and mildly abnormal sensation. The disease is progressive, and hand deformities may occur later.

CMT disease usually presents in patients aged 10 to 20 years. The development of upper limb symptoms frequently lags behind lower limb involvement. Initial hand involvement is characterized by loss of intrinsic muscle function and symmetrical atrophy of forearm musculature. In advanced stages, intrinsic paralysis occurs in both the median and ulnar nerves, with severe clawing. The progressive muscular atrophy is more severe peripherally than centrally. As the fingers become severely clawed, the thumb assumes a supinated, flattened position.

The progressive course of CMT paralysis has historically limited enthusiasm for tendon transfers. Although ulnar and median paralysis will progress, however, radial nerve involvement is rare. Transfer of radial innervated donors, in combination with selected arthrodeses and tenodeses, can provide long-term benefit. One group reported that the majority of their patients with CMT disease had slow motor conduction velocities of the median nerve. Release of the transverse carpal ligament was not helpful in their experience. Tendon transfers can be helpful in selected patients with CMT disease. In patients with advanced CMT disease, thumb paralysis can be managed with fusion of the carpometacarpal joint, transfer of the extensor carpi ulnaris to EPB for opposition, transfer of the EIP around the middle metacarpal into the adductor pollicis for power pinch, and prolongation of the APL with a tendon graft transferred into the first dorsal interosseous for index finger abduction. Finger clawing can be managed with either a lasso procedure or MCP capsulodesis.

Annotated Bibliography

Principles of Tendon Transfer

Almquist EE: Principles of tendon transfers, in Gelberman RH (ed): *Operative Nerve Repair and Reconstruction.* Philadelphia, PA, JB Lippincott, 1991, pp 689–696.

The development of tendon transfer principles is reviewed, with emphasis on application of biomechanical concepts.

Brand PW: Biomechanics of tendon transfers. *Hand Clin* 1988; 4:137–154.

This chapter explains the application of strength and excursion in developing optimal redistribution of musculotendinous units in the disabled hand.

Brand PW: Mechanics of tendon transfer, in Hunter JM, Mackin E, Callahan AD (eds): *Rehabilitation of the Hand: Surgery and Therapy,* ed 4. St. Louis, MO, Mosby-Year Book, 1995, pp 715–728.

In this lucid and concise discourse on the fundamental mechanics of tendon transfer, the author explains the relationship between tendon excursion and joint moment arm or leverage and emphasizes the importance of methods of measurement in determining relative effectiveness of various procedures.

Karev A: Principles of tendon transfers, in Peimer CA (ed): *Surgery of the Hand and Upper Extremity.* New York, NY, McGraw-Hill, 1996, pp 1217–1221.

In this general review of the principles of tendon transfer, the author recommends that the choice for donor tendon be determined by an algorithm. Annotated references are provided.

Smith RJ (ed): *Tendon Transfers of the Hand and Forearm.* Boston, MA, Little, Brown and Company, 1987.

This valuable monograph describes the many tendon transfers available for hand surgeons in comprehensive detail. The author outlines a variety of choices for the management of many conditions.

Radial Nerve Paralysis

Green DP: Radial nerve palsy, in Green DP, Hotchkiss RN (eds): *Operative Hand Surgery,* ed 3. New York, NY, Churchill-Livingstone, 1993, vol 2, pp 1401–1417.

This chapter provides a comprehensive review of the history and techniques of tendon transplantation for radial nerve palsy.

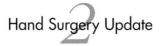

Schneider LH: Tendon transfer for radial nerve palsy, in Gelberman RH (ed): *Operative Nerve Repair and Reconstruction.* Philadelphia, PA, JB Lippincott, 1991, pp 697–709.

In this review of the history and indications for tendon transfer in radial palsy, the author describes the comprehensive approach to the patient and details his preferences. Flexor carpi ulnaris is his first choice as a transfer for digital extension.

Strickland JW, Kleinman WB: Tendon transfers for radial nerve paralysis, in Strickland JW (ed): *The Hand.* Philadelphia, PA, Lippincott-Raven, 1998, pp 303–318.

The authors outline reconstructive techniques for radial paralysis, and provide superb descriptions and illustrations of their preferred surgical technique.

Wheeler DR: Reconstruction for radial nerve palsy, in Peimer CA (ed): *Surgery of the Hand and Upper Extremity.* New York, NY, McGraw-Hill, 1996, vol 2, pp 1363–1379.

An up-to-date comprehensive review of the subject is clearly outlined. An extensive bibliography is provided with selected annotated references.

Restoring Thumb Opposition

Burkhalter WE: Median nerve palsy, in Green DP, Hotchkiss RN (eds): *Operative Hand Surgery,* ed 3. New York, NY, Churchill-Livingstone, 1993, vol 2, pp 1419–1448.

In this comprehensive review of opponensplasty, the author outlines surgical options and specific indications for each option.

Cooney WP: Tendon transfer for median nerve palsy. *Hand Clin* 1988;4:155–165.

This is an excellent review of tendon transfers in median paralysis, using biomechanical concepts to develop specific rationale for tendon transfer.

Eversmann WW: Median nerve palsy, in Gelberman RH (ed): *Operative Nerve Repair and Reconstruction.* Philadelphia, PA, JB Lippincott, 1991, pp 711–728.

This superb review of median nerve palsy adds emphasis on opposition as well as the problem of sensory deficit.

Restoring Intrinsic Muscle Function to the Fingers

Burkhalter WE: Ulnar nerve palsy, in Gelberman RH (ed): *Operative Nerve Repair and Reconstruction.* Philadelphia, PA, JB Lippincott, 1991, pp 729–746.

This excellent chapter stresses the loss of pinch and grip strength in ulnar paralysis. In order to improve strength in intrinsic paralysis, ECRL or FCR rather than FDS should be used as a motor. The muscle tendon unit is prolonged with tendon grafts through the lumbrical canals inserted into the base of the proximal phalanges.

Green SM: Reconstruction for ulnar nerve palsy, in Peimer CA (ed): *Surgery of the Hand and Upper Extremity.* New York, NY, McGraw-Hill, 1996, vol 2, pp 1399–1409.

A general description of the deficits of ulnar paralysis precedes a discussion of treatment options for extrinsic and intrinsic ulnar paralysis.

Hastings H: Ulnar nerve paralysis, in Strickland JW (ed): *The Hand.* Philadelphia, PA, Lippincott-Raven, 1998, pp 335–350.

A refined technique for digital intrinsic reconstruction in ulnar paralysis is described and illustrated. A wrist extensor is used to increase grip strength.

Hastings H II, Davidson S: Tendon transfers for ulnar nerve palsy: Evaluation of results and practical treatment considerations. *Hand Clin* 1988;4:167–178.

Standard tendon transfers are described, and results compared. The goals of different transfers are clearly described. The difference between transfers for balance and those for strength is emphasized.

Proximal Median, Ulnar, and Combination Paralyses

Eversmann WW Jr: Tendon transfers for combined nerve injuries. *Hand Clin* 1988;4:187–199.

Recommended schemes for tendon transfers are described for common and rare combinations of nerve deficit. The limited expectations for these severe injuries are emphasized. The planning logic is excellent, and makes this article valuable reading for all surgeons who do tendon transfers.

Imbriglia JE, Hagberg WC, Baratz ME: Median nerve reconstruction, in Peimer CA (ed): *Surgery of the Hand and Upper Extremity.* New York, NY, McGraw-Hill, 1996, vol 2, pp 1381–1397.

This current and complete review of the topic includes an extensive bibliography with selected annotated references.

Omer GE Jr: Tendon transfers in combined nerve lesions. *Orthop Clin North Am* 1974;5:377–387.

Based on the author's experience with 204 extremities with combined nerve lesions, tendon transfer schemes are recommended for all pairs of forearm nerve injuries. Treatment complications such as scarring, stiffness, and contracture are described.

Omer GE Jr: Tendon transfers for median nerve paralysis, in Strickland JW (ed): *The Hand.* Philadelphia, PA, Lippincott-Raven, 1998, pp 319–334.

The author clearly outlines available alternatives, and presents his preferred approach to low and high median nerve deficits. Reconstruction of sensory deficits with digital nerve translocation and neurovascular cutaneous island pedicle flaps are thoroughly described.

Omer GE Jr: Ulnar nerve palsy, in Green DP, Hotchkiss RN (eds): *Operative Hand Surgery,* ed 3. New York, NY, Churchill-Livingstone, 1993, vol 2, pp 1449–1466.

This comprehensive review of reconstruction for ulnar paralysis includes the author's preferences and describes a specific patient-oriented approach.

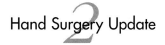

Tendon Transfers in Systemic Disease

Anderson GA, Lee V, Sundararaj GD: Opponensplasty by extensor indicis and flexor digitorum superficialis tendon transfer. *J Hand Surg* 1992;17B:611–614.

This group, focusing on opponensplasty in Hansen's disease, suggests that EIP provides the best results in supple hands. In stiffer hands, the FDS provides added force. Harvest of the FDS through a palmar oblique incision is recommended to minimize complications in the donor finger.

Brandsma JW, Brand PW: Claw-finger correction: Considerations in choice of technique. *J Hand Surg* 1992;17B:615–621.

The authors review the subtle details of the techniques used for intrinsic replacement and encourage replacement of active metacarpal flexion. In Hansen's disease patients, passing a tendon transfer through the carpal tunnel does not jeopardize the median nerve.

Brandsma JW, Ottenhoff-De Jonge MW: Flexor digitorum superficialis tendon transfer for intrinsic replacement: Long-term results and the effect on donor fingers. *J Hand Surg* 1992;17B:625–628.

Good or excellent results were obtained in 59 of 76 FDS claw hand reconstructions and 68 of 82 FDS opponensplasties. Problems in the donor finger included swan-neck deformity, distal IP flexion contracture, proximal IP flexion contracture, and loss of active flexion; causes of these complications are discussed.

Wood VE, Huene D, Nguyen J: Treatment of the upper limb in Charcot-Marie-Tooth disease. *J Hand Surg* 1995;20B:511–518.

The types of Charcot-Marie-Tooth disease and results of treatment are outlined. Tendon transfers can be helpful in selected patients. For patients with advanced CMT disease, they recommend fusion of the MCP joint of the thumb, transfer of extensor carpi ulnaris to EPB for opposition, transfer of EIP around the third metacarpal into the adductor pollicis for pinch, and transfer of 1 slip of APL using a tendon graft into the first dorsal interosseous for index finger abduction. If clawing is severe, palmaris longus extended with palmar fascia as a lasso about the A1 pulley is an option.

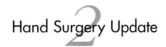

Section IV
Nerve

American Society for Surgery of the Hand

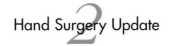

Chapter 17
Peripheral Nerve Biology

Thomas M. Brushart, MD

Functional Anatomy

Epineurium

The external epineurium is a layer of collagenous connective tissue that forms the outer covering of peripheral nerve (Fig. 1). The internal epineurium, an extension of this tissue, surrounds individual fascicles within the nerve. Internal epineurium cushions the fascicles from external pressure, allowing them to move against each other; both layers absorb longitudinal stress before it is transmitted to the perineurium. The percentage of nerve cross-sectional area occupied by epineurium varies along each nerve, from nerve to nerve, and from individual to individual. Near joints, where extra padding is needed, as much as 75% of the nerve is epineurium. Epineurial fibroblasts respond vigorously to injury; much of the scar formed after nerve transection results from brisk proliferation of these cells.

Perineurium

Perineurium is the tissue layer surounding individual fascicles (Fig. 1). As many as 10 concentric layers of flattened cells with prominent basement membranes are dovetailed together and linked with tight junctions. Longitudinally and obliquely oriented collagen fibers occupy the space between layers. The perineurium is an extension of the blood-brain barrier, controlling the intraneural environment by limiting diffusion, blocking the ingress of infection, and maintaining a slightly positive intrafascicular pressure. The perineurium is also the neural component most resistant to longitudinal traction; as long as it remains intact, the elastic properties of the nerve are retained.

Endoneurium

The endoneurium is the collagenous packing that surrounds individual axons within the perineurium (Fig. 1). Endoneurium is also a component of the Schwann cell tube, or endoneurial tube, the cylindrical structure that contains the myelinated axon and its associated Schwann cells. Larger myelinated axons are surrounded by 2 layers of collagen. The outer layer is longitudinally oriented; the inner layer is arranged randomly and associated with carbohydrate-rich reticulin. Small myelinated axons have only the outer, longitudinal layer.

Vascular Supply

Segmental nutrient vessels supply longitudinally oriented vascular networks in the epineurium (Fig. 1). These networks in turn feed similar plexi within the perineurial lamellae. Perineurial vessels often enter the endoneurium at an oblique angle, placing them at risk for occlusion if endoneurial pressure is raised. The endoneurial space is devoid of lymphatics. A longitudinal network of capillaries, arterioles, and venules extends throughout the endoneurium of each fasicicle; the direction of flow in any portion can rapidly be changed in response to injury. The longitudinal orientation and dynamic flexibility of its vascular supply allows uninjured peripheral nerve to be mobilized over long distances without risk of ischemia.

Fascicles

A fascicle is a group of axons packed within endoneurial connective tissue and contained by a sleeve of perineurium. The fascicle is the smallest unit of nerve structure that can be manipulated surgically. The number of fascicles within a

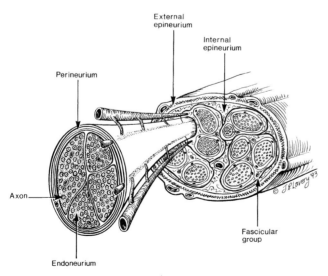

Figure 1

The macroscopic and gross microscopic organization of peripheral nerve. (Copyright ©1993 JP Lavery)

nerve varies throughout its course; the median nerve contains as few as 3 and as many as 36. Fascicles interconnect to form an intraneural plexus. Plexus formation is most prominent in nerves to the proximal extremity, such as the musculocutaneous nerve, and occurs less frequently in the distal median and ulnar nerves. In many areas of peripheral nerve, fascicles are clustered into fascicular groups of 3 to 6 fascicles bound together by condensations of the inner epineurium (Fig. 1). Fascicular groups can be isolated over much greater distances than individual fascicles, and may still be identified and matched after several centimeters of nerve substance have been lost. Although fascicular interconnections may be common within a group, fascicles from different groups rarely interconnect.

The degree to which axons destined for a terminal nerve branch are grouped together in proximal portions of the nerve has been the subject of recent controversy. Although studies based on anatomic dissection have not detected functional localization at proximal levels, these studies are inherently limited by assumptions that are forced on the dissector. The dissector functionally identifies a fascicle by its distal termination and then works proximally, separating the fascicle from its neighbors (Fig. 2). When an intrafascicular plexus is encountered, however, it must be assumed that all proximal components contribute equally to the single distal fascicle being traced. As fascicular interconnections are repeatedly encountered, a large number of fascicles are traced, most of which do not actually contribute to the fascicle under study. Maps based on dissection thus represent the sum of all potential axon sources; their failure to detect localization cannot be used as evidence that it does not exist.

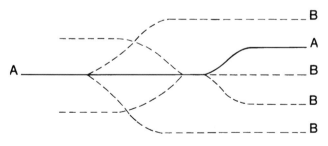

Figure 2

The formation of interfascicular plexi within peripheral nerve. Distal is to the left, proximal to the right. The solid line (**A**) represents the true course of a group of axons through this segment of nerve. The fascicles (**B**) on the proximal end will all be identified by the dissector as potential sources of the axons in A because of interfascicular connections. Dissection produces a map of all potential axon sources. (Reproduced with permission from Brushart, TM: Peripheral nerve biology, in Manske PR (ed): *Hand Surgery Update*. Rosemont, IL, American Academy of Orthopaedic Surgeons, 1996, pp 209–220.)

Greater precision has recently been achieved by histochemical tracing of primate axons, and by intrafascicular microstimulation studies in awake human subjects. Primate digital nerve axons were traced with horseradish peroxidase (HRP) and were found to occupy only one third to one sixth of the median nerve cross-section as it entered the brachial plexus. In early microstimulation studies, 42% of human median nerve fascicles in the upper arm projected only to skin; of these, 67% projected only to a single digital interspace. At the wrist level, 87% of fascicles projected even more discretely to a single digital nerve. With refinements in technique, somatotopic arrangement of axons has also been demonstrated within individual fascicles. This evidence strongly suggests that axons terminating in a peripheral median nerve fascicle travel near one another even at proximal levels; they are not widely separated by interfascicular plexus formation, as suggested by earlier dissection studies. Consequently, the long-accepted view of intraneural chaos, which reflects the limitations of dissection technique, is replaced by one of partial localization of distal function at proximal levels.

Longitudinal Excursion

Peripheral nerve is loosely anchored by nutrient vessels and terminal branches and rarely crosses a joint at the axis of motion; limb movement accordingly causes sliding of the nerve along its bed. The resulting longitudinal excursion of upper extremity peripheral nerves has been studied electrophysiologically and anatomically. Study of action potentials showed wrist and digital flexion-extension to produce 7.4 mm of median nerve excursion, with an additional 4.3 mm resulting from elbow flexion. Displacement of the median nerve during wrist and digital flexion was 2 to 4 times greater at the wrist than in the upper arm. Anatomic dissection revealed a brachial plexus excursion of 15 mm in the frontal plane during abduction of the arm. The median and ulnar nerves moved an average of 7.3 and 9.8 mm, respectively, through a full range of elbow motion. Full wrist flexion-extension produced the greatest excursion—15.5 mm of the median nerve and 14.8 mm of the ulnar nerve, as measured at the proximal edge of the carpal tunnel. The excursion was much lower in the palm and digits.

Cellular Components

The Neuron

The "wires" in peripheral nerve are the axonal processes of parent neurons, associated with Schwann cells as they course distally (Fig. 3). Motor neurons lie in the anterior horn of the spinal cord, sensory neurons within the dorsal

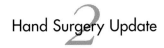
root ganglia, and autonomic neurons within paravertebral ganglia. Synthesis of structural components and transmitters occurs within the neuron, the location of ribosomes, endoplasmic reticulum, and the Golgi apparatus. In contrast, the axon contains mostly axoplasm, neurofilaments, and microtubules. Neurofilaments, polymers of cytokeratin protein, are approximately 10 nm in diameter, are longitudinally oriented, and form the major skeletal component of the axon. Microtubules are cylindrical polymers of tubulin, 25 to 30 nm in diameter and up to 0.1 mm long. They are also arranged longitudinally, but are found in only one third to one tenth the concentration of neurofilaments. They participate in axoplasmic transport.

Products of synthesis originate within the neuron, but must be transported to the periphery within the axon. Three major types of axoplasmic transport have been described. Fast anterograde (away from the neuron) transport moves membrane-enclosed subcellular organelles, such as synaptic vesicles, down the "railroad track" of microtubules at speeds of up to 400 mm/day. The motor for this process is kinesin, an adenosine triphosphatase (ATPase) that links the traveling organelles to the underlying microtubules. In contrast, slow anterograde transport carries cytoskeletal elements and soluble proteins at 0.2 to 5 mm/day. The volume of neurofilament components being transported in this way helps determine the caliber of the axon. Material is also transported from the periphery back to the neuron. Fast retrograde (to the neuron) transport is linked to microtubules in a fashion similar to that of the anterograde direction. However, it is driven by the ATPase dynein and travels only about half as fast as the anterograde transport driven by kinesin. Retrograde transport returns scavenged components to the cell body for recycling, and also carries messages regarding end-organ connections from the periphery to the cell body. Best-characterized of these messages is nerve growth factor (NGF), a protein manufactured by the targets of developing sensory and sympathetic axons. Axons that make end-organ contact take up NGF and transport it back to the cell body, where it promotes neuronal survival. This relationship is termed neurotrophic, or nutritive, and NGF is termed a neurotrophic factor. Axons without appropriate connections cannot provide NGF to their neurons, which subsequently die.

The Schwann Cell

The Schwann cell is the glial cell of the peripheral nervous system. Its phenotype is largely determined by the type of axon it encircles. The nonmyelinating phenotype is expressed when the Schwann cell envelops several small (< 1 μm in diameter) axons within invaginations of its cytoplasm. In this state, the Schwann cell expresses NGF receptors and the adhesion molecules L1 and neural cell adhesion molecule (NCAM). Myelinating Schwann cells, in contrast, are each associated with a single axon. During development, this axon is surrounded by the mesaxon (Fig. 3), a tongue of Schwann cell membrane that progressively elongates as it spirals around the axon in concentric circles. The cytoplasm is squeezed from between these layers, which condense into the lamellae of compact myelin. The larger the axon, the thicker is the myelin sheath. Myelin is 70% lipid, largely cholesterol and phospholipid, closely resembling the composition of the cell membrane from which it is made; the remaining 30% is protein. The adhesion molecule myelin-associated glycoprotein (MAG), a member of the immunoglobulin superfamily, is found predominately at the edge of the developing myelin sheath, and is thought to participate in the process of myelin formation. Protein zero (Po), also a member of the immunoglobulin superfamily, is the major structural protein of myelin. Po bridges the adjacent layers of membrane, and may play a role in myelin compaction by interacting with receptors on the opposing surfaces. Additional protein constituents include the family of myelin basic proteins (MBP). The myelinating Schwann cell thus expresses MAG, Po, and MBP.

Electrical Properties

Ion Channels

The electrical activity of peripheral nerve is mediated by ion channels, glycoprotein molecules that bridge the inner and outer surfaces of the cell membrane and provide a pathway

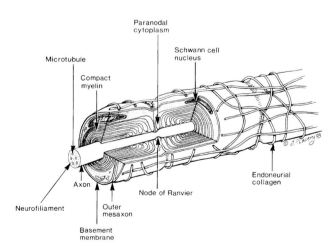

Figure 3

The contents of the Schwann cell tube. (© 1993 JP Lavery)

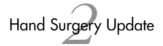
for movement of ions in and out of the cell. Channels are specific for a particular ion. Channels that remain open at all times are termed nongated, and are responsible for the cell membrane's passive electrical properties. Other channels can be opened selectively, or gated, and participate in rapid ion fluxes during impulse conduction. Gated channels open in response to a change in voltage, the presence of a chemical transmitter, or mechanical deformation.

Resting Potential

The neural membrane functions as a capacitor, separating a positive charge on its external surface from a negative internal charge. The result of this charge separation—the resting membrane potential—is normally between –60 and –70 millivolts (mV), and is determined by the relative concentration of ions on both sides of the membrane. Na^+ and Cl^- are more concentrated outside the cell, and K^+ and organic ions are more concentrated inside. The organic ions, largely organic acids and proteins, cannot diffuse through the membrane and are permanently contained within the cell. The resting potential is determined by the relative concentration of nongated channels for K^+, Na^+, and Cl^-. The more numerous the channels, the more rapid is the diffusion of a specific ion across the membrane. Nongated K^+ channels far outnumber those for Na^+ and Cl^-; consequently, the resting membrane potential is largely determined by the activity of the K^+ ion. K^+ tends to diffuse down its concentration gradient and out of the cell, leaving the large, nondiffusable organic anions (– charge) inside. However, as the outside of the cell becomes more positively charged, the resulting electrical potential tends to drive K^+ back into the cell, against its diffusion gradient. The membrane potential at which the 2 factors reach equilibrium was first calculated by Nernst in 1888, and is called the Nernst potential. If nongated channels permitted only K^+ to pass, this potential would be –75 mV. However, the membrane is also permeable to Na^+, which follows its concentration gradient into the cell and is driven into the cell by the positive external charge established by K^+. The resting potential is thus slightly more positive than the Nernst potential of K^+ alone. Equilibrium is maintained by the Na^+/K^+ pump, which expends ATPase to counteract the K^+ and Na^+ fluxes.

The Action Potential and Its Conduction

The interaction of gated axon channels to produce the action potential was described in 1952. Voltage-gated Na^+ channels open, allowing Na^+ to move down its concentration gradient into the cell. The resulting decrease in membrane potential produces the rising phase of the action potential. The falling phase is then produced by 2 simultaneous events: the Na^+ channels are closed, halting the influx of Na^+; and

voltage-gated K^+ channels are opened, allowing more K^+ to diffuse out of the cell. The membrane potential then returns to its resting value. The action potential generated in one segment of membrane supplies the depolarizing current to the adjacent segment, activating the voltage-gated channels and depolarizing the membrane. The depolarization of adjacent membrane, and thus axon conduction, however, is slowed by the electrical resistance of the axoplasm. The time required for spread of depolarization varies inversely with the product of axon resistance and capacitance over a given length; accordingly, 2 strategies are available for speeding axonal conduction. Increasing axon diameter, and thus volume, will increase the supply of available ions (charge carriers) and decrease the resistance to current flow. This strategy is limited by the large number of axons that must be contained within peripheral nerve. Production of myelin to decrease capacitance is a more efficient solution to the problem. Myelin dramatically increases effective thickness of the membrane, thereby decreasing its capacitance and enabling a small amount of current to discharge the membrane and propagate the action potential passively. However, myelin also interferes with the flux of ions across the cell membrane, blocking the normal mechanism for active propagation of the action potential. If the myelin sheath were continuous, the action potential would eventually die out. This problem is solved by the node of Ranvier (Fig. 3), the small exposed portion of axonal membrane at the juncture between Schwann cells. This area contains a high concentration of voltage-gated Na^+ channels, and amplifies the signal by generating a strong inward Na^+ current when stimulated by the more passive spread of depolarization from within the myelinated segment. The brief slowing of conduction during this amplification process at the node of Ranvier results in the impulse jumping from node to node, or saltatory conduction.

Neuromuscular Transmission

As the motor axon potential nears muscle, it is distributed to several terminal axon branches, each of which ends in a synaptic bouton (Fig. 4). The bouton is structurally adapted for transmitter release. Acetylcholine (ACh), the neuromuscular transmitter, is contained within synaptic vesicles that have been transported from the neuron by rapid axoplasmic transport. The active zone, the distal portion of the bouton membrane, is designed for transmitter release. The terminal portion of the bouton also contains voltage-gated Ca^+ channels. These respond to the action potential by allowing influx of Ca^+, which triggers fusion of synaptic vesicles and release of their contents. The ACh released from the bouton diffuses across the synaptic cleft to interact with specific ACh receptors in the muscle basement membrane. These

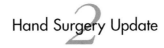
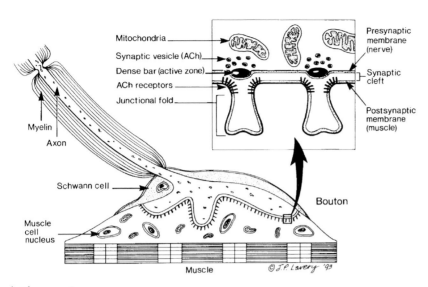

Figure 4

Light microscopic and electron microscopic views of the motor end plate. (© 1993 JP Lavery)

receptors are transmitter-gated ion channels that respond to ACh by opening and allowing passage of Na^+ ions across the muscle membrane. Na^+ influx depolarizes the membrane, resulting in a small end-plate potential; its magnitude is limited by the volume of ACh released. However, Na^+ influx also activates voltage-gated Na^+ channels adjacent to the end plate. The additional Na^+ is sufficient to depolarize the membrane and result in an action potential and muscle contraction.

The Motor Unit

The term "motor unit" was introduced in 1925 to describe the smallest unit of neuromuscular function—a single motoneuron and the muscle fibers innervated by it. The number of muscle fibers in the motor unit is called the innervation ratio. This count varies from 80 to 100 in the intrinsic muscles to 1,000 to 2,000 in the large muscles of the leg. Smaller innervation ratios allow more precise muscular control. Muscle fibers, initially classified as either slow (type I) or fast (type II) on the basis of contractile properties, have been further characterized from both functional and histochemical perspectives. Slow fatigable (type I) muscle contracts slowly and is highly resistant to fatigue. This muscle type is histochemically characterized as slow oxidative, with high concentrations of mitochondria, oxidative enzymes, and the myoglobin responsible for its dark color. However, slow fatigable muscle can generate only a tenth the force of the most powerful fibers—the fast fatigable fibers (type IIB), which contract and relax quickly

but are also quick to fatigue. Histochemically identified as fast glycolytic, high levels of myosin ATPase correlate with their rapid contraction rate. High concentrations of glycogen and glycolytic enzymes, and a paucity of mitochondria, similarly reflect their anaerobic metabolism. These extremes are bridged by fast fatigue resistant (type IIA, fast oxidative-glycolytic) and fast fatigue intermediate (type IIC, fast intermediate) muscle fiber, representing relatively slow and intermediate types of fast muscle. It is important to realize that these functional and histochemical grades overlap significantly, and correlate generally but not precisely with one another. Each muscle contains a mixture of the various fiber types, which are present in varying proportions depending on the muscle's function. Slow units are usually deep within the muscle; fast units are superficial. The individual fibers of each motor unit are dispersed within the muscle rather than existing directly adjacent to one another.

Within an individual motor unit, neuronal properties correlate effectively with muscle fiber characteristics. Fast fatigable fibers are supplied by large, rapidly conducting axons from large motoneurons and slow fatigable fibers by smaller, slower axons from smaller motoneurons, so that conduction speed and contraction speed are matched. Motor units are recruited in an orderly, reproducible pattern as increasing increments of force are required of a muscle. The smallest motoneurons are discharged first because they have the lowest threshold for activation. Motoneurons serving a given muscle are grouped together in a motoneuron pool within the anterior horn of the spinal cord. As the impulse to the motoneuron pool increases in strength, progressively larger motoneurons with larger axons and faster muscle fibers are activated. This size principle is a basic concept of neuromuscular integration. A direct consequence is simplified control of muscular force; progressively stronger input to the motoneuron pool as a whole will result in progressively stronger force generation, without the need for specific activation of different fiber types.

Touch

Peripheral Receptors

Glabrous (nonhairy) skin has 3 types of mechanoreceptors that transduce components of touch into neural action potentials—the Merkel cell complex, the Meissner corpuscle, and the Pacinian corpuscle. All 3 transmit these action potentials through A-beta, small myelinated fibers 6 to 12 μm in diameter. The Merkel cell complex is clustered around the sweat duct as it enters the undersurface of the intermediate dermal ridge. This complex consists of several receptors served by branches of a single axon. In each receptor, the axon terminal synapses directly with an epithelial cell transducer. The receptor is slowly adapting, and continues to fire as long as the stimulus is present. The receptive field, the area of skin through which appropriate stimuli will fire the receptor, is well-circumscribed at 2 to 4 mm. The Merkel cell is thus equipped to respond to small areas of steady skin indentation, and is probably the principle mediator of static 2-point discrimination.

The Meissner corpuscle is located at the sides of the intermediate ridge, to which it is attached by thin strands of connective tissue. The encapsulated receptor contains stacks of flattened disks—the lamellar cells—and is served by 2 to 8 terminal axon branches. In contrast to the Merkel cell, the Meissner corpuscle is rapidly adapting; it fires briefly at the beginning of a stimulus, and occasionally at the end, but not throughout. Its maximum sensitivity is to flutter vibration at 30 cps. Like the Merkel cell, the Meissner corpuscle has a small receptive field. The Meissner corpuscle is thus well-suited to the analysis of motion, and may provide the information that results in moving 2-point discrimination.

The Pacinian corpuscle lies within subcutaneous tissue. It is visible to the naked eye during surgery, resembling a small grain of rice. A single axon is surrounded by 40 to 60 concentric lamellae, giving it the appearance of an eliptical onion on cross-section. The Pacinian corpuscle is rapidly adapting, responding maximally to vibration at 250 cps. However, it cannot precisely localize these stimuli because of its large receptive field, often several centimeters in diameter.

Degeneration and Regeneration

Wallerian Degeneration

When the axon is severed, the distal stump undergoes wallerian degeneration (Fig. 5). This process clears degraded myelin and axoplasm from the Schwann cell tube and provides an environment that is attractive to regenerating axons. The sequence begins with breakdown of axoplasm and cytoskeleton into granular material, an event triggered by injury-induced calcium influx. This granular disintegration occurs within 24 to 48 hours in rodents, the subjects of most experimental evidence. However, the slower pace of granular disintegration in humans can be inferred from electrophysiologic studies. Motor amplitudes decrease by

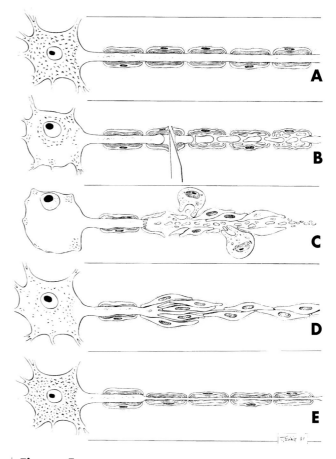

Figure 5

Degeneration and regeneration of a myelinated nerve fiber: **A,** Normal appearance. **B,** Axon transection is followed by disintegration of the cytoplasm. The cell body swells and the nucleus becomes eccentric. **C,** Macrophages enter the distal segment, and phagocytose myelin along with the dividing Schwann cells. **D,** Schwann cells have proliferated to form the band of Büngner, now the principal contents of the Schwann cell tube. The proximal axon sends out multiple sprouts, the regenerating unit, which course distally between basement membrane and Schwann cells within the Schwann cell tube. **E,** At the completion of regeneration a single nerve fiber remains. It is smaller in diameter, less well-myelinated, and conducts less rapidly than the axon that it replaces. (Reproduced with permission from Lundborg G: *Nerve Injury and Repair.* New York, NY, Churchill Livingstone, 1988, p 151.)

50% 3 to 5 days after injury, and are absent by 9 days. Sensory amplitudes are reduced by 50% at 7 days, and are absent by 11 days.

A major advance in the understanding of wallerian degeneration has been the identification of the macrophage as the primary phagocyte of myelin. Some macrophages are recruited from the small population resident within the nerve, but most originate in the circulation. Macrophages are present in the endoneurium in significant numbers 2 to 3 days after injury,

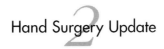
when they express Ia (the major histocompatability marker) and complement receptor 3 (CR3). They lose these markers as they pass through the basement membrane of the Schwann cell tube, but continue to express interleukin 1 (IL-1), a potent stimulus to Schwann cell NGF production. Schwann cells then break down myelin, first into ovoids and then into disorganized whorls that are phagocytosed and removed by macrophages. This process cannot occur when macrophage invasion is blocked. Individual Schwann cells become metabolically active and proliferate, forming a continuous chain of cells—the band of Büngner—that remains within the confines of the original Schwann cell tube. These Schwann cells produce neurotrophic (nourishing) factors that support regenerating axons. They also express the neural adhesion molecules L1 and NCAM, which provide a favorable surface for axon elongation. Conversely, components of mature myelin (MAG, Po and MBP) are downregulated until axons return. Additional cellular changes include leakiness of endoneurial capillaries, which results in endoneurial edema and breakdown of the blood-nerve barrier, and proliferation of endoneurial fibroblasts.

A potent tool for the analysis of wallerian degeneration has recently become available. In the Ola mutant of the C57Bl6 mouse, the distal stump of transected peripheral nerve survives intact for several weeks. This observation indicates that Wallerian degeneration is not an immediate consequence of axotomy. The defect in the Ola results from delayed axonal recruitment of macrophages. A better understanding of its mechanism may lead to clinical strategies for the modification of Wallerian degeneration.

Cell Body Reaction

The neuron responds to axotomy by returning to its developmental program. Production of growth associated proteins (GAPs) is increased 100-fold. These axonally transported phosphoproteins, found on the inner surface of the developing and regenerating neuronal membrane, are substrates for protein kinase C and are thought to participate in growth cone extension. Production of actin, another protein crucial to growth cone function, and tubulin, a component of microtubules, are also increased after axotomy. Neurofilament protein, the skeletal subunit normally made in development of the organism only after axons have contacted their targets, is downregulated. The volume of available neurofilaments can regulate axon caliber; regenerating axons are thus smaller than the axons they replace. The stimulus for the neuronal response to axotomy is probably the interruption of trophic support from the periphery. In NGF-dependent neurons, the neuron reaction to axotomy is blocked by NGF administration and mimicked by administration of antibodies to NGF.

The Axon

Transected axons form regenerative sprouts within hours of injury. The initial sprouts are often resorbed; more durable ones, with internal cytoskeletons, are present after the first 24 hours. Sprouts are generated at the most distal node of Ranvier, which remains intact. Although this node will be directly adjacent to a sharp transection, it may be far proximal to more diffuse trauma with crush or blast components. Multiple collateral sprouts from each axon advance distally as the regenerating unit. As a result, myelinated axon counts in the distal stump are elevated by a factor of 1.5 to 5 for several months after nerve transection and repair. In a recent sequential study of rat sciatic nerve regeneration, the number of myelinated distal stump axons was almost twice normal at 3 months, then gradually diminished until normal numbers were reached at 24 months. The collateral sprouts from a single regenerating unit may enter separate, and often unrelated, Schwann cell tubes in the distal nerve stump. Once entered, these pathways usually confine axons and guide them to the end-organ served by the original axon. Collaterals of a single motoneuron may reinnervate separate muscles, and collaterals of a single sensory axon may supply separate receptive fields. Ultimately, collateral survival is determined by successful reestablishment of end-organ contact. Even in the final survivors, axon caliber, and hence conduction velocity, will not return to normal. The myelin sheath will also be thinner, reflecting Schwann cell response to the shorter internodal distance in regenerated axons.

The rate of axon elongation within the environment of the distal stump is species-dependent. Rodent axons may reach speeds of 2 to 3.5 mm/day, while the maximum rate in humans is 1 to 2 mm/day. This rate slows progressively as the periphery is neared. The rate of axon outgrowth may be increased by a prior "conditioning" lesion. By 7 days after an initial injury, slow transport of structural protein in the rat sciatic nerve is increased from 3.6 ± 0.5 mm/day to 5.1 ± 0.5 mm/day; this correlates directly with an increased outgrowth rate. Changes in fast transport do not appear to be involved. Conditioning was initially described in response to axon transection, but has subsequently been found to result from a variety of insults, including crush, chronic nerve compression, freeze, or inflammation in the area of the parent neuron. At this time, conditioning has not yet been found to influence the final outcome of axon regeneration.

Injury and regeneration also affect the proximal axon, adjacent to the neuron. Neurofilament protein synthesis controls axonal caliber and is downregulated during regeneration. As neuronal supplies of neurofilament are depleted, the proximal axon shrinks, and this atrophy spreads distally

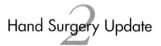

from the neuron at the speed of slow axoplasmic transport. This shrinkage is later reversed when contact with the periphery is reestablished.

Growth Cone and Pathway

The growth cone—the tip of the regenerating axon—is the locomotive of regeneration. It is designed to sample the surrounding terrain, integrate its findings, and pull the axon into the most suitable environment. Fingerlike extensions, the filopodia, actively extend and sample; they are followed by lamellipodia, larger expansions of the membrane. These processes extend on a framework of actin filaments, backed by microtubules that enter the base of the growth cone. As the axon grows, membrane components are supplied by anterograde (cell to periphery) transport of vesicles that fuse with the growth cone surface. The growth cone membrane is rich in GAP-43, a molecule involved in both growth cone motility and intracellular signaling. Protein kinase C and the tyrosene kinases also signal peripheral events to the cell's interior. The growth cone is active in the endocytosis of molecules from the environment, eg, NGF, which is transported back to the cell body to perform its neurotrophic function.

The regenerating axon propagates distally within the Schwann cell tube, between basement membrane and Schwann cell surfaces (Fig. 6). This optimal location provides adhesive interactions between axon and basal lamina and between axon and Schwann cell, as well as trophic support from factors produced by the Schwann cell. The Schwann cell is crucial to peripheral growth cone elonga-

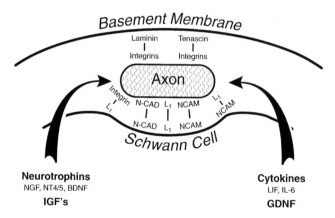

Figure 6

The regenerating axon benefits from 3 types of interaction as it proceeds distally within the Schwann cell tube between Schwann cell and basement membrane. Axonal integrins bind to laminin and tenascin within the basement membrane. Adhesion molecules on axonal and Schwann cell surfaces participate in both homophilic and heterophilic interactions with one another. The Schwann cell also produces neurotrophic factors that support neuron survival and growth.

tion. Acellular environments, such as tubular nerve guides or muscle basement membrane grafts, must be populated with Schwann cells before axons can pass. If Schwann cell migration is blocked by cytotoxins, regeneration will not occur. Axons regenerating in culture prefer the inner surface of the basal lamina tube; those navigating outside the tube in vivo suffer growth arrest after short distances. Laminin is the basal lamina constituent that most vigorously promotes axon outgrowth. Its 3 subunits—the alpha, beta, and gamma chains—may be altered to produce laminin isoforms that differ in location and function. Laminin 2 in Schwann cell basement membrane promotes axon regeneration, while laminin 3 (S-laminin) acts as a stop signal at the neuromuscular junction. Axonal adhesion to laminin is mediated by the integrins, a class of surface molecules that also bind extracellular matrix components such as Tenascin.

Schwann cell L1 and NCAM, members of the immunoglobulin superfamily, bind homophilically (molecule to like molecule) with L1 and NCAM on the axon surface (Fig. 6). They also bind heterophilically with other cell adhesion molecules or to the integrins. L2, another member of the immunoglobulin superfamily of adhesion molecules, is displayed only by Schwann cells within motor pathways and may contribute to their preferential reinnervation by motor axons. Axon to Schwann cell adhesion is also mediated by the cadherins through homophilic interactions.

A variety of trophic factors participate in regeneration. Members of the neurotrophin family (NGF, neurotrophin [NT]-3, NT-4/5, brain-derived neurotrophic factor [BDNF]) bind avidly to tyrosine kinase (Trk) receptors on the axon. NGF binds preferentially to Trk A, BDNF and NT-4/5 to Trk B, and NT-3 to Trk C. Production of all but NT-3 is upregulated by Schwann cells during wallerian degeneration. NGF prevents the death of axotomized sensory neurons, while BDNF and NT-3 most effectively support motoneurons. Experimental application of NGF to injured nerve has no effect on the regeneration of sensory or motor axons, but increases the rate of regeneration across enclosed gaps by stimulating angiogenesis and glial activity. The cytokines—ciliary neurotrophic factor (CNTF), leukocyte inhibitory factor (LIF), and IL-6—bind to similar receptors and activate JAK/STAT pathways. In contrast to the neurotrophins, CNTF production by Schwann cells is downregulated after injury, and the CNTF molecule lacks a sequence needed for secretion from the cell. If endogenous CNTF has any function in regeneration, it is as an injury factor released by damaged cells early in wallerian degeneration. However, experimental application of exogenous CNTF increases regeneration rate and may improve ultimate function in some models. Although less is known about LIF and IL-6, both are upregulated after injury and support motoneurons in vitro.

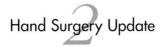

The fibroblast growth factors, similar to CNTF, are down-regulated after injury, but enhance regeneration across a gap through their effects on angiogenesis and glial function. The insulin-like growth factors (IGFs) rescue motoneurons in culture, are upregulated by denervated Schwann cells, and increase the rate of regeneration when applied to the injured sciatic nerve. Experimental inhibition of regeneration with antibodies to the IGFs confirms their crucial role in the support of regeneration. Glial-derived neurotrophic factor (GDNF), a factor identified only recently, is upregulated by Schwann cells after injury and is the most potent promoter of motoneuron survival yet described.

Recent experimental work has identified pathway deterioration, rather than muscle atrophy, as a primary cause of poor outcome when muscle reinnervation is delayed. In the rat sciatic model, long-term denervated muscle was able to accept regenerating axons; compensatory motor unit enlargement resulted in total muscle reinnervation when only 35% of motoneurons regenerated. Older microscopic studies of pathway failure describe Schwann cell atrophy, disruption of the basal lamina, and fibrosis. Recent work at the molecular level has shown prolonged denervation to result in loss of the B1 subunit of the integrins, receptors for laminin and cell adhesion molecules; loss of the p75 low-affinity neurotrophin receptor; and downregulation of glial growth factor (GGF), a soluble member of the neuregulin family of growth factors. Unlike the neurotrophins, GGF is produced by axons to regulate glial survival. Manipulation of these factors in denervated peripheral nerve to maintain Schwann cell responsiveness to reinnervation may soon improve the outcome of peripheral nerve repair.

Regeneration Specificity

The specificity of axon regeneration has profound functional consequences. Axons may regenerate in normal numbers, but little or no useful function will result if they reach inappropriate targets. For example, motor axons may enter sensory Schwann cell tubes and be directed to skin, while cutaneous axons may enter motor Schwann cell tubes and be directed to muscle. These misdirected axons will usually fail to establish functional connections and may exclude appropriate axons from the pathways they occupy.

The specificity of axon regeneration may be viewed in a hierarchical framework, proceeding from gross through progressively finer discriminations. The most basic form of specificity involves growth of regenerating axons to other nervous tissue (instead of bone or tendon) and is termed tissue specificity. Tissue specificity probably reflects the action of neurotropism (not to be confused with neurotrophism),

or directed axon growth up a gradient of a diffusable substance produced by the target. The action of neurotropism can only be proven if the axons are seen en route to the target; once target contact is made, specificity may be generated by selective neurotrophic support of these axons at the expense of those that have reinnervated other, inappropriate targets.

Several experiments in the last decade have been interpreted as showing specificity at the level of the nerve trunk. This work, largely performed in the rat sciatic nerve model, involved preferential growth of tibial or peroneal nerve axons back to the appropriate distal stump. However, this would occur only in a Y tube, and when only 1 stump was present as axon source. Recently, it has been shown that the size of the distal fascicle, not its specific identity, is responsible for the number of axons attracted to it. There appears to be no inherent nerve trunk specificity.

Recent work has evaluated the possibility of sensory-motor specificity. This has demonstrated that motor axons regenerating in mixed nerve preferentially reinnervate distal motor branches and/or muscle, a process called preferential motor reinnervation (PMR). Collaterals of a single motor axon often enter both sensory and motor Schwann cell tubes of the distal stump; specificity is generated by pruning collaterals from sensory pathways while maintaining those in motor pathways, even when the pathway ends blindly in a silicon tube. Motor pathways thus differ from sensory pathways in ways that survive wallerian degeneration, and that can be used by regenerating motor axons as a basis for collateral pruning to save only appropriate distal connections. The carbohydrate epitope L2/HNK-1, present in motor pathways but not in sensory pathways, selectively enhances motor axon regeneration in tissue culture. The interaction of motor axons with this molecule to produce regeneration specificity in vivo is currently under investigation.

Within both sensory and motor systems, there is a potential for topographic and/or end-organ specificity. Topographic specificity describes reinnervation of the correct muscle within the motor system or the correct patch of skin within the sensory system; end-organ specificity involves reinnervation of the correct type of sensory end organ within the sensory system, and the correct fiber type (fast versus slow, motor end plate versus muscle spindle) in the motor system. In the sensory system, topographic specificity can be generated only by surgical axon alignment. The consequences of failure to control topographic specificity are readily apparent when the cortical projections of reinnervated skin are mapped. Early experiments on end-organ reinnervation were interpreted as providing evidence for inherent end-organ specificity. However, they were performed in the sural nerve, where a limited receptor population made appropriate reinnervation likely. In a larger mixed nerve, where more receptor types are available, sensory end-organ reinnervation was found to be random. Recent evidence also suggests that modality-specific information may be transmitted by regenerating axons that have not made end-organ contact. The degree to which sensory axons and end organs must be matched to provide meaningful function thus remains unclear. The topography of motor innervation is not restored in adult mammals after most nerve lesions. However, reinnervation of the diaphragm and serratus anterior, muscles innervated by multiple spinal levels, is topographically specific in the adult rat. This is consistent with recent observations that muscles display surface markers of their spinal level of origin. Motor axons do not selectively reinnervate muscle fiber types in the adult. Instead, the motoneuron converts the muscle fiber type. This conversion is accomplished to varying degrees, however, so that a reinnervated motor unit will contain an admixture of hybrid myofiber types. In neonatal rats, soleus motoneurons selectively reinnervate slow muscle fibers, providing evidence of a developmental cue that is present on neonatal muscle; however, the cue is lost, or axons become insensitive to it, in the adult.

Overall, there is only limited evidence for inherent regeneration specificity of sufficient magnitude to influence the outcome of nerve repair. The principal exception is PMR, which shapes the outcome of routine nerve suture and is strong enough to overcome the effects of stump malalignment or an interstump gap. Mechanical alignment of proximal and distal stumps by the surgeon remains the only determinant of topographic specificity in both motor and sensory systems. End-organ specificity remains an elusive goal.

Annotated Bibliography

General

Kandel ER, Schwartz JH, Jessell TM (eds): *Principles of Neural Science,* ed 3. New York, NY, Elsevier, 1991.

Chapters 5 through 10 provide a highly-readable discussion of ion channels, membrane potential, conduction of the action potential, and synaptic transmission.

Functional Anatomy

Brushart TM: Central course of digital axons within the median nerve of Macaca mulatta. *J Comp Neurol* 1991;311:197–209.

HRP-WGA was used to continuously trace digital nerve axons throughout the median nerves of monkeys. These axons were more tightly grouped than the dissection studies of Sunderland would suggest, occupying 1/3 to 1/6 the cross-section of the nerve at the entrance to the brachial plexus. Axon tracing techniques map actual axon location; dissection can only infer location, and is limited in its accuracy by interfascicular plexus formation.

Hallin RG: Microneurography in relation to intraneural topography: Somatotopic organisation of median nerve fascicles in humans. *J Neurol Neurosurg Psychiatry* 1990;53:736–744.

Recordings were made from the proximal median nerves of awake human subjects with a new concentric needle electrode. Myelinated axons are not randomly distributed within a fascicle, but are arranged somatotopically into microbundles that supply limited areas of skin.

Lundborg G: The intrinsic vascularization of human peripheral nerves: Structural and functional aspects. *J Hand Surg* 1979; 4A:34–41.

Fascicles are vascularized segmentally by epineurial vessels, and each fascicle presents a well-defined vascular organization composed of endoneurial and perineurial microvascular systems in combination.

Wilgis EF, Murphy R: The significance of longitudinal excursion in peripheral nerves. *Hand Clin* 1986;2:761–766.

This study of fresh cadaver arms documented mean longitudinal excursion of nerves to be: brachial plexus, 15.3 mm; median nerve proximal to carpal tunnel, 14.5 mm; radial sensory nerve at wrist, 5.8 mm; common digital nerves, 7.0 mm; and digital nerves proximal to PIP, 3.1 to 3.6 mm. Interference with this mobility by scar tethering can focus longitudinal stress on the injured and often painful area.

Cellular Components

Jessen KR, Mirsky R: Schwann cell precursors and their development. *Glia* 1991;4:185–194.

A homogeneous pool of embryonic Schwann cells gives rise to two adult phenotypes. Myelin-forming Schwann cells are associated with axons of larger diameter, and express Po, MAG, and MBP. Nonmyelin-forming Schwann cells are associated with smaller diameter axons, and express NCAM, L1, GFAP, and NGF receptor. In vivo, the timing of myelination appears to be linked to signals that suppress proliferation and increase Schwann cell cAMP levels.

Electrical Properties

Chaudhry V, Cornblath DR: Wallerian degeneration in human nerves: Serial electrophysiological studies. *Muscle Nerve* 1992;15:687–693.

Motor-evoked amplitudes were reduced by 50% at 3 to 5 days after injury; the response was absent by day 9. Sensory-evoked amplitudes were reduced by 50% at 7 days after injury; the response was absent by day 11. Wallerian degeneration proceeds more slowly in humans than in rodent experimental models.

Mendell LM, Taylor JS, Johnson RD, Munson JB: Rescue of motoneuron and muscle afferent function in cats by regeneration into skin: II. Ia-motoneuron synapse. *J Neurophysiol* 1995;73:662–673.

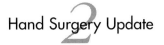

Synaptic efficacy is severly reduced by target depletion, partially rescued by cross-reinnervation into skin, and reversed almost completely by regeneration into native muscle. Improvement of motoneuron properties by regeneration into skin may reflect uptake of neurotrophins that support both motoneurons and sensory neurons, eg, BDNF, from cutaneous receptors that produce them.

Rafuse VF, Gordon T: Self-reinnervated cat medial gastrocnemius muscles: I. Comparisons of the capacity for regenerating nerves to form enlarged motor units after extensive peripheral nerve injuries. *J Neurophysiol* 1996;75:268–281.

Transected motor axons have the capacity to form enlarged motor units, provided that the regenerating axons grow along the distal endoneurial nerve sheath. As a result, all denervated muscle fibers become reinnervated if 35% of the muscle's normal complement of motor axons make functional connections.

Degeneration and Regeneration

Brushart TM: Motor axons preferentially reinnervate motor pathways. *J Neurosci* 1993;13:2730–2738.

Motor axons regenerating after transection of mixed nerve preferentially reinnervate distal motor branches and/or muscle, a process called preferential motor reinnervation (PMR). Collaterals of a single motor axon often enter both sensory and motor Schwann cell tubes of the distal stump; specificity is generated by pruning collaterals from sensory pathways while maintaining those in motor pathways. This occurs even if the pathways end blindly. Motor pathways thus differ from sensory pathways in ways that can be used by regenerating motor axons as a basis for collateral pruning and specificity generation.

Brushart TM, Mathur V, Sood R, Koschorke GM: Dispersion of regenerating axons across enclosed neural gaps. *J Hand Surg* 1995;20A:557–564.

Axons tend to grow straight across a tubular gap, with dispersion increasing as a factor of distance when correct fascicular alignment is maintained. When alignment is reversed, axonal dispersion is controled by fascicular size rather than by fascicular identity. These experiments produce evidence against regeneration specificity at the fascicular or nerve trunk level.

Dahlin LB, Kanje M: Conditioning effect induced by chronic nerve compression: An experimental study of the sciatic and tibial nerves of rats. *Scand J Plast Reconstr Surg Hand Surg* 1992;26:37–41.

Silicon tubes were chronically implanted around the sciatic nerves of rats. After a subsequent nerve crush, regeneration as measured by the pinch reflex test was more rapid in nerves that had been compressed than in those that had only been mobilized and crushed. Chronic compression may thus serve as a conditioning lesion.

Diamond J, Foerster A, Holmes M, Coughlin M: Sensory nerves in adult rats regenerate and restore sensory function to the skin independently of endogenous NGF. *J Neurosci* 1992; 12:1467–1476.

The ability of crushed axons to regrow and to restore functional recovery of three sensory modalities in adult rat skin (A-α-mediated touch, A-δ-mediated mechanonociception, and C-fiber-mediated heat nociception) was totally unaffected by anti-NGF treatment. NGF clearly affects axon regeneration in culture, but its presumed role in sensory axon regeneration in vivo must be questioned.

Doolabh VB, Hertl MC, Mackinnon SE: The role of conduits in nerve repair: A review. *Rev Neurosci* 1996;7:47–84.

This review summarizes 20 years of research on the bridging of nerve gaps with enclosed conduits or nerve guides. Gaps of up to 4 cm may be bridged successfully in primates. However, axon dispersion increases with distance, probably limiting the specificity of axon regeneration and thus clinical utility.

Fu SY, Gordon T: Contributing factors to poor functional recovery after delayed nerve repair: Prolonged axotomy. *J Neurosci* 1995;15:3876–3885.

The primary cause of poor recovery after long-term denervation is a profound reduction in the number of axons that successfully regenerate through deterioriating intramuscular nerve sheaths, rather than inability of denervated motor end plates to accept returning axons.

Fu SY, Gordon T: The cellular and molecular basis of peripheral nerve regeneration. *Mol Neurobiol* 1997;14:67–116.

This recent work is a comprehensive review of the cellular and molecular factors that influence peripheral nerve regeneration.

Glass JD, Brushart TM, George EB, Griffin JW: Prolonged survival of transected nerve fibres in C57BL/Ola mice is an intrinsic characteristic of the axon. *J Neurocytol* 1993;22:311–321.

The onset of wallerian degeneration is markedly retarded in the C57BL6/Ola mouse. Nerve segments were exchanged between standard C57BL6 and C57BL6/Ola mice, allowing regeneration of host axons through grafts containing donor Schwann cells. These nerves were then transected and the time course of axonal degeneration was observed. Fast or slow degeneration was found to be a property of the host axon, not the graft Schwann cells.

Goodman CS: Mechanisms and molecules that control growth cone guidance. *Annu Rev Neurosci* 1996;19:341–377.

Secreted and cell surface ligands in the growth cone's environment bind to receptors on the growth cone surface, trigger second-messenger signals, and lead to appropriate steering decisions. Growth cones respond to contact-mediated attraction, chemoattraction, contact-mediated repulsion, and chemorepulsion.

Luckenbill-Edds L: Laminin and the mechanism of neuronal outgrowth. *Brain Res Brain Res Rev* 1997;23:1–27.

This review summarizes the structure of the laminin molecule and its role in development, pathfinding, and regeneration in the vertebrate nervous system.

Mackinnon SE, Dellon AL, O'Brien JP: Changes in nerve fiber numbers distal to a nerve repair in the rat sciatic nerve model. *Muscle Nerve* 1991;14:1116–1122.

Myelinated axon counts in the distal rat sciatic nerve were evaluated between 1 and 24 months after proximal repair. Axon counts were

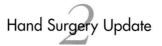

highest at 3 months, and did not return to normal until 24 months. Even in the rat, notorious for its rapid regeneration, 2 years must pass before final results of nerve repair can be assessed.

Martini R, Schachner M, Brushart TM: The L2/HNK-1 carbohydrate is preferentially expressed by previously motor axon-associated Schwann cells in reinnervated peripheral nerves. *J Neurosci* 1994;14:7180–7191.

The L2/HNK-1 carbohydrate is normally found in muscle nerve but not in cutaneous nerve. During regeneration of mixed nerve, L2/HNK-1 is upregulated only when a motor axon reinnervates a muscle pathway. This selective upregulation may form the molecular basis for the preferential reinnervation of muscle pathways by regenerating motor axons.

Scheidt P, Friede RL: Myelin phagocytosis in Wallerian degeneration: Properties of millipore diffusion chambers and immunohistochemical identification of cell populations. *Acta Neuropathol (Berl)* 1987;75:77–84.

Mouse nerve, within millipore filters that did not allow passage of macrophages, were placed in the peritoneal cavity. Schwann cells did not proliferate, and myelin was not phagocytosed. When the pores were large enough to let macrophages in, these macrophages actively consumed myelin. The macrophage, not the Schwann cell, is the primary myelin phagocyte.

Skene JH, Jacobson RD, Snipes GJ, McGuire CB, Norden JJ, Freeman JA: A protein induced during nerve growth (GAP-43) is a major component of growth-cone membranes. *Science* 1986;233:783–786.

Axonal development and regeneration are both accompanied by high levels of the growth-associated protein GAP-43. This protein has been found to be a major component of growth cone membranes. The growth cone is a specialized structure at the tip of growing axons that is essential to their elongation and guidance.

Totosy de Zepetnek JE, Zung HV, Erdebil S, Gordon T: Motor-unit categorization based on contractile and histochemical properties: A glycogen depletion analysis of normal and reinnervated rat tibialis anterior muscle. *J Neurophysiol* 1992;67:1404-1415.

There is reasonable, but not complete, correspondence in normal muscle between physiologic classification of motor units and histologic classification of fiber types. In reinnervated muscle there is less correspondence between the 2 classifications, consistent with incomplete respecification of muscle fiber properties by the motoneurons that reinnervate them.

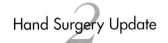
Chapter 18
Nerve Compression Syndromes

Robert M. Szabo, MD, MPH

Epidemiology

Typical presentation of an upper extremity compression neuropathy has historically been either posttraumatic, or gradual onset of paresthesias and pain in late middle-aged women. In the first population-based study of carpal tunnel syndrome, the mean age at diagnosis was 50 years for men and 51 years for women; women accounted for 78.5% of the cases. Younger industrial workers of both sexes are now being diagnosed with apparent compressive neuropathies from work-related repetitive motions. The Bureau of Labor and Statistics reported 92,576 cases of repetitive-motion disorder of the upper extremity in 1994 that resulted in lost days of work; nearly 41% were carpal tunnel syndrome.

Task-related factors that contribute to carpal tunnel syndrome include repetitiveness, force, mechanical stress, posture, vibration, and temperature. Occupational factors, however, are not so clearly defined and the mechanisms by which they produce neuropathy are not well known. Further complicating the matter, neuropathy that is believed to be causally related to work activities is usually accompanied by other upper extremity tendon or muscle symptoms that are poorly characterized and difficult to label with a precise diagnosis. In several recent studies, investigators concluded that carpal tunnel syndrome is more closely correlated with health habits and lifestyle (eg, obesity, and use of tobacco and caffeine) than to workplace activities. The association of carpal tunnel syndrome with work-related risk factors is a recurring theme of causation voiced by workers, ergonomists, lawyers, and physicians; however, the majority of the literature that tries to establish this as a causal association fails to meet standards of epidemiologic validity. To conclude that carpal tunnel syndrome is a repetitive motion disorder, the significance of repetition as a risk factor in the development of carpal tunnel syndrome must be determined. This involves consideration of the interaction of job exposures (extrinsic risk factors) with various innate anatomic, physiologic, or behavioral characteristics of the worker (intrinsic risk factors) that render the worker more likely to develop carpal tunnel syndrome. Clearly documented intrinsic risk factors for compressive neuropathies are female sex, pregnancy, diabetes, hypothyroidism, and rheumatoid arthritis. Occupational risk factors alone do not explain the occurrence of carpal tunnel syndrome; rather, carpal tunnel syndrome is the culmination of many distinct converging causal links. Repetition may be considered a risk factor in typing, for example, but neither extreme wrist flexion, extension, or forceful grasping are involved. Some epidemiologic studies have found that keyboarding appears to have a relative protective effect from developing symptoms of median nerve compression when compared to other occupations. Although no relationship between exposure to keyboard work and median nerve deficit has been reported, several keyboard manufacturers are involved in highly publicized product liability cases, defending charges that their products caused carpal tunnel syndrome and cubital tunnel syndrome in workers.

This work-related focus of epidemiology requires a compensatory change in the physician's approach to managing the condition. An early discussion with patients about different risk factors for their syndrome is warranted, without automatically attributing the cause to the workplace. A successful outcome is more likely if the patient takes an active role in rehabilitation and is encouraged not to pass blame onto an employer. As with industrial low back pain, it is best to pursue nonsurgical management if specific objective evidence of a compression neuropathy is lacking.

Pathophysiology

The term compression neuropathy implies an etiology; the nerve is compressed by some adjacent anatomic structure. Between the cervical spine and the wrist there are a number of specific sites where nerve compression is common, and these give rise to various well-known nerve compression syndromes. A careful history and physical examination can identify these syndromes; for most, surgical procedures to decompress the nerve have been established. This concept of the etiology of nerve compression syndromes, however, is oversimplified; several other factors play integral roles in the pathophysiology.

Systemic Conditions
Diabetes, alcoholism, hypothyroidism, or exposure to industrial solvents may cause a systemic depression in peripheral

nerve function that lowers the threshold for manifestation of a compression neuropathy. In many people, aging has a similar systemic effect. Indicative of the importance of systemic conditions is the high prevalence of bilateral occurrence or multiple-nerve involvement, even if only one extremity is used in an activity that provokes symptoms. Children with mucopolysaccharidosis or mucolipidosis frequently have carpal tunnel syndrome and benefit from early carpal tunnel release.

Ischemia/Mechanical Processes

The dramatic reversal of symptoms that sometimes occurs following surgical decompression suggests an ischemic etiology to many compression neuropathies. The earliest manifestation of low-grade peripheral nerve compression is reduced epineurial blood flow, which occurs at 20 to 30 mm mercury compression. Axonal transport becomes impaired at 30 mm mercury; with extended pressure at this level, endoneurial fluid pressure increases. Neurophysiologic changes and symptoms of paresthesias have been induced in human volunteers with 30 to 40 mm mercury compression on the median nerve. Experimental compression at levels of 50 mm mercury for 2 hours caused epineural edema and axonal transport block. Pressures greater than 60 mm mercury caused complete intraneural ischemia with complete sensory block, followed by complete motor block. Morphologic examination after severe compression in animals has shown nodal displacement with invagination of compressed areas toward uncompressed nerve segments. In extended cases of nerve compression, recovery following decompression may be very slow, or progression of the condition may halt but without improvement of symptoms. In these cases, the initial vascular etiology is superseded by other mechanical processes, particularly fibrosis of the nerve, which diminish potential for recovery. These findings suggest that nerve compression lesions occur as a spectrum, which can be divided into early, intermediate, and late categories. Early stages of low-grade compression respond most favorably to conservative management, such as steroid injection and splinting in the case of carpal tunnel syndrome. Intermediate stages of nerve compression involve patients who have persistent interference with intraneural microcirculation and symptoms of constant paresthesias and numbness. These patients respond best to decompression of the nerve; in the case of carpal tunnel syndrome, they predictably do well with carpal tunnel release. In advanced cases, persistent endoneurial edema induces fibroblast proliferation and endoneurial fibrosis. Patients in this late stage of carpal tunnel syndrome, for instance, have permanent sensory loss and thenar atrophy; carpal tunnel release alone may not eliminate all symptoms. These patients were once treated with internal neurolysis, but recent studies have shown no benefits from neurolysis.

Traction Injuries

Nerves of the upper extremity have considerable mobility throughout their lengths. Compression may tether the nerve, restricting its mobility, and thereby cause traction (stretching) in response to joint motion. Anatomic studies comparing carpal tunnel syndrome patients to normal volunteers with dynamic ultrasound or magnetic resonance imaging (MRI) have shown that the dimensions of the carpal tunnel change as a function of wrist position. When the wrist is flexed, the median nerve is compressed between the flexor tendons and the flexor retinaculum. Because the path of the median nerve lies palmar to the centers of rotation of the joints of the hand, flexion of the wrist and fingers will shorten the bed of the nerve, allowing it to slide proximally. Similarly, extension of the wrist and fingers lengthens the course of the median nerve in the hand, causing it to slide distally. To the extent that the normal sliding of the median nerve is restricted, eg, as a result of adhesions or compressive entrapments, lengthening of the nerve bed in response to joint motion must be accommodated by focal, excessive elongation of a short nerve segment. This type of nerve traction can result in temporary or permanent disruption of action potential propagation, causing impairment of sensory and motor function. In response to simulated active finger flexion, proximal sliding of the median nerve occurs consistently at 43% of the rate of proximal sliding of the finger flexor tendons, suggesting that there are shear forces between the median nerve and adjacent tendons. In addition to longitudinal sliding, displacement of the median nerve in the palmar-dorsal direction and radial-ulnar direction in response to hand motion has been observed in dynamic ultrasound and MRI studies. Many upper-extremity compression neuropathies likely include traction on the nerve as an element of pathophysiology.

Double Crush Phenomenon

The nerve cell body synthesizes enzymes, polypeptides, polysaccharides, free amino acids, neurosecretory granules, mitochondria, and tubulin subunits, which are necessary for survival and normal function of the axon. These substances travel distally along the axon, and metabolized products resulting from their breakdown return in a proximal direction by fast and slow axoplasmic transport mechanisms. Any

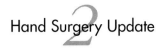

disruption of the synthesis or blockage of the transport of these materials may increase susceptibility of the axons to compression. A compression lesion at one point on a peripheral nerve may lower the threshold for occurrence of a compression neuropathy at another site on the same nerve, possibly by restricting axonal transport kinetics. In such a case, the outcome of surgical decompression may be disappointing, unless both entrapments are treated. Less compression of the median nerve at the carpal tunnel level, as manifested by distal sensory latency, is found to produce symptoms when a proximal cervical lesion is present. Coexistent cervical root compression is one of the reasons cited for persistent residual symptoms following carpal tunnel release. The authors who first coined the term "double crush" acknowledged that the term is too restrictive because there could be more than 2 areas involved along the course of the nerve; a proximal focal disturbance could be due to traction, and a generalized subclinical polyneuropathy could act as the proximal site of compression. Recently other authors proposed that the double crush hypothesis is offered clinically far more often than warranted. They cite the lack of good experimental evidence to prove its existence, and note that the prerequisites for use are often ignored. For instance, the tenet that there be anatomic continuity of nerve fibers between two or more lesion sites is most often breached. Two focal nerve disorders along the same pathway only fulfill this criteria if the same axons are compromised at both sites. Accordingly, lesions within the intraspinal canal should not be able to interfere with axoplasmic transport mechanisms when they involve sensory fibers because they injure sensory fibers proximal to their cell bodies of origin in the dorsal root ganglion, in contrast to the more distally situated lesions that damage the postganglionic sensory fibers. The pre- and postganglionic sensory fibers are not anatomically continuous; injury to one of them has no effect on the other unless there is concomitant damage to their common cell body.

Clinical Presentation and Diagnosis

Upper extremity nerve compression is normally gradual in onset and chronic. Presentation generally falls into 2 groups—dynamic or exertional, with symptoms appearing in response to a specific provocative activity and resolving when the activity is stopped, and insidious, with symptoms that develop gradually with no notable relationship to activity and often worsen at night. It is important to differentiate these by obtaining a careful history.

Only rarely will an upper extremity nerve compression syndrome develop rapidly in the context of trauma. Acute presentation, analogous to compartment syndrome, should be considered an emergency requiring prompt surgical decompression. Acute carpal tunnel syndrome, for example, may be seen following a distal radius fracture; spontaneous bleeding in a patient on anticoagulation therapy; or secondary to a variety of infectious, rheumatologic, or hematologic disorders. These situations mandate immediate carpal tunnel release.

The diagnosis of an upper extremity compression neuropathy is a 2-part process—demonstration of a specific nerve lesion, and determination of the underlying cause. Although the cause may be purely mechanical, it is frequently potentiated by a coexisting systemic disorder or sometimes a more proximal lesion of the same nerve (double crush phenomenon). It is important to avoid tunnel vision early in the diagnostic process; the possibility of additional causes must be considered. Some of the factors associated with development of carpal tunnel syndrome are listed in Outline 1. A patient with a Pancoast tumor compressing the brachial plexus may have complaints that mimic ulnar nerve symptoms, underlining the importance of casting a wide diagnostic net.

A number of tests are available to characterize nerve compression syndromes in the upper extremity. Diagnostic tests for carpal tunnel syndrome are listed in Table 1. The carpal tunnel compression test has been shown to be more sensitive and specific than the traditional provocative tests of nerve percussion (Tinel) and wrist flexion (Phalen). Direct compression of the median nerve at the carpal tunnel is performed with both thumbs of the examiner. If paresthesias are elicited within 30 seconds, the test is positive. A device is available that allows quantification of the amount of pressure to be applied. There is a trade-off between tests that have only modest accuracy but are easily performed (eg, Phalen's test), and tests that have high accuracy but are difficult, expensive, or invasive (eg, electrodiagnostic tests). Liquid crystal thermography has received some attention, but sensitivity is quite low and its usefulness in the diagnosis of nerve compression is questionable.

Although electrodiagnostic testing remains the diagnostic gold standard, it still has a number of pitfalls. Highly operator-dependent, the test should be conducted with the same equipment and operator each time. Nerve conduction velocities and latencies can be compared to published population norms, to the contralateral nerve, to other nerves in the same extremity, or to previous tests in the same patient. Systemic conditions (including age-dependent alterations in nerve conduction) or

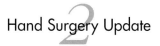
Outline 1
Factors in the pathogenesis of carpal tunnel syndrome

I. Anatomy
  A. Decreased size of carpal tunnel
    1. Bony abnormalities of the carpal bones
    2. Thickened transverse carpal ligament
    3. Acromegaly

  B. Increased contents of canal
    1. Neuroma
    2. Lipoma
    3. Myeloma
    4. Abnormal muscle bellies
    5. Persistent median artery (thrombosed or patent)
    6. Hypertrophic synovium
    7. Distal radius fracture callus
    8. Posttraumatic osteophytes
    9. Hematoma (hemophilia, anticoagulation therapy)

II. Physiology
  A. Neuropathic conditions
    1. Diabetes
    2. Alcoholism
    3. Proximal lesion of median nerve (double crush syndrome)

  B. Inflammatory conditions
    1. Tenosynovitis
    2. Rheumatoid arthritis
    3. Infection
    4. Gout

C. Alternations of fluid balance
  1. Pregnancy
  2. Eclampsia
  3. Myxedema
  4. Long-term hemodialysis
  5. Horizontal position and muscle relaxation (sleep)
  6. Raynaud's disease
  7. Obesity

D. Congenital
  1. Mucopolysaccharidosis
  2. Mucolipidosis

III. Position and use of the wrist
  A. Repetitive forceful flexion/extension (manual labor)

  B. Repetitive forceful squeezing and release of a tool, or repetitive forceful torsion of a tool

  C. Vibration exposure

  D. Weightbearing with wrist extended
    1. Paraplegia
    2. Long-distance bicycling

  E. Immobilization with the wrist flexed, ulnarly-deviated
    1. Casting after Colles' fracture
    2. Awkward sleep position

(Adapted with permission from Szabo RM: Carpal tunnel syndrome: General, in Gelberman RH (ed): *Operative Nerve Repair and Reconstruction.* Philadelphia, PA, JB Lippincott, 1991, pp 869–888.)

failure to control limb temperature may confound the comparisons. Repetition of studies of a particular nerve over time can document progression or resolution of a neuropathy. Inching techniques are useful in localizing a lesion. Nerve conduction studies often provide the only objective evidence of the neuropathic condition.

Radiographic information has only modest value in diagnosis of upper extremity compression neuropathies. Unless there is a history of trauma, rheumatoid arthritis, or findings of limited wrist motion on physical examination, radiography has been shown to be a low-yield diagnostic test for carpal tunnel syndrome. Plain radiographs in 2 orthogonal planes can be useful to rule out posttraumatic deformity, neoplasm, cervical ribs, or other possible bony causes of the nerve condition. A chest radiograph should be obtained whenever the patient history includes smoking, ulnar nerve symptoms, and shoulder pain. Although MRI can be helpful in assessing the extent of a soft-tissue mass in a posterior interosseous nerve syndrome, MRI and computed tomography rarely play a role in diagnosis.

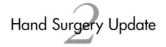
Table 1

Diagnostic tests for carpal tunnel syndrome

Name of Test	How Performed	Condition Measured	Positive Result	Interpretation of Positive Result
Phalen's test	Patient places elbows on table, forearms vertical, wrists flexed	Paresthesias in response to position	Numbness or tingling on radial side digits within 60 seconds	Probable carpal tunnel syndrome (sensitivity 0.75, specificity 0.47)
Percussion test (Tinel's)	Examiner lightly taps along median nerve, at the wrist, proximal to distal	Site of nerve lesion	Tingling response in fingers at site of compression	Probable carpal tunnel syndrome if response is at the wrist (sensitivity 0.60, specificity 0.67)
Carpal tunnel compression test	Direct compression of median nerve by examiner	Paresthesias in response to pressure	Paresthesias within 30 seconds	Probable carpal tunnel syndrome (sensitivity 0.87, specificity 0.90)
Hand diagram	Patient marks sites of pain or altered sensation on an outline diagram of the hand	Patient's perception of site of nerve deficit	Signs on palmar side of radial digits without signs in the palm	Probable carpal tunnel syndrome (sensitivity 0.96, specificity 0.73), negative predictive (value of a negative test = 0.91)
Hand volume stress test	Hand volume measured by water displacement. Repeat after 7-minute stress test and 10-minute rest	Hand volume	Hand volume increased by 10 mL or more	Probable dynamic carpal tunnel syndrome
Direct measurement of carpal tunnel pressure	Wick or infusion catheter is placed in carpal tunnel; pressure measured	Hydrostatic pressure: resting, and in response to position or stress	Resting pressure 25 mmHg or more (This number is variable and may be technique-related.)	Hydrostatic compression at wrist is cause of probable carpal tunnel syndrome
Static 2-point discrimination	Determine minimum separation of 2 points perceived as distinct when lightly touched to palmar surface of digit	Innervation density of slowly adapting fibers	Failure to discriminate points more than 6 mm apart	Advanced nerve dysfunction
Moving 2-point discrimination	As above, but with points moving	Innervation density of quickly adapting fibers	Failure to discriminate points more than 5 mm apart	Advanced nerve dysfunction

(Continued)

Table 1
Continued

Name of Test	How Performed	Condition Measured	Positive Result	Interpretation of Positive Result
Vibrometry	Vibrometer head is placed on palmar side of digit; amplitude at 120 Hz increased to threshold of perception; compare median, ulnar nerves, both hands	Threshold of quickly adapting fibers	Asymmetry with contralateral hand or radial versus ulnar	Probable carpal tunnel syndrome (sensitivity 0.87)
Semmes-Weinstein monofilaments	Monofilaments of increasing diameter touched to palmar side of digit until patient can tell which digit is touched	Threshold of slowly adapting fibers	Value greater than 2.83 in radial digits	Median nerve impairment (sensitivity 0.83)
Distal sensory latency and conduction velocity	Orthodromic stimulus and recording across wrist	Latency, conduction velocity of sensory fibers	Latency greater than 3.5 mm/sec or asymmetry of conduction velocity greater than 0.5 mm/sec versus contralateral hand	Probable carpal tunnel syndrome
Distal motor latency and conduction velocity	Orthodromic stimulus and recording across wrist	Latency, conduction velocity of motor fibers of median nerve	Latency greater than 4.5 mm/sec or asymmetry of conduction velocity greater than 1.0 mm/sec	Probable carpal tunnel syndrome
Electromyography	Needle electrodes placed in muscle	Denervation of thenar muscles	Fibrillation potentials, sharp waves, increased insertional activity	Very advanced motor median nerve compression

(Adapted with permission from Szabo RM: Common hand problems. *Orthop Clin North Am* 1992;23:105.)

Median Nerve

Carpal Tunnel Syndrome

Compression of the median nerve at the wrist is the most common and well-known compression neuropathy of the upper extremity. Each year an estimated 1 million adults in the United States report carpal tunnel syndrome requiring medical treatment. The clinical picture of pain and paresthesias on the palmar-radial aspect of the hand, often worse at night and/or exacerbated by repetitive forceful use of the hand, is readily recognized. A variety of diagnostic tests are described. Threshold tests such as Semmes-Weinstein monofilament or vibrometry tests, which measure a single nerve fiber innervating a group of receptors, are most sensitive at evaluating sensibility. Nerve conduction studies can provide objective evidence of impaired conduction. Phalen's wrist flexion test, Tinel's test, the carpal tunnel nerve compression test, and the hand diagram (in which the patient

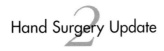
marks the location of pain, numbness, or tingling on an outline of the dorsal and palmar aspects of the hand) are easily performed to support the diagnosis.

The outcome movement in medicine has encouraged the development of patient questionnaires as measures of well-being. A disease-specific questionnaire for carpal tunnel syndrome was introduced in 1993. The developers reported a high correlation between functional status scores and severity of symptoms; moderate correlation between each subscale and measurements of grip and pinch strength; and weak correlations for sensibility testing with 2-point discrimination, Semmes-Weinstein monofilaments, or median nerve sensory nerve conduction velocity. Subsequent investigations have explored the use of outcome instruments, focusing on their importance while downgrading the value of physical examination. One group appraised the value of various clinical and questionnaire measures for the assessment of outcome after carpal tunnel surgery with the Medical Outcomes Study 36-item short form health survey, the Arthritis Impact Measurement Scale, the Brigham and Women's Hospital carpal tunnel questionnaire, wrist range of motion, power pinch grip strength, pressure sensibility, and dexterity. This study found standardized questionnaires to be more sensitive to the clinical change produced by carpal tunnel surgery than the common physical measures of outcome. Another group evaluated the Brigham and Women's Hospital carpal tunnel questionnaire in 156 consecutive new patients presenting with pain, numbness, or tingling of the upper extremity. They concluded that outcome measures must be distinguished from diagnostic tests; these measures are not useful in clinical diagnosis. Diagnosis of carpal tunnel syndrome must be made independent of any outcome score. Symptoms measured with the carpal tunnel syndrome outcome instrument are similar in many causes of pain, numbness, and tingling and are indistinguishable from many other upper extremity nerve compression symptoms.

Carpal tunnel syndrome should be considered in the context of the patient's overall health before narrowing focus on the mechanical problems at the wrist. Particularly if the condition is bilateral, metabolic abnormalities or other systemic causes should be sought. The surgeon should be alert to the possibility of coexisting nerve compression more proximal, particularly cervical radiculopathy, thoracic outlet compression syndrome, and pronator syndrome. Patients with poliomyelitis or other paralysis requiring ambulatory aids are predisposed to carpal tunnel syndrome. This group of patients is particularly difficult to treat, as surgery is less predictable and recurrent problems are common.

Conservative therapy includes splinting the wrist in neutral position, oral anti-inflammatory drugs to reduce synovitis, diuretics to reduce edema, and management of underlying systemic diseases. Steroid injection will offer transient relief to 80% of patients; however, only 22% will be symptom-free after 12 months. Steroid injection is most effective in patients who have had symptoms for less than 1 year, and also have diffuse and intermittent numbness; normal 2-point discrimination; no weakness, thenar atrophy, or denervation potentials on electromyography (EMG) examination; and only 1- to 2-millisecond prolongation of distal motor and sensory latencies. Forty percent of this latter group will remain symptom free longer than 12 months. In a more recent study of 57 younger (mostly female) patients in the labor force, steroid injection resolved symptoms in only 13%. This study suggests that most of this young female working population probably did not have true carpal tunnel syndrome; the injection can be useful in diagnosis. Pyridoxine (vitamin B$_6$) does not appear to modify the natural history of this disease. Cold laser therapy, acupuncture, transcutaneous electrical nerve stimulation (TENS) units, yoga, and chiropractic carpal tunnel manipulations have all been proposed recently as treatments for carpal tunnel syndrome; however, no scientific evidence of their effectiveness exists. This quest for new nonsurgical remedies has stemmed in part from the failure of carpal tunnel syndrome surgery in the so-called repetitive trauma patient, who is often incorrectly diagnosed to begin with.

Failure of nonsurgical treatment in the properly diagnosed patient is an indication for surgical release of the transverse carpal ligament. New information suggests that earlier intervention leads to better results. One study showed that patients who had surgery 3 or more years after initial diagnosis of carpal tunnel syndrome were less than half as likely to have symptom resolution than were patients who had surgery within 3 years of diagnosis. Another study demonstrated that patients with intermittent preoperative numbness and paresthesias had a much better sensory recovery than patients with constant symptoms.

The controversy between open versus endoscopic carpal tunnel release continues. Several devices are available for endoscopic ligament release. Proponents of this technique cite a smaller scar and possible transient acceleration of rehabilitation as advantages. Pillar pain has not been reduced and palmar tenderness has not been eliminated. Grip strength has been shown to return to preoperative level by 3 months after open release, and pinch strength within 6 weeks. Endoscopic carpal tunnel release has had minimal effect on this recovery period. Although there was an initial frenzy of enthusiasm for these new endoscopic techniques, recent independent controlled studies have demonstrated little or no difference in surgical results between conventional and endoscopic groups. Endoscopic release has the significant disadvantage of poor or absent visualization, with the attendant risk of iatrogenic injury to the neurovascular structures. Endoscopic technique has prompted other surgeons to describe minimally invasive incisions, or to invent instrumentation to facilitate transverse carpal ligament sectioning via a small incision. Because of its reliability and good visualization, open release remains the preferred technique, particularly for the surgeon who does not perform this surgery frequently.

In the past, internal neurolysis was commonly performed during carpal tunnel surgery. Several clinical studies have failed to demonstrate any benefit to neurolysis; consequently, it is no longer recommended. Recently, 3 different prospective randomized comparative studies have addressed the role of epineurotomy in the treatment of carpal tunnel syndrome. All 3 studies concluded that the use of epineurotomy as an adjunctive procedure during carpal tunnel release offered no additional benefit.

The etiology of pillar pain—pain at the base of the hand after carpal tunnel release—is still unknown. One group developed a technique for dividing the radial attachments of the transverse carpal ligament under direct visualization, using the flexor carpi radialis as a guide. Using this technique in 87 hands, they reported that 79 obtained complete or partial relief of preoperative symptoms and quick resolution of pillar tenderness. This technique does not permit visualization of the motor branch of the median nerve, can result in hypertrophy of the wrist scar, and puts the palmar branch of the median nerve more at risk than ulnar-based incisions. Additional complications of flexor pollicus longus (FPL) adhesions requiring manipulation under sedation were reported in 2 cases.

Patients with carpal tunnel symptoms occasionally have sensory symptoms in the little finger. In the past, surgeons have recommended release of Guyon's canal; however, this is no longer recommended. Recent MRI evidence shows that the dimensions of Guyon's canal enlarge with carpal tunnel release alone. This finding has been substantiated clinically; if patients' ulnar nerve symptoms truly come from Guyon's canal compression, they will improve after carpal tunnel release alone.

The flexor retinaculum at the wrist serves as a pulley, restraining the digital flexor tendons when the wrist is flexed. Concern that division of this pulley during carpal tunnel surgery may permit bowstringing of the tendons, entrapment of the median nerve in scar, or wound dehiscence is the principal motivation for splinting the wrist after carpal tunnel surgery. Eighty-one percent of American hand surgeons splint patients' wrists for 2 to 4 weeks following carpal tunnel surgery. In a prospective randomized study of 50 consecutive patients undergoing surgery for idiopathic carpal tunnel syndrome, neither bowstringing of tendons

nor wound problems were observed in splinted or unsplinted wrists. Patients who were splinted experienced significant delays in return to activities of daily living, return to work at light and full duty, and in recovery of grip and key pinch strength. Patients with splinted wrists also had increased pain and scar tenderness in the first month after surgery. Other than these factors, there was no difference between groups in the incidence of complications. Based on these findings, splinting for 2 weeks after carpal tunnel surgery is largely detrimental and should not be routine. If used at all, splinting should be limited to 1 week as a precaution against complications of tendon bowstringing and nerve entrapment in scar. A home physiotherapy program is encouraged, in which the wrist and fingers are exercised separately to avoid simultaneous finger and wrist flexion, the position most prone to cause bowstringing.

Pronator Syndrome

The median nerve is vulnerable to compression at several sites around the elbow: between a supracondylar process and a ligament of Struthers, beneath the bicipital aponeurosis, deep to the arch of origin of the pronator teres, and under the origin of the flexor digitorum superficialis. The principal symptoms of thenar weakness and numbness in the radial 3.5 digits and may be incorrectly attributed to carpal tunnel syndrome. Sensory symptoms may also be present over the thenar eminence in the distribution of the palmar cutaneous nerve. Diagnostic features of pronator syndrome include pain in the anterior aspect of the proximal forearm, a positive nerve percussion sign in the forearm, and a negative Phalen's test. Unlike carpal tunnel syndrome, symptoms of pronator syndrome typically are absent at night. Specific provocative maneuvers that reproduce the pain and distal paresthesias are used to localize the site of compression. Resisted elbow flexion with the forearm in supination implicates compression by the bicipital aponeurosis. Resisted forearm pronation with the elbow in full extension suggests compression between the two heads of the pronator. Isolated proximal interphalangeal joint flexion of the middle finger producing paresthesias in the radial 3 digits or local pain suggests entrapment under the fibrous origin of the flexor digitorum superficialis. Palpation of the medial humeral condyle and distal diaphysis may reveal a bony prominence that is a supracondyloid process; anteroposterior, lateral, and oblique radiographs of the distal humerus should be obtained before surgery to rule out its presence. Surgical decompression through the 4 sites mentioned above will yield rapid recovery in most cases.

Nerve conduction velocity measurement of the median nerve in the proximal forearm is misleading; reduced velocity of conduction in the forearm has been noted in 20% to 32%

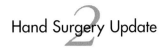

of patients with carpal tunnel syndrome. Standard nerve conduction velocity tests measure the forearm segment in combination with the distal latency, and this may not represent an accurate assessment of conduction in the proximal portion of the nerve. Forearm median nerve conduction velocities in patients with carpal tunnel syndrome are significantly slower than in normal subjects. Retrograde degeneration of nerve axons may result from entrapment in the carpal tunnel. Electrophysiologic findings, especially needle EMG when positive, may be more definitive than findings from clinical examination. The EMG diagnosis depends on observance of fibrillations, positive sharp waves, and reduced interference patterns in the FPL and pronator quadratus muscles. However, EMG cannot distinguish a median nerve lesion at the pronator teres from a more proximal lesion. Electrodiagnostic studies were found to be a poor predictor of the results of surgical decompression in a series of 36 patients.

Anterior Interosseous Nerve Syndrome

Compression of the anterior interosseous nerve (AIN) results in loss of motor function without sensory involvement. The patient is unable to end-pinch between index finger and thumb, and often complains of a nonspecific aching pain in the anterior forearm. In this syndrome, the index finger extends at the distal interphalangeal joint with compensatory increased flexion at the proximal interphalangeal joint during pinch. The thumb hyperextends at the interphalangeal joint and displays increased flexion of the metacarpophalangeal joint. Involvement of the pronator quadratus can be evaluated by testing the strength of resisted forced supination with the elbow maximally flexed. This eliminates the effect of the humeral head of the pronator teres, which is responsible for 75% of the rotational strength of this muscle. Bilateral involvement suggests Parsonage-Turner syndrome (brachial neuritis) or symmetrical polyneuropathy. The onset of symptoms is usually spontaneous, and electrophysiologic examination is valuable in confirming diagnosis.

One pair of investigators reported that the literature is divided between describing AIN syndrome as a compression neuropathy and as a peripheral nerve manifestation of a brachial plexus neuropathy. Surgical exploration was conducted in 46 of 100 cases reported in surgical literature, and 4 of 32 cases in medical specialty literature; outcome analysis revealed good results in both groups. If a patient presents with a history of acute spontaneous pain in the forearm, followed within a few days or weeks by AIN palsy, Parsonage-Turner syndrome is possible; observation for 3 months is warranted. Failure of conservative management indicates surgery. Any of a variety of anomalous structures may be the mechanical cause of compression; consequently, exploration

of the full length of the nerve is appropriate, with release of all constricting structures encountered.

Presentation of this syndrome may be incomplete, with only one finger involved; in such cases, misdiagnosis as tendon rupture is possible.

Ulnar Nerve

Pathologic compression of the ulnar nerve occurs most commonly at the elbow (cubital tunnel syndrome) or at the wrist where the ulnar nerve passes through the confines of the canal of Guyon (ulnar tunnel syndrome). The patient may report numbness along the little finger and the ulnar half of the ring finger, often accompanied by weakness of grip (particularly in activities in which torque is applied to a tool). The site of the compression may be determined by careful physical examination; pain at the medial aspect of the elbow, a positive percussion test at the cubital tunnel, or exacerbation of symptoms by full flexion of the elbow suggest cubital tunnel syndrome. Sensory involvement on the ulnar dorsal aspect of the hand also suggests cubital tunnel syndrome, as the dorsal cutaneous branch of the ulnar nerve originates proximal to the canal of Guyon. Weakness of the deep flexors to the ring and little fingers, as well as weakness of the flexor carpi ulnaris, signal proximal ulnar nerve entrapment.

A worrisome occurrence is unexpected onset of ulnar neuropathy after an unrelated surgery, suggesting improper patient positioning as a cause. Most patients in this category had a preexisting neuropathy.

Cubital Tunnel Syndrome

Cubital tunnel syndrome may be caused by constricting fascial bands, soft-tissue structures (hypertrophied synovium, tumor, ganglion, anconeus epitrochlearis muscle), bony abnormalities (cubitus valgus, bone spurs), or by subluxation of the ulnar nerve over the medial epicondyle with elbow flexion. Although work-related activities involving repetitive elbow flexion and extension may aggravate cubital tunnel syndrome, there are no scientific data supporting work as a causal risk factor.

Examination of the patient with symptoms of ulnar nerve compression should begin at the neck, searching for cervical disk disease or arthritis. Provocative maneuvers such as Adson's, hyperabduction, military brace positioning, and 3-minute elevation should be used to screen for thoracic outlet syndrome, while keeping in mind the frequent false positives these tests can yield. Range of motion of the elbow should be observed, and the ulnar nerve should be palpated during flexion–extension to elicit subluxation. Percussion over the ulnar nerve can be performed, looking for a positive Tinel sign. The elbow flexion test is much like the wrist flexion test (Phalen's test) for diagnosing carpal tunnel syndrome; it is performed by maximally flexing the elbow with forearm supination and wrist extension. Symptoms of paresthesias in the ulnar nerve distribution within 1 minute constitute a positive test. The pressure provocative test is performed by applying pressure for 60 seconds proximal to the cubital tunnel, with the elbow in 20° flexion and the forearm supinated. The test is positive if symptoms are reported in the ulnar nerve distribution. Combining the pressure and flexion provocative test has been shown to produce sensitivity of 0.91 compared to the sensitivity of the Tinel sign (0.70), the pressure provocative test alone (0.55), and the elbow flexion test alone (0.32). Sensory examination of the hand, including the dorsum, should be performed using Semmes-Weinstein monofilaments. Decreased dorsal ulnar sensation is found when a lesion is proximal to the wrist. Motor examination should carefully grade the flexor carpi ulnaris, flexor digitorum profundus to the little and ring fingers, and the intrinsic muscles of the hand. Median nerve fibers may supply some of the intrinsic hand muscles in 7.5% of limbs via a Martin-Gruber connection. The flexor carpi ulnaris and flexor digitorum profundus are often spared; their innervation may arise proximal to the cubital tunnel, or the axons innervating these muscles may be less vulnerable to compression due to their posterolateral location in the cubital tunnel.

Cubital tunnel syndrome may be treated either conservatively or surgically. In mild cases, nonsurgical therapy is effective. The use of elbow splints (particularly at night), pads, and steroid injections have been recommended; however, there is no published evidence confirming any added value of steroid injections over splinting alone.

Options for surgical treatment of cubital tunnel syndrome include simple decompression, subcutaneous transposition, intramuscular transposition, submuscular transposition, and medial epicondylectomy. These techniques can be expected to provide 80% to 90% good results, with return of function within 6 months. All of these techniques have recurrence rates or poor results ranging from 25% to 33% in moderate or severe degrees of compression. Simple decompression, achieved by releasing the arch of origin of the flexor carpi ulnaris, may be appropriate if a localized nerve percussion sign suggests isolated entrapment at this site. Postoperative subluxation is a statistically significant cause of failure of simple decompression. Anterior transposition is preferred for cases with bony deformity, subluxation or dislocation of the nerve, or severe cases with motor involvement, especially in a younger patient. The sites of compression that should be explored and released

from proximal to distal include the arcade of Struthers, the medial intermuscular septum, the medial epicondyle, the cubital tunnel, and the deep flexor-pronator aponeurosis. Anterior submuscular transposition is the most popular procedure for reoperation of an unsuccessful decompression or transposition. Some surgeons routinely perform medial epicondylectomy for cubital tunnel syndrome; however, medial epicondylectomy is best suited for nonunion of an epicondylar fracture with ulnar nerve symptoms. If a medial epicondylectomy is performed, the dissection should be extended proximally and distally to ensure mobility of the nerve. Disadvantages of medial epicondylectomy include nerve vulnerability, bone tenderness, elbow joint instability, flexor forearm muscle weakness, and ectopic bone formation. Most authors seem unconcerned by the risk of injury to the ulnar collateral ligament with this procedure. In one recent study, the authors recommended repair of the medial collateral ligament after observing valgus instability in 4 elbows in 46 patients who had medial epicondylectomies. One investigator demonstrated that the amount of bone that can be removed without violating the anterior medial collateral ligament is only 1 to 4 mm, approximately 20% of the overall width of the epicondyle.

In a review of 50 reports published between 1898 and 1988, one author suggested that little more than personal bias is available for guidance in selecting treatment. Reinterpreting published data based on contemporary concepts of the pathophysiology of chronic nerve compression, he concluded that for minimal compression, excellent results can be achieved in 50% of patients with conservative treatment, and in nearly 100% by any of the accepted surgical approaches. For moderate compression, the anterior submuscular transposition yields the most excellent results with the fewest recurrences. For severe compression, the anterior intramuscular transposition yielded the fewest excellent results and the most recurrences; the submuscular transposition gave the best results.

Several new techniques have been introduced for cubital tunnel surgery. One author recommends simple decompression with endoscopic assistance, while another advocates submuscular transposition with musculofascial lengthening of the flexor-pronator mass. In a cadaver model, simple decompression and medial epicondylectomy result in significantly lower intraneural pressures than either the Learmonth submuscular or the subcutaneous transposition. Each of these 4 techniques, however, results in elevated intraneural pressures. The musculofascial lengthening technique for submuscular transposition was the only one that reduced intraneural ulnar pressure for all degrees of elbow flexion.

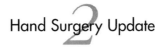

Failure can often be traced to inadequate decompression, inadequate mobilization of the nerve distally and proximally with the creation of new iatrogenic compression, or scarring in the surgical bed causing traction neuropathy. Mobility of the nerve should be verified intraoperatively for 10 to 12 cm proximal to the cubital tunnel to clear the arcade of Struthers, and 5 to 10 cm distally to clear the deep flexor-pronator aponeurosis. Failure due to tethering of the nerve in its new bed may be avoided by instituting early mobilization. Even a very limited arc of elbow motion with the forearm pronated and the wrist flexed is sufficient to prevent tethering of the transposed nerve. For a failed decompression of the ulnar nerve at the elbow, reoperation with anterior submuscular transposition of the nerve can be expected to result in improvement in 75% of cases, although with residual symptoms.

Ulnar Tunnel Syndrome

The anatomy of Guyon's canal has been redefined by one group who determined that the roof of Guyon's canal does not directly connect to the hamate bone; rather, it extends radially to the hook of hamate and attaches to the flexor retinaculum. The ulnar artery and sensory component of the ulnar nerve course radially to the hook of hamate and lie on the flexor retinaculum, sometimes directly palmar where they are exposed to risk of injury, particularly during carpal tunnel surgery. The roof and radial border consist of a proximal segment that begins near the pisiform and extends distally to the level of the hook of hamate, a central segment that contains only adipose tissue, and a distal fascial layer that includes the palmaris brevis muscle. The floor is comprised of the flexor retinaculum and muscles of the hypothenar eminence with their fibers of origin.

Patients with entrapment at this level may present with pure motor, pure sensory, or mixed symptoms, depending on the precise location of entrapment. Pain is usually less prominent than in carpal tunnel syndrome. The distal ulnar tunnel is divided into 3 zones. Zone 1 is the area proximal to the bifurcation of the nerve. Beginning at the edge of the palmar carpal ligament, it is about 3 cm in length. Compression in zone 1 causes combined motor and sensory deficits, and is most likely due to ganglions or fractures of the hook of the hamate. Zones 2 and 3 travel alongside each other from the bifurcation of the ulnar nerve to just beyond the fibrous arch of the hypothenar muscles. Zone 2 surrounds the deep motor branch; compression in this region will produce motor deficits without sensory disturbances. Again, ganglions and fractures of the hook of the hamate are the most likely causes. Zone 3 surrounds the superficial branch of the ulnar nerve; compression in this zone will produce pure sensory deficits. Synovial inflammation has been reported to cause compression in zone 3. More frequently, however, compression in zone 3 is due to a vascular lesion resulting from thrombosis or aneurysm of the ulnar artery. The Allen test and Doppler studies are useful in determining this diagnosis. Fractures of the hook of the hamate causing compression of the ulnar nerve in the ulnar tunnel can best be identified by computerized tomographic scans; however, carpal tunnel radiographs and oblique views of the wrist frequently yield a diagnosis.

Radial Nerve

Radial Nerve Entrapment in the Arm

In rare situations, the radial nerve can be compressed proximal to the elbow. Reported cases have been both acute and chronic in onset. The condition often follows strenuous muscular activity. Compression is associated with a fibrous arch from the lateral head of the triceps. Clinical examination will reveal weakness of distal muscles and radial sensory symptoms. Electromyography helps establish the diagnosis. Recovery typically occurs in 1 month. If there are no signs of recovery by 3 months, surgical decompression is indicated.

Posterior Interosseous Nerve Compression Syndrome

The radial nerve bifurcates proximal to the elbow; the posterior interosseous nerve (PIN) is vulnerable to entrapment just distal to this point, where it passes between the 2 heads of the supinator muscle. As the PIN lacks cutaneous nerve fibers, this syndrome causes weakness and pain but not sensory disorders. The muscles innervated by the PIN include the extensor carpi radialis brevis, supinator, extensor carpi ulnaris, extensor digitorum communis, extensor indicis proprius and digiti quinti, abductor pollicus longus, and the extensor pollicus longus and brevis. The onset is typically insidious; the patient may not initially notice weakness of finger and wrist extension, or a tendency toward radial drift of the hand with wrist extension. Active wrist extension in radial deviation is still possible, because the extensor carpi radialis longus is innervated proximally by the radial nerve. The syndrome may be incomplete. When only the ring and little fingers are involved, the posture of the hand has been referred to as pseudo-ulnar claw. In rheumatoids, rupture of the extensor communis tendons may present a picture similar to PIN syndrome. To add to the confusion, chronic proliferative rheumatoid synovitis can distend the elbow capsule and compress the

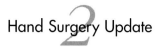
PIN. The first fibers to be affected are those to the extensors of the little and ring fingers, the same fingers affected first by extensor tendon ruptures. A careful examination will distinguish these; EMG studies are usually diagnostic as well. Routine elbow radiographs should be taken to rule out unreduced radial head dislocations that may have resulted in childhood, as well as fractures of the proximal radius or radial head pathology.

Gradual, painless loss of function may be due to a slow growing mass (typically a lipoma or ganglion) at the elbow. A preoperative MRI is very useful in planning surgery in these cases.

If there is no improvement after 4 to 12 weeks of observation from the onset, surgical decompression of the PIN may be undertaken, with an expectation of good to excellent results in 85% of patients. Possible anatomic sites of compression include thickened fascial tissue superficial to the radiocapitellar joint, a leash of vessels from the radial recurrent artery (the leash of Henry), the fibrous edge of the extensor carpi radialis brevis, the proximal edge of the supinator (the arcade of Frohse), and the distal edge of the supinator. All actual or potential sites should be released. Recovery of strength may continue progressing for up to 18 months.

Radial Tunnel Syndrome

Radial tunnel syndrome is often found in a work-related setting, with repetitive forceful elbow extension or forearm rotation as an inciting factor. A typical complaint is deep and aching pain on the lateral aspect of the elbow. Passive pronation with wrist flexion and active supination with wrist extension against resistance will aggravate symptoms. Night pain may be a significant complaint of some patients. The primary differential diagnosis is lateral epicondylitis. These conditions can coexist; 5% of patients with lateral epicondylitis will also have radial tunnel syndrome. In isolated radial tunnel syndrome, tenderness is more distal, over the radial tunnel rather than over the lateral epicondyle. A middle finger test is performed with the elbow and middle finger completely extended and the wrist in neutral position. Firm pressure is applied by the examiner to the dorsum of the proximal phalanx of the middle finger. The test is positive if it produces pain at the edge of the extensor carpi radialis brevis in the proximal forearm. Electrodiagnostic studies are not useful for this syndrome. Diagnosis is confirmed by injection of anesthetic into the radial tunnel, which both produces a complete PIN palsy and relieves symptoms. Reviewing 10 years of experience at the Mayo Clinic, one group had only 51% good results with surgery. Outcome in workers' compensation patients was often unsatisfactory. The worst results of decompression have been reported in patients who have work-related injuries, chronic pain, and poor localization of symptoms on physical examination. Finding success rates in the literature ranging from 10% to over 90%, another group concluded that the symptoms and signs used as diagnostic criteria for radial tunnel syndrome may be unreliable, and the results of surgery unpredictable.

Wartenberg's Syndrome

The sensory branch of the radial nerve may be compressed by a scissors-like action of the tendons of the extensor carpi radialis longus and the brachioradialis as the forearm is pronated. The nerve can also emerge from under the fascia between 2 slips of a split brachioradialis tendon, a variation found in 7 of 143 operative cases in one published report. The patient complains of pain, numbness, or tingling over the dorsal radial aspect of the hand, exacerbated by wrist movement or by making a tight pinch with the thumb and index finger. Elicitation of symptoms within 30 to 60 seconds of forcefully pronating the forearm is a useful provocative test. A positive nerve percussion sign is found over the radial sensory nerve as it exits the deep fascia in the forearm in 96% of patients. Relief of symptoms by injection of anesthetic dorsal to the musculotendinous junction of the brachioradialis confirms the diagnosis. Diagnostic injection, in addition to careful sensory testing, can distinguish Wartenberg's syndrome from de Quervain's stenosing tendovaginitis. Differential anesthetic blocks are also useful in distinguishing entrapment of the sensory branch of the radial nerve from compressive neuropathy of the lateral antebrachial cutaneous nerve. Nonsurgical treatment including splinting, anti-inflammatory drugs, and changes in work activities should be attempted before surgical decompression is recommended. In one reported series of 52 patients, conservative treatment achieved 71% excellent and good results and surgery yielded 74%.

Lateral Antebrachial Nerve Compression

The lateral antebrachial nerve is vulnerable to compression at the level of the elbow as it emerges lateral to the bicipital tendon and medial to the brachioradialis muscle. This is a sensory nerve, and motor deficits are not involved. Typical symptoms are pain and dysesthesias of the radial forearm, incited by repetitive forceful hand motions with the elbow extended. Nerve block with local anesthetic and sensory conduction velocity studies between the elbow and axilla aid in the diagnosis. Failure of nonsurgical treatment may indicate surgical decompression in selected patients; a wedge of the lateral edge of the biceps tendon is removed.

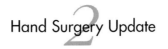

Thoracic Outlet Syndrome

There are two types of thoracic outlet syndrome (TOS)—vascular and neurogenic. Vascular TOS is secondary to large vessel disease, leads to subclavian artery intimal damage or aneurysm, and is easily diagnosed by clinical and imaging studies. Neurogenic TOS is infrequent; diagnosis is usually clinical, substantiated by physical findings. Electrophysiologic studies are rarely helpful. Symptoms include headaches; neck pain; and disabling pain, weakness, and paresthesias of the upper extremity. Patients often exhibit a strong underlying emotional component to their illness, displayed as depression or changes in personality. Psychological testing and psychotherapy have been as controversial as surgery in the treatment of this disorder.

Physical findings manifested by arterial compression include a decrease or absence of the radial pulse, or a drop in systolic blood pressure of 20 mm mercury on extension and abduction of the shoulder. Unfortunately, 92% of normal people obliterate their radial pulse in at least one asymptomatic extremity. Adson's test is performed by palpating the radial pulse with the head turned toward the affected side. Obliteration of the pulse indicates compression from the scalenus anticus muscle. A costoclavicular maneuver, upward and backward shrugging of the shoulders, may obliterate the radial pulse by compression from the pectoralis minor, clavicle, or scalenus medius muscle in symptomatic individuals. The Roos elevation test is performed as the patient abducts the shoulders and arms to 90°, and opens and closes the hand slowly for 3 minutes. A positive result occurs if the patient cannot complete this task due to pain or a feeling of profound heaviness.

Physical therapy should be prescribed, including active strengthening of the upper extremity and neck, shoulder shrugging to strengthen the trapezius, shoulder and scapula adduction and abduction exercises, instruction on proper body mechanics, and posturing and relaxation techniques. If a true congenital anomaly is causing TOS, these exercises may actually aggravate symptoms. Poor overall outcome of conservative therapy has been found to be related to obesity, workers' compensation, and associated carpal or cubital tunnel syndrome. Numerous procedures have been advocated—supraclavicular, infraclavicular, and transaxillary approaches for scalenotomy; scalenectomy; resection of fibrous bands; and cervical or first rib resections. Transaxillary first rib resection is the favored procedure, with 90% good to excellent results reported. Complication rates are significant, however, and include irreversible injury to the brachial plexus, causalgia, intercostal brachial nerve pain, painful snapping scapula, and recurrent symptoms.

Annotated Bibliography

Epidemiology and Pathophysiology

Mackinnon SE, Novak CB: Repetitive strain in the workplace. *J Hand Surg* 1997;22A:2–18.

The January 1997 issue of the *Journal of Hand Surgery* was devoted to repetitive strain. Mackinnon and Novak presented a case for repetitive stress injuries being work-related, but noted that carpal tunnel syndrome is implicated in only 2% of all repetitive-motion cases. Hadler followed with an article titled "Repetitive upper-extremity motions in the workplace are not hazardous." The letters to the editor in ensuing months are worth pursuing for readers interested in this debate.

Szabo RM: Occupational carpal tunnel syndrome, in Kasdan ML (ed): *Occupational Hand & Upper Extremity Injuries & Diseases*. Philadelphia, PA, Hanley & Belfus, 1998, pp 113–127.

This chapter explores the epidemiology of carpal tunnel syndrome as it relates to occupation. A good glossary of epidemiologic terms is included for those who need a crash course in the language necessary to understand this body of literature.

Szabo RM, Madison M: Carpal tunnel syndrome as a work-related disorder, in Gordon SL, Blair SJ, Fine LJ (eds): *Repetitive Motion Disorders of the Upper Extremity*. Rosemont, IL, American Academy of Orthopaedic Surgeons, 1995, pp 421–434.

This chapter is the product of a workshop on repetitive motion disorders of the upper extremity held in 1994. The book covers epidemiologic, pathophysiologic, and clinical issues related to repetitive trauma, and is mandatory reading for anyone interested in this controversial topic.

Vender MI, Kasdan ML, Truppa KL: Upper extremity disorders: A literature review to determine work-relatedness. *J Hand Surg* 1995;20A:534–541.

The authors reviewed the literature to establish possible validation of a causal relationship between upper extremity disorders and work activities. They concluded that there is insufficient evidence to prove that work is the sole cause of cumulative trauma. Letters to the editor in subsequent issues of the *Journal of Hand Surgery* continued this debate.

Double Crush Phenomenon

Wilbourn AJ, Gilliatt RW: Double-crush syndrome: A critical analysis. *Neurology* 1997;49:21–29.

The authors revisit the concept of double crush lesions, offering some excellent arguments that tear down traditional concepts.

Carpal Tunnel Syndrome

Amadio PC, Silverstein MD, Ilstrup DM, Schleck CD, Jensen LM: Outcome assessment for carpal tunnel surgery: The relative responsiveness of generic, arthritis-specific, disease-specific, and physical examination measures. *J Hand Surg* 1996; 21A:338–346.

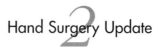

196   Nerve Compression Syndromes

Standardized questionnaires and outcome studies are currently flooding the literature, prompted by a need to prove to insurance companies and HMOs that what we do in the practice of medicine is worthwhile for patients. Expect to see more studies like this until the environment changes.

Atroshi I, Breidenbach WC, McCabe SJ: Assessment of the carpal tunnel outcome instrument in patients with nerve-compression symptoms. *J Hand Surg* 1997;22A:222–227.

This outcome study makes a distinction between diagnostic tests and outcome measures. This difference must be understood before using and interpreting questionnaires.

Blair WF, Goetz DD, Ross MA, Steyers CM, Chang P: Carpal tunnel release with and without epineurotomy: A comparative prospective trial. *J Hand Surg* 1996;21A:655–661.

In this study, 117 involved hands were evaluated by an extensive preoperative questionnaire, a detailed physical examination, and preoperative neurophysiologic testing. The physical findings, neurophysiologic findings, and patient perceptions of outcome after surgery were similar with or without epineurotomy.

Bowers WH, Berner SH: Limited-incision carpal tunnel release: *Techn Hand Upper Extremity Surg* 1997;1:15–20.

Several authors have described their limited-incision techniques over the last few years. This article details the technique and reviews a comparative study with conventional release by an author who abandoned the single portal endoscopic method in favor of limited incision.

Cook AC, Szabo RM, Birkholz SW, King EF: Early mobilization following carpal tunnel release: A prospective randomized study. *J Hand Surg* 1995;20B:228–230.

Fifty consecutive patients undergoing surgery for carpal tunnel syndrome were prospectively randomized to determine the value of splinting of the wrist following open carpal tunnel release. Patients were either splinted for 2 weeks following surgery or began range of motion exercises on the first postoperative day. Splinted patients had significant delays in return to activities of daily living, return to work at light and full duty, and in recovery of grip and key pinch strength, as well as increased pain and scar tenderness in the first month after surgery; otherwise there was no difference between the groups in the incidence of complications. The authors' recommendations for postoperative home physical therapy are detailed.

DeStefano F, Nordstrom DL, Vierkant RA: Long-term symptom outcomes of carpal tunnel syndrome and its treatment. *J Hand Surg* 1997;22A:200–210.

This population-based study proves that carpal tunnel syndrome surgery is highly effective. For the best results, surgery should be performed earlier.

Foulkes GD, Atkinson RE, Beuchel C, Doyle JR, Singer DI: Outcome following epineurotomy in carpal tunnel syndrome: A prospective, randomized clinical trial. *J Hand Surg* 1994; 19A:539–547.

Thirty-six wrists were prospectively randomized into epineurotomy and nonepineurotomy treatment groups. Extensive sensory testing showed overall improvement within both groups postoperatively, but no difference between the 2 groups at 6 and 12 months postoperatively. Motor testing revealed no improvement in the grip strength or pinch of either group at 12 months when compared to preoperative levels.

Jacobsen MB, Rahme H: A prospective, randomized study with an independent observer comparing open carpal tunnel release with endoscopic carpal tunnel release. *J Hand Surg* 1996; 21B:202–204.

This report is one of several comparative studies that show little relative benefit from endoscopic carpal tunnel release. This study was designed with return to work as the primary outcome measure. All study participants were employed in Sweden, and had clinical and electrical signs consistent with carpal tunnel syndrome. With a power of 85%, the authors found no significant difference in sick leave between open and endoscopic release. There were no complications in the open group. In the endoscopic group, 18% suffered transient numbness on the radial side of their ring fingers.

Leinberry CF, Hammond NL III, Siegfried JW: The role of epineurotomy in the operative treatment of carpal tunnel syndrome. *J Bone Joint Surg* 1997;79A:555–557.

Fifty hands were randomized into 2 groups with either a release of the transverse carpal ligament alone, or a release and adjuvant epineurotomy of the median nerve. The authors found no detectable differences between the 2 groups with regard to symptoms, objective findings, or electrophysiologic findings.

Rosen B, Lundborg G, Abrahamsson SO, Hagberg L, Rosen I: Sensory function after median nerve decompression in carpal tunnel syndrome: Preoperative vs postoperative findings. *J Hand Surg* 1997;22B:602–606.

The longer a patient has carpal tunnel syndrome, the more likely irreversible structural changes will occur and therefore the results of surgery will not be as good.

Sanders WE: Letter: Flexor carpi radialis approach for carpal tunnel release. *J Hand Surg* 1997;22A:950–951.

Anyone interested in the approach described in the previous article should read the authors' subsequent corrections in this letter to the editor.

Tanaka S, Wild DK, Seligman PJ, Behrens V, Cameron L, Putz-Anderson V: The US prevalence of self-reported carpal tunnel syndrome: 1988 national health interview survey data. *Am J Public Health* 1994;84:1846–1848.

This population data is from the Occupational Health Supplement of the 1988 National Health Interview Survey. Based on a response rate of 91.5% in a sample of over 44,000 households, an estimated 1.55% (2.65 million) of 170 million adults self-reported carpal tunnel syndrome. Of 127 million adults who worked during the 12 months before the survey, 0.53% (0.68 million) reported that their hand discomfort was called carpal tunnel syndrome by a health care provider.

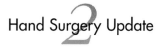
Weber RA, Sanders WE: Flexor carpi radialis approach for carpal tunnel release. *J Hand Surg* 1997;22A:120–126.

The authors describe their technique for carpal tunnel release and the results in 87 hands. This method may be appropriate for the carpal tunnel syndrome patient with coexisting carpometacarpal arthritis who is being considered for a ligament replacement tendon interposition procedure at the time of carpal tunnel release. The lack of good visualization of the entire median nerve and the added risk of complications when operating on the radial side of the median nerve are cause for concern.

Weiss AP, Sachar K, Gendreau M: Conservative management of carpal tunnel syndrome: A reexamination of steroid injection and splinting. *J Hand Surg* 1994;19A:410–415.

This article is an update of Gelberman's classic study published in 1980. Apply caution before accepting the conclusions regarding workers' compensation patients; a power analysis of the authors' data indicates that they would be unlikely to find a difference between workers' compensation and nonworkers' compensation patients in their study.

Pronator Syndrome

Olehnik WK, Manske PR, Szerzinski J: Median nerve compression in the proximal forearm. *J Hand Surg* 1994;19A:121–126.

This is the largest recent experience (36 cases) detailing preoperative, intraoperative, and postoperative findings in patients who underwent surgical decompression of the median nerve in the proximal forearm.

Anterior Interosseous Nerve Syndrome

Wong L, Dellon AL: Brachial neuritis presenting as anterior interosseous nerve compression: Implications for diagnosis and treatment. A case report. *J Hand Surg* 1997;22A:536–539.

Is anterior interosseous nerve syndrome a compression syndrome or a form of brachial plexus neuritis? This detailed review of the medical and surgical literature notes that opinion and treatment may depend on whether one is a medical specialist or a surgeon. This article belongs in everyone's library.

Cubital Tunnel Syndrome

Dellon AL, Chang E, Coert JH, Campbell KR: Intraneural ulnar nerve pressure changes related to operative techniques for cubital tunnel decompression. *J Hand Surg* 1994;19A:923–930.

The authors determined intraneural ulnar nerve pressure in 50 cadavers after simple decompression, medial epicondylectomy, subcutaneous transposition, and submuscular transposition by the Learmonth and by the musculofascial lengthening technique. Based on these laboratory measurements, they believe that the flexor/pronator muscle mass should be Z-lengthened to reduce potential pressure on the ulnar nerve during submuscular transposition. Simple decompression and medial epicondylectomy were associated with a smaller increase in intraneural pressure than either the subcutaneous or Learmonth submuscular transposition.

Nathan PA, Keniston RC, Meadows KD: Outcome study of ulnar nerve compression at the elbow treated with simple decompression and an early program of physical therapy. *J Hand Surg* 1995;20B:628–637.

Simple decompression has not been as popular as anterior transposition or medial epicondylectomy among hand surgeons. The good results presented in this study should at least stimulate consideration of "maybe less is better."

Novak CB, Lee GW, Mackinnon SE, Lay L: Provocative testing for cubital tunnel syndrome. *J Hand Surg* 1994;19A:817–820.

Provocative testing is exhaustively described in the literature for carpal tunnel syndrome, but is not as well documented for cubital tunnel syndrome. The authors present the results of their comparison of 4 provocative tests—Tinel's sign, elbow flexion, pressure provocation, and combined elbow flexion and pressure provocation. The reported specificity of these tests ranged from 0.95 to 0.98, illustrating a common problem when using normal healthy asymptomatic individuals as controls for a study evaluating diagnostic tests.

Tada H, Hirayama T, Katsuki M, Habaguchi T: Long term results using a modified King's method for cubital tunnel syndrome. *Clin Orthop* 1997;336:107–110.

Patient series of medial epicondylectomy rarely document the problems of medial collateral ligament insufficiency. This one does, and warns us that the results of medial epicondylectomy are inconsistent with stability of the elbow.

Tsai TM, Bonczar M, Tsuruta T, Syed SA: A new operative technique: Cubital tunnel decompression with endoscopic assistance. *Hand Clin* 1995;11:71–80.

This is an excellent article for those interested in the triumph of technique over reason.

Ulnar Tunnel Syndrome

Cobb TK, Carmichael SW, Cooney WP: Guyon's canal revisited: An anatomic study of the carpal ulnar neurovascular space. *J Hand Surg* 1996;21A:861–869.

This is a current and accurate anatomical study of Guyon's canal, with new insight regarding position of the ulnar sensory nerve and the ulnar artery in relation to the hook of the hamate, which has significant clinical implications.

Radial Tunnel Syndrome

Atroshi I, Johnsson R, Ornstein E: Radial tunnel release: Unpredictable outcome in 37 consecutive cases with a 1-5 year followup. *Acta Orthop Scand* 1995;66:255–257.

Radial tunnel syndrome is predominantly a clinical diagnosis of pain and is most commonly found in the workers' compensation population. Not surprisingly, this study found that preoperative and operative findings do not correlate to the outcome. Perhaps this diagnosis should be made with extreme caution until we have more reliable or objective diagnostic tests.

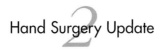

Wartenberg's Syndrome

Lanzetta M, Foucher G: Entrapment of the superficial branch of the radial nerve (Wartenberg's syndrome): A report of 52 cases. *Int Orthop* 1993;17:342–345.

Conservative treatment for Wartenberg's syndrome is successful in 71% of the authors' cases. De Quervain's disease was associated with 50% of their cases. Because these 2 conditions can coexist, it is important to diagnose both before surgery, to avoid unexpected postoperative complications.

Turkof E, Puig S, Choi SS, Zoch G, Dellon AL: The radial sensory nerve entrapped between the two slips of a split brachioradialis tendon: A rare aspect of Wartenberg's syndrome. *J Hand Surg* 1995;20A:676–678.

This article details an anatomic variation that has direct clinical significance.

Thoracic Outlet Syndrome

Novak CB, Collins ED, Mackinnon SE: Outcome following conservative management of thoracic outlet syndrome. *J Hand Surg* 1995;20A:542–548.

The majority of thoracic outlet syndrome (TOS) cases involve conservative treatment, most notably physical therapy. This study by authors who have a particular interest in TOS details the results of physical therapy in 42 patients. With symptomatic improvement in only 25 (60%), the outlook for patients is guarded.

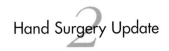

Chapter 19
Peripheral Nerve Injuries

Susan E. Mackinnon, MD, FRCSC

Peripheral nerve injury is common and frequently disabling. In spite of the frequency and importance of nerve injuries in upper extremity and hand injuries, results following nerve repair and grafting are generally considered poor. The large volume of traumatic nerve injuries treated during World War II provided an important foundation for surgeons interested in the treatment of nerve-injured patients. Although the functional results achieved with the early repairs were generally poor, the clinical material and surgical techniques used at that time provided an important reference point from which current surgical management has evolved.

Classification of Nerve Injury

There are several patterns of nerve injury which may vary from fascicle to fascicle and along the longitudinal axis of the nerve. The 2 main systems for classifying these injuries were developed by Seddon in 1943 and by Sunderland in 1951. An understanding of these classifications is critical for a surgeon planning to repair injured nerves.

Seddon described 3 types of nerve injury: neurapraxia, axonotmesis, and neurotmesis. Sunderland expanded this classification to include 2 degrees of nerve injury intermediate between axonotmesis and neurotmesis. Neurapraxia (Sunderland first-degree injury) involves a localized area of conduction block. Histologic changes, if noted, are those of segmental demyelination. Because there is no axonal abnormality, a Tinel's sign will not be present, and function will be completely restored with correction of the conduction block or remyelination. Axonotmesis (Sunderland second-degree injury) involves an injury to the axons such that wallerian degeneration will occur distal to the level of the injury. A Tinel's sign progresses distally at the rate of 1 in per month, corresponding to axonal regeneration. These axons usually will regenerate along their original endoneurial tubes to their original distal receptors. Recovery should be complete unless the level of the injury is so far from the sensory or motor targets that time of denervation becomes a factor in influencing ultimate end-organ function. Sunderland's third- and fourth-degree injuries were included as

extensions of axonotmesis and neurotmesis, respectively, in Seddon's classification. These are common and important injury patterns.

Sunderland's third-degree injury in which axonal injury is associated with endoneurial scarring yields the most variable ultimate recovery. The amount of scar tissue and the type of fascicle involved influence ultimate recovery. If the fascicle contains both sensory and motor fibers, then a mixing or mismatching of motor and sensory fibers can occur, resulting in a poorer functional result than if the injury involved a "pure" motor or sensory fascicle. This is the type of injury most frequently seen in the medical-legal arena when some, but not complete, recovery occurs following an iatrogenic nerve injury.

In a Sunderland fourth-degree injury, the nerve is in continuity, but at the level of the injury there is complete scarring across the nerve, such that regeneration cannot occur. A Tinel's sign will be present at the level of the injury, but will not proceed distally. Neurotmesis (Sunderland fifth-degree injury) involves complete transection of the nerve with no functional recovery anticipated.

To these must be added the concept of a mixed injury, which I have termed a sixth-degree injury or neuroma in continuity. This injury combines various injury patterns from fascicle to fascicle and along the longitudinal length of the nerve (Fig. 1). It provides the greatest surgical challenge in that normal fascicles or those with potential for good recovery must be protected while fascicles with Sunderland fourth- and fifth-degree injuries are reconstructed using repair or grafting techniques (Table 1).

Compression neuropathy is a common problem managed by the hand surgeon; thus, its histopathology is important to understand. Chronic nerve compression spans a broad spectrum of nerve injury from initial breakdown in the blood nerve barrier to fibrosis within the nerve to isolated nerve fiber pathology of segmental demyelination to diffuse nerve fiber changes and finally to wallerian degeneration. The patient's symptoms and clinical findings will parallel these histopathologic changes (Fig. 2).

Electrodiagnostic studies are extremely useful in determining the degree and treatment of a given nerve injury. A

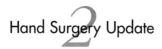
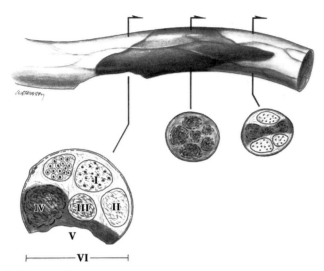

Figure 1

A cross-section of the sixth-degree (mixed, neuroma in continuity) injury. A first-degree injury (neurapraxia) is noted (I) with segmental demyelination. A second-degree injury with axonal injury (II) is noted (axonotmesis). In the center of the nerve, a fascicle demonstrates a third-degree injury (III) with a significant amount of scarring in the endoneurium. A fourth-degree injury is noted (IV) with complete scarring of the fascicle such that no regeneration can occur. A fifth-degree injury (neurotmesis) with division of the fascicle is noted (V) in the lower portion of the nerve. The diagram demonstrates that the nerve injury can vary in a longitudinal as well as transverse extent. (Adapted with permission from Mackinnon SE: Comparative analysis of nerve injury of the face and hand, implications for surgical treatments. *Oral Maxillofacial Surg Clin North Am* 1992;4:483–502.)

few points should be emphasized. The myelin will affect conduction velocity and distal latency, and the number of axons conducting is reflected in the amplitude of the resulting response. A demyelination injury (neurapraxia) will be associated with a decrease in the conduction velocity and an increase in distal latency. Any injury involving the axon will be associated with a decrease in amplitude because fewer axons are conducting.

False positives are easily generated in electrodiagnostic testing. For example, a 1° C decrease in temperature will decrease the conduction velocity by approximately 5% and increase distal latency by 0.2 to 0.3 ms per degree. Similarly, when 2-needle electrotomyography is performed, a temperature reduction will increase both polyphasic units and the duration of waveforms, giving the impression of a neurogenic injury.

A neurapraxic process will resolve with remyelination over a period of days to 3 months. When the axon is injured, it may be possible to stimulate distal to the injury for 7 days. After this time, there will be loss of response to motor and sensory nerve stimulation, but fibrillations are not seen until approximately 3 weeks after the axonal injury. If the muscle is completely denervated and is not reinnervated these fibrillations generally dissipate within a year. Fibrillations may be seen for years in incompletely denervated muscle.

Table 1

Relationship of injury to recovery

Degree of Injury	Tinel Sign Present/Progresses Distally	Recovery Pattern	Rate of Recovery	Surgical Procedure
I. Neurapraxia	– / –	Complete	Fast, days to 12 weeks	None
II. Axonotmesis	+ / +	Complete	Slow (1 in/month)	None
III.	+ / +	Great variation*	Slow (1 in/month)	None or neurolysis
IV.	+ / –	None	No recovery	Nerve repair or nerve graft
V. Neurotmesis	– / –	None	No recovery	Nerve repair or nerve graft
VI. Mixed, neuroma in continuity	Varies with each fascicle, depending on the combination of injury patterns as noted above.			

*Recovery is at least as good as a nerve repair but can vary from excellent to poor depending on the degree of endoneurial scarring and the amount of sensory or motor axonal misdirection within the injured fascicle. (Adapted with permission from Mackinnon SE, Dellon AL: *Surgery of the Peripheral Nerve.* New York, NY, Thieme Medical Publishers, 1988, p 74.)

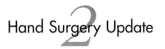

Recovery from partial muscle denervation will start with collateral axons sprouting from remaining viable axons as they send small sprouts to the denervated muscle fibers. This results in increased duration and polyphasia of the remaining motor units but the main body of these motor units will retain a normal amplitude. These changes generally are seen 4 to 6 weeks after axonal injury. Polyphasic motor units are a sign of reinnervation, and if they have a large amplitude suggest collateral sprouting. Short duration, low voltage, immature polyphasic units are evidence of axonal regrowth and reinnervation, not collateral sprouting. They can generally be recorded approximately 2 months before any clinical evidence of reinnervation is noted. As the reinnervation process continues and more muscle fibers are reinnervated, motor units will increase in size over a period of months to years. As the amplitude increases, the number of polyphasic units decreases. Fibrillations will dissipate as the muscle is reinnervated. Ultimately, the reinnervation process will be complete, and large motor units greater than 5 millivolts and frequently 8 to 12 millivolts will be present. Thus, in a closed injury, electrodiagnostic studies done approximately 6 weeks after injury should show evidence of reinnervation if the injury pattern will allow collateral sprouting. Surgical intervention is indicated if there is no evidence of reinnervation by 3 months after closed injury. Intraoperative electrodiagnostic testing will be done to confirm preoperative findings.

How to Examine the Nerve-Injured Patient

Preoperative evaluation of neurologic function is critical in planning surgical intervention. If the nerve is completely divided, there is no motor or sensory function in the distribution of the nerve involved. Outline 1 lists the critical points of the physical examination for each of the 3 major nerves in the upper extremity. Assessment of pinch, grip, and individual muscle function is recommended. Strength assessment measures not only function of the 3 major nerves but also patient motivation.

Significant effort has been directed toward developing tests to evaluate sensory function in the hand. These tests and the correlation between test results and fiber-receptor systems are well developed. A simple analogy has been useful to describe and understand the relationship between innervation density and threshold and the various tests currently used to measure sensibility (Fig. 3). Two-point discrimination reflects the innervation density and provides an indication of the number of innervated receptors. Static 2-point discrimination, which reflects the slowly adapting receptor function, is evaluated by holding 2 points against the skin for several seconds and asking the individual whether he or she feels 1 or 2 prongs. The smallest spacing at which 2 of 3 trials are correctly identified is recorded in millimeters. Moving 2-point discrimination is assessed by slowly moving the 2 prongs longitudinally along the distal portion of the finger pulp with just enough pressure to elicit a response, repeating the query, and recording the smallest spacing in millimeters.

A more sensitive test of receptor function uses a vibrometer to quantify the threshold of the quickly adapting fibers. The vibrating portion of the vibrometer is placed against the skin, and the smallest stimulus perceived is identified as the baseline vibration threshold and recorded in microns of motion.

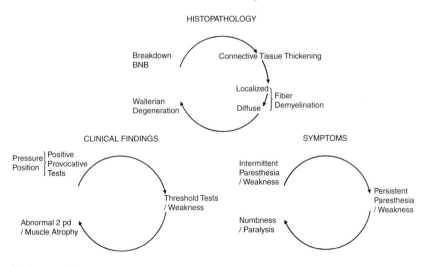

Figure 2

The histopathology of chronic nerve compression parallels the patient's symptoms and clinical findings. It spans a broad spectrum from simple changes of blood-nerve barrier (BNB) function to actual wallerian degeneration. (Reproduced with permission from Mackinnon SE: Upper extremity nerve injuries: Primary repair and reconstruction, in Cohen ML (ed): *Mastery of Plastic and Reconstructive Surgery*. Boston, MA, Little, Brown and Co, 1994, p 1609.)

Outline 1
Critical physical examination points in diagnosis of nerve injury

I.   Muscles to test for unambiguous diagnosis of motor nerve injury

    A.   Radial nerve: extrinsic
      1.   Wrist extension
      2.   Extension of fingers at metacarpophalangeal joints
      3.   Extension of thumb

    B.   Median nerve: intrinsic
      1.   Thumb-palmar abduction

    C.   Median nerve: extrinsic
      1.   All flexor sublimi
      2.   Flexor profundus to index
      3.   Flexor pollicis longus
      4.   Flexor carpi radialis

    D.   Ulnar nerve: intrinsic
      1.   First dorsal interossei
      2.   Hypothenar muscles

    E.   Ulnar nerve: extrinsic
      1.   Flexor profundus to little finger
      2.   Flexor carpi ulnaris

II. Areas to test for unambiguous diagnosis of sensory nerve injury

    A.   Radial nerve: dorsal radial aspect of hand toward the first web
    B.   Median nerve: pulp of thumb and index finger
    C.   Ulnar nerve: pulp of the little finger
    D.   Palmar cutaneous branch of median nerve: proximal palm near thenar eminence
    E.   Dorsal cutaneous branch of ulnar nerve: dorsal ulnar surface of hand
    F.   Digital nerve: not the tip of the finger (overlap), but the proximal third of the distal phalanx and distal third of middle phalanx, adjacent to the distal skin crease

(Reproduced with permission from Mackinnon SE, Dellon AL (eds): *Surgery of the Peripheral Nerve.* New York, NY, Thieme Medical Publishers, 1988, p 74.)

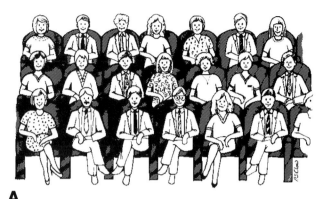

A

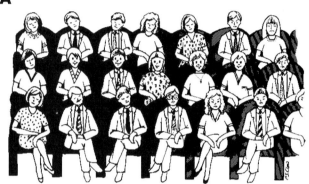

B

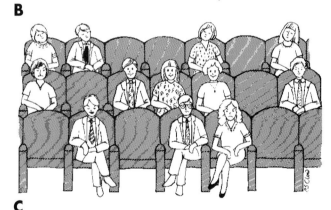

C

Figure 3
A simple analogy helps to describe the relationship between innervation density and threshold. **A,** If each person in the audience is considered as a single fiber/sensory receptor unit, then the number of people present in the audience can be considered the innervation density. The "status, health, or well-being" of the individuals can be considered their threshold. If all the seats in the audience are full and the individuals in the audience are "awake and content" then all testing for fiber receptor function will be normal (both innervation density and threshold tests). **B,** The threshold testing will be abnormal (vibration and Semmes-Weinstein monofilaments) if the individuals are not "awake and content" but are "asleep or unhappy." It will take more effort (ie, greater pressure, larger amplitude) to "wake up" these sleepy receptors. Moving and static 2-point discrimination will be normal because all the people in the audience are present. **C,** If individuals in the audience vacate the auditorium, the innervation density test (2-point discrimination) will be abnormal. If the remaining individuals are other than "happy and content," the threshold tests will be abnormal as well. (Reproduced with permission from Mackinnon SE: Peripheral nerve injuries in the hand, in Vistnes LM (ed): *How They Do It: Procedures in Plastic and Reconstructive Surgery.* Boston, Little, Brown and Co, 1991, p 625.)

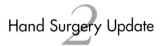

Pressure thresholds are assessed quantitatively using Semmes-Weinstein monofilaments. The nylon monofilaments are applied perpendicular to the cutaneous surface, and the pressure is increased until bending of the monofilament is observed. The probes are sequentially applied to each of the test sites. The number of the probe on the filament represents the logarithm of the force in 0.1 mg required to bow the monofilament. The number of the lightest probe that can elicit perception is recorded. There are several problems with the use of the Semmes-Weinstein filaments. Monofilaments can be damaged and invalidate the test, and the method of testing can alter the patient's perception and response. As the contact time on the fingertip increases, the amount of force required to perceive the presence of a filament also increases. Because the number on the filament is a logarithm, the difference between filament numbers is disproportionately discontinuous, and therefore, measurements cannot be summed and averaged. Although several quantitative evaluation systems are available, the results of the testing have not altered our patient management.

Nerve Repair

The use of microneurosurgical technique to reconstruct injured nerves is now generally accepted. Several key points can be emphasized: (1) Microsurgical technique with appropriate magnification, instrumentation, and suture material should be used. (2) A nerve repair must be relatively tension free (Fig. 4). (3) The proximal and distal extent of the nerve injury must be carefully assessed so that damaged nerve, which will heal with scar tissue, is resected (Fig. 5). (4) When a tension-free repair is not possible, an interposition nerve graft should be used (Fig. 6). (5) Extreme postural positioning of the extremity to facilitate an end-to-end repair is discouraged. Both a nerve repair and a nerve graft must be carried out without tension at the repair site. (6) When clinical and surgical conditions permit, a primary nerve repair should be performed. (7) An epineurial repair should be performed unless the intraneural topography of the peripheral nerve dictates a group fascicular repair. (8) Postoperative motor and sensory reeducation and rehabilitation may maximize the potential of the surgical result.

Most acute nerve injuries can be repaired primarily. The nature of the injury suggests its longitudinal extent. If the patient has sustained a relatively clean injury, then a primary repair with an end-to-end epineurial or group fascicular technique is preferred. The surgeon trims back the divided proximal and distal ends of the nerve (with a sharp instrument). For ulnar nerve injuries in the region of the cubital tunnel, primary transposition of the ulnar nerve decreases

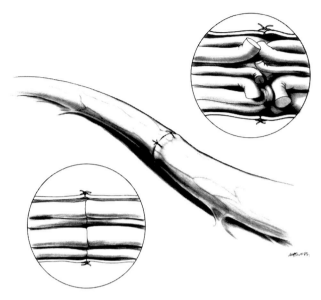

Figure 4

The surgeon must take care that the proximal and distal faces of the fascicles are not turned back on themselves (upper circle). A satisfactory appearance on the exterior surface can belie poor fascicular alignment. (Reproduced with permission from Mackinnon SE: Peripheral nerve injuries, in Manske PR (ed): *Hand Surgery Update*. Rosemont, IL, American Academy of Orthopaedic Surgeons, 1996, pp 233–241.)

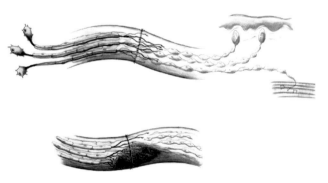

Figure 5

The top of the drawing demonstrates the ideal nerve repair coapting healthy proximal and distal nerve. The bottom diagram emphasizes that if the nerve repair is performed between damaged proximal and distal nerve, then nerve regeneration will be inhibited even when perfect microtechnique is used. (Reproduced with permission from Mackinnon SE: Peripheral nerve injuries, Manske PR (ed): in *Hand Surgery Update*. Rosemont, IL, American Academy of Orthopaedic Surgeons, 1996, pp 233–241.)

tension on the nerve repair. The surgeon gains approximately 2 to 3 cm of "length" with this technique. When the ulnar nerve is injured at the level of the midforearm, its muscular attachments tether the ulnar nerve such that transposition is not helpful in gaining length and decreasing nerve repair tension.

For injuries at the level of the wrist, decompression of the carpal tunnel and Guyon's canal distally is recommended for median and ulnar injuries, respectively, so nerve regeneration proceeds uninhibited by superimposed compression. Decompression also facilitates confirmation of motor-sensory orientation in the distal part of the nerve. Appropriate magnification and fine instrumentation is critical in effecting a good nerve repair. When the nerve injury is acute, the fascicular orientation of the proximal and distal surfaces are easily matched.

If there is any concern about the motor-sensory orientation on the proximal side of the nerve injury, then awake electrical stimulation can be used. When the longitudinal extent of the injury is unknown, a simple disposable nerve stimulator can be used to touch the nerve at the level of the proximal cut nerve. If the patient perceives sensation, the nerve at this level obviously is healthy. If the patient perceives no sensation, the stimulator can be tapped along the nerve in a proximal direction until the patient perceives a sensation, suggesting the level of healthy nerve. In secondary reconstruction, awake stimulation is most useful in determining motor and sensory fascicular grouping in the proximal stump. Compliance by the patient and support by the anesthetist are critical in the success of this technique. Initial dissection is carried out with neurolept and local regional anesthesia technique. A short-acting anesthetic hypnotic agent must be used when the proximal portion of the nerve is sharply transected because this is painful.

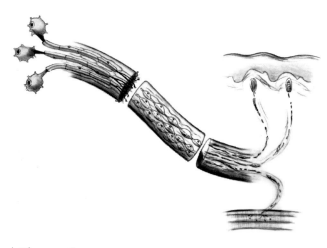

Figure 6

A nerve graft will serve as a conduit to direct nerve regeneration. (Reproduced with permission from Mackinnon SE: Upper extremity nerve injuries: Primary repair and reconstruction, in Cohen ML (ed): *Mastery of Plastic and Reconstructive Surgery.* Boston, MA, Little, Brown and Co, 1994, p 1605.)

A disposable nerve stimulator usually does not deliver a discrete enough stimulus to reliably separate motor and sensory fascicles, and more sophisticated electrical equipment that allows the stimulus to be gradually increased is required. Stimulation of sensory fascicles is interpreted by the patient as significant burning or "electrical" pain in a specific cutaneous distribution. By contrast, stimulation of the motor fibers, which contain some afferent sensory fibers, is interpreted by the patient as a dull, nonspecific stimulus that usually is localized to the midportion of the muscle belly of the corresponding motor nerve.

Chemical staining of the nerve is less practical. Several chemical staining techniques have been used to identify motor (acetylcholinesterase, cholineacetyltransferase) and sensory (carbonic anhydrase) fibers. The incubation technique for processing tissue has been decreased to 1 hour; however, the enzyme staining technique requires assistance from a pathologist or a trained technician and is not yet universally available.

During the nerve repair the surgeon moves the digits and extremity and determines the amount of movement of the extremity that is acceptable at the nerve repair. It is recommended that the nerve repair be protected with a splint for approximately 3 weeks, and protected movement begun in the early postoperative period. For example, a median nerve repaired at the wrist would be managed with a splint to hold the wrist in neutral and the metacarpophalangeal joints flexed. If necessary, a small amount of wrist flexion is acceptable in a primary repair. The patient is encouraged to begin active movement of the fingers immediately after surgery. This allows the adhesions that form between the median nerve and the surrounding tendons and soft tissue to be long adhesions that facilitate subsequent gliding of the nerve.

Nerve Grafting

When a nerve repair without tension is not possible, a nerve graft is used. The ability to align the motor and sensory fascicles in the proximal and distal stumps is critical to improving results after nerve grafting. If the nerve grafts are placed between the proximal and distal ends of the nerve gap without consideration for both proximal and distal sensory-motor topography, then the probability of inappropriate sensory-motor alignment increases dramatically. Several techniques can be used to aid in identification of sensory and motor fascicles in the proximal nerve stump. These include anatomic clues (surgical identification of fascicles going to specific muscles or cutaneous territories), topography maps, awake stimulation, and enzyme staining. Distally, it is not possible to use awake stimulation

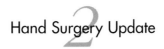

or enzyme staining, and the surgeon relies on anatomic surgical dissection aided by topography maps. These maps are best learned by stimulating the surface of normal nerves with a disposable nerve stimulator whenever the surgical opportunity arises. Over time the surgeon will become familiar with which portions of various nerves are motor. This stimulation is very specific; for example, stimulation of a discrete fascicle of the radial nerve in the axilla results in specific thumb extension.

Median nerve injuries at the distal forearm and wrist level that require nerve grafting are usually treated at a time after injury that would preclude recovery of muscle function (Fig. 7). In these cases, the incision is extended into the hand to anatomically distinguish the fascicles destined for specific digits and the motor branch to the thenar muscles. Proximally, awake stimulation theoretically could be used to separate most of the sensory fascicles from the few fascicles that innervate the thenar and lumbrical muscles. From a practical point of view, the distal dissection is used to exclude motor fascicles to the thenar muscle, whereas the "contamination" of the motor fibers from the proximal nerve stump is accepted. The nerve grafts attach the proximal median nerve to the distal median nerve with exclusion of distal motor fascicles. In the distal extremity there is a paucity of plexus formation between fascicles, thus orthotopic alignment of the grafts from the proximal stump to the distal stump should result in recovery of sensation with good localization (Fig. 8).

The ulnar nerve at the wrist is composed of a significant number (40%) of motor fibers. The sensory and motor fascicular groups are located in distinct positions in the ulnar nerve; thus, the opportunity exists for excellent functional recovery if the sensory-motor alignment is correct or for no functional recovery if the proximal or distal stump is misaligned by 180° (Fig. 9). The topography of the ulnar nerve in the forearm has been well described. Proximally, the motor group is located between the sensory groups to the dorsal cutaneous territory and those to the glabrous skin of the hand. After the dorsal cutaneous branch has separated from the main nerve in the midforearm, the alignment remains such that the motor group is medial and slightly dorsal to the sensory group. This topography is constant until the region of Guyon's canal, where the motor group passes dorsal and radial to the cutaneous group. Orientation of the distal stump in an ulnar nerve

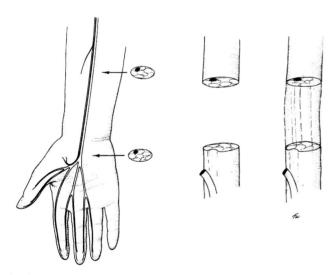

Figure 7

Reconstruction of established median nerve injuries in the distal forearm and hand in which recovery of motor function is not anticipated can include exclusion of the distal motor branch, determined by anatomic dissection. Proximally, the motor fascicles theoretically could be identified with awake stimulation, but from a practical point of view satisfactory sensibility will be recovered even if this motor component is not excluded. (Reproduced with permission from Mackinnon SE: Upper extremity nerve injuries: Primary repair and reconstruction, in Cohen ML (ed): *Mastery of Plastic and Reconstructive Surgery.* Boston, MA, Little, Brown and Co, 1994, p 1616.)

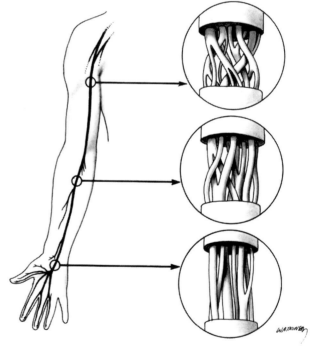

Figure 8

A schematic diagram of the internal topography of the median nerve. The degree of plexus formation that occurs between fascicles decreases in the distal portion of the extremity. (Reproduced with permission from Mackinnon SE, Dellon AL (eds): *Surgery of the Peripheral Nerve.* New York, NY, Thieme Medical Publishers, 1988, p 6.)

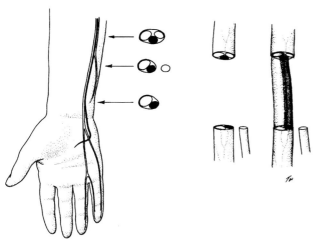

Figure 9

Reconstruction of ulnar nerve injuries when the surgeon anticipates both sensory and motor recovery includes identification of the motor (black) and sensory (white) fascicular groups in the hand. Proximally, the motor group is located between the sensory components to the glabrous skin and the dorsal skin of the hand. Awake stimulation and nerve-staining techniques can be used to identify the sensory and motor groups in the proximal portion of the ulnar nerve. The surgeon expects the motor group to be slightly smaller than the sensory group and located medial to the main sensory bundle. (Reproduced with permission from Mackinnon SE: Upper extremity nerve injuries: Primary repair and reconstruction, in Cohen ML (ed): *Mastery of Plastic and Reconstructive Surgery.* Boston, MA, Little, Brown and Co, 1994, p 1617.)

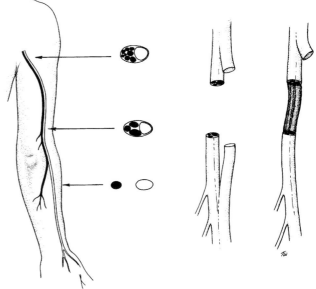

Figure 10

Reconstruction of the radial nerve injury is directed at reconstruction of the motor fascicles (black). Distally, the radial sensory nerve (white) should be excluded from the distal nerve repair. Proximally, awake stimulation can be used to separate motor from sensory which are located in discrete areas of the proximal nerve. (Reproduced with permission from Mackinnon SE: Upper extremity nerve injuries: Primary repair and reconstruction, in Cohen ML (ed): *Mastery of Plastic and Reconstructive Surgery.* Boston, MA, Little, Brown and Co, 1994, p 1617.)

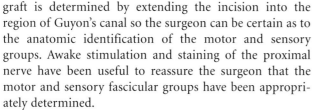

graft is determined by extending the incision into the region of Guyon's canal so the surgeon can be certain as to the anatomic identification of the motor and sensory groups. Awake stimulation and staining of the proximal nerve have been useful to reassure the surgeon that the motor and sensory fascicular groups have been appropriately determined.

Radial nerve grafting can be viewed from a similar perspective (Fig. 10). Proximally, in the arm, approximately 70% of the radial nerve consists of motor fibers. Distally, the radial sensory nerve can be identified and followed proximally to the site of the distal stump. The radial sensory nerve can then be excluded from the distal nerve repair to ensure that no motor fibers regenerate into the cutaneous nerve distribution. If necessary, the radial sensory nerve can be used as nerve graft material. Proximal motor fibers will be directed into the distal motor branches of the radial nerve. A redundant triceps branch can be included in the proximal repair to ensure additional good motor input. This does not compromise overall triceps function. If nerve graft material is at a premium, the branches to the brachioradialis can be excluded because they do not provide important motor function in isolated radial nerve injuries.

Donor Nerve Grafts

Donor nerve grafts in the upper extremity are useful to the hand surgeon. The traditional nerve harvested for donor nerve graft is the sural nerve, which will provide 30 to 40 cm of useful graft material. The sural nerve is found adjacent to the lesser saphenous vein just posterior to the lateral malleolus; a longitudinal incision follows its course. The lateral antebrachial cutaneous nerve is found adjacent to the cephalic vein in the forearm. This nerve is located on the ulnar border of the brachioradialis muscle. There are usually 2 branches at this level. A maximum of 8 cm of nerve graft can be harvested. The diameter of the nerve graft is suitable for digital nerve reconstruction and the loss of sensibility is minimal; however, the scar on the forearm is prominent. The medial antebrachial cutaneous nerve is found adjacent to the basilic vein in the groove just medial to the biceps muscle. There are 2 branches, 1 on either side of the basilic vein. The anterior branch is recommended because the sensory loss will not be on the important ulnar border of the elbow and forearm. Because of its location in the medial aspect of the arm, the scar from harvesting the medial antebrachial cutaneous nerve is more acceptable than that associated with harvesting the lateral antebrachial nerve. If necessary, 18 to 20 cm of nerve graft material can be harvested from the medial antebrachial cutaneous nerve. Both anterior and posterior branches have been harvested when harvesting a sural nerve graft was contraindicated.

When nerve grafting is considered for median and ulnar nerve injuries frequently an expendable portion of the median or ulnar nerve often is used to reconstruct more critical components of these nerves. For example, proximal and distal to a median nerve injury, the nerves destined to the third web space of the hand can be harvested as donor nerve grafts (Fig. 11). Twenty-four centimeters of nerve graft material can be obtained from this source before reaching a major plexus formation in the proximal forearm. Thus, in the patient who has no sensation in the median nerve distribution, the 5 lateral digital nerves can be reinnervated using nerve graft material that would otherwise provide sensation to the 2 digital nerves to the third web space. The patient has no added sensory morbidity from harvesting this donor nerve graft. Similarly, in established ulnar nerve injury in which it is not functioning, the dorsal cutaneous branch of the ulnar nerve can be used as donor nerve material to reconstruct the remainder of the ulnar nerve. Upper extremity nerves have a more favorable neural-to-connective tissue ratio than lower extremity nerves, which may enhance nerve regeneration.

Obtaining the donor nerve graft from the extremity with the nerve injury is also beneficial. In several patients, the terminal branch of the anterior interosseous nerve has proven to be a satisfactory nerve graft. It is harvested through a distal forearm longitudinal incision. The nerve is identified proximal to where it enters the pronator quadratus and is followed into the midportion of the muscle. It is a good size match for a digital nerve repair or for when a partial median or ulnar nerve injury requires just a short segment of nerve graft. This donor graft is associated with no motor or sensory deficit.

Neuroma in Continuity

Neuroma in continuity or sixth-degree injury is the most challenging of all surgical peripheral nerve problems. Careful clinical evaluation will allow the surgeon to preoperatively determine which fascicular groups are normal, and which are partially or completely injured. The challenge of sixth-degree injuries is to repair the damaged components of the nerve (fourth- and fifth-degree injury) and, at the same time, not "downgrade" normal fascicles or those with potential for recovery.

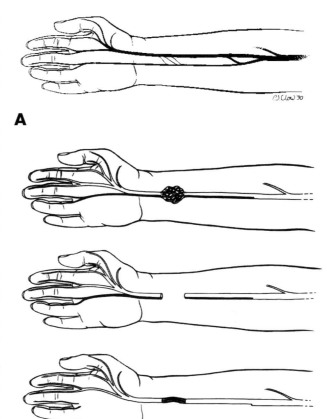

A

B

Figure 11

A, Schema of the internal topography of the fascicles to the third digital web space. A microinternal neurolysis of the fascicles to the third web space can be carried out proximally to a level of approximately 145 mm proximal to the radial styloid to meet a large plexus, which precludes further dissection. (Reproduced with permission from Mackinnon SE: Peripheral nerve injuries, in *Hand Surgery Update.* Rosemont, IL, American Academy of Orthopaedic Surgeons, 1996, pp 233–241.) **B,** In a fourth-degree injury of the median nerve (**top**), the neuroma in continuity is resected (**center**), and the fascicles to the third digital web space are dissected both proximal and distal to the injury site to facilitate reconstruction of the nerve injury using the third web space fascicles as the donor nerve graft (**bottom**). (Reproduced with permission from Ross DO, Mackinnon SE, Chang YZ: Internal topography of the median nerve facilitates nerve sharing procedures. *J Reconst Microsurgery* 1992;8:225–232.)

Recently, a simple technique was described for treatment of the neuroma in continuity in a situation in which functioning motor fibers must be maintained during identification and reconstruction of sensory fibers that either are not functioning or are producing disabling pain. Once the neuroma in continuity is identified, a simple disposable nerve stimulator can be used to identify the motor fascicles proximal and distal to the level of injury. These motor fibers are protected, then the electrically silent sensory fascicles, both proximal and distal to the neuroma in continuity, are divided and reconstructed with a nerve graft. In this way, a tedious and potentially "down-grading" dissection through the neuroma in continuity itself is avoided (Fig. 12). In the reverse situation when sensory fascicles need to be protected and motor function reconstructed, depending on the duration of denervation, tendon transfers are appropriate. If reconstruction of the nerve is more appropriate, then nerve-to-nerve fascicular recordings will be necessary to identify and protect functioning sensory fascicles.

Nerve Transfers

The concept of nerve-to-nerve transfer is not new, but in general has been reserved for problems relating to brachial plexus injuries. With more hand surgeons involved in brachial plexus reconstruction, this concept of nerve transfers recently has been extrapolated from brachial plexus to upper extremity injuries involving the forearm and hand. The principle of a nerve transfer is to change a proximal high-level nerve injury to a more distal lower-level problem. In general, a nearby, expendable, pure motor nerve is transferred to the denervated recipient nerve. For example, the loss of pronation associated with a proximal injury such as seen in a mononeuritis of the median nerve is treated by transfer of an expendable (flexor carpi ulnaris) nerve from a portion of the ulnar nerve at the level of the proximal forearm. If some motor branches of the median nerve are functioning (eg, to the palmaris longus or superficialis), then these nerve branches can be transferred to the nonfunctioning nerve of the pronator teres. Similarly, a high ulnar nerve injury will be treated with a transfer of the distal portion of the anterior interosseous nerve innervating the pronator quadratus muscle to the deep motor branch of the ulnar nerve in the distal forearm level. Sensory nerve transfers are also used for high injuries. An upper brachial plexus injury with sensory loss in the thumb and index finger will be treated with a nerve transfer of the third or fourth web space digital nerves to the radial digital nerve of the index finger and the ulnar digital nerve of the thumb.

The experiences with nerve transfer techniques in the brachial plexus, combined with the ability to do intraneural dissection of the peripheral nerve to identify expendable motor fascicles allow for a totally new way of treating proximal nerve injuries. The surgeon can select healthy, normal, nearby expendable motor fascicles to reconstruct the injury more distal in the extremity and much closer to the muscle end plates. Long nerve grafts can be avoided, and the time for reinnervation is decreased by many months. The surgeon

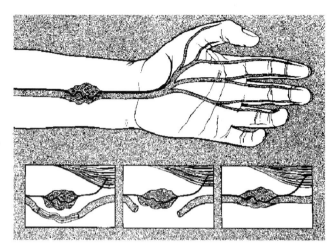

Figure 12

Schema of the bypass operation for management of the neuroma in continuity of the median nerve in which the motor fascicles (black) are protected and preserved and the sensory component of the median nerve is reconstructed with a nerve graft. (Reproduced with permission from Mackinnon SE: Peripheral nerve injuries, in Manske PR (ed): *Hand Surgery Update.* Rosemont, IL, American Academy of Orthopaedic Surgeons, 1996, pp 233–241.)

is not obliged to carry out the reconstruction in the proximal extremity at the level of the injury.

Results of Nerve Repair and Grafting

In spite of the large number of nerve repairs, very little has been published on results of nerve repair or grafting. Most surgeons who do not actively treat a large number of patients with peripheral nerve problems perceive that the results of nerve surgery are poor. This perception arises, in part, from the published results dealing with nerve injuries during World War II. In a 5-year follow-up of 3,656 nerve injuries, nerve grafting was used in only 30 cases. Seddon's report of the war experience demonstrated equally poor results. Although these injuries would now be treated differently, with microneurosurgical technique and nerve grafting, surgeons' attitudes towards peripheral nerve surgery have been significantly influenced by these large series of patients with long-term follow-up.

In general, the results following nerve repair and grafting are improving. In 1995, Kline and Hudson reported on their personal results of nerve repair in a textbook on nerve injuries. However, nothing has been published in the peer reviewed literature since 1980 on the results of high median nerve injuries treated with nerve repair. There have been 5 published papers documenting results of low median nerve repairs. Using sensory reeducation, the author in 1992

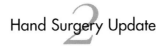
reported 80% of patients recovering as S3+ following median nerve grafting. Since 1980, there have been only 6 reports of results of repair of low ulnar nerve injuries and only 2 reports on function following high ulnar nerve repair. The results of motor recovery varied from only 10% to 91% of patients recovering M4 or M5 motor function. No patients recovered M5 function, and only 9% of patients in one study recovered M4 function.

Children recover better neurologic function after nerve injury than do adults. This difference likely relates to central plasticity rather than to significant differences in peripheral nerve regeneration or motor-sensory recovery. It needs to be stressed that the accepted rating scales for both sensory (Highet's) and motor (British Medical Research Council) grading are imperfect. However, at the moment, there is no uniformity among surgeons as to alternative sensory-motor grading systems. Review of published series should provide stimulus for all surgeons to accept better follow-up and consider independent evaluation of patient results as well as the possibility of establishing a nerve repair and graft patient registry.

Postoperative Rehabilitation

In the postoperative period, maintenance of range of motion of all joints is critical in determining potential outcome after motor recovery. There has been long-term interest in the potential effect of electrical stimulation of denervated muscles. It is hypothesized that even in the absence of neurotrophic influence, contractile activity produced by electrical stimulation would ultimately be beneficial to functional motor recovery. When this experimental question was investigated in a number of research studies, it was found that implantable electrodes and pulse generators with continuous stimulation were required if any effect was to be seen. The same investigators currently are supervising a multicenter clinical trial of the use of electrical stimulation for major nerve injuries in the upper extremity and are gratified with the early results.

Motor reeducation is useful after nerve regeneration, especially when a less than perfectly synergistic nerve has been transferred or when significant motor-sensory fiber mixing has occurred. Late-phase motor reeducation emphasizes motions or activities that mimic the patient's job activities. Having the patient work in a workshop or with a work simulator is useful before returning the patient to the work place.

Sensory Reeducation

After nerve regeneration there may be a misdirection of sensory fibers such that aberrant localization of sensation is experienced. Sensory reeducation assists the patient with such a sensory impairment to reinterpret an altered profile of neural impulses. Experiments in independent laboratories have demonstrated cortical changes following nerve injury and regeneration in adult monkeys. An improvement in cortical mapping is seen when the primates are forced to use their reinnervated digits frequently (a form of sensory reeducation).

Patients may be taught the basics of sensory reeducation even before their surgery so they are familiar with the techniques in the postoperative period. In the very early postoperative period, desensitization is a form of sensory reeducation as the patient is trained to perceive altered stimuli as nonpainful. As soon as the patient perceives any touch in the reinnervated area, the early phase of sensory reeducation is started. The goals are to reeducate specific perceptions such as movement versus constant touch and to begin to reeducate incorrect localization. The patient is encouraged to perform the sensory reeducation exercises frequently. As the sensibility improves, more challenging sensory tasks are included in the reeducation program. Sensory tasks that are too difficult should not be introduced before the patient is capable of working with them. Late-phase sensory reeducation includes exercises to identify and recognize objects, beginning with large objects and progressing to smaller ones. This continues until appropriate functional sensibility has returned, and the patient is using the hand to the extent that he or she essentially is performing sensory reeducation on a continuing basis.

Annotated Bibliography

Classification of Nerve Injury

Mackinnon SE, Dellon AL (eds): *Surgery of the Peripheral Nerve.* New York, NY, Thieme Publishing, 1988.

These surgeons present a comprehensive textbook outlining the investigation and management of peripheral nerve disorders; surgical techniques are described in detail.

Omer GE, Spinner M, Van Beek A (eds): *Management of Peripheral Nerve Problems,* ed 2. Philadelphia, PA, WB Saunders, 1998.

Over 100 authors contributed to this textbook, presenting their various perspectives on surgical management of nerve injuries.

How to Examine the Nerve-Injured Patient

Kimura J (ed): *Electrodiagnosis in Diseases of Nerve and Muscle: Principles and Practice,* ed 2. Philadelphia, PA, FA Davis, 1989.

This is an excellent review of the role of electrodiagnostic studies in evaluating nerve injuries.

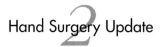

Nerve Repair

Brandt KE, Mackinnon SE: Microsurgical repair of peripheral nerves and nerve grafts, in Aston SJ, Beasley RWA, Thorne CHM (eds): *Grabb and Smith's Plastic Surgery*, ed 5. Philadelphia, PA, Lippincott-Raven, 1997, pp 79–90.

This is a comprehensive review of nerve injuries and reconstructions.

Mackinnon SE: Techniques of nerve repair, in Tindall GT, Cooper PR, Barrow DL (eds): *The Practice of Neurosurgery*. Baltimore, MD, Williams & Wilkins, 1996, vol 3, pp 2879–2908.

The authors provide a detailed review of peripheral nerve reconstruction.

Watchmaker GP, Mackinnon SE: Nerve injury and repair, in Peimer CA (ed): *Surgery of the Hand and Upper Extremity*. New York, NY, McGraw-Hill Health Professions Division, 1996, pp 1251–1275.

This is a review of the basis for nerve reconstruction and an overview of surgical techniques in nerve repair.

Nerve Grafting

Mackinnon SE: Surgical approach to the radial nerve. *Techniques in Hand and Upper Extremity Surgery*. 1999, in press.

This is an overview of the surgical management of radial nerve injuries.

Mackinnon SE: Upper extremity nerve injuries: Primary repair and reconstruction, in Cohen M (ed): *Mastery of Plastic and Reconstructive Surgery*. Boston, MA, Little, Brown & Co, 1994.

The techniques for treatment of nerve injuries in the upper extremity are described, including techniques of reconstruction.

Donor Nerve Grafting

Mackinnon SE: Evaluation of nerve gaps: Upper and lower extremities, in Omer GE, Spinner M, Van Beek A (eds): *Management of Peripheral Nerve Problems*, ed 2. Philadelphia, PA, WB Saunders, 1998, pp 328–339.

The author outlines the surgical management and options for nerve injuries associated with a significant gap.

Watchmaker GP, Mackinnon SE: Advances in peripheral nerve repair. *Clin Plast Surg* 1997;24:63–73.

A discussion of surgical options for complex nerve reconstruction in the hand.

Nerve Transfers

Nath RK, Mackinnon SE, Shenaq SM: New nerve transfers after nerve injury, in Lee WPA (ed): *Innovations in Hand Surgery*. Philadelphia, PA, WB Saunders, 1998, pp 2–11.

An overview of nerve transfer techniques in upper extremity reconstruction.

Results of Nerve Repair and Grafting

Kline DG, Hudson AR (eds): *Nerve Injuries: Operative Results for Major Nerve Injuries, Entrapments, and Tumors*. Philadelphia, PA, WB Saunders, 1995.

These authors present their philosophy on the management of nerve injuries and their personal results from reconstruction of peripheral nerve injuries.

Postoperative Rehabilitation

Williams HB: A clinical pilot study to assess functional return following continuous muscle stimulation after nerve injury and repair in the upper extremity using a completely implantable electrical system. *Microsurgery* 1996;17:597–605.

A discussion of the early results of muscle electrical stimulation is provided.

Williams HB: The value of continuous electrical muscle stimulation using a completely implantable system in the preservation of muscle function following motor nerve injury and repair: An experimental study. *Microsurgery* 1996;17:589–596.

The author outlines the status of muscle stimulation for improvement of functional recovery.

Sensory Reeducation

Merzenich MM, Jenkins WM: Reorganization of cortical representations of the hand following alterations of skin inputs induced by nerve injury, skin island transfers and experience. *J Hand Surg* 1993;6:89–104.

The importance of the cortical influence on nerve injury is discussed.

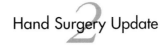

Chapter 20
Brachial Plexus Injuries

211

Vincent R. Hentz, MD

Brachial Plexus Injuries: Nonobstetric

Introduction

Since the publication of the initial volume of *Hand Surgery Update* in 1993, there have been significant advances in the diagnosis and treatment of injuries to the brachial plexus. The following sections will present background information from the initial volume where necessary and review newer ideas published since 1993.

Before modern microneurosurgical techniques, there was little enthusiasm for operating on the injured brachial plexus. If the palsy was complete, amputation of the arm was recommended. Today, with modern surgical techniques, useful function frequently can be restored, even to completely paralyzed limbs. Key developments include recommendations for additional sources of motor axons and extension of the principles of microvascular innervated free-muscle transfers to the severely paralyzed limb.

Pathology of the Lesion

Patient demographics have changed little over the last decade. The typical patient remains a young man thrown from a motorcycle. The extent of the injury reflects the amount of energy absorbed and, to some degree, the direction of the force relative to the limb and shoulder. These high-energy injuries are associated with significant nerve pathology, including rupture of plexal segments at any level (Sunderland grade V) or avulsions of nerve roots from the spinal cord. Because more injuries now are explored surgically, the high incidence of simultaneous lesions at several anatomic levels is better known by surgeons. Low-energy injuries, such as a fall onto the shoulder, typically cause mostly reversible injuries such as neurapraxia (Sunderland grade I) or various degrees of axonotmesis (Sunderland grades II through V). Because of its anatomy, the lower structures of the brachial plexus suffer more significant injuries, such as root avulsion, than do the more proximally located roots, trunks, and cords (Table 1). Essentially every Sunderland grade of injury plus root avulsion can occur in the same patient (Fig. 1).

Table 1

Surgical findings for each root from a series of 114 adult patients with total or near total brachial plexus palsy

Root	Ruptured	Avulsed	Other
C5	59	14	40
C6	44	35	35
C7	39	53	20
C8	11	67	31
T1	11	61	37

(Reproduced with permission from Hentz VR: Brachial plexus injuries, in *Hand Surgery Update*. Rosemont, IL, American Academy of Orthopaedic Surgeons, 1996, pp 243–251.)

Evaluation of the Patient

The goal is to determine the extent of the nerve injury and, from this, to decide whether the patient is a candidate for early surgical reconstruction of the brachial plexus or for a period of further observation.

Significant Physical Signs A Horner's sign indicates severe injury to the C-8 and T-1 roots and has been strongly correlated with avulsion of one or both of these roots. Severe pain in an anesthetic extremity is also a sign of poor prognosis, indicating some degree of deafferentiation of the limb, again strongly correlated with root avulsion injuries.

Motor and Sensory Examination Two important indicators of the level of injury for the patient with near total palsy are the presence or absence of activity of the rhomboids and serratus anterior muscles.

Diagnostic Imaging Tests Plain radiographs of the cervical spine, chest, clavicle, and scapula are necessary. The chest

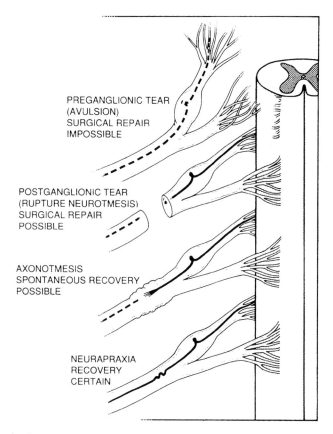

Figure 1

In the same patient, a severe traction injury to the brachial plexus may cause nerve injuries of varying severity, including avulsion of the nerve rootlets from the spinal cord (non-reparable), extraforaminal rupture of the root or trunk (surgically reparable), or an intra-neural rupture of fascicles or axons within fascicles (some spontaneous recovery possible). (Reproduced with permission from Hentz VR: Microneural reconstruction of the brachial plexus, in Green DP (ed): *Operative Hand Surgery*, ed 3. New York, NY, Churchill Livingstone, 1993, vol 2, pp 1223–1252.)

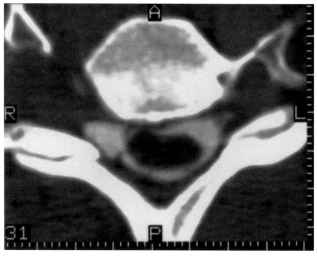

Figure 2

Computed tomography of the cervical spine with contrast demonstrates avulsion of a part of the transverse process and absence of a right root shadow at the C6 level. The left root shadow is clearly outlined. This appearance suggests that the C6 root has been avulsed. (Reproduced with permission from Hentz VR: Microneural reconstruction of the brachial plexus, in Green DP (ed): *Operative Hand Surgery*, ed 3. New York, NY, Churchill Livingstone, 1993, vol 2, pp 1223–1252.)

radiograph should include inspiration and expiration antero-posterior views to determine the activity of the diaphragm. A paralyzed diaphragm is an indicator of severe injury to the upper roots of the plexus. Fractures of the transverse processes are also strong evidence of a high-energy injury.

Modern imaging techniques have improved the clinician's ability to predict what the microneurosurgeon will find at exploration. Traditional myelography using metrizimide contrast has been largely supplanted by computed tomography (CT) or magnetic resonance imaging (MRI) examinations performed with and without contrast agents (Fig. 2). Both CT and MRI may be useful, although contrast CT myelography appears to be the current benchmark examination. MRI reformatting provides a better picture of the soft tissues. The T2-weighted images highlight the fat content of the cervical spinal cord and nerve roots, and the T1

image highlights the water content associated with a pseudomeningocele. The presence of a pseudomeningocele has been strongly correlated with avulsion of the corresponding root. Other evidence of significant injury includes empty-appearing root sleeves or a shift of the cord away from the midline.

When these tests are performed within a few days of injury, especially with contrast, there may be a higher incidence of false positive interpretations because the contrast agent may leak through small tears in the dura, which may occur without root avulsion. Two recent publications document the predictive ability of MRI in assessing presence or absence of root avulsion. For the C5 and C6 roots, the axial and axial oblique planes proved more useful than coronal or sagittal reformats. The accuracy of MRI was equal or superior to that of more invasive techniques such as myelography. Avulsion of lower rootlets was more difficult to confirm by MRI. Another MRI format, fast-spin echo MRI, appears to be an excellent alternative to contrast CT myelography, especially in evaluating infants with presumed root avulsions.

Sensory and Motor Evoked Potentials Standard electromyography is not as helpful for severe injuries as are sensory evoked potentials, corticosensory evoked potentials, and spinograms. Stimulating over Erb's point in the supraclavicular fossa and recording from the cortex using scalp electrodes may provide

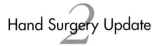

evidence that some roots are still in continuity with the spinal cord. The spinogram can provide information about the level of intact innervation of the paraspinous muscles. Because they are innervated by the posterior primary rami of the plexus, paralysis of these muscles indicates a very proximal injury but does not tell the examiner whether the injury is associated with avulsion, rupture, or axonotmesis. The role of noninvasive electromagnetic stimulation of the motor cortex by powerful electromagnetic field generators to produce a motor action potential at a peripheral site is being assessed.

No single test can be the conclusive basis for surgical decision making. All the information must be assimilated and, most importantly, be viewed within the context of the presumed energy of the trauma.

Indications for Surgery

Most modern series describing brachial plexus reconstruction attest to the inverse relationship between time from injury to operation and outcome. In cautious and skilled hands, exploration seldom results in extension of the injury. Even when total palsy exists, less than 20% of patients demonstrate avulsions of all 5 roots of the plexus. For the great majority, the surgeon will find something to repair or graft and, if this is not possible, to reinnervate by nerve transfer from an extraplexal source of motor and sensory axons. If nerve transfer is included, virtually 100% of patients might theoretically benefit from microneural reconstruction. These factors imply that when there is a strong suspicion of significant damage to the plexus, in the form of root avulsions and nerve ruptures, surgical exploration is warranted.

Timing of Surgery

Immediate Surgery Immediate surgery is indicated for any patient with a plexus injury secondary to a penetrating injury, such as a stab wound, or following iatrogenic injury to the plexus at the time of first rib resection for the treatment of thoracic outlet syndrome. There are many good arguments against immediate reconstruction of the plexus after traction injuries. Most surgeons feel that some period of time must pass to permit delineation of injured from noninjured nerve.

Early Surgery Early surgery (3 weeks to 3 months) is indicated for patients who present with total or near total palsy, or an injury associated with high-energy levels. It is also indicated for gunshot wounds to the plexus. For those injuries associated with lower levels of energy and those associated with partial upper-level palsy, it is preferable to follow the course of recovery for 3 to 6 months, leaning toward surgery if recovery seems to plateau as determined by several successive evaluations carried out at monthly inter-

vals. The presence or absence of an advancing Tinel's sign can be a useful guide. The absence of a Tinel's sign in the supraclavicular fossa in the face of a nearly complete C5–C6 level palsy is a poor prognostic sign for spontaneous recovery and warrants early exploration, with the likelihood that C5 and C6 nerve roots may be avulsed. In this case, nerve transfer will be necessary.

Controversial Indications The occasional patient who presents with a partial C8 and complete T1 lesion, with some finger flexors working but with intrinsic palsy and anesthesia in the C8 and/or T1 distribution, represents a dilemma in decision making, because it is almost impossible to recover intrinsic muscle function in the adult. When injured, the C8 and T1 nerve roots are so often avulsed from the spinal cord that it is unlikely that anything reparable will be found.

Surgical Findings

Unless the injury is clearly limited to a single area of the plexus, as for example following a stab wound, the entire plexus, from neck to axilla, may need to be exposed. A variety of problems may be seen. If the upper roots are avulsed, the rootlets and swollen dorsal root ganglion may be found twisted and lying either behind the clavicle or slightly above it in the region of the C8 root. If the upper roots or superior trunk and/or the middle trunk has ruptured, the distal ends typically lie behind the clavicle. The avulsed (often) or ruptured (infrequently) C8 and T1 structures are usually found much closer to their respective foramina than is the case with C5 or C6 structures. Essentially any combination of injuries may occur, including avulsion, rupture, and a neuroma-in-continuity. The supraclavicular dissection usually allows this assessment. However, it is critical to complete the remainder of the dissection if the findings above favor some type of reconstruction by nerve grafting. Lesions often occur at 2 levels, for example, rupture of the superior trunk in combination with avulsion of the axillary nerve from the deltoid, or rupture of the musculocutaneous nerve at the level of the shoulder.

Intraoperative Evoked Potentials

These potentials (Fig. 3) are helpful in determining when, for example, an intraforaminal avulsion (uncommon) rather than a rupture has occurred, or to determine whether there exists only an empty root sleeve; that is, only connective tissue with no axons therein (more common). The technique is not foolproof, because if sensory rootlets remain in continuity while the motor rootlets are avulsed, a cortical signal may still be produced. To avoid this dilemma, one author has described using electromagnetic stimulation of the motor cortex while recording from the cervical root.

By 2 to 3 months after injury, evoked potentials across a neuroma-in-continuity are reliable in assisting in decision

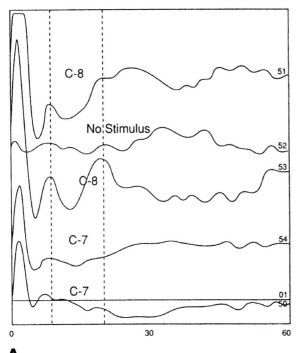

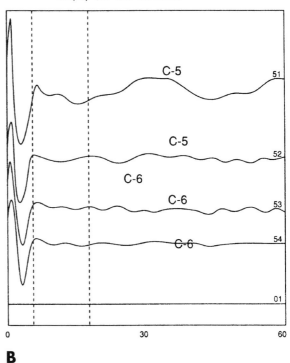

A   **B**

Figure 3

The results of intraoperative corticosensory evoked potentials are demonstrated in a patient with a C5, C6, C7 palsy. At exploration, all roots could be found exiting their foramina but the C5, C6, and C7 roots were somewhat firmer than the C8 root. **A,** The 3 upper tracings are the result of stimulating (or recording but not stimulating) the C8 root, recording from scalp electrodes. With C8 root stimulation, a large corticosensory response could be measured with the scalp electrodes. Stimulation of the C7 root (lower 2 tracings) and sequential stimulation of C5 and then C6 roots (**B**) resulted in no measurable brain response indicating probable avulsion of these roots within the bony canal. (Reproduced with permission from Hentz VR: Microneural reconstruction of the brachial plexus, in Green DP (ed): *Operative Hand Surgery*, ed 3. New York, NY, Churchill Livingstone, 1993, vol 2, pp 1223–1252.)

making. When stimulating and recording across a neuroma-in-continuity, it is unnecessary to average a large number of stimulations. If there is no easily discernible response above the noise level without averaging, the neuroma and adjacent damaged nerve are resected using the microscope to assist in determining when debridement is adequate, and nerve grafts are placed in the resultant defect. If a clear signal is identified above the noise, then only a neurolysis under magnification is performed.

Intraoperative Decisions and Priorities of Repair
When the patient presents with total brachial plexus palsy, the priorities of repair include: (1) provisions for elbow flexion by biceps/brachialis muscle reinnervation; (2) provisions for shoulder stabilization, abduction, and external rotation by axillary and/or suprascapular nerve reinnervation; (3) provisions for brachiothoracic pinch (adduction of

the arm against the chest) by reinnervation of the pectoralis major muscle; (4) provisions for sensation below the elbow in the C6–C7 area by reinnervation of the lateral cord; and (5) provisions for wrist extension and finger flexion by reinnervation of the lateral and posterior cord.

These priorities have been chosen for 3 reasons. The first is their functional significance, the second relates to the likelihood of obtaining the chosen function by nerve reconstruction (more proximal muscles will be reinnervated more successfully than very distal muscles), and the third relates to the degree of difficulty in achieving the individual functions listed above by secondary surgery.

Surgical Techniques for Plexoplexal Nerve Reconstruction
The surgeon should take advantage of the knowledge gained by others in internally mapping the plexus. At the root level,

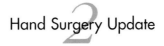
axons destined for posterior and anterior divisions are delineated in an attempt to guide these axons to appropriate target nerves. Next, the distal targets are dissected. These usually include the suprascapular nerve, which is frequently difficult to find, the lateral cord, and the posterior cord. Typically, there are far more targets for nerve grafts than proximal resources.

There is recently published enthusiasm for applying one of several enzyme histochemical techniques as an aid in determining the relative health of the proximal stump. Techniques to analyze the location of motor axons have been suggested, including the staining method of Scabolcz and a rapid analysis acetylcholinesterase technique. Simpler intraoperative histologic tests, such as use of Masson trichrome stain to define axon versus scar ratios, have also been useful.

Choice of Nerve Grafts The typical first choice are the sural nerves. Other donor sites for standard grafts include both medial brachial and medial antebrachial cutaneous nerves. Standard microsuture techniques typically are used, although some surgeons now use autologous derived fibrinogen as a tissue adhesive to glue together nerve ends more rapidly, apparently with equal success.

Vascularized Nerve Grafts The principal reason to consider a vascularized nerve graft in plexus reconstruction is to maximize the length and diameter of nerve graft available. The best indication for a vascularized graft is a case involving proven avulsion of C8 and T1 in association with large root stumps of the remaining plexus. There is no possibility of spontaneous recovery of the ulnar nerve innervated structures and it makes little sense to waste precious proximal axons to recover some sensibility in the ulnar side of the hand. (Intrinsic muscle recovery is essentially never seen in the adult when C8 and T1 have been badly injured.) In this instance, the best source of a vascularized nerve graft is the ulnar nerve itself, based in the upper arm on 1 of several branches of the brachial artery, usually the superior ulnar collateral artery. Some surgeons use the ulnar nerve as a vascularized graft in a 2-stage procedure employing intercostal nerves as a source of motor axons.

Surgical Techniques for Nerve Transfer In the most severe injuries, there are insufficient numbers of proximal axon resources from the remaining parts of the plexus still in continuity with the spinal cord. Currently, researchers are investigating the possibility of novel surgical means to correct functional deficits after spinal root injuries. Success with animal studies confirming the possibility of reestablishing continuity between severed roots and the damaged spinal cord segment has prompted early clinical application.

Most surgeons turn to extraplexal sources of especially motor and also sensory axons. Many different nerves have been advocated. Until recently, the most common sources of extraplexal motor axons have been the spinal accessory nerve and the intercostal nerves from C3 to C6. Nagano and associates have demonstrated better outcomes when the intercostal nerve is transferred to the musculocutaneous nerve without the use of an interpositional nerve graft. This requires a more anterior and distal dissection of the intercostal nerve.

Contemporary surgeons have suggested additional extraplexal sources of motor and sensory axons. One group described the use of a motor fascicle from the ulnar nerve crossed to the biceps muscle for patients with C5–C6 avulsions. Another has successfully used pectoralis major branches crossed to the musculocutaneous nerve and recommends an additional surgical step whenever the musculocutaneous nerve is reinnervated. This step involves sectioning the cutaneous continuation of the musculocutaneous nerve in the distal upper arm and implanting the proximal stump directly into the biceps muscle to avoid wasting any motor axons that might grow down the cutaneous portion of the nerve. In addition, motor branches of the cervical rami or even cross chest branches of the contralateral plexus, such as a branch from the lateral pectoral nerve, are used.

Perhaps the greatest contemporary interest is in the role of contralateral C7 transfer. This technique has been suggested both for the adult following traumatic plexus injury and for the infant suffering avulsions following birth trauma. In a preliminary communication, Chuang describes little to no persistent functional deficit in the donor extremity. In 1995, Chuang reviewed neurotization procedures for brachial plexus injuries and recommended this transfer for patients with total root avulsion injuries, elongating the contralateral C7 root with either a vascularized or nonvascularized ulnar nerve interpositional graft. The target is the median nerve, followed 2 years later by free-muscle transfer using the now reinnervated median nerve as the motor axon source.

The most appropriate targets for nerve transfer had been the suprascapular nerve (shoulder abduction and external rotation), the musculocutaneous nerve (elbow flexion), or the lateral pectoral nerve (thoracohumeral pinch). More recently, surgeons have been more aggressive in their application of extraplexal nerve transfer procedures. One group describes several different strategies to simultaneously reconstruct elbow and finger flexion using free or pedicled latissimus dorsi muscle transfer and innervation by spinal accessory, with intercostal transfer to the radial nerve and sensory intercostal transfer to the median nerve. Others also recommend sensory innervation by sensory intercostal to median nerve transfer. Another group reports restoring limited sensibility (up to

S2+) in 12 of 15 patients. The addition of shoulder fusion has improved the function of the elbow.

Nerve Transfer in the Neglected Plexus Injury It is possible to combine microneural reconstruction with free vascularized functional muscle transfers for neglected cases of total brachial plexus palsy. In these cases, the time since injury is too long (in the adult, certainly beyond 2 years) for successful nerve transfer or reinnervation of previously denervated muscles. The opposite latissimus dorsi, the gracilis, or another muscle is transferred to the shoulder and arm by microvascular free transfer. The motor nerve of the transferred muscle is joined to the donor motor nerve, which usually is an extraplexal motor nerve, such as the spinal accessory or intercostal nerve. It seems that there is no significant difference whether 2 or 3 intercostal nerves are used to reinnervate the free-muscle transfer. Several very aggressive surgical strategies have been recommended for these patients with the goal of restoring function to the elbow and hand, as mentioned above.

Postoperative Care At the completion of the operation, a cervical collar is fitted about the neck to restrict neck motion. The shoulder and elbow are immobilized, the shoulder in adduction and the elbow in 90° of flexion, for 2 weeks; range-of-motion exercises are then renewed without restrictions. After initial healing, the progress of nerve regeneration is assessed about every 3 months. At least 2 and perhaps 3 years are necessary before the results of nerve reconstruction can be assessed.

Results of Nerve Reconstruction by Graft and Nerve Transfer

During the last several years greater numbers of surgeons, particularly Asian colleagues from countries where motorized bicycles are a common mode of transportation, have reported results of reconstruction in large series of patients. New information is available about specific reconstructive goals. One group described their results in restoring shoulder abduction in 99 patients using several different reconstructive strategies. More reliable results were obtained if both suprascapular and axillary nerve were targeted. They also reported 80% success in restoring useful elbow flexion (M4 level) using functioning free-muscle transfers. In patients with C5–C6 avulsion who underwent surgery before 6 months, intercostal transfer to the musculocutaneous nerve resulted in 67% with grade M4 level elbow flexion. Other authors have demonstrated equally good results with spinal accessory to musculocutaneous transfer, a much less time-consuming and technically less demanding procedure.

Analysis of published series (Tables 2 and 3) leads to several conclusions. Repair does improve the prognosis. Infraclavicular injuries have a better prognosis than do supraclavicular

Table 2
Results of reconstruction

Author	Patients	Developed Useful Function
Total supraclavicular palsy		
Millesi	20	10*
Sedel	26†	22
Partial palsy (infraclavicular)		
Millesi	11 supraclavicular	9
	12 infraclavicular	10
Sedel/Narakas	23	20

* Shoulder 5/8, elbow flexion 9/18, wrist/finger 2/18
† MRC grade 3, 11; grade 4, 12; grade 5, 3
(Adapted with permission from Hentz VR: Microneural reconstruction of the brachial plexus, in Green DP (ed): *Operative Hand Surgery,* ed 3. New York, NY, Churchill Livingstone, 1993, vol 2, pp 1223–1252.)

Table 3
Results of nerve transfer for elbow flexion

Nerve	Author	Patients	Results Good %	Results Poor %
Spinal accessory	Allieu	15	20	80
	Narakas	3	67	33
	Merle	7	42	58
	Songcharoen	184	75	25
Intercostal	Millesi	22	50	50
	Narakas	24	38	62
	Nagano	117	68	32
	Chaung	66	80	20

(Adapted with permission from Hentz VR: Microneural reconstruction of the brachial plexus, in Green DP (ed): *Operative Hand Surgery,* ed 3. New York, NY, Churchill Livingstone, 1993, vol 2, pp 1223–1252.)

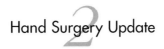
injuries. Supraclavicular injuries associated with at least 2 reparable roots have a better prognosis, especially when there are partial injuries. The results of nerve transfer have been more mixed.

Microneural Reconstruction for Obstetric Palsy

The approach to the infant who has suffered a traction injury of the brachial plexus differs somewhat from the approach to the adult although the mechanism of injury is similar; that is, excessive direct traction on the brachial plexus associated with a difficult delivery or perhaps by compression of the plexus by the first rib. In most cases a similar set of circumstances prevails, including a high birth weight, usually greater than 4 kg (frequently associated with maternal diabetes or short, heavy mothers); a difficult presentation (shoulder dystocia); cephalopelvic disproportion; or forceps delivery. Since the first reported attempts at repair in 1903, the role of surgical reconstruction has been far more controversial than for the adult cases and remains so to this day. The principal reason behind the controversy regarding the role of microneural reconstruction lies in the lack of a uniform system of evaluation. Most studies lack reliable data on the initial clinical picture, and there is no consensus on what constitutes a good result. For most studies, a good result translates into a well-functioning hand regardless of the condition of the shoulder, which frequently lacks normal external rotation and abduction. However, the hand frequently is spared because a majority of lesions involve C5 and C6 (plus or minus C7) roots (Fig. 4). Renewed interest in operating on infants has been stimulated primarily by a better understanding of the natural history of spontaneous evolution following injury, which was provided by longitudinal studies that determined that (1) complete recovery seems possible only if the biceps and deltoid demonstrate some level of function by the second month; (2) the results, although still good, are nevertheless incomplete if initial contracting of these 2 muscles requires 3 to 3.5 months; and (3) if the biceps is not contracting strongly by 5 months, the results will be highly unsatisfactory.

Gilbert recommended using the rate of biceps recovery as a means of determining which baby should have early plexus exploration (3 to 4 months of age). More recently published and presented longitudinal studies have questioned whether the rate of recovery of the biceps is sufficiently predictive. One study found that biceps recovery incorrectly predicted recovery in 13% of patients. Another recommends combining scores for elbow flexion with scores for wrist, finger, and thumb extension. These were predictive in almost 95% of 61 patients allowed to evolve without nerve surgery.

Preoperative Evaluation

The posture of the newborn is frequently diagnostic, with either a flail limb, indicating complete palsy, or an internally rotated, adducted limb with the forearm pronated and the wrist flexed, indicating an upper root problem (Fig. 4). A simple muscle-testing scheme for these infants has been used in which M0 is no contraction; M1 represents contraction without movement; M2, slight movement; and M3, complete movement. A somewhat more complicated analysis has been recommended in which 7 grades are used for each muscle (Table 4).

The sensory examination is even less precise; the examiner tests the reaction to pinching the skin only. Other signs to be

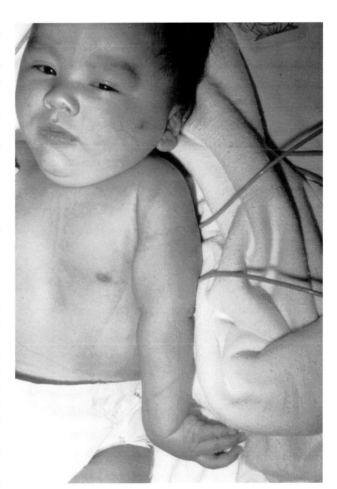

Figure 4

A typical appearance of an infant with an upper (C5–C6) plexus obstetrical palsy. The most frequently used eponym is Erb's palsy. The arm is held by the side, with the elbow extended, the forearm held in pronation, and the wrist in flexion. Depending on the status of the C7 root, the fingers may be held in flexion (injured C7 root) or the infant may demonstrate active extension (probably a healthy C7 root). Wrist and finger flexors and hand intrinsic muscles are typically strong. (Reproduced with permission from Hentz VR: Microneural reconstruction of the brachial plexus, in Green DP (ed): *Operative Hand Surgery*, ed 3. New York, NY, Churchill Livingstone, 1993, vol 2, 1223–1252.)

Table 4
Hospital for Sick Children Muscle Grading system

Observation	Muscle Grade
Gravity eliminated	
No contraction	0
Contraction, no motion	1
Motion ≤ 1/2 range	2
Motion > 1/2 range	3
Full motion	4
Against gravity	
Motion ≤ 1/2 range	5
Motion > 1/2 range	6
Full motion	7

(Adapted with permission from Michelow BJ, Clarke HM, Curtis CG, Zuker RM, Seifu Y, Andrews DF: The natural history of obstetrical brachial plexus palsy. *Plast Reconstr Surg* 1994;93:675–681.)

observed include evidence of trophic changes, such as differences in hair growth or color, and the presence of a Horner's sign. Electromyelograms (EMGs) are not obtained until later.

The infant is reexamined at 1 month of age. Recovery may already be evident and if present will probably ultimately be complete. For the remaining babies, several factors are evident: if the palsy is still total and is associated with a Horner's sign, the outlook for spontaneous recovery is poor and early surgery is indicated; or if the hand is recovering but no biceps or shoulder recovery is evident, there is still a chance for spontaneous recovery. A third evaluation prior to 3 months of age will be necessary to determine indications for surgery.

At 3 months of age, the child is retested. If any biceps function is evident, surgery is not recommended. For those without biceps function, an EMG is scheduled, although EMG results have been difficult to correlate with final outcome. However, total absence of electrical evidence of reinnervation at this time indicates avulsion of the corresponding roots. Cervical myelography was previously recommended. Today less invasive MRI, when skillfully performed, can give almost equivalent sensitivity and reliability.

Gilbert firmly adheres to his previously published guidelines regarding early surgery depending on biceps recovery. Others wait until 6 months or later to make a decision. No firm consensus exists today.

Surgical Approach
The supraclavicular part of the incision alone will usually suffice for C5, C6, and C7 palsies. Otherwise, the dissection is the same as that for the adult. The surgical findings (Table 5) differ from those in the adult in that a neuroma-in-continuity is far more frequently encountered in the infant, typically at the level of the superior trunk. If C7 is affected, it is usually adherent to this neuroma. The clavicle can be lifted up off the plexus, allowing exposure of the divisions and the proximal cords. The suprascapular nerve can frequently be found exiting the neuroma. When all roots have been identified, they are sequentially stimulated and the evoked potentials measured. It is rare to find a root that is both injured extraforaminally and avulsed from the cord. Even C8 and T1 can be seen from the supraclavicular approach. In cases of total palsy, if these roots are normal by electrical studies, then an infraclavicular injury must be suspected and the infraclavicular portion of the incision made. If grafting from a supraclavicular to infraclavicular location is to be done, the clavicle is sectioned obliquely. When fibrous scar extends into the subclavicular region, the surgeon can expect to find 1 or 2 avulsed roots curled within the scar.

Surgical Decision Making
With the presence of a neuroma, it is tempting to perform only a neurolysis. This has led to disappointing results. In most instances, a purposeful decision to resect the neuroma and perform interpositional nerve grafts is made. Frequently, essentially no healthy appearing nerve fibers are found in the distal neuroma on serial histology.

In summary, for subtotal lesions, lesions of C5, C6, and C7 are nearly always extraforaminal ruptures, frequently in-continuity lesions. The lesions are all above the clavicle and

Table 5
Anatomic lesions of upper roots in 75 cases of subtotal obstetrical palsy

Nerve Root	Rupture	Avulsion	Avulsion and Rupture
C5, C6	38	1	1
C5, C6, C7	19	1	5

(Adapted with permission from Michelow BJ, Clarke HM, Curtis CG, Zuker RM, Seifu Y, Andrews DF: The natural history of obstetrical brachial plexus palsy. *Plast Reconstr Surg* 1994;93:675–681.)

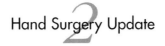
may be repaired through limited incisions. For complete palsy, C8 and T1 are almost always avulsed, and there is always at least 1 root available for reconstruction. This justifies systematic surgical intervention. No isolated lower root injuries without injury to the upper roots were found.

Gilbert has reported on his experience with obstetrical palsy associated with breech delivery. He believes that this mechanism results frequently in intraforaminal rootlet injury. The extraforaminal plexus may be essentially normal in appearance yet no corticosensory potentials can be evoked.

Table 6
Gilbert's results after plexus reconstruction—Mallet scale

Injury	Time Postinjury	Grade	Good to Excellent Results
C5-C6	2 years	>IV	52%
		III	40%
		II	8%
	4 years*	>IV	80%
		III	20%
C5-C6-C7	2 years	>IV	36%
		III	46%
		II	18%
	4 years†	>IV	61%
		III	29%
		II	10%
Complete paralysis	4 years	>IV	49%
		III	29%
		II	22%

* One third had second shoulder surgical procedure
† One fourth had second shoulder surgery
(Adapted with permission from Michelow BJ, Clarke HM, Curtis CG, Zuker RM, Seifu Y, Andrews DF: The natural history of obstetrical brachial plexus palsy. *Plast Reconstr Surg* 1994;93:675–681.)

Postoperative Care
The infant is placed into a clam-shell splint for approximately 3 weeks. Exercises aimed at maintaining good shoulder external rotation and abduction, elbow extension, and forearm rotation are initiated at 3 weeks.

Results of Surgery
The results of surgery must be categorized according to the severity of the initial presentation and surgical findings. Table 6 outlines the results following reconstruction in subtotal palsy in the largest series published to date. The Mallet scheme is used as the basis for determining the postoperative grade (Fig. 5). These results indicate that two thirds of the surgically treated group achieved a more functional

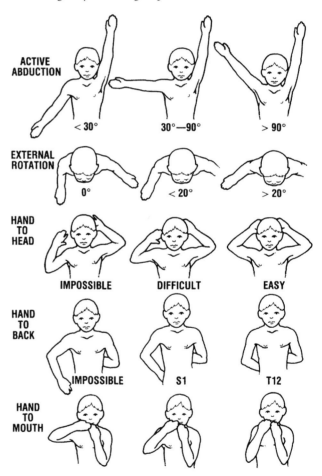

Figure 5
Mallet's scheme for assessing shoulder function forms the basis for Gilbert's method of grading functional outcome following reconstruction for obstetric palsy. Illustrated from left to right are Mallet grades II through IV. The assessment includes a grade I, which signifies any activity less than grade II, and a grade V, which implies normal movement. Grades I and V are not illustrated here. (Reproduced with permission from Mallet J: Paralysie obstetricale du plexus brachial symposium: Traitement des sepuelles: Primaute du traitement de l'e'paule - methode d'expression des resultats. *Rev Chir Orthop Reparatrice Appar Mot* 1972;58:166–168.)

shoulder than if they had been allowed to evolve spontaneously. Reconstruction of the infant plexus also seems to result in improved growth of the affected limb, but not to normal. For infants operated on with complete palsies, the results are less impressive, in part because some part of the upper plexus may be used to reinnervate the lower plexus. However, in contrast to the adult situation, it is possible in more than 50% of cases to recover some intrinsic muscle activity and in 90%, some active digital flexion is obtained. When compared to the group allowed to evolve spontaneously, the results of surgery are fundamentally improved. These hands are functional and are used.

Summary

The typical palsy is a traumatic traction injury caused by forced lowering of the shoulder during delivery. While the lesion may affect all roots, the upper roots usually are ruptures whereas the lower roots frequently are avulsed. Spontaneous recovery is possible but its quality depends greatly on how early recovery begins. Microneural reconstruction is always possible, usually by grafting or by neurotization. The results of surgery are better than the results of spontaneous evolution in similar injury patterns. Palliative treatment of the sequellae of birth palsies is difficult, and the results obtained are rarely totally satisfactory.

For these reasons, the initial surgical intervention should be on the plexus itself in those cases meeting the criteria described above. It is important to make this decision as quickly as possible before neuroplasticity is diminished and joint contractures have occurred.

Annotated Bibliography

Alnot JY: Traumatic brachial plexus lesions in the adult: Indications and results. *Hand Clin* 1995;11:623–631.

The author discusses his experience with 810 patients who underwent surgery from 1975 to 1994.

Becker MH, Lassner F, Schaller E, Berger A: Enzymhistochemical evaluation of ulnar nerve grafts in brachial plexus lesions. *Microsurgery* 1993;14:440–443.

The authors describe a histochemical technique for determining the distribution of motor axons within a nerve.

Brandt KE, Mackinnon SE: A technique for maximizing biceps recovery in brachial plexus reconstruction. *J Hand Surg* 1993;18A:726–733.

The authors describe cadaveric anatomic studies of the intramuscular anatomy of the musculocutaneous nerve, demonstrating that nearly 50% of axons entering the nerve are sensory. They recommend a procedure to capture any motor axons that become misdirected toward cutaneous receptors.

Carlstedt TP: Spinal nerve root injuries in brachial plexus lesions: Basic science and clinical application of new surgical strategies. A review. *Microsurgery* 1995;16:13–16.

This article reviews studies aimed at developing novel surgical means to correct functional deficits after spinal nerve root injuries in brachial plexus lesions. Animal studies show that functional connections can be created by implanting a severed root stump into a damaged area of spinal cord.

Clarke HM, Curtis CG: An approach to obstetrical brachial plexus injuries. *Hand Clin* 1995; 11:563–581.

This review of the experience from the Hospital for Sick Children in Toronto describes their methods of evaluation, rationale, and indications and timing for surgical treatment.

Chuang DC, Epstein MD, Yeh MC, Wei FC: Functional restoration of elbow flexion in brachial plexus injuries: Results in 167 patients (excluding obstetric brachial plexus injury). *J Hand Surg* 1993;18A:285–291.

The authors describe a large series of reconstructed patients. They noted better results with intercostal transfer than with spinal accessory transfer.

Chuang DC, Lee GW, Hashem F, Wei FC: Restoration of shoulder abduction by nerve transfer in avulsed brachial plexus injury: Evaluation of 99 patients with various nerve transfers. *Plast Reconstr Surg* 1995;96:122–128.

The authors describe the outcome of reconstruction of shoulder function in 99 patients with upper root avulsion injuries. Best results were obtained when suprascapular and axillary nerves were simultaneously reinnervated. Donor nerves included intercostal, phrenic, spinal accessory, and cervical plexus.

Chuang DC: Functioning free muscle transplantation for brachial plexus injury. *Clin Orthop* 1995;314:104–111.

Sixty-four cases of functioning free muscle transplantation to reconstruct brachial plexus injuries were reviewed for the years 1986 to 1991. Free-muscle transfer for shoulder abduction was ineffective. Useful elbow function was restored in 80%. New strategies to restore function distal to the elbow are suggested.

Chuang D, Wei F, Noordhoff M. Cross-chest C7 nerve grafting followed by free muscle transplantations for the treatment of total avulsed brachial plexus injuries: A preliminary report. *Plast Reconstr Surg* 1993;92:717–727.

The authors describe novel treatment strategies using contralateral C7 in 15 patients with total root avulsions. This is a very preliminary report but the early results are hopeful. The donor limb suffers little long-lasting effect.

Chuang DC: Neurotization procedures for brachial plexus injuries. *Hand Clin* 1995;11:633–645.

This is an excellent up-to-date review of the various extraplexal nerve transfers for avulsion injuries of the brachial plexus. A treatment algorithm for various patterns of injury is also presented.

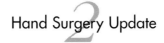
Doi K, Sakai K, Kuwata N, Ihara K, Kawai S: Reconstruction of finger and elbow function after complete avulsion of the brachial plexus. *J Hand Surg* 1991;16A:796–803.

The authors describe several aggressive treatment protocols with the goal of simultaneously restoring function to the elbow and hand. This preliminary but promising report involves extraplexal nerve transfers and free functioning muscle transfers.

Francel PC, Koby M, Park TS, et al: Fast spin-echo magnetic resonance imaging for radiological assessment of neonatal brachial plexus injury. *J Neurosurg* 1995;83:461–466.

Fast spin echo MRI provides a high-speed noninvasive image that allows evaluation of preganglionic root injuries. Its use in 3 cases is illustrated.

Gilbert A: Long-term evaluation of brachial plexus surgery in obstetrical palsy. *Hand Clin* 1995;11:583–595.

The author reviews his rationale for managing infants with obstetrical palsy and reviews his surgical experience and functional outcome. His work represents the largest surgical experience to date.

Geutjens G, Gilbert A, Helsen K: Obstetric brachial plexus palsy associated with breech delivery: A different pattern of injury. *J Bone Joint Surg* 1996;78B:303–306.

This is a review of 36 babies who suffered a brachial plexus injury in association with a breech delivery. As opposed to babies with plexus injuries secondary to shoulder dystocia, these babies have upper root avulsions that frequently are intraforaminal. Their prognosis is much worse.

Ihara K, Doi K, Sakai K, Kuwata N, Kawai S: Restoration of sensibility in the hand after complete brachial plexus injury. *J Hand Surg* 1996;21A:381–386.

Twenty-one patients with complete palsy secondary to avulsions were treated by nerve crossing to the median nerve with supraclavicular or intercostal nerve. Twelve of 15 recovered useful sensation, a few to the S2+ level.

Laurent JP, Lee RT: Birth-related upper brachial plexus injuries in infants: Operative and nonoperative approaches. *J Child Neurol* 1994;9:111–118.

The authors describe surgical experience with 70 infants, 50 followed for more than 18 months. Surgical and nonsurgical approaches are reviewed.

Mehta VS, Banerji AK, Tripathi RP: Surgical treatment of brachial plexus injuries. *Br J Neurosurg* 1993;7:491–500.

The authors describe their experience with 99 consecutive patients who had various procedures including neurolysis, grafting, and nerve transfer.

Michelow BJ, Clarke HM, Curtis CG, Zuker RM, Seifu Y, Andrews DF: The natural history of obstetrical brachial plexus palsy. *Plast Reconstr Surg* 1994;93:675–681.

In this review of 66 patients with obstetric palsy, 61 patients recovered spontaneously. A better indicator of the degree of spontaneous recovery (95% accuracy) was a scoring system that combined strength of elbow flexion with scores for wrist, finger, and thumb extension.

Nagano A, Ochiai N, Okinaga S: Restoration of elbow flexion in root lesions of brachial plexus injuries. *J Hand Surg* 1992;17A:815–821.

The authors describe their surgical techniques for intercostal innervation of the musculocutaneous nerve. They establish that better outcome is associated with avoidance of an interpositional nerve graft.

Oberlin C, Béal D, Leechavengvongs S, Salon A, Dauge MC, Sarcy JJ: Nerve transfer to biceps muscle using a part of ulnar nerve for C5–C6 avulsion of the brachial plexus: Anatomical study and report of four cases. *J Hand Surg* 1994; 19A:232–237.

The authors describe a new technique for nerve transfer to restore elbow flexion. There is much to recommend this procedure: the shortest possible reinnervation time and little to no long-term donor deficit.

Ochi M, Ikuta Y, Watanabe M, Kimori K, Itoh K: The diagnostic value of MRI in traumatic brachial plexus injury. *J Hand Surg* 1994;19B:55–59.

The authors document 34 patients having myelography, MRI, and surgical exploration. Only the axial and axial oblique MRI planes were useful. C5 and C6 avulsions were recognized equally well by MRI and myelography. Lower roots were not as clearly seen.

Ogino T, Naito T: Intercostal nerve crossing to restore elbow flexion and sensibility of the hand for a root avulsion type of brachial plexus injury. *Microsurgery* 1995;16:571–577.

Motor branches from intercostal nerves were transferred to the musculocutaneous nerve to restore elbow flexion. Sensory rami were transferred to the median nerve to restore protective sensation in the hand.

Smith SJ: The role of neurophysiological investigation in traumatic brachial plexus lesions in adults and children. *J Hand Surg* 1996;21B:145–147.

This is a review of the current status of neurophysiologic testing in determining the magnitude of injury in adult and obstetric brachial plexus palsy.

Songcharoen P, Mahaisavariya B, Chotigavanich C: Spinal accessory neurotization for restoration of elbow flexion in avulsion injuries of the brachial plexus. *J Hand Surg* 1996; 21A:387–390.

This is a report of 216 patients treated with spinal accessory to musculotaneous nerve transfer to restore elbow flexion. By 17 months, 73% had recovered M3 or better biceps. Poor results were obtained if surgery was delayed later than 9 months after injury. This is a technically easier procedure than intercostal nerve transfer.

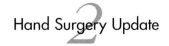

Chapter 21
Painful Upper Extremity

L. Andrew Koman, MD

Physiology of Pain

The conscious perception of pain following trauma and cellular damage is adaptive, appropriate, and protective. In the absence of ongoing cellular injury and/or ischemia, persistent pain is pathologic, may delay recovery, may prevent optimal outcome, and impacts negatively on health-related quality of life. Conscious pain depends on an appropriate balance between afferent and efferent information and is modulated by individual physiologic capacity during acute and chronic "painful" events. Nociceptive input during or after peripheral injury is perceived consciously as pain and reflects cellular compromise, produces a primary and secondary inflammatory response, and activates polymodal afferent nerves.

Nociceptors and Pain Pathways

Terminal polymodal nociceptors may be activated by mechanical, thermal, chemical, or ischemic events. Nociceptive information is transmitted by a small myelinated (A-delta) and unmyelinated (C) afferent peripheral fibers. Central recognition of nociceptive input is related to the magnitude, duration, and frequency of insult. Nociceptors may be sensitized by repetitive stimuli, by chemical mediators released by injured cells (eg, histamine), or by locally synthesized enzymes (eg, prostaglandins). Afferent nociceptive information is relayed through peripheral nerves to the dorsal root ganglion and spinal cord where internuncial neurons within the dorsal horn transmit ascending and descending information to cortical centers and to reflex pathways that affect both the ipsilateral and contralateral extremity (Fig. 1).

Nociceptive pain is modulated by descending pathways from the cerebral cortex, brain stem, and spinal cord by incompletely understood mechanism(s). Descending pathways are

The author or the department with which he is affiliated has received something of value from a commercial or other party related directly or indirectly to the subject of this chapter.

within the periaqueductal gray region of the midbrain, the nucleus magnus raphae of the pons, and the dorsal horn of the spinal cord. Endogenously produced neuropeptides, beta endorphins, and dynorphins affect the magnitude of the nociceptive stimulus (Fig. 2).

Perception of Pain

The conscious perception of pain is complex, requires cortical interpretation of nociceptive data, and is affected by physiologic events and psychological factors. The cortical (central nervous system) perception of nociceptive information is a protective mechanism. Polymodal nociceptor activity warns the host of danger and initiates the release of peptides and neuromodulators that promote the inflammatory process and initiate repair. A variety of mediators participate in the transmission of information interpreted as pain. Nonneurogenic mediators include bradykinin, serotonin, histamine, acetylcholine, prostaglandins E_1 and E_2, and leukotrienes. Neurogenic mediators (biologically active peptides produced by primary afferent neurons) potentiate or inhibit nociceptive information and include substance P, vasoactive intestinal peptide, calcitonin gene-related peptide, gastrin-releasing peptide, dynorphin, enkephalin, galanin, cholecystokinin-like substance, somatostatin, gamma aminobutyric acid, dopamine, glycine, and cholecystokinin. Alpha adrenergic agonists participate in the control of the microcirculation and modulate the peripheral and central nervous system. Recent data confirm the role of adrenergic transmitter/receptors in skin hyperalgesia. Abnormal adrenoreceptor function and/or modulation in both the neural and vascular structures supports the concept that some forms of chronic regional pain are "a receptor disease."

The "gate theory," developed by Melzack and Wall, is an appropriate aid in the conceptualization of pain. The dorsal horn of the spinal cord is the "gate," and the volume of peripheral information received at cortical levels that may pass through this area is assumed to be finite. Thus, painful information can be displaced or modified by innocuous data passing simultaneously through the gate.

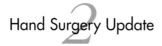

Ascending   **Descending**

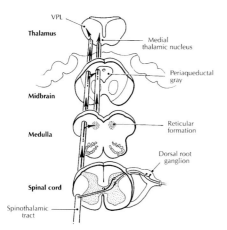
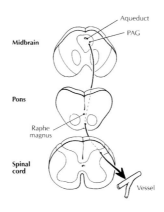

Figure 1

Ascending and descending pathways. (Adapted with permission from Koman LA (ed): *Orthopaedic Workbook*. Winston-Salem, NC, Wake Forest University Press, 1998, p 1.)

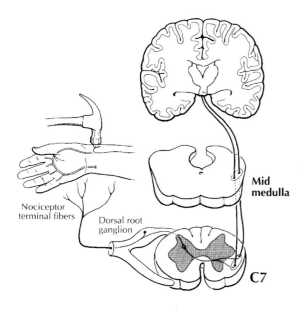
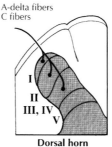

Figure 2

A nociceptive peripheral stimulus is relayed through peripheral nerves to the dorsal root ganglion and then into the dorsal horn of the spinal cord. (Adapted with permission from Koman LA (ed): *Orthopaedic Workbook*. Winston-Salem, NC, Wake Forest University Press, 1998, p 2.)

Acute Versus Chronic Pain

Acute pain accompanying tissue injury is normal. Acute pain may be both beneficial and harmful. Pain warns the host of danger and facilitates the repair process but may initiate inadvertently harmful effects (eg, excessive hypertension). When it occurs in the absence of ongoing tissue destruction, chronic pain that inappropriately reflects the intensity, magnitude, and/or duration of nociceptive input is detrimental. Following trauma or surgery, a transient period of altered (dystrophic) extremity function is expected. However, prolonged pain in the absence of ongoing tissue damage may result in hyperpathia, allodynia, vasomotor disturbances, and functional deficiencies. Over time, prolonged dystrophic events may damage or compromise arteriovenous shunt mechanisms, produce arthrofibrosis, cause excessive osteopenia, alter neuro-receptor function, and/or result in central pain imprinting.

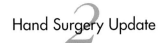
Neuroma and Neuroma in Continuity

The formation of a neuroma following peripheral nerve injury is normal. Axonal regeneration, stimulated by target-derived neurotrophic factors, results in successful reinnervation if the distal endoneural tissue (nerve stump) is reached. In the absence of a distal endoneural tube, a disorganized mass of neurons, fibroblasts, and connective tissue form a neuroma. Neuromas may be painful or not painful. Phantom sensation (the conscious impression of the amputated or injured part) is normal and occurs in most patients following amputation. Phantom "pain" exists in 50% of amputees.

The size of a neuroma depends on the distance of the injury from the anterior horn cell, the percentage of connective tissue in the injured nerve, and/or the age of the patient. The mechanism(s) producing a painful neuroma are unclear. However, neuromas may be sensitive to local irritation and mechanical deformation, may become a nociceptive focus by generalizing spontaneous action potentials, and/or may contribute to complex regional pain syndromes.

A neuroma in continuity occurs after an incomplete nerve injury if transected axons are unable to reach the distal stump. Both pure neuromas and neuromas in continuity may produce pain, cold sensitivity, and impaired function. The diagnosis of a neuroma is based on history and physical examination. The history of blunt or open trauma is common. Symptoms include dysesthesia, hyperalgesia, burning pain, cold sensitivity, and specific areas of point tenderness. Dystrophic symptoms of hyperpathia, allodynia, autonomic dysfunction, and excessive pain may occur. Signs include a palpable mass (trigger point), positive percussion test (Tinel's Sign), and decreased discomfort after local injection with a neural blocking agent (ie, lidocaine). Treatment is based on location and type of neuroma. Neuromas associated with chronic pain require simultaneous treatment of both processes. It may be necessary to manage the dystrophy in order to identify the exact location of the neuroma.

Nonsurgical treatments include oral medications, desensitization, transcutaneous nerve stimulators, and local or regional injections. A combination of these techniques may be necessary. If nonsurgical treatment fails, surgical intervention is indicated. Surgical options include alteration of the proximal nerve and neuroma by physical or chemical methods, alteration of the neuroma's environment by rerouting or relocating the neuroma, and modification of the neuronal environment by nerve repair, nerve wrap, or implantable nerve stimulators. Often 2 or more of these methods are employed simultaneously. A painful stump neuroma may be prevented by use of neurovascular island pedicle flaps and diminished by infusion of local anesthetic in the perioperative period. Treatments of painful neuromas include resection of the neuroma; mobilization of the neuroma by placing it within muscle, bone, or fat; covering the neuroma with a rotational or free flap; nerve-to-vein anastomosis and/or neuroneural anastomosis; or an implantable nerve stimulator (Outline 1).

Outline 1
Management of painful neuroma

I. Nonsurgical

    A. Oral medications
    B. Desensitization
    C. TENS unit
    D. Local injections

II. Surgical

    A. Alteration of proximal nerve
        1. Physical transection, crush, cauterization
        2. Proximal ligation
        3. Epineural ligation
        4. Capping

    B. Neural rerouting
        1. Neuroneural anastomosis
        2. Nerve-vein anastomosis
        3. Centrocentral anastomosis

    C. Relocation
        1. Muscle implantation
        2. Bone implantation

    D. Environmental modification
        1. Muscle flap
        2. Skin flap
        3. Vein wrap

    E. Neurorrhaphy
        1. End to end
        2. Nerve graft
        3. Nerve to vein

    F. Nerve wrap

    G. Nerve stimulator-implanted

(Reproduced with permission from Koman LA: Painful upper extremity, in Manske PR (ed): *Hand Surgery Update*. Rosemont, IL, American Academy of Orthopaedic Surgeons, 1996, pp 253–259.)

The management of a neuroma in continuity requires a patient-oriented approach and should address the location of the injury, the type of nerve involved, the size of the neuroma, and the functional impairment. Painful neuromas in continuity involving mixed motor-sensory nerves (eg, median nerve in forearm with intact fascicles providing innervation to thenar intrinsics and thumb sensory dermatomes) have a significant risk of additional functional loss if internal dissection and nerve grafting are performed. Acceptance of the neural deficit and management of the pain by nonsurgical or surgical means, including implantable stimulators, may produce less morbidity than attempts at nerve repair or grafting. Alternatively, intraneural dissection and neurorrhaphy will decrease symptoms and have the potential to restore function.

Complex Regional Pain Syndrome

Complex regional pain syndrome (CRPS) types I and II has been introduced to replace the term reflex sympathetic dystrophy (RSD) and the myriad synonyms that confound the existing taxonomy. CRPS requires the presence of regional pain following a noxious event. CRPS eliminates the implied but unproven sympathetic etiology in the diagnosis. Type I corresponds to classic RSD and occurs without an identifiable nerve injury. CRPS type II, "causalgia," is used to describe posttraumatic pain that occurs after an identifiable neural injury. CRPS type I or II may be sympathetically maintained or sympathetically independent. Over time, sympathetically maintained pain (SMP) may become sympathetically independent pain (SIP).

Altered extremity physiology after trauma is normal. Abnormal prolongation of this normal response is pathologic and, over time, may produce irreversible changes in end organ anatomy and function. CRPS is an abnormally severe and inappropriately prolonged manifestation of a series of normal postinjury responses. Clinical findings are pain out of proportion to the identifiable injury, diminished function, stiffness, and atrophy. Burning pain and restlessness are often early symptoms. CRPS is a dynamic physiologic process and varies related to extremity adaptation, peripheral and central nervous system modulation, and alterations in natural history secondary to partial treatment. The natural history of RSD is based on arbitrary staging and grading systems defined by time, clinical signs, and/or symptoms.

Although children and adolescents may develop CRPS, most patients are between 30 and 55 years of age. The incidence of cigarette smoking is statistically higher in patients with CRPS than in others. Women are affected more frequently than men. Structural nociceptive injury (eg, nerve damage) is identified in approximately 50% of cases. In the upper extremity, fracture of the distal radius and ulna is the most common injury associated with CRPS type I (over 30% in 1 prospective series). CRPS type II is associated with injury to the palmar cutaneous branch of the median nerve, damage to the superficial branch of the radial nerve, trauma to the dorsal branch of the ulnar nerve, and partial injury to the median and ulnar nerves. CRPS has been reported to occur more frequently after simultaneous median nerve decompression at the wrist and partial palmar fasciectomy for Dupuytren's disease.

Patients with CRPS do not have psychological or emotional disorders. However, factitious syndromes may mimic CRPS and are associated with severe psychological disturbances. Early treatment of CRPS is the most important variable in predicting pain relief and functional recovery. Eighty percent of patients treated within 1 year of injury show significant improvement, but fewer than 50% of those treated after 1 year will improve significantly. Early diagnosis and prompt intervention portend the best prognosis for recovery.

The clinical diagnosis of CRPS requires pain, atrophic changes, vasomotor and autonomic dysfunction, and functional impairment. Diagnosis is strengthened if subjective complaints are quantified by standardized or validated instruments and by objective measures of autonomic vasomotor and/or functional deficits. Physical findings include allodynia, hyperpathia, changes in nails and skin texture, and abnormal sudomotor activity (eg, sweating and piloerection). Partial treatment may produce variant forms of CRPS that challenge clinical diagnosis. Standardized testing using monofilaments, dolorimetry, and/or computer-controlled stimuli to quantify pain or allodynia objectively define pain thresholds.

Objective testing provides important insights into the physiologic events associated with or precipitating CRPS and may support clinical impressions. Changes in alpha 1 and alpha 2 receptor sensitivity have been implicated in CRPS, and improvement following adrenergic blockade defines SMP. Skin blood flow abnormalities and neural abnormalities have been recognized both in the central nervous system and in the periphery. Arteriovenous shunting in both the skin and deeper tissues affects

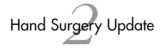

microvascular performance, disrupts normal sudomotor function, and increases bone turnover (osteopenia). Vasomotor and autonomic control abnormalities occur in the vast majority of patients. Functional impairment may require standardized assessments of hand function such as the Moberg pick-up test or the use of computerized testing instruments.

Diagnostic tests include plain radiographs, 3-phase bone scan, and evaluation(s) of microcirculatory function, autonomic control, and/or endurance. The radiographic evaluation of RSD typically demonstrates patchy osteopenia, which is periarticular initially and then becomes diffuse. Osteopenia occurs early in the process, involves trabecular and cortical bone, and is related to arteriovenous shunting.

Five patterns of resorption have been described by Genant and associates: (1) irregular resorption of trabecular bone in the metaphysis creating a patchy appearance; (2) subperiosteal bone resorption; (3) intercortical bone resorption; (4) endosteal bone resorption; and (5) surface erosions in subchondral and juxtachondral bone. Although quantifiable osteopenia is not always clinically apparent, it occurs in untreated complex regional pain syndrome type I or II. Plain radiographs have indicated that 20% of patients with RSD are without bony resorption; however, quantitative scintigraphy in patients following fracture of the distal radius demonstrates significant abnormalities in bone density in patients with CRPS compared to comparably immobilized fractures in patients without CRPS.

Three-phase bone scan analysis may be useful in CRPS. However, current data do not support third-phase bone scintigraphy as necessary to verify CRPS. Bone scan data do not address the physiologic mechanism of pain, limit the diagnosis, and do not correlate with clinical symptoms or prognosis. Bone scan data are specific in confirming clinical CRPS (75% to 98%), but lack sensitivity (50% or less). The role of bone scans in variant forms of RSD has not been evaluated. Bone scans of the upper extremity do not correlate with the existing stages or phases of CRPS, do not predict recovery, and have no demonstratable prognostic implications.

Qualitative and quantitative evaluation of peripheral autonomic regulation and physiologic estimations of microcirculatory function provide valuable information. The extent of upper extremity microcirculatory abnormalities associated with CRPS requires evaluation of both components of total flow, which are thermoregulatory and nutritional. Abnormal thermoregulatory and nutritional flow is documented in CRPS and, in part, explains the existence of similar pain in both the hot and cold phases of the CRPS process. In the normal state, total flow is primarily thermoregulatory (80% to 95%) and nutritional flow is 5% to 20%. Control of extremity flow is a dynamic process and requires stress to be evaluated fully. A combination of temperature, laser Doppler fluxmetry, vital capillaroscopy, and sympathetic skin response allows evaluation of vasomotor and autonomic control. Sudomotor activity may be evaluated by resting sweat output, quantitative sudomotor axon reflex test, galvanic skin response, and peripheral autonomic surface potential reflex response and sympathetic skin response. Unstressed evaluation of microcirculatory and myoneural function may be misleading. Stress may be induced by thermal, psychologic, physiologic, or ischemic methods.

Sympathetically Maintained Pain Versus Independent Pain

The concept of SMP becoming, over time, SIP is now recognized. CRPS type I or II may be sympathetically maintained or sympathetically independent. The response to intravenous phentolamine mesylate (a mixed alpha-1, alpha-2 antagonist), stellate ganglion block, or continuous peripheral or epidural block supports the diagnosis of a sympathetically maintained component of CRPS. Continuous epidural infusion of drug and/or continuous axillary blocks may provide relief when a stellate block does not.

Treatment

The treatment of CRPS is complex and depends on the clinical course, identification of a persistent nociceptive focus, pre- and postmorbid anatomy, and physiologic adaptations. In general, a combination of interventions is necessary. Treatment options include physical and occupational therapy, oral pharmacologic agents, transcutaneous medications, injected pharmacologic agents, surgical or ablative interventions, and biofeedback (Table 1).

In general, amputation for CRPS is not appropriate and should be reserved for patients with intractable infection and severe physical impairment secondary to stiffness or mass effect. Pain alone is not an indication for amputation. After amputation, the probability that a prosthesis will be used is low.

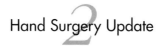

Table 1
Treatment options for complex regional pain syndrome

Physical modalities

    Occupational therapy

    Stress loading

    Contrast baths

    Continuous passive motion

    Intermittent pressure

Pharmacologic options

    Calcium channel blockers

    Antidepressant

    Membrane stabilizing agent

    Anticonvulsants

    Adrenergic agents

    Corticosteroid

    Intravenous regional anesthetics

Continuous autonomic blockade

Neurolytic blockade

Surgical sympathectomy

Surgical correction nociceptive focus

Neurologic procedures

Dorsal column stimulator

Thalamic stimulator

Periventricular gray matter stimulators

Peripheral nerve stimulators

Annotated Bibliography

General

Covington EC: Psychological issues in reflex sympathetic dystrophy, in Jänig W, Stanton-Hicks M (eds): *Reflex Sympathetic Dystrophy: A Reappraisal.* Seattle, WA, IASP Press, 1996, pp 191–215.

This is an excellent critical review of the psychological issues in CRPS (RSD). It concludes that there is no documentation of a predisposing psychological link to RSD.

Koman LA, Poehling GG, Smith TL: Complex regional pain syndrome: Reflex sympathetic dystrophy and causalgia, in Green DP, Hotchkiss RN, Pederson WC (eds): *Operative Hand Surgery*, ed 4. New York, NY, Churchill Livingstone, 1999, pp 636–666.

This overview of CRPS includes a detailed description of pharmacologic and surgical management. Extensive tables of the mechanism and side effects of pharmacologic agents are provided.

Koman LA, Smith TL, Smith BP, Li Z: The painful hand. *Hand Clin* 1996;12:757–764.

This is an overview of the evaluation and management of the painful upper extremity.

Kurvers HA, Jacobs MJ, Beuk RJ, et al: Reflex sympathetic dystrophy: Evolution of microcirculatory disturbances in time. *Pain* 1995;60:333–340.

A new physiologic staging system based on microcirculatory flow characteristics using temperature, laser Doppler, and vital capillaroscopy is presented in a 120-patient series.

Melzack R, Wall PD: Pain mechanisms: A new theory. *Science* 1965;150:971–979.

This is the classic article on the gate theory of pain.

Stanton-Hicks M, Jänig W, Hassenbusch S, Haddox JD, Boas R, Wilson P: Reflex sympathetic dystrophy: Changing concepts and taxonomy. *Pain* 1995;63:127–133.

This is a revised taxonomic system for disorders previously called RSD and causalgia. Based on the conclusions of a consensus conference, CRPS is defined by the history, presenting symptoms, and findings at diagnosis. Following a noxious event, CRPS requires the presence of regional pain and sensory changes, autonomic dysfunction (eg, abnormal skin color, temperature change, abnormal sudomotor activity), or edema and functional impairment. CRPS type I, traditional RSD, occurs without a definable nerve lesion and type II, causalgia, requires the presence of a nerve lesion.

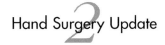

Neuroma and Neuroma in Continuity

Gould JS: Treatment of the painful injured nerve in-continuity, in Gelberman RH (ed): *Operative Nerve Repair and Reconstruction.* Philadelphia, PA, JB Lippincott, 1991, vol 2, pp 1541–1550.

This is an excellent discussion of the management of the painful incomplete nerve injury.

Irwin MS, Gilbert SE, Terenghi G, Smith RW, Green CJ: Cold intolerance following peripheral nerve injury: Natural history and factors predicting severity of symptoms. *J Hand Surg* 1997;22B:308–316.

This is a retrospective review of 814 patients, with 398 (57%) answering an initial questionnaire. Incidence of cold intolerance in the respondents was 83%, and a severity score was presented.

Kurvers HA, Jacobs MJ, Beuk RJ, et al: The spinal component to skin blood flow abnormalities in reflex sympathetic dystrophy. *Arch Neurol* 1997;53:58–65.

This evaluation of microcirculation in 54 patients compared involved extremities to contralateral uninvolved extremities and normal controls. Traumatic excitation of a clinically affected peripheral nerve appears to initiate spinal cord level antidromic vasodilator mechanisms in patients with stage I (stationary warmth) RSD.

Rose J, Belsky MR, Millender LH, Feldon P: Intrinsic muscle flaps: The treatment of painful neuromas in continuity. *J Hand Surg* 1996;21A:671–674.

The authors report the technique and results in 8 patients with painful neuroma in continuity treated with local muscle flaps and dissection of the nerve.

St-Laurent JY, Duclos L: Prevention of neuroma in elective digital amputations by utilization of neurovascular island flap. *Ann Chir Main Memb Super* 1996;15:50–54.

The authors discuss prevention of painful neuroma in elective amputations by burying distal nerve loop between adjacent metacarpal or using the pulp flap to cover the proximal stump.

Wartan SW, Hamann W, Wedley JR, McColl I: Phantom pain and sensation among British veteran amputees. *Br J Anaesth* 1997;78:652–659.

This is the report of a mail survey of 590 veteran amputees. Of the 89% of respondents, 55% report phantom limb pain.

Complex Regional Pain Syndrome—Diagnosis

Genant HK, Kozin F, Bekerman C, McCarty DJ, Sims J: The reflex sympathetic dystrophy syndrome: A comprehensive analysis using fine-detail radiography, photon absorptiometry, and bone and joint scintigraphy. *Radiology* 1975;117:21–32.

This is a classic description of the radiographic findings in patients with RSD (CRPS).

Kozin F, Soin JS, Ryan LM, Carrera GF, Wortmann RL: Bone scintigraphy in the reflex sympathetic dystrophy syndrome. *Radiology* 1981;138:437–443.

The sensitivity (60% versus 69%) and specificity (92% versus 79%) of bone scans versus radiography, was assessed in 64 patients with RSD in this classic article.

Mackinnon SE, Holder LE: The use of three-phase radionuclide bone scanning in the diagnosis of reflex sympathetic dystrophy. *J Hand Surg* 1984;9A:556–563.

This is a retrospective analysis of 3-phase bone scans in 145 patients with a diagnosis of hand pain (n = 102) and RSD (n = 23). This study shows a high sensitivity (96%) and specificity (98%) for the third (delayed image) phase of bone scanning.

Pollock FE Jr, Koman LA, Smith BP, Poehling GG: Patterns of microvascular response associated with reflex sympathetic dystrophy of the hand and wrist. *J Hand Surg* 1993;18A:847–852.

Positive 3-phase technetium bone scans did not correlate with vasomotor disturbances in 28 RSD patients.

Werner R, Davidoff G, Jackson MD, Cremer S, Ventocilla C, Wolf L: Factors affecting the sensitivity and specificity of the three-phase technetium bone scan in the diagnosis of reflex sympathetic dystrophy syndrome in the upper extremity. *J Hand Surg* 1989;14A:520–523.

Three-phase bone scans were found to have low sensitivity (50%), modest positive predictive value (67%), high specificity (92%), and negative predictive value (84%) in 63 patients diagnosed with RSD. The sensitivity is lower than reported in previous studies.

Complex Regional Pain Syndrome (Type I, Traditional RSD)

Wilder RT, Berde CB, Wolohan M, Vieyra MA, Masek BJ, Micheli LJ: Reflex sympathetic dystrophy in children: Clinical characteristics and follow-up of seventy patients. *J Bone Joint Surg* 1992;74A:910–919.

Seventy patients younger than 18 years of age are presented. The differences in the clinical course of RSD in children and adults are outlined. The prognosis for complete relief of symptoms, in spite of a multidisciplinary treatment approach, is poor, with 38 of 70 manifesting residual pain and dysfunction at follow-up.

Complex Regional Pain Syndrome (Type II, Causalgia Secondary to a Nerve Lesion)

Galer BS, Jensen MP: Development and preliminary validation of a pain measure specific to neuropathic pain: The neuropathic pain scale. *Neurology* 1997;48:332–338.

This article describes the development and preliminary validation of the Neuropathic Pain Scale (NPS), which is designed to assess distinct pain qualities associated with neuropathic pain. Results support the discriminate and predictive validity of the NPS items and support its use in evaluating outcome.

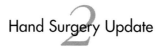

Jupiter JB, Seiler JG III, Zienowicz R: Sympathetic maintained pain (causalgia) associated with a demonstrable peripheral-nerve lesion: Operative treatment. *J Bone Joint Surg* 1994; 76A:1376–1384.

The authors discuss the importance of surgical management of peripheral-nerve lesions that created a nociceptive focus and produced CRPS type II. Nine patients underwent continuous sympathetic block and surgical management of their nerve lesion followed by rotation of a muscle flap, resulting in maintained pain relief at 48 months after surgery.

Complex Regional Pain Syndrome—Treatment

Czop C, Smith TL, Rauck R, Koman LA: The pharmacologic approach to the painful hand. *Hand Clin* 1996;12:633–642.

This article outlines the pharmacologic options available to treat dystrophic pain, provides an overview of mechanisms-of-action, and defines relative indications for administration of pharmacologic agents.

Dielissen PW, Claassen AT, Veldman PH, Goris RJ: Amputation for reflex sympathetic dystrophy. *J Bone Joint Surg* 1995; 77B:270–273.

Clinical experience after 34 amputations in 31 limbs with RSD is presented. Pain relief occurred in 2 limbs. Twenty-eight of 34 had recurrence of RSD, and prosthesis use was unlikely.

Hassenbusch SJ, Stanton-Hicks M, Schoppa D, Walsh JG, Covington EC: Long-term results of peripheral nerve stimulation for reflex sympathetic dystrophy. *J Neurosurg* 1996; 84:415–423.

This is the report of a prospective clinical trial involving implantable peripheral nerve stimulators. There was long-term good or fair relief in 19 of 30 patients at 2 to 4 years.

Sotereanos DG, Giannakopoulos PN, Mitsionis GI, Xu J, Herndon JH: Vein-graft wrapping for the treatment of recurrent compression of the median nerve. *Microsurgery* 1995; 16:752–756.

The indications, surgical technique, and 2-year results of vein wrapping in 3 patients are presented.

Watson HK, Carlson L: Treatment of reflex sympathetic dystrophy of the hand with an active "stress loading" program. *J Hand Surg* 1987;12A:779–785.

A program of active traction and compression exercises without joint motion is described in 41 RSD patients. Long-term (2 year) results of symptoms, signs, and function are presented.

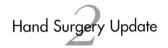

Hand Surgery Update 2

Section V
Skin and Soft Tissues

American Society for Surgery of the Hand

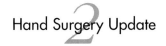
Chapter 22
Physiology of Wound Healing

233

Dennis P. Orgill, MD, PhD

The science of wound healing has advanced dramatically over the last 5 years. Molecular techniques have clarified mechanisms of wound healing, and advances in tissue engineering have led to development of entirely new methods of treating wounds. Because the hand has such diverse tissues—bone, ligaments, tendons, nerves, blood vessels, and skin—a thorough knowledge of the healing mechanisms of each tissue is essential. Hand surgeons must also understand the impact of time and age on wound healing.

Mammals respond to tissue injury in a predictable pattern of wound contraction and scarring. The biochemical and cellular events associated with these phenomena can be altered by genetics, disease, or environmental influences. Results of tissue repair range from a lack of wound healing (eg, diabetic ulcers) to excessive scarring (Fig. 1).

Tissue injury evokes several common pathways of host response. Injury can be caused by trauma, infection, neoplasm, congenital defects, or irradiation. After traumatic injury, the initial host response is to stop the bleeding. Exposed collagen activates the coagulation cascade, vessels constrict, platelets aggregate and degranulate, and a fibrin clot forms. A number of cytokines are then released to initiate tissue repair. Growth factors attract inflammatory cells that stimulate blood vessel formation. Roughly 12 hours after injury, the surrounding epidermis begins to proliferate, migrating centrally to close the wound. Wound closure is assisted by wound contraction, which usually begins 4 to 5 days after injury and appears to be driven by myofibroblasts in the wound. During wound contraction, exuberant red tissue, often referred to as granulation tissue, forms in the center of the wound. Granulation tissue is composed of a high density of capillary loops and inflammatory cells; these cells produce enzymes that can digest overlying necrotic tissue. The presence of granulation tissue is predictive of wound healing. Granulation tissue provides the underlying structure for closure with epithelium. Because the epidermis of skin is not directly vascularized, it relies on diffusion from a rich bed of capillaries in the dermis or underlying tissue. However, granulation tissue is

also a precursor of scar tissue; many experienced surgeons excise it before closing a wound.

Time Sequence of Healing Processes

Collagen synthesis begins between day 4 and 6, first as a gel-like substance and later with substantial remodeling and strengthening (Fig. 2). Fiber orientation begins to develop parallel to lines of stress within the wound. Concurrently, metalloproteinases are capable of degrading necrotic collagen, gelatin, and other matrix components in the wound. Collagen synthesis progresses rapidly into the third week and then slows down until the sixth week. After that time, wound strength increases for at least 2 years, due to continuing reorganization of the collagen fibrils within the wound. Despite the dramatic changes that occur in the wound during healing, the final biomechanical properties of healed skin include decreased tensile strength and increased stiffness (Young's modulus of elasticity) compared to normal skin. Scar tissue develops very high levels of stress with much less elongation (stretching) of the skin.

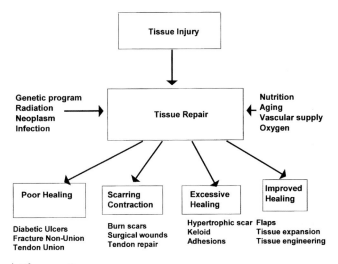

Figure 1

Mechanisms of tissue repair. (Adapted with permission from Davidson JM: Wounds: Cellular mechanisms and clinical correlates. *Wounds* 1995;7(suppl A):2A–12A.)

The author or the department with which he is affiliated has received something of value from a commercial or other party related directly or indirectly to the subject of this chapter.

Factors Influencing Wound Healing

Several factors influence basic wound healing mechanisms. Patients with peripheral vascular disease, for example, have a lower perfusion pressure, reducing nutrient transport. Restoration of perfusion pressure to the wounded area is essential for wound healing. Patients who have received radiation therapy often have severe wound healing problems, which may be related to the reduced ability of irradiated tissues to form new blood vessels. Hyperbaric oxygen can stimulate the production of new capillary growth in irradiated patients and may enhance wound healing.

Drugs such as steroids or antimetabolites block inflammatory processes in the wound. Diseases can also lead to poor wound healing. In malnutrition, critical amino acids or cofactors are absent. The serum albumin level, a first-order approximation of the nutritional state of the patient, has been directly correlated as an independent risk factor for morbidity and mortality following elective surgery.

Metabolic disorders, such as diabetes mellitus, contribute to poor wound healing by a variety of mechanisms (Fig. 3). It is estimated that 1 in 10 people in the United States will develop diabetes in their lifetime. High glucose levels decrease the chemotactic response of leukocytes, decreasing local inflammation and reducing the ability of the local environment to resist infection. Patients with diabetes mellitus also have a high incidence of peripheral vascular disease, which reduces wound perfusion. Perhaps the most severe complication of diabetes is the peripheral neuropathy that makes patients unaware of ulcerations on their extremities. Patients with diabetic retinopathy often have difficulty seeing their extremities clearly. Fortunately, diabetic ulcers are much less common in upper limbs than lower limbs, probably because of less repetitive trauma. Renal failure patients, who often have diabetes mellitus, can exhibit digital necrosis following arteriovenous shunting for hemodialysis. This problem can be very difficult to solve; it may involve both arterial hypotension and venous hypertension. Frequently ligation of the arteriovenous fistula is required. A combination of modalities will be helpful in managing the various complications of diabetes patients.

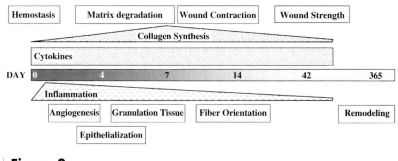

Figure 2

Typical time sequence of healing processes in a normal wound.

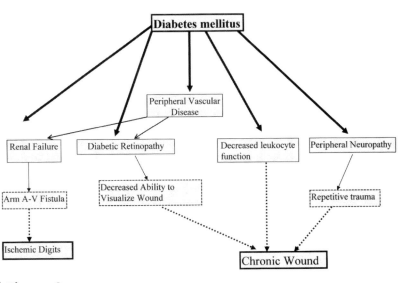

Figure 3

Pathogenesis of ulcers in diabetes mellitus.

Scarring

Scarring is a normal result of the healing process. Although the degree of scarring can be affected by surgical technique, the amount of eventual scar is often more strongly dictated by genetics. Wounds closed with careful dermal approximation generally heal with a flat, narrow scar. Skin flaps heal with scarring only at the wound edges. Sutures that pass through the epidermis and are left in for more than 7 days often result in "railroad tracks" across the line of closure. Certain patients seem to be genetically inclined to form excessive

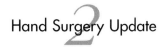
scar tissue as hypertrophic scarring or keloids. Hypertrophic scarring occurs frequently in burn patients and also in scars involving the anterior chest wall. Hypertrophic scars lie within the confines of the original wound but are raised above the wound surface. Studies of hypertrophic scars have shown that mast cells and plasma histamine levels were increased compared to normal skin. Hypertrophic scarring appears to result from an imbalance between collagen production and collagen degradation. Keloids extend beyond the borders of the original scar and are raised above normal skin even higher than hypertrophic scars. There is a strong genetic predisposition toward keloids; they are more frequent among dark-skinned individuals. Treatment for both hypertrophic scars and keloids can be difficult. Recent studies indicate that silicone sheeting may be effective in treating hypertrophic scarring; however, the mechanism of action has not been clarified. Although compression garments are frequently used to combat hypertrophic scars, their efficacy has not been definitively demonstrated. Steroid injection is probably the most common method of treating hypertrophic scars and keloids. Other promising treatments under investigation include tamoxifen and interferon.

A variety of surgical methods can be employed to reduce the amount of scar present in wounds lacking adequate skin. Tissue expansion provides adjacent skin of similar texture and color while eliminating the need for skin grafts. Skin, fasciocutaneous, and myocutaneous flaps can also provide large areas of cutaneous coverage with scars limited to the borders of the wound and donor defect.

Early Development and Wound Healing

Wound healing is directed by the genetic program of the organism and the environment in which that program is expressed. The sequence of limb formation and differentiation begins as small buds form on the lateral body wall at 4 weeks of gestation. Over the next 4 weeks, shaping of the upper limb takes place. Changes in basic limb morphology do not occur after the fiftieth day. The molecular genetics involved in bone development have been defined for many congenital syndromes. The genes responsible for defining limb-bud differentiation, such as the sonic hedgehog gene, have been studied extensively. The sonic hedgehog gene is expressed in the zone of polarizing activity and can act as either an endoprotease or a cholesterol transferase. Targets for this gene include transcription factors such as HOXD13, which is responsible for synpolydactyly. Further investigation has determined the molecular mechanism for synpoly-

dactyly. Hox genes regulate patterning during limb development, and may play a role in determining the timing and extent of local growth rates. Synpolydactyly, an inherited human abnormality of the hands and feet, is caused by expansions of a polyalanine stretch in the aminoterminal region of HOXD13. Expression of the phenotype results in transformation of metacarpal bones to carpal-like bones.

The use of knockout mouse has greatly facilitated the study of wound healing mechanisms. Deleting genes for metalloelastase in the macrophage and for cathepsin G in the neutrophil prevented normal migration of macrophages and decreased the breaking strength of wounds. Given the rapid advances in genetics, the next 5 years will likely further define molecular mechanisms responsible for many other inherited disorders related to fetal development and wound healing.

The expression of genes in fetal wound healing is dramatically different from that of adults. Early gestational animals seem to heal incisional wounds with little or no scarring. At some time late in gestation, the healing ability changes and scar tissue forms in the repair process. The study of fetal wounds in a variety of animals has elucidated many of the mechanisms of wound healing. The formation of scar appears to be both temporally and organ-specific. Incisions in the diaphragm or stomach heal with scar and without regeneration, independent of the gestational age. In contrast, depending on the species studied, skin wounds and bone defects heal with minimal scar early in gestation. The inflammatory and cytokine response, as well as the dermal architecture, may be determinants of the degree of scarring in a wound. The cytokine most studied is transforming growth factor beta (TGF-β). In one series of experiments, antibodies to TGF-$\beta_{1,2}$ were applied in rodent wounds and improved the observed scar in healed wounds. A proper balance of cytokines in the wound bed is likely necessary to reduce scarring, because antibodies to TGF-$\beta_{1,2,3}$, platelet-derived growth factors (PDGFs), or basic fibroblast growth factors do not reduce scarring in adult rodent wounds.

Growth Factors

The discovery of numerous factors has enhanced our ability to understand wound healing. One of the most useful systems for studying the mechanism of growth factors has been in a polyvinyl wound chamber. This model demonstrates the temporal elaboration of multiple growth factors in the healing of experimental wound. By adding epidermal growth factor (EGF) in concentrations of 10 to 1,000 ng/ml, wound closure by epithelialization was stimulated in partial-thickness wounds.

Despite the promise of growth factors in animal trials, their application in humans has been disappointing. In one series of burn patients, the authors reported a small but positive effect of EGF in combination with silver sulfadiazine. However, another study demonstrated no difference in the healing of split-thickness wounds treated with EGF and silver sulfadiazine compared to a silver sulfadiazine control group. A recent trial of PDGF showed a 48% healing of diabetic ulcers over a 20-week period, compared to 25% healing in control wounds. In this study, adequate debridement of the ulcer proved critical to healing. It appears that PDGF may have a useful effect in nonhealing diabetic ulcers; however, final results of the clinical study have not yet been published. Despite their potential therapeutic effect, the high costs of growth factors are likely to limit their application.

Angiogenesis

The development of new blood vessels is a requirement for healing of any wound. Granulation tissue, fine loops of capillaries seen in many wounds, suggests the ability of wounds to spontaneously heal over time. Angiogenic factors in selected wounds are extremely important to clinical wound healing. Angiogenic peptides may critically alter wound healing kinetics. There appear to be angiogenic factors that both promote and block the formation of new blood vessels. Clinical work with angiogenic factors has already shown promise in treating malignancy and vascular malformations. Alpha interferon has been shown to reduce the proliferating capacity of hemangiomas, and antiangiogenic drugs are being used to control the growth of tumors.

Hyperbaric oxygen appears to act as a mechanism to stimulate angiogenesis in wounds. After decades of research, clinical indications for hyperbaric oxygen have been clearly defined. Indications related to wound healing include radiation-induced tissue injury, acute traumatic ischemic injury, salvage of ischemic flaps or skin grafts, and nonhealing chronic wounds.

Skin Replacement

Skin performs many essential functions. With its stratum corneum, the epidermis provides a protective layer against bacterial invasion and water loss. The dermis, rich in collagen and elastin, protects the body from mechanical trauma. Autologous, full-thickness, and split-thickness skin grafts provide reasonable coverage to wounds with a good vascular supply; however, grafts are often in short supply and cause obligate donor site scarring. The challenge is to provide effective closure of large wounds with a functional physiologic skin replacement. Most investigators believe that an optimal skin replacement requires both a dermal and epidermal component. A fully differentiated epidermis with a keratin layer is necessary to protect the body from bacterial invasion and moisture loss. Significant progress has been made using epidermal sheets grown from small biopsies. Improved results have been reported in burn centers where epidermal sheets have been combined with dermal allografts. The dermal allograft incorporates into the wound without significant rejection. The epidermis of the allograft is removed and then covered with the cultured sheets. Because of an expansion factor of up to 10,000 times the size of the biopsy, skin culture holds promise for patients with large areas of skin loss.

Clinical trials of a collagen gel–epidermal composite show some benefit in chronic wounds, even though allogeneic keratinocytes are used. The cells from these composite grafts may produce a number of growth factors that accelerate closure of chronic wounds.

Although allodermis is an effective dermal substitute, it is often in short supply and also carries some risk of disease transmission. Production of an extracellular matrix analog from animal proteins or synthetic materials holds promise for treating large wounds. A collagen-glycosaminoglycan matrix was recently approved for clinical use in burn patients. After excision of the burn, the material is applied and allowed to vascularize for 2 to 6 weeks; a very thin epidermal autograft can then be placed over the matrix to close the wound. To avoid the second operative step, the collagen-glycosaminoglycan membrane can be seeded with either cultured or uncultured keratinocytes before application. Application of semisynthetic membranes to burn victims usually results in good skin quality with substantial long-term elasticity.

A biosynthetic skin substitute consisting of human neonatal fibroblasts was recently evaluated for temporary coverage of excised burn wounds in a multicenter clinical trial. Patients tolerated the biosynthetic membrane better than cryopreserved human cadaver skin.

Contracture

Contractures continue to present challenges for surgeons. Although skin grafts have been the mainstay of treatment of contractures, more recent evidence suggests that normal skin in the form of a flap provides much more resistance to contraction. Flaps often provide a better cosmetic appearance as well. Aesthetically pleasing results have been obtained using large fasciocutaneous flaps on human neck contractures.

Tendon Healing

Our understanding of the mechanisms of tendon healing has been enhanced by biomechanical testing, and by analysis of growth factors present at the time of healing. Electrical stimulation has been shown to reduce adhesions and promote healing of cut tendons in an animal model. Cyclic stresses applied to the healing tendon may also hasten the repair process.

Nerve Healing

Advances in peripheral nerve healing continue to trigger changes in clinical practice. Nerve conduits such as silicone, vein graft, or arterial grafts have been shown to be effective in bridging small gaps in peripheral nerves; however, results have not been any better than nerve grafting. Recent research on end-to-side neurorrhaphy has called many of the basic tenets of nerve healing in question. Although end-to-side neurorrhaphy remains a controversial topic, better understanding could significantly alter basic concepts of nerve repair.

Bone Healing

Distraction osteogenesis is currently applied to traumatic and congenital bone defects in the hand; several recent studies have refined our understanding of this process. Electrical stimulation has aided bone healing in both animal studies and clinical trials. Bone morphogenic proteins (BMPs) have been shown to stimulate bone formation in vitro and in vivo. BMPs have just become available in quantities for critical-sized bone defects and fractures. An unresolved clinical problem is a delivery method that allows the proteins to remain at the site of repair over a critical length of time.

Summary of Advances

Advances in biology have provided investigators with new tools for the study of wound healing. A better understanding of the human genome is clarifying the basis of inherited deformities and wound healing deficiencies. Molecular techniques have also been applied to better understand the various cytokines associated with normal and abnormal wound healing. Increased knowledge of host–biomaterial interactions has led to improved biomaterials compatible with surrounding tissues. The ability to replicate cells outside of the body allows tissue replacement while minimizing donor sites.

Annotated Bibliography

Factors Influencing Wound Healing

Corral CJ, Wesselschmidt RL, Ley TJ, et al: Altered wound healing in macrophage metallo-elastase and neutrophil cathepsin G knockout mice. Proceedings of the Plastic Surgery Research Council 41st Annual Meeting, St. Louis, MO, 1996.

The authors describe the methodology of knockout mice in the study of wound healing.

Davidson JM: Wounds: Cellular mechanisms and clinical correlates. Wounds 1995;7(suppl A):2A–12A.

This article provides an excellent and current introduction to wound healing. Other articles in this issue discuss specific aspects of wound healing in depth.

Mackinnon SE: What's new in plastic surgery. J Am Coll Surg 1996;182:150–161.

The author reviews new literature (published during 1995) on plastic surgery.

Phillips LG: What's new in plastic surgery. J Am Coll Surg 1997;184:187–195.

Phillips summarizes 1996 publications in plastic surgery.

Tibbles PM, Edelsberg JS: Hyperbaric-oxygen therapy. N Eng J Med 1996;334:1642–1648.

This review article summarizes papers written on hyperbaric oxygen therapy, and reviews the approved uses of hyperbaric oxygen.

Early Development and Wound Healing

Mulliken JB, Warman ML: Molecular genetics and craniofacial surgery. Plast Reconstr Surg 1996;97:666–675.

This is an excellent review of craniofacial syndromes and the rapidly developing field of genetics. The authors describe linkage analysis, other molecular techniques, and many of the recently discovered genes for craniofacial disorders.

Muragaki Y, Mundlos S, Upton J, Olsen BR: Altered growth and branching patterns in synpolydactyly caused by mutations in HOXD13. Science 1996;272:548–551.

This important work demonstrates the genetic basis for synpolydactyly. The authors show that sympolydactyly is caused by expansions of a polyalanine stretch in the amino-terminal region of HOXD13.

Weed M, Mundlos S, Olsen BR: The role of sonic hedgehog in vertebrate development. Matrix Biol 1997:16:53–58.

This article presents basic research findings on the sonic hedgehog gene, important in limb development. The authors also highlight the importance of cholesterol metabolism in development.

Growth Factors

Breuing K, Andree C, Helo G, Slama J, Liu PY, Eriksson E: Growth factors in the repair of partial thickness porcine skin wounds. *Plast Reconstr Surg* 1997;100:657–664.

The authors describe the methodology for measuring soluble growth factors in a porcine wound model. They show the temporal changes in concentration of important growth factors.

Brown GL, Nanney LB, Griffen J, et al: Enhancement of wound healing by topical treatment with epidermal growth factor. *N Engl J Med* 1989;321:76–79.

This is the first published study demonstrating a clinical difference in wound healing using growth factors. The study compares epidermal growth factor with silver sulfadiazine cream.

Cohen IK, Crossland MC, Garrett A, Diegelmann RF: Topical application of epidermal growth factor onto partial-thickness wounds in human volunteers does not enhance re-epithelialization. *Plast Reconstr Surg* 1995;96:251–254.

In this randomized controlled trial, epidermal growth factor was used in normal volunteers. No effect of epidermal growth factor was seen in these partial-thickness wounds; there was no difference between epidermal growth factor and silver sulfadiazine cream.

Steed DL, Donohoe D, Webster MW, Lindsley L: Effect of extensive debridement and treatment on the healing of diabetic foot ulcers: Diabetic ulcer study group. *J Am Coll Surg* 1996;183:61–64.

These investigators describe a randomized prospective double-blind trial treating diabetic wounds with platelet-derived growth factors. They also emphasize the importance of wound care including periodic debridement.

Scarring and Contraction

Ahn ST, Monafo WW, Mustoe TA: Topical silicone gel for the prevention and treatment of hypertrophic scar. *Arch Surg* 1991;126:499–504.

This article reviews the use of topical silicone sheeting in the treatment of hypertrophic scars.

Ferguson MW, Whitby DJ, Shah M, Armstrong J, Siebert JW, Longaker MT: Scar formation: The spectral nature of fetal and adult wound repair. *Plast Reconstr Surg* 1996;97:854–860.

In this review of the field of fetal wound healing, the authors describe differences in gestational age and species on scar formation.

Morris DE, Wu L, Zhao LL, et al: Acute and chronic animal models for excessive dermal scarring: Quantitative studies. *Plast Reconstr Surg* 1997;100:674–681.

Morris and associates describe a new animal model using a rabbit ear for dermal scarring. They were able to modulate scar formation by intralesional corticosteroid treatment.

Shah M, Foreman DM, Ferguson MW: Neutralising antibody to TGF-beta1,2 reduces cutaneous scarring in adult rodents. *J Cell Sci* 1994;107:1137–1157.

The authors describe the effect of an antibody to TGF-$\beta_{1,2}$ on scarring in animals. The architecture of the neodermis of wounds treated with neutralizing antibody to TGF-β more closely resembled uninjured skin.

Angiogenesis

Butler CE, Orgill DP, Compton C, Yannas IV: Effects of cell culturing on keratinocyte-seeded collagen glycosaminoglycan matrix skin replacement in full-thickness porcine wounds. *Surg Forum* 1996;47:752–754.

The authors describe a tissue engineering approach to skin regeneration using a biodegradable membrane and cultured keratinocytes. This shows simultaneous regeneration of dermis and epidermis in an animal model.

Folkman J: Seminars in Medicine of the Beth Israel Hospital, Boston: Clinical applications of research on angiogenesis. *N Engl J Med* 1995;333:1757–1763.

This is an excellent review article on the field of angiogenesis. Folkman describes the research and clinical applications in areas of cancer therapy and vascular malformations.

Purdue GF, Hunt JL, Still JM Jr, et al: A multicenter clinical trial of biosynthetic skin replacement, Dermagraft-TC, compared with cryopreserved human cadaver skin for temporary coverage of excised burn wounds. *J Burn Care Rehabil* 1997;18:52–57.

This article describes the clinical trial of a promising biosynthetic membrane, Dermagraft-TC.

Bone Healing

Kessler I, Hecht O, Baruch A: Distraction-lengthening of digital rays in the management of the injured hand. *J Bone Joint Surg* 1979;61A:83–87.

Kessler and associates describe distraction lengthening in hand surgery.

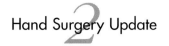

Chapter 23
Burn Injuries

John O. Kucan, MD

Introduction

Hands are burned more often than any other part of the body. Although the hands comprise only about 5% of the total body surface area, their functional importance sets them apart. The American Burn Association has categorized hand burns as major thermal injuries. While such a classification might be viewed initially as an exaggeration, closer scrutiny permits an appreciation of the singular importance of the hand and the debilitating consequences of burns. Burns of the hand require specialized care to maximize the potential for restoration of optimal function.

Viewed from the perspectives of etiology and severity, the spectrum of burn injuries to the hands is broad. Bilateral injuries are common. A 1958 report from the Brooke Army Medical Center indicated that 75% of patients had sustained hand burns; 80% were bilateral. In the civilian population, the incidence of hand burns in conjunction with other burn injuries exceeds 50%. The frequency of hand burns, coupled with a variety of etiologies and severity, presents a wide array of functional impairments. Treatment assumes a significant role in minimizing or aggravating functional impairment. The basic philosophy that guides treatment is to "circumvent the need for future reconstruction and rehabilitation;" incorporating this tenet as the foundation of treatment for burned hands optimizes function. The primary goal of treatment is the attainment of stable, pliable soft-tissue coverage, through which preservation or restoration of optimal function can be realized.

Analysis of the Problem

Proper care of the burned hand requires an accurate analysis of the problem and development of an organized and systematic treatment plan. The first component is a complete history. The history should include a thorough recounting of the injury event, with emphasis on the mechanism, and a general review of the patient's medical condition. The patient's occupation, special activities or hobbies, dominant hand, and age should be recorded. A complete physical examination should be obtained, and necessary physiologic stabilization achieved.

The burned hand is examined to determine the severity of the injury. An understanding of the mechanism of injury is a major aid in ascertaining the severity. The essential elements of this evaluation are the depth of the burn wound, extent or distribution of the burn wound, presence and degree of edema, circulation, sensation, range of motion, and involvement of underlying structures.

The first priority is restoration or preservation of circulation to the hand. Circumferential burn wounds of the upper extremity, partial thickness and full thickness alike, may result in compartment syndrome and subsequent cessation of nutrient blood flow. The obligatory edema of burn injury that occurs beneath a nonyielding circumferential eschar results in rapidly increasing interstitial pressure and impairment of nutrient blood flow. Although most circumferential upper extremity burns can be treated by escharotomy alone, charred full-thickness (fourth degree) burns or burns resulting from high-voltage electrical injury will likely require fasciotomy. The only accurate determinant of the need for escharotomy or fasciotomy is direct compartment pressure measurement. Physical examination and Doppler examination can be misleading. Pressures in excess of 30 mm Hg necessitate decompression to restore nutrient blood flow to nerves and muscles (Fig. 1).

Pathophysiology

Thermal injury causes cellular death directly and indirectly because injured cells liberate vasoactive products that produce edema, vasoconstriction, and tissue necrosis. The vasoactive substances liberated from damaged cells include histamine, seratonin, kinins, thromboxane, prostaglandins, free oxygen radicals, and lipid peroxides. Bacterial colonization with subsequent multiplication can further contribute to tissue destruction (Fig. 2).

Treatment of Acute Burns

Treatment of the burned hand depends on the extent of the injury. First-degree (redness only) burns require only symptomatic treatment as an outpatient. Patients with

Circumferential Extremity Burn

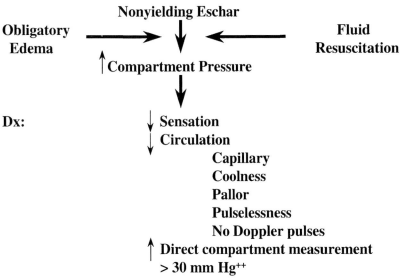

Figure 1

Pathophysiology, signs, symptoms, and treatment of the circumferential extremity burn. (Reproduced with permission from Kucan JO: Burn injuries, in Manske PR (ed): *Hand Surgery Update*. Rosemont, IL, American Academy of Orthopaedic Surgeons, 1996, pp 413–419.)

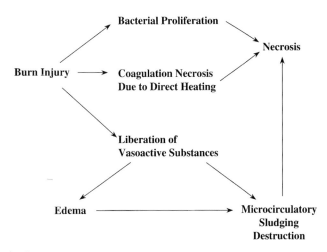

Figure 2

Mode of tissue destruction following thermal injury. (Reproduced with permission from Kucan JO: Burn injuries, in Manske PR (ed): *Hand Surgery Update*. Rosemont, IL, American Academy of Orthopaedic Surgeons, 1996, pp 413–419.)

small circumscribed partial-thickness and full-thickness burns of the hand are admitted at the physician's discretion. With the exception of very minor injuries, burns of the hand are best treated in the hospital. Hospitalization is standard for bilateral hand burns.

The basic principles of treatment of the burned hand include protection from further injury, maintenance of circulation, prevention of infection, attainment of expeditious wound closure, preservation of motion, and achievement of functional rehabilitation.

Prevention of Further Damage

Burn wounds have 3 zones: the zone of coagulation, an area of irreversible injury; the zone of stasis, the intermediate region of damaged but potentially salvageable cells; and the zone of hyperemia, the peripheral, transiently affected area that is destined to heal. Cooling of the burn wound within 30 minutes of injury may help limit injury to the zone of stasis and prevent further damage. The prevention of wound maceration or desiccation is essential. Blisters should be aspirated or debrided to remove fluid; this fluid contains high levels of thromboxane and other mediators known to be deleterious to the microcirculation within the zone of stasis.

Maintenance of Circulation

Control of edema can be achieved by elevating the injured hand above the level of the heart. The circumferentially burned hand and upper extremity must be observed for the development of compartment syndrome. Because clinical signs and symptoms may be misleading, delayed, or misinterpreted, direct compartment measurement with a handheld, portable compartment measuring device will provide accurate, reliable, and meaningful information. Prompt decompression by surgical or chemical escharotomy is indicated when compartmental pressures exceed 30 mm Hg.

Surgical escharotomy is performed by incision of the offending circumferential eschar, thus achieving decompression of the hand or arm. This technique requires meticulous hemostasis to prevent potentially exsanguinating hemorrhage. Lysis of the eschar by the application of proteolytic enzymes eliminates surgical incisions and may be an effective alternative to surgical decompression in selected patients. The advantages of

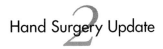

the chemical technique over surgical escharotomy include the elimination of surgical incisions, decreased morbidity, improved estimation of burn wound depth, and earlier preparation of the wound for definitive wound closure. Chemical escharotomy with the papain-urea ointment Accuzyme® may be effective in selected patients, but monitoring compartment pressures during treatment is critical. Chemical escharotomy should not be employed for charred full-thickness burns, high-voltage electrical injuries, or in the presence of elevated compartment pressures more than 4 to 6 hours after injury.

Prevention of Infection

Infection of the burned hand, although uncommon, can occur. During the initial edema phase, inactivation of antistreptococcal fatty acids of the skin may increase the likelihood for development of streptococcal cellulitis. Administration of a specific antistreptococcal drug, such as penicillin or erythromycin, may be indicated during the edema phase. Topical antimicrobial therapy is indicated in deep partial-thickness and full-thickness burns to control bacterial proliferation and prevent wound sepsis. Silver sulfadiazine cream is most commonly applied either in a hand dressing or in conjunction with Gore-Tex® bags, which permit motion but prevent maceration.

Attainment of a Closed Wound

Autologous skin provides the only permanent wound cover. Adequate, durable, stable, supple cover is essential to normal function. Prompt closure of the burn wound facilitates a decrease in wound infection rates, scar formation, and contractures, and markedly reduces pain and length of hospitalization. Therapy and rehabilitation can be initiated sooner, and the likelihood of additional reconstructive procedures is substantially reduced. Wound closure options in the hand are primarily determined by the depth of the wound. Closure options include spontaneous healing (< 14 days), early wound excision and split-thickness skin grafting (STSG), delayed spontaneous healing (> 14 days), delayed STSG (> 14 days), and delayed excision and STSG (Fig. 3).

Superficial burn wounds that are expected to heal within 14 days should be protected from desiccation. Topical antimicrobials are generally not required. A semisynthetic skin substitute (Biobrane®) glove is used. Alternative treatments include application of

nonadhering gauze dressings and ointments, calcium alginate dressings, or biologic dressings such as porcine xenografts. The primary management requirements are control of pain and maintenance of active motion. Uncomplicated healing and full functional recovery can be expected.

Full-thickness and intermediate depth partial-thickness wounds of the hands are managed best by early surgical excision and skin grafting. The depth of the burn wound is the primary determinant of healing. Wounds that require healing times in excess of 2 to 2.5 weeks frequently heal with dense scarring inhibiting motion and rehabilitation. Accordingly, the sooner the depth of the wound can be determined, the sooner definitive treatment can be initiated. Although numerous methods of determining burn wound depth have been described, investigated, and applied in the clinical setting, there is no single universally accepted, reliable tool to determine depth. The judgment of an experienced surgeon, coupled with a thorough history of the injury and clinical examination, provides the best means for predicting or determining the depth of the burn. Enzymatic debridement, by eliminating a significant amount of devitalized tissue, may provide additional useful information and increase the accuracy of the estimation of burn depth.

Burns can be debrided by either tangential excision or excision to fascia. Full-thickness burns of the dorsum of the hand are often managed by excision to fascia and STSG. The dorsal veins and paratenon should be preserved and sheet grafting employed whenever possible. Although excision to

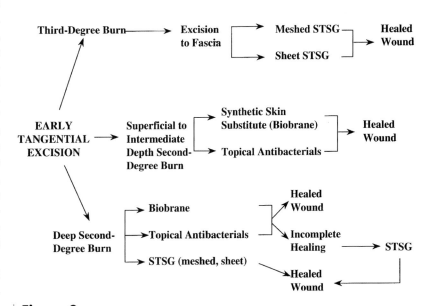

Figure 3

Wound closure options for burn injuries. (Reproduced with permission from Kucan JO: Burn injuries, in Manske PR (ed): *Hand Surgery Update*. Rosemont, IL, American Academy of Orthopaedic Surgeons, 1996, pp 413–419.)

fascia provides a viable bed for grafting, the resultant edema and cosmetic defect secondary to loss of the subcutaneous tissue is undesirable. Intradermal debridement (tangential excision) is more tedious than fascial excision, but less edema and cosmetic deficits are created. The nonviable tissue is shaved with a dermatome until obviously viable dermis or fat is encountered. Hemostasis is achieved with pneumatic tourniquets, hemostatic agents, and firm hemostatic wraps. Skin grafts are applied when hemostasis is complete and a viable recipient bed attained. Delayed grafting may be indicated if recipient bed hemostasis is incomplete or questionable. Sheet grafts provide a better appearance than meshed autografts, with no difference in the rate of "take."

Full-thickness burns to the palmar surface are much less common than injuries to the dorsum. Palmar wounds are more difficult to excise and close, and functional outcomes are frequently less successful than with dorsal wounds. Circumferential burns of the hands provide great therapeutic challenges, characterized by relatively poor functional outcomes and the need for secondary reconstructive procedures. There is a dearth of published information on optimal treatment for circumferential injuries. However, full-thickness or thick partial-thickness skin grafts to the palmar surface seem to provide skin surface superior to that of very thin grafts, and may improve long-term function. Early intervention, use of thicker grafts, and proper postoperative splinting and therapy appear to produce results that are considerably better than those in wounds managed by delayed grafting onto a granulating wound bed.

The predominant burn injuries to the hands are deep dermal burns of the dorsum. Optimal treatment was somewhat controversial until recent research data and clinical reports validated the concept of early excision and grafting as most appropriate. This treatment results in good function, while substantially decreasing pain, length of hospitalization, and frequency of secondary procedures.

Fourth-degree burns of the hands are rare but devastating injuries. Wound closure via skin grafting is often impossible; exposure of tendon, bone, joints, nerves, or even arteries frequently dictates complex and challenging methods of wound closure. Flap coverage is often necessary; regional flaps and free-tissue transfers are the primary techniques. Amputation, either primary or delayed, is often required. However, due to advances in reconstructive surgery—especially reconstructive microsurgery—over the past 2 decades, overall functional outcomes have improved dramatically.

Partial-thickness burn wounds to the palmar surface of the hand are infrequently excised; most heal spontaneously. If excision is undertaken, absence of a defined surgical plane and production of significant blood loss complicate the task. Bleeding can be minimized by use of a tourniquet. The arm

and hand should not be exsanguinated prior to tourniquet inflation, because the pooled blood aids in the recognition of the viable tissue plane in debridement of dorsal and palmar burns. Splinting of the palm in the antideformity position, to maintain palmar width and breadth, is critical to success.

Satisfactory results have been demonstrated with both operative and nonoperative treatment for dorsal partial-thickness burns of the hand. Effective mobilization, proper splinting, edema control, and a carefully orchestrated hand therapy program are the determinants of success.

Skin grafting of the burned hand should be carried out in accordance with established guidelines to ensure success. (1) The recipient bed must be viable and devoid of eschar or infection. (2) Hemostasis must be complete. (3) Sheet grafts should be used whenever possible. (4) The maximum amount of skin should be provided by placing the hand in extreme positions, thereby accentuating the defect. (5) Immobilization and splinting are necessary to prevent mechanical disruption of the graft from the recipient bed. (6) Darting or interposition of skin grafts with unburned skin are recommended to reduce the likelihood of linear contractures or syndactyly.

Preservation of Motion

To preserve motion, splinting and positioning must be initiated as soon as possible after injury. Elevation of the injured part to minimize edema formation is also important. Gentle active range of motion should be encouraged under the supervision of a hand therapist.

The hand should be splinted in the intrinsic-plus position with the wrist in mild dorsiflexion, metacarpophalangeal joint flexion of 70° to 80°, and interphalangeal joint extension—the position of safety. The thumb should be abducted and slightly circumducted into the palm.

On the fifth day after excision and grafting, gentle active range of motion exercises should be initiated. Active assisted and passive range of motion should be started gradually. Splints and continuous passive motion machines may be helpful in achieving full motion. If early grafting is not performed, hand therapy is critical to optimal results. Range of motion should be documented. Failure to progress should prompt reappraisal of the therapy program.

Achievement of Functional Rehabilitation

Restoration of optimal function is the primary goal in treating the burned patient as a whole and the burned hand in particular. Functional results may not be apparent immediately following wound closure, because complete wound healing and scar maturation take several months. During this period, close supervision, scar pressure, exercise, massage, and edema control are critical. Assessment of functional recovery must be based on objective measurement and the

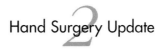

patient's ability to perform specific tasks. Work evaluation and functional capacity testing are frequently necessary to determine the degree and permanence of disability.

Recent data suggest that commercially available computer-assisted impairment evaluation systems provide a useful and accurate adjunct in the total rehabilitative process. These systems offer ease of operation, reproducibility, and reduced examination times. Implementation of a personalized, comprehensive, and closely supervised therapy program is essential to successful rehabilitation. Therapy is initiated shortly after the patient's admission and frequently continues for months and in some cases years.

Reconstruction of the Burned Hand

Reconstruction of the burned hand often presents a formidable challenge. The need for reconstruction is influenced by many contributing factors acting independently or in various combinations. These factors include severity of initial injury, specific areas of involvement, adequacy of initial care, prior management of the burn wound, postoperative management, quality of hand therapy, and motivation and reliability of the patient and caregivers. Frequently, reconstruction must address established deformities and their functional sequelae, which in turn affect the ultimate success or failure of reconstruction.

The global goal of reconstructive surgery is the restoration of form and function. In the hand, function translates into power, delicacy, mobility, dexterity, and tactile sensibility. Because the hand must operate in concert with the more proximal regions of the upper limb, proximal deficits must be addressed and successfully managed to optimize hand function.

The spectrum of deformities and problems requiring reconstruction varies widely in severity. Some problems can be solved with straightforward methods, while others defy satisfactory resolution. A thoughtful delineation of the deformity and the involvement of tissues and structures and a thorough assessment of function are the cornerstones of any reconstructive effort. Photographs, radiographs, scans, and vascular studies may be required. Thorough and realistic discussion with the patient, family, employer, and insurance carrier are necessary.

While many problems and techniques for late reconstruction are beyond the scope of this chapter, a few basic rules apply to any reconstructive effort. (1) Adhere to the reconstructive ladder, from simple to complex. (2) Choose the best reconstruction for the patient. (3) Plan alternatives and "lifeboats" in advance. (4) Review options with the patient, and let the patient participate in the decision process. (5) Do not let pride distort the objective. (6) Amputation can be a

reasonable alternative. (7) The simplest solution may not be the best solution. (8) Always consider the patient's emotional needs, daily living requirements, and occupation.

Insufficiency or instability of skin mandates the provision of adequate, stable skin coverage. The original defect must be recreated by removal of the entire scar. Skin grafts may be inadequate for coverage; local, regional, or distant flaps may be needed. Fixed deformities of subcutaneous structures, both soft and hard, may require releases, bone fusions, amputations, transpositions, or grafts.

Peripheral compression neuropathies involving the median and ulnar nerves have been described in as many as 30% of burned patients. Compression neuropathies often resolve with conservative treatment. If resolution does not occur, however, surgical decompression should be performed. Neuromata of cutaneous or digital nerves following excision, grafting, or amputation may require treatment.

Application of moisturizing agents to the spontaneously healed or grafted burn wound will help control dryness, itching, and fissure formation, thereby improving comfort, skin pliability, and ultimately function. Splints, pressure garments, custom inserts, or silicone gel sheeting can help minimize the frequency or severity of scar formation and its sequelae. Mechanical compression for chronic recalcitrant hand edema following burn injuries is usually beneficial.

Electrical Injuries

High-voltage electricity produces devastating injuries to the hand. Injuries to the dominant hand predominate, and frequently result in amputation (incidence of 33% to 50%). Patients rarely recover sufficient function to resume the same work. At the sites of entrance and exit, high temperatures are generated and thermal injury results. In addition, all intervening tissues may be affected to varying degrees by the flow of current. Low-voltage injuries can produce small circumscribed burns, resulting in localized tissue necrosis or occasionally loss of a digit.

The severity of an electrical injury depends on physical factors such as voltage, amperage, resistance, type of current, duration of contact, and the pathway of the current through the body. Voltage is the amount of electromotive force; amperage is the current flow; and resistance is the quality of any material that resists the flow of electrons. The highest resistance is at the skin surface and depends on thickness, cleanliness, and moisture. The greatest heat is generated at the sites of entry and exit from the body, resulting in implosive and explosive injuries, respectively. Although a gradation in resistance among body tissues has been described, with nerve offering the least resistance and bone offering the greatest resistance, the flow of electrical current through the body is essentially uniform throughout all tissues once skin resistance has been overcome. Cross-sectional area is a significant determinant of current density and, thus, the severity of injury. In the hand, wrist, and forearm, because of the small cross-sectional areas, relatively high concentrations of current exist and cause a greater degree of tissue damage.

Electrical energy produces tissue injury by 1 of 3 mechanisms—direct current effect at the point of contact and intervening body tissues, arc burn, or ignition of clothing and flame burn. The effect of high-voltage electrical injury has been likened to that of crush injury. A large volume of tissue is affected, unlike the pure surface injury characteristic of thermal burns.

The precise method by which deep tissues sustain damage has not been clearly defined. The most commonly accepted pathogenesis is the conversion of electrical energy to heat. However, recent data challenge this theory as the sole explanation for electrical injury. One computer modeling study demonstrated that the heat generated depends on whether the conducting layers are arranged in series or in parallel; if arranged in series, the layer with the greatest tissue resistance generates the most heat; if arranged in parallel, however, the layer with the highest conductivity (least resistance) generates the highest temperature. Other experimental data described the phenomenon of electroporation as a significant component in the pathogenesis of high-voltage electrical injury. Many authors believe that the extent of tissue necrosis is determined at the time of the initial injury. Other investigators demonstrated experimentally that some progression of injury may be the consequence of release of potent vasoconstrictors such as thromboxane after high-voltage electrical injury.

Initial Management

The initial management of high-voltage electrical injury to the hand must be undertaken within the framework of total patient care. Adherence to the principles of resuscitation and care of the multiply traumatized patient is fundamental. Assessment for possible systemic injuries should be conducted. Adequate fluid replacement to maintain urine output in excess of 100 ml/hr and alkalinization of the urine are critical. Mannitol, tetanus prophylaxis, and prophylactic antibiotics (including penicillin for clostridia) should be administered. Renal function, heart function, cardiac and liver enzymes, and electrolytes should be evaluated and followed carefully. Regular determinations of myoglobin and hemoglobin breakdown products are also necessary. Once stabilization has been achieved and life-threatening problems managed, attention can be focused on the wound.

High-voltage electricity produces wounds of various sizes; the extent of injury may not be apparent during the initial examination. In most cases, the severity of the injury can be ascertained by the posture of the hand, inability to passively extend the wrist or digits from their extremely flexed position, and tenderness of forearm musculature. Charring of skin, marked edema, or frank necrosis may also be apparent. The presence of large amounts of myoglobin or hemoglobin in the urine is an additional indicator of the severity of injury. Further evidence of severity may be obtained from careful examination of the neurovascular status of the hand and upper extremity.

Treatment

Injuries involving the hand and upper extremity should be treated as surgical emergencies. Initial management usually requires prompt surgical decompression. Following stabilization, the patient should be taken to the operating room for fasciotomy of involved muscle compartments and release of nerves at known sites of compression. Surgery provides an opportunity for direct examination of the injured tissues so that the extent and severity of injury, diagnostic and prognostic information, and treatment can be determined. Surgical decompression may, to varying degrees, preserve nutrient blood flow to nerves and muscle compartments. It should be undertaken after a thorough assessment and documentation of the patient's neurologic and circulatory status. Some patients who have been exposed to electrical current may not require surgical management and decompression. Only those who demonstrate signs of neurosensory deficits and circulatory embarrassment in the presence of obvious cutaneous or subcutaneous injury should undergo surgical decompression and exploration. In marginal cases, direct measurements of compartment pressures should be taken. After fasciotomy and initial debridement, the wound should be dressed with a topical antimicrobial. The topical antimicrobial of choice following high-voltage electrical injury is mafenide acetate cream (Sulfamylon®), because it penetrates tissues to a greater degree than other topical antimicrobial agents and is effective against anaerobic species. In addition, because of the activity of mafenide as a carbonic anhydrase inhibitor, it acts in concert with alkalinizing agents to produce a desirable alkaline urine. Following initial debridement and dressing, the hand should be splinted in the intrinsic-plus position. Proximal areas of involvement should be similarly dressed and splinted to optimize restoration of function.

Technetium-99 pyrophosphate scanning within the first 3 to 5 days after injury will accurately predict the extent of occult muscle damage. The patient should be returned to the operating room until all devitalized tissue has been debrided. Because of the severity of these injuries, debridement frequently results in amputations. When nerve,

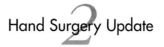
tendon, bone, or joint are exposed and in need of vascularized durable coverage, biologic dressings may prevent desiccation and allow additional time for planning of definitive reconstruction procedures. Split-thickness skin grafts are usually inadequate for satisfactory closure and permanent coverage of the exposed structures. In many instances, distant flaps are necessary; local or regional flaps may not be feasible due to extensive regional injury. In the presence of small defects, local flaps provide ideal coverage for small and important structures such as flexor tendons and digital nerves. For larger defects, options include groin, abdominal, pectoralis major island, latissimus dorsi muscle, and myocutaneous flaps, or a variety of free-tissue transfers. Selection of the best flap requires thoughtful planning and must encompass the needs of the patient, technical concerns inherent to the procedure, and functional considerations.

Amputation and Prosthetics

Although amputation is rarely indicated at the initial treatment stage of high-voltage electrical injury, amputations are common in the later stages to avoid sepsis or to address a nonfunctional and insensate extremity. Decisions to amputate are difficult; consultation with an experienced colleague can help restore objectivity. Clearly, the patient and family must be thoroughly apprised.

Chemical Burns

Chemical burns to the hand are generally localized but often require admission to a burn center and produce variable degrees of tissue necrosis. A key difference in chemical burns is that the causative agent may remain in contact with the skin for a prolonged period. Prolonged contact produces extensive and progressive tissue damage or destruction. The degree and extent of damage depend on the chemical agent, quantity, concentration, skin contact duration, and the type of chemical reaction. In general, acids cause coagulation necrosis; alkalis produce liquefaction; and vesicants result in ischemic and anoxic injury. Most chemical agents produce a thermal burn as a result of an exothermic reaction, which is short-lived. Tissue damage from a chemical agent will continue relentlessly until it is washed away from the skin, neutralized, or its toxicity is spent by reaction with the tissues. Certain chemical agents may produce systemic toxicity by absorption.

First Aid

Effective first aid treatment is immediate and continuous irrigation with tap water to remove heat. In addition, water dilutes or totally removes the offending agent. Irrigation should continue until pain has subsided. Water irrigation is preferable to neutralizing agents, which can produce an exothermic reaction and further thermal injury. Subsequent management of chemical injuries is similar to that of thermal burns and includes topical antimicrobial agents, debridement, and wound closure.

Hydrofluoric Acid Burns

Burns caused by hydrofluoric acid mandate special attention. Hydrofluoric acid is a strong inorganic acid used in many industries as a cleaning agent and solvent. It is highly corrosive and penetrates tissue, producing cytotoxic injury at the cellular level. It creates liquefaction necrosis of the soft tissues and bony erosion. The severity and onset of symptoms are directly related to the area of skin exposure, the concentration of the acid, and duration of exposure. The patient presents with swelling, a yellowish-white area of necrosis, associated blistering, erythema, and severe pain. Treatment consists of immediate irrigation with copious amounts of water, followed by attempts to neutralize or eliminate the free fluoride ions that are responsible for tissue damage. When injuries involve the fingertips, 2.5% calcium gluconate gel may be applied topically; placing the hand in a rubber glove will provide sufficient contact between the calcium gluconate and the hydrofluoric acid. The glove and gel also relieve pain; the calcium combines with the fluoride ion and the combination precipitates as an insoluble complex. When larger areas of the hand are involved, 10 cc of calcium gluconate and 40 cc of normal saline are infused via the radial or ulnar artery over a 4-hour period. (The intraarterial method has replaced previously recommended subcutaneous injections of 10% calcium gluconate.) In the event that the forearm and hand are involved, 20 cc of 20% calcium gluconate and 80 cc of normal saline are infused via the brachial artery over a 4-hour period.

Annotated Bibliography

American Burn Association: Guidelines for service standards and severity classifications in the treatment of burn injury. *Bull Am Coll Surg* 1984;69:24–28.

A concise description of the standards for providing care to the burned patient is provided.

Ause-Ellias KL, Richard R, Miller SF, Finley RK Jr: The effect of mechanical compression on chronic hand edema after burn injury: A preliminary report. *J Burn Care Rehabil* 1994;15:29–33.

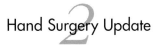

246   Burn Injuries

The authors review the numerous treatment protocols that address the issue of chronic hand edema following burn injuries to the hand. Compression therapy is presented, and its overall impact discussed.

Dimick AR: Experience with the use of proteolytic enzyme (Travase) in burn patients. *J Trauma* 1977;17:948–955.

The author describes the concept and practical application of enzymatic debridement in management of the burned patient.

Drueck C III: Emergency department treatment of hand burns. *Emerg Med Clin North Am* 1993;11:797–809.

Drueck reviews the assessment, types, and treatment of burns presenting in the emergency room. Information on pain management and wound care is provided. Criteria for admission versus outpatient treatment are also outlined.

Edstrom L, Robson MC, Macchiaverna JR, Scala AD: Management of deep partial thickness dorsal hand burns: Study of operative vs nonoperative therapy. *Orthop Rev* 1979;8:27–33.

This prospective randomized study addresses the issue of spontaneous healing versus delayed excision and grafting. The study supports the notion that surgical and nonsurgical results are comparable for deep partial-thickness burn wounds of the hand.

Gant TD: The early enzymatic debridement and grafting of deep dermal burns to the hand. *Plast Reconstr Surg* 1980;66:185–190.

Gant describes a useful technique for enzymatic debridement and early grafting of deep dermal burns to the hands.

Goodwin CW, Maguire MS, McManus WF, Pruitt BA Jr: Prospective study of burn wound excision of the hands. *J Trauma* 1983;23:510–517.

This prospective evaluation of 164 burned hands indicates that early or late excision and grafting of deep dermal burns offers no distinct functional advantage over physical therapy and primary healing.

Grobbelaar AO, Harrison DH: The distally based ulnar artery island flap in hand reconstruction. *J Hand Surg* 1997;22B:204–211.

The authors provide an excellent description of the distally-based ulnar artery island flap, which can be used for a variety of situations in reconstruction of the hand. This is a useful reference for various applications, as either a fasciocutaneous fascial or composite skin flap.

Hammond J, Ward CG: The use of Technetium-99 pyrophosphate scanning in management of high voltage electrical injuries. *Am Surg* 1994;60:886–888.

The authors evaluate the efficacy of Technetium-99 pyrophosphate scanning following high-voltage electrical injury. The impact on clinical outcome is also presented.

Harvey KD, Barillo DJ, Hobbs CL, et al: Computer-assisted evaluation of hand and arm function after thermal injury. *J Burn Care Rehabil* 1996;17:176–180.

Measurements of extremity function with computer-assisted methods are described, and compared to conventional methods.

Heggers JP, Ko F, Robson MC, Heggers R, Craft KE: Evaluation of burn blister fluid. *Plast Reconstr Surg* 1980;65:798–804.

This article provides a concise description of the content of burn blister fluid and its protective effect against bacterial contamination.

Janzekovic Z: A new concept in the early excision and immediate grafting of burns. *J Trauma* 1970;10:1103–1108.

This landmark article describes early intradermal debridement and grafting of burn wounds, setting the stage for modern aggressive burn wound management.

Krizek TJ, Flagg SV, Wolfort FG, Jabaley ME: Delayed primary excision and skin grafting of the burned hand. *Plast Reconstr Surg* 1973;51:524–529.

The rationale for delayed primary excision and skin grafting of the hands is presented in this historic article.

Kurtzman LC, Stern PJ: Upper extremity burn contractures. *Hand Clin* 1990;6:261–279.

This is a concise and practical overview of the various upper extremity burn scar contractures and their management.

Lee KS, Park SW, Kim HY: Tendocutaneous free flap transfer from the dorsum of the foot. *Microsurgery* 1994;15:882–885.

This article exemplifies the creative and innovative aspects of reconstructive microsurgery in dealing with difficult wound problems. The authors describe the use of a tendocutaneous free tissue transfer when skin and tendon replacement are required. The operation, risks, benefits, and complications are clearly described.

Lee RC, Gottlieb LJ, Krizek TJ: Pathophysiology and clinical manifestations of tissue injury in electrical trauma. *Adv Plast Reconstr Surg* 1992;8:1–29.

This interesting article provides another theory on the pathogenesis of high-voltage electrical injury.

Nuchtern JG, Engrav LH, Nakamura DY, Dutcher KA, Heimbach DM, Vedder NB: Treatment of fourth-degree hand burns. *J Burn Care Rehabil* 1995;16:36–42.

This report of a 10-year experience with deep thermal burns involving the hand describes the difficulty and complexity of treatment, and provides a good overview.

Pribaz JJ, Eriksson E, Smith DJ: Acute management of the burned hand. *Plast Reconstr Surg* 1989;209–225.

The authors present a broad overview of management of the acutely burned hand.

Richard R, Staley M, Daugherty MB, Miller SF, Warden GD: The wide variety of designs for dorsal hand burn splints. *J Burn Care Rehabil* 1994;15:275–280.

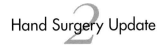
This is a valuable resource on the various methods of splint fabrication. The authors describe the wide degree of variability among splints used for the treatment of dorsal hand burns.

Robson MC, Smith DJ Jr, VanderZee AJ, Roberts L: Making the burned hand functional. *Clin Plast Surg* 1992;19:663–671.

This article provides an overview and an algorithm for management and treatment of the acutely burned hand.

Schwanholt C, Greenhalgh DG, Warden GD: A comparison of full-thickness versus split-thickness autografts for the coverage of deep palm burns in the very young pediatric patient. *J Burn Care Rehabil* 1993;14:29–33.

In a useful review of patients with difficult deep burns of the palms, full-thickness skin grafts are compared to split-thickness skin grafts.

Sheridan RL, Hurley J, Smith MA, et al: The acutely burned hand: Management and outcome based on a ten-year experience with 1047 acute hand burns. *J Trauma* 1995;38:406–411.

A retrospective analysis of 1,047 acute hand burns describes the surgical approach to management of the acutely burned hand and includes a clear analysis of outcomes. This useful review article provides 30 references.

Simpson RL, Flaherty ME: The burned small finger. *Clin Plast Surg* 1992;19:673–682.

This is a detailed and useful analysis of the pathogenesis and correction of problems associated with burns of the fifth finger.

Smith DJ, McHugh TP, Phillips LG, Robson MC, Heggers JP: Biosynthetic compound dressings: Management of hand burns. *Burns Incl Therm Inj* 1988;14:405–408.

Clinical experience with 218 burns managed with the biosynthetic dressing Biobrane is described. Advantages and cost-effectiveness are compared to standard wound management.

Stern PJ, Neale HW, Graham TJ, Warden GD: Classification and treatment of postburn proximal interphalangeal joint flexion contractures in children. *J Hand Surg* 1987;12A:450–457.

This article provides a classification system based on severity of burn contractures, and an assessment of treatment results.

Terrill PJ, Kedwards SM, Lawrence JC: The use of GORE-TEX bags for hand burns. *Burns* 1991;17:161–165.

Clinical and laboratory assessments of water vapor permeable Gore-Tex® bags are provided, and their application in the treatment of burned hands is described. This alternative method of treatment may be useful in selected patients.

Upton J, Rogers C, Durham-Smith G, Swartz WM: Clinical applications of free temporoparietal flaps in hand reconstruction. *J Hand Surg* 1986;11A:475–483.

This article is an anatomic and practical description of the applications of free temporoparietal flaps in reconstruction of a variety of hand defects.

Weinzweig N, Chen L, Chen ZW: The distally based radial forearm fasciosubcutaneous flap with preservation of the radial artery: An anatomic and clinical approach. *Plast Reconstr Surg* 1994;94:675–684.

This is an excellent anatomic study of the distally based radial forearm fasciocutaneous flap with preservation of the radial artery. Clinical application is also presented. This important article should be reviewed when considering coverage of soft-tissue defects of the hand.

Yotsuyanagi T, Yokoi K, Omizo M: A simple and compressive splint for palmar skin grafting in young children with burns. *Burns* 1994;20:55–57.

This description of a simple and easily applied splinting technique is particularly useful in the palmar burns of pediatric patients. Some useful tips and thoughts for treating burns in uncooperative patients are provided.

Zeller J, Sturm G, Cruse CW: Patients with burns are successful in work hardening programs. *J Burn Care Rehabil* 1993;14:189–196.

In an evaluation of patients who were enrolled in a work-hardening program following burns, 91% returned to work. This report is useful in evaluating the goals and approaches to work rehabilitation.

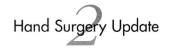

Chapter 24
Soft-Tissue Coverage of the Hand

W. Bradford Rockwell, MD

Wounds of the hand are usually the result of trauma but may result from tumor excision or extensive reconstructive surgery. All but the smallest wounds are closed with skin grafts or flaps. The type of wound coverage depends on the structures exposed in the base of the wound, the availability of local and regional tissue, and the general health of the patient. The reconstructive choices proceed from direct closure to skin grafts to local flaps to regional flaps and, finally, to free flaps. The simplest method that provides adequate, stable coverage is best. Thorough evaluation of the wound and surrounding structures is important. Evaluation of the vascularity, function, and type of tissue in the wound base is mandatory. Wounds with adequately vascularized soft tissue may be appropriate for skin grafts. The indications for flap coverage are (1) a bed containing bone, cartilage, or tendon that cannot revascularize a free skin graft and/or (2) a location in which a free skin graft would impair function, later reconstruction, or would be likely to undergo repeated ulceration.

Local or regional flaps are appropriate for most hand wounds (Table 1). They are composed of skin similar to that originally occupying the area of the wound and they inflict no injury on distant parts of the body. However, these flaps are limited in availability. The larger the primary defect created by injury or excision, the less local tissue is available for flap coverage. Use of local flaps also inflicts further injury to a hand or finger. The resultant compound wound may cause a greater functional deficit than existed from the original injury.

Regional and distant pedicle flaps provide additional tissue for wound coverage. Distant pedicle flaps create an additional vascular demand on the traumatized area and usually require that the hand be dependent during attachment. Dependency may be uncomfortable, and the lack of exercise may result in joint stiffness.

Free flaps have a permanent pedicle and do not create increased vascular demands on the already compromised limb. Free flaps are available in virtually any area and thickness. They can be tailored to fit the wound with precision and may cover areas on any portion of the limb. They permit elevation of the limb and early mobilization. Random movement is possible in infants and disoriented patients.

Preoperative Assessment

A complete examination of the limb is mandatory. The examination should encompass 6 general areas of the limb, with 3 being important for immediate reconstruction and 3 important for subsequent function of the hand. Adequate skin cover, adequate blood supply, and a stable bony skeleton are necessary for initial limb reconstruction. Mobile joints, intact muscle-tendon units, and functioning nerves produce a useful limb after reconstruction is complete.

Specific characteristics of a wound are also important to evaluate. Area, depth, and special requirements of the wound help determine the type of coverage. Initially, wound approximation may reduce the size of the soft-tissue defect. However, increased skin tension may result, with its accompanying adverse effects of delayed wound healing, edema, and limitation of early motion. Importation of additional tissue can reduce skin tension and the bulk of the flap can fill dead space.

The skeleton should be evaluated radiographically. Rigid fixation of fractures is an essential prerequisite to early motion because motion and unstable fractures create dead space in which infection may develop. If indicated, the vascular tree should be studied by Doppler ultrasound to determine the direction of flow and the possible presence of an occlusion in the radial-ulnar arch system. The flow distal to the wound in a recently injured limb may require assessment both before surgery and after fracture reduction and fixation.

Wound Preparation

Some wounds may require excision of scarred or injured tissue. Debridement ideally should include all devitalized or injured tissue. Ulcerated skin and immobile tissue fixed to deeper tissues should be removed. Debridement may produce a wound considerably larger than that initially seen; thus, the final pattern for the flap should not be made until wound excision has been completed. Soft-tissue coverage should be applied to a wound with an underlying stable skeleton. Ideally, the wound would not contain contamination or tissue with a compromised blood supply. For flap

Table 1

Coverage options for hand wounds*

Region	Coverage
Fingertip	Skin graft
	V-Y advancement
	Cross finger
	Thenar
	Vascular island
Dorsal digit	STSG
	Rotation or transportation
	Reversed cross finger
Palmar digit	FTSG
	Rotation or transposition
	Cross finger
	Axial flag
	Vascular island
Dorsal hand	STSG
	Rotation or transposition
	Axial flag
	Vascular island
	Fillet
	Dorsal metacarpal artery
	Posterior interosseous
Palmar hand	FTSG
	Rotation or transposition
	Axial flag
	Vascular island
	Fillet
	Radial forearm
Thumb	V-Y advancement
	Moberg
	First dorsal metacarpal artery
	Standard and reversed cross finger
	Neurovascular island

*This list does not include distant, pedicled flaps (groin, infraclavicular) or free-tissue transfers
STSG, split-thickness skin graft; FTSGA, full-thickness skin graft

coverage, the wound should present as flat a bed as possible. Radical debridement of the wound will produce such a bed. However, the surgeon must know that adequate soft-tissue coverage is available if debridement is undertaken. Significant hand wounds are debrided under tourniquet control, with the debridement margins incised in normal tissue. The exceptions to radical debridement are longitudinal structures that carry potential for function. Intact tendons, nerves, or functioning major vessels should not be debrided.

With the exception of highly specialized areas, such as fingertips or the palm, all marginally viable skin should be removed because it may harbor infection and heal with significant scarring. If questions remain regarding retained tissue, tissue samples may be taken for rapid Gram stain and quantitative cultures. Once adequate debridement has been completed, the skin margins are considered. Margins should be made by excising any irregularities that lack functional importance. The resulting wound becomes ready for coverage.

Skin Grafts

Skin grafts are appropriate for wounds that do not require significant soft-tissue bulk and that have well-vascularized wound beds without exposed tendons, cartilage, or bones. Generally split-thickness skin grafts (STSG) are used for dorsal wounds, whereas full-thickness skin grafts (FTSG) are used for palmar wounds. FTSG may provide more durable coverage but their size is limited by the need for primary closure or STSG of the donor site. The beds beneath FTSG contract less than those beneath STSG, although wound contraction will still occur. Postoperative splinting and compression garments are required for larger grafts to maximize hand function.

Satisfactory donor sites for smaller skin grafts are the ulnar side of the hypothenar area or the proximal ulnar forearm. Larger full-thickness grafts are harvested from the inguinal crease lateral to all hair. Split-thickness grafts are generally harvested from the lateral buttock and proximal thigh.

Flaps

Hand injuries may be covered with local, regional, or distant flaps. In addition to the anatomic description, flaps may be described as either random or axial, depending on their blood supply. Axial flaps import tissue that contains its own vascularity. Random flaps import tissue without significant additional blood flow and consequently may place further vascular demands on the injured tissue.

Digits

Fingertip injuries more frequently involve the palmar side. When more skin is lost dorsally or the amputation is trans-

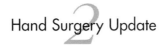

verse, V-Y advancement flaps will provide coverage (Fig. 1). A single palmar flap may be raised with its proximal apex at the distal interphalangeal flexion crease. This flap is partially elevated off of the underlying bone. Its blood supply courses through the soft tissue deep to the skin incisions. Fibrous septae deep to the skin incisions must be divided to permit flap advancement. Neurovascular elements remain intact. Bilateral V-Y advancement flaps based on the proper digital neurovascular bundles will also close distal wounds. Advancement may require division of the distal phalangeal nerve branches to the palmar pad.

When more skin is lost from the palmar surface, a regional flap is required. A cross-finger flap from the dorsal middle phalanx of the adjacent finger (Fig. 2) or a thenar flap is appropriate. A cross-finger flap requires leaving the extensor paratenon of the donor site intact so a skin graft will take. The thenar flap allows immediate closure of the donor site. Both flaps require significant proximal interphalangeal (PIP) joint flexion for the 14 days of pedicle flap attachment. PIP flexion contracture may result. The thenar flap donor site is less visible and consequently may be preferred in female patients. In patients with less supple joints, a cross-finger flap is preferred

because this flap requires less PIP flexion during pedicle attachment. A neurovascular island flap from an adjacent digit will provide immediate wound coverage without the need for pedicle protection and consequent immobilization. A neurovascular island flap may also be harvested from a toe and applied to the injured digit as a free-tissue transfer.

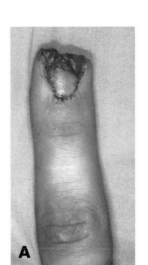
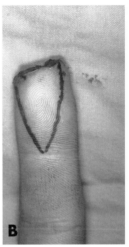
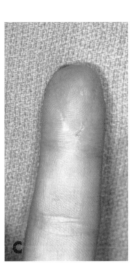

Figure 1

V-Y advancement flap. **A,** This flap is best suited for transverse or dorsally angulated fingertip wounds. **B,** The flap is designed with a width equal to that of the open wound and a length extending from the wound to the distal interphalangeal joint. The skin and the underlying fibrous septae are divided, allowing the flap to advance distally. **C,** The flap maintains reasonable sensation while providing a cosmetically acceptable wound closure.

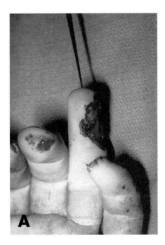
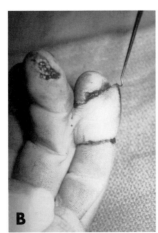
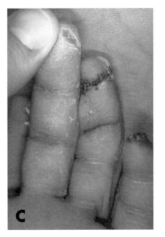
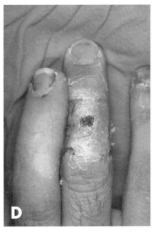

Figure 2

Cross-finger flap. **A,** This exposed wound on the radial side to the distal middle finger was not suitable for skin grafting and required flap coverage. **B,** The flap was raised from the dorsum of the middle phalanx of the adjacent ring finger with the margins of the flap being at the midaxial line on either side and the proximal and distal interphalangeal joints. **C,** After 2 weeks of attachment, the flap is ready for division and final insetting. **D,** Preservation of the paratenon is essential at the donor site. A split-thickness skin graft provides coverage of this area.

Dorsal wounds that cannot be closed with a local rotation or transposition flap will require a reversed (inverted) cross-finger flap. The dimensions of this flap are the same as for a standard cross-finger flap. The deepithelialized flap is applied to the dorsum of the injured digit and covered with a split-thickness skin graft. PIP joint wounds are covered with conventional cross-finger flaps for palmar wounds and reversed cross-finger flaps for dorsal wounds. Small defects on the palmar aspect of the proximal phalanx are readily closed with local transposition flaps from the lateral or dorsal skin. Larger defects solely on the palmar surface can be covered with an extended cross-finger flap. However, kinking of the pedicle may occur if the defect extends onto the lateral aspect. These wounds are best treated with an axial flag flap (Fig. 3). Again, a skin graft is required for the donor site. The axial flag flap is based on a dorsal digital artery that originates from either the proper digital artery or the dorsal metacarpal artery. Its existence is fairly reliable in the index-middle web space allowing reliable blood supply to an axial flag flap on the index or middle fingers. The vessel supplying these flaps is not always reliable in the third and fourth web spaces. Consequently Doppler examination is mandatory to ensure adequate axial blood flow to the flap. Margins of the flap are the metacarpophalangeal (MCP) and PIP dorsal creases and the midaxial lines on either side of the finger. If an axial flag flap cannot be raised, a standard or reversed cross-finger flap from the proximal phalanx is used.

Metacarpophalangeal Area and Palm

Wounds in the MCP area are generally treated with either an axial flag flap, a vascular island flap, or a dorsal metacarpal artery flap. Palmar defects preferentially are covered with an axial flag flap, assuming the injury did not damage the vascular pedicle. If preoperative Doppler evaluation does not indicate an intact pedicle, a vascular island flap, based on the proper digital artery of an adjacent uninjured finger, provides coverage. Dorsal defects in this area are treated similarly. Because the vascular pedicle for the axial flag flap is more reliable in the index-middle web space, the flap is more reliable for coverage involving these 2 fingers. The vascular island, in general, is more reliable for the ring and little fingers. A reversed second dorsal metacarpal artery, pedicled at the index-middle MCP joint and based on the second dorsal metacarpal artery, may reach the fifth MCP joint. Preoperative Doppler examination will also indicate the presence of the dorsal metacarpal artery. The first and second dorsal metacarpal arteries are fairly reliable. The third and fourth are variably present. These flaps may include tissue from the carpometacarpal joint to the MCP joint. In general, their width is restricted by the desire to primarily close the donor site. However, wider flaps may be harvested if skin grafting of the donor site is acceptable.

Injuries over the palmar or dorsal metacarpal area are covered with skin grafts if bone or tendon is not exposed and a graft would provide stable coverage. If flap coverage is required, multiple local or regional flaps may cover one large defect. Flaps suitable for this kind of coverage are axial flag flaps, vascular island flaps, fillet flaps if a vascularized digit is deemed to be of no functional value, or random rotation or transposition flaps. Certain wounds may be suitable for coverage by syndactylization of the fingers. After cutaneous coverage is

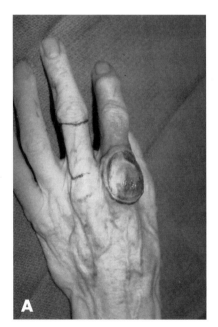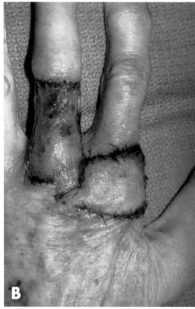

Figure 3

Axial flag flap. **A,** An ulcer over the dorsal index metacarpophalangeal (MCP) joint had eroded to the tendon and bone. An axial flag flap from the middle finger was used for coverage. The margins of the flap are the MCP and proximal interphalangeal joints and the midaxial lines radial and ulnar. **B,** Ten days after flap elevation, the flap provides satisfactory wound coverage, while the split-thickness skin graft covers the donor site.

ensured with adequate healing, the syndactalized digits are divided and skin grafted.

Larger defects on the palm or dorsum may be covered with a radial forearm flap (Fig. 4). Adequate preoperative blood flow to the hand through the ulnar artery must be documented with Allen's test or a Doppler study. Patency of the vascular arches of the hand with continued reverse flow into the radial artery must also be ascertained. A fasciocutaneous radial forearm flap tends to be bulky after it has completely healed. The flap may be raised as a fascia only flap and covered with a split-thickness skin graft. Using fascia only also avoids the unsightly forearm skin graft required for the fasciocutaneous flap. A posterior interosseous fasciocutaneous flap is distally based on perforators from the posterior interosseous artery. Primary closure of the donor site is possible as is coverage of some wounds on the dorsum of the hand or wrist area.

Distant pedicled flaps can also be used for coverage of metacarpal wounds. The groin flap is preferentially used for larger defects (Fig. 5). This flap is axial to the level of the anterior superior iliac spine and based on the superficial circumflex iliac artery. Extension of the flap lateral to the anterior superior iliac spine is as a random flap with a 1:1 ratio. Subcutaneous tissue makes the groin flap bulky, especially in its axial portion. The flap also requires an attachment of the injured extremity to the groin for 2 to 3 weeks before flap division and insetting. Smaller defects in the metacarpal area or fingertips can be covered with a pedicled infraclavicular flap. Concerns regarding flap bulk and extremity immobilization are the same as those for the groin flap. A cross-arm flap or random thoracoepigastric flap are other options with similar concerns.

Free-tissue transfer may be a preferential choice for larger wounds in this area. The lateral arm free flap may be harvested as a fasciocutaneous flap or as a fascia only flap. The donor site in general is better accepted than that of a radial forearm flap. The specifics of free-tissue transfer for wound coverage are discussed in chapter 29.

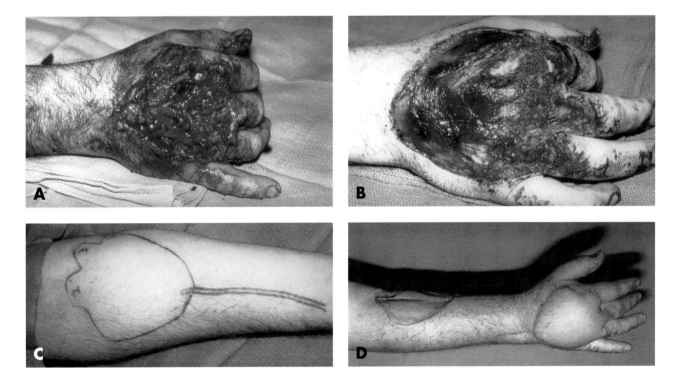

Figure 4

Radial forearm flap. **A,** Avulsion injury to the dorsal hand created a wound requiring significant debridement. **B,** Immediate radical debridement was performed, removing all devitalized tissue and burring exposed bone. **C,** A radial forearm flap was designed with a wound template. The pedicle point was the radial artery at the wrist. **D,** The radial forearm flap provided complete coverage of the wound although it is bulkier than normal dorsal hand skin. The donor site is covered with a split-thickness, nonmeshed skin graft. The appearance of the donor site may be unacceptable to some patients.

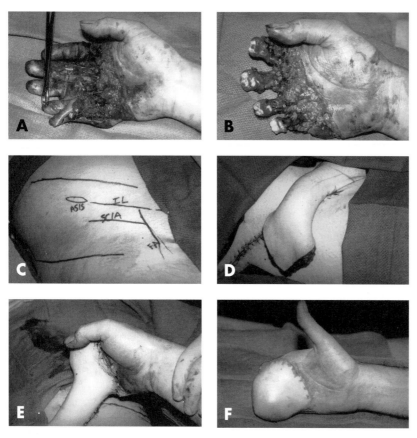

Figure 5

Pedicled groin flap. **A,** A printing press injury caused degloving of the hand from the mid-palm distally. **B,** Devascularization of the finger required amputation at the proximal interphalangeal joints. **C,** A pedicled groin flap contained an axial portion, based on the superficial circumflex iliac artery, and a random portion lateral to the anterior superior iliac spine. The vascular supply to the flap courses parallel and inferior to the inguinal ligament. **D,** After raising the flap, the proximal portion is tubed while the donor site is closed primarily. **E,** The distal portion of the flap is sutured to the palmar side of the wound. The dorsum of the wound was covered with a split-thickness skin graft. **F,** After 3 weeks, the flap was divided and inset. This flap created a syndactyly of the 4 fingers. They were subsequently divided in 2 separate operations and reasonable phalangeal motion was achieved.

Thumb

Adequate stable coverage of thumb wounds is of added importance because of the functional importance of the thumb to the hand. Local flaps for thumb coverage include V-Y advancement flap, Moberg advancement flap, first dorsal metacarpal artery flap, and cross-finger flap. Random distant pedicle flaps can provide coverage for larger wounds on the thumb.

Distal tip wounds with more loss dorsal than palmar are well covered with a V-Y advancement flap created by tissue distal to the interphalangeal (IP) crease (Fig. 1). The V-Y

flap for the thumb is raised and advanced in a manner identical to that on fingers. A Moberg advancement flap is suitable for distal wounds with more loss palmar than dorsal (Fig. 6). The tissue loss must be less than two thirds of the palmar pulp. The Moberg flap is raised just superficial to the flexor tendon sheath and includes both neurovascular islands with the palmar skin and subcutaneous tissue. The flap is elevated to about the level of the MCP joint. The flap is then advanced distally and sewn in to cover the wound. IP joint flexion is frequently necessary to allow coverage of the entire wound. The IP joint flexion may be relieved by making a transverse incision at the base of the flap while preserving the intact neurovascular bundles. The resulting exposed area is then covered with a skin graft. The advantage of the Moberg flap is that it provides well-vascularized, sensate tissue for the distal pulp of the thumb. A Moberg flap is suitable for the thumb because the larger dorsal artery supplies adequate blood flow for the remainder of the thumb. The Moberg flap is not suitable for the other digits because an adequately large dorsal artery is not reliably present.

Wounds on the dorsal distal thumb can be covered with an axial flap from the index finger, which is lengthened by including the entire first dorsal metacarpal artery. The flap is pedicled on an axis at the carpometacarpal area and can be transposed with a portion of skin over the artery or it can be tunneled subcutaneously, with the flap skin from the dorsal index proximal phalanx being used to cover the wound on the thumb. The axial flap is also suitable for palmar wounds on the thumb. It may be made sensate if a branch of the radial sensory nerve is located in the region of the flap. The flap requires skin grafting of the dorsal proximal phalanx of the index finger while primary closure of the dorsal hand donor site is accomplished.

Total pulp loss on the thumb is covered either with a neurovascular island flap or with a radially supplied cross-finger flap from the index finger. The neurovascular island flap is preferentially harvested from a toe. If microsurgical skills are not available, the neurovascular island flap can

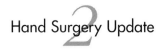

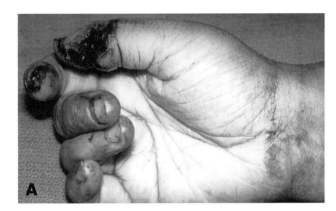

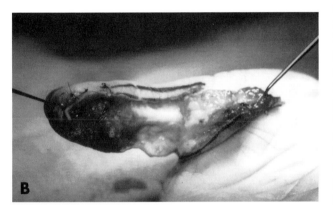

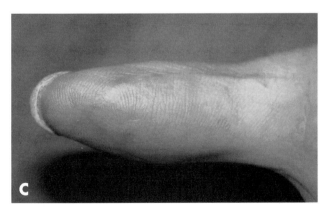

Figure 6

Moberg advancement flap. **A,** A wound to the distal phalanx of the thumb presents an open wound with devitalized tissue. **B,** Following debridement, the proximal two thirds of the palmar distal phalanx was exposed. The Moberg flap was raised with a width equal to that of the original wound. The flap is elevated superficial to the flexor tendon sheath and includes both neurovascular bundles. **C,** The interphalangeal joint was flexed and the flap was sutured into position. With postoperative therapy, full range of motion of the thumb was achieved, and the flap provided sensate covering for the wound.

be transposed as a pedicle flap from an adjacent uninjured finger. The radial side of the middle finger is the donor site of choice if other considerations do not exist. A cross-finger flap from the middle or proximal phalanx of the index finger will also cover palmar thumb wounds; a reversed cross-finger flap will cover dorsal thumb wounds as with cross-finger flaps to fingers. Cross-finger flaps require at least 10 days of immobilization and a second surgery to divide and fully inset the flap.

Larger wounds on the thumb cannot be adequately covered by local flaps; such wounds require coverage with a pedicled random flap from the infraclavicular or groin region. The groin flap can be designed as an axial flap (Fig. 5). However, the axial portion of the flap is not suitable for coverage of tip injuries because the subcutaneous bulk is unacceptable. The aforementioned flaps also require 2 to 3 weeks of immobilization to protect the attached flap and subsequent surgery for division and insetting. The infraclavicular flap will cover smaller regions, whereas the groin flap can cover circumferential wounds on the thumb. The groin flap also has the advantage that the pedicle may be tubed, thus decreasing exposed soft tissue during the attachment phase. If bony loss has also occurred with thumb injuries, a subsequent toe to hand transfer or pollicization may be indicated. In certain instances, additional soft tissue is necessary to provide coverage for a toe to hand transfer or pollicization. In very large defects, the pedicled groin flap will cover the original wound and supply initially excessive soft tissue. The excess tissue can be tailored during a subsequent procedure.

Wrist, Forearm, Elbow

Wounds in these areas tend to be large. If there are no exposed bone, tendon, or neurovascular structures, skin grafts are appropriate. If flap coverage is necessary, free-tissue transfer is usually the procedure of choice.

Annotated Bibliography

General Reference

Lister GD: Skin flaps, in Green DP, Hotchkiss RN (eds): *Operative Hand Surgery*, ed 3. New York, NY, Churchill Livingstone, 1993, vol 2, pp 1741–1822.

This is a complete review of flap options and surgical techniques for hand coverage.

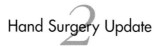

256   Soft-Tissue Coverage of the Hand

Rockwell WB, Lister GD: Soft tissue reconstruction: Coverage of hand injuries. *Orthop Clin North Am* 1993;24:411–424.

This is an overview of wound assessment and preparation with a description and algorithm of flap options.

Strauch B, Vasconez LO, Hall-Findlay EJ, Grabb WC (eds): *Grabb's Encyclopedia of Flaps.* Boston, MA, Little, Brown & Co, 1990.

This 3-volume resource provides a thorough description of the various upper extremity flaps with details of surgical techniques.

Local Flaps

Gebhard B, Meissl G: An extended first dorsal metacarpal artery neurovascular island flap. *J Hand Surg* 1995;20B:529–531.

This is an anatomic and technique description of the innervated first dorsal metacarpal artery flap.

Goitz RJ, Westkaemper JG, Tamaino MM, Sotereanos DG: Soft-tissue defects of the digits: Coverage considerations. *Hand Clin* 1997;13:189–205.

This article provides a thorough overview of local flaps for hand coverage.

Hallock GG: The random fasciocutaneous flap for upper extremity coverage. *J Hand Surg* 1992;17A:93–101.

This is a report of random, local fasciocutaneous flaps used to cover upper extremity wounds.

Hynes DE: Neurovascular pedicle and advancement flaps for palmar thumb defects. *Hand Clin* 1997;13:207–216.

The author provides a comprehensive review of flaps available for thumb coverage.

Karacalar A, Ozcan M: A new approach to the reverse dorsal metacarpal artery flap. *J Hand Surg* 1997;22:307–310.

Distally based metacarpal artery flaps are described.

Regional, Distant Flaps

Brown DM, Upton J, Khouri RK: Free flap coverage of the hand. *Clin Plast Surg* 1997;24:57–62.

This article provides a comprehensive description of free flap coverage options for the hand.

Koshima I, Moriguchi T, Etoh H, Tsuda K, Tonaka H: The radial artery perforator-based adipofascial flap for dorsal hand coverage. *Ann Plast Surg* 1995;35:474–479.

The authors describe a variant of the radial artery forearm flap that preserves the blood flow to the hand.

Chapter 25
Fingertip and Nail-Bed Injuries

Richard E. Brown, MD

Introduction

Fingertip and nail-bed injuries are 2 of the most common injuries encountered by hand surgeons. As such, they cause time lost from work and other activities. Many of these injuries can be repaired or reconstructed simply; however, others require more technically demanding procedures to avoid chronic deformity and disability.

Anatomy

The anatomy of the fingertip and nail bed has been well described (Fig. 1). However, replantations at a very distal level and reconstructions with various local axial island flaps have led to studies of the arterial and venous anatomy of the tip and nail bed. The ulnar digital artery is usually larger in the thumb, index, and long fingers, whereas the radial digital artery is almost always larger in the ring and small fingers. The paired digital arteries form 3 major palmar arches. The first is located just proximal to the proximal interphalangeal joint, the second is located just proximal to the distal interphalangeal (DIP) joint, and the most distal and important arch with regards to fingertip reconstruction is located just distal to the insertion of the profundus tendon. The diameter

of the vessel in the most distal arch averages 0.85 mm; generally, 3 longitudinal vessels with diameters averaging 0.58 mm arise off this arch. The longitudinal vessels travel to the tip of the pulp and then turn dorsally to communicate with a vascular arch overlying the sterile matrix. Branches arise on either side of the digit and course dorsally to form a proximal matrix arch near the lunula. These 2 dorsally coursing branches are about 0.48 mm in diameter.

Most of the venous drainage occurs over the dorsum of the fingers. There are a series of dorsal venous arches, one over each phalanx, which are connected through multiple longitudinal veins. A valvular system in these small veins directs the flow from distal to proximal, palmar to dorsal, and radial to ulnar.

There is a consistent branching of the digital nerve at about the eponychial level. One branch supplies the skin just proximal to the nail bed. The second branch generally supplies the lateral border of the nail bed, as well as the nail bed itself. The third, and largest branch, goes into the pad of the fingertip. Therefore, the digital nerve can be repaired out to the level of the lunula.

Fingertip Injuries

Fingertip injuries may involve loss of varying amounts of skin, fat, and bone. The amount and orientation of the tissue loss usually dictates the type of soft-tissue coverage needed. The 3 main types of coverage are healing by secondary intention, skin grafts, and flaps. Skin grafts may be split or full thickness. Flaps include local, regional, free, and replantation. In choosing the type of reconstruction, the surgeon must remember the nail bed requires bony support to prevent secondary hooking of the nail.

Healing By Secondary Intention
Healing by secondary intention has been recommended by many, especially in children and when no bone is exposed. Some even claim that the tip will "regenerate." However, radiographic studies have not shown regeneration. Nevertheless, healing by secondary intention is reasonable if there is adequate bony support for the nail and mostly soft-tissue loss. The patient must, however, be willing to do dressing

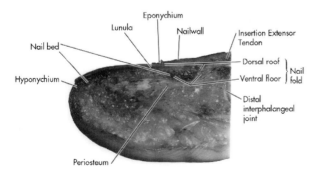

Figure 1

Anatomy of the nail bed. (Reproduced with permission from Zook EG: Nail Bed and Fingertip Injuries, in Manske PR (ed): *Hand Surgery Update*. Rosemont, IL, American Academy of Orthopaedic Surgeons, 1996, pp 289–293.)

changes over a period of 4 to 6 weeks. Opsite™ or Adaptic™ are alternatives to daily dressing changes; weekly changes decreased the pain in the healing tip. A finger cap made of Hyphecan, a substance made from chitin, has been used in Hong Kong as a 1-time dressing to allow healing by secondary intention. Although excellent results were reported, I am unsure if Hyphecan is available in the United States.

Grafts

Graft reconstruction of an injured fingertip may be by split- or full-thickness skin, from either the amputated part or another donor site. The amputated part may also be replaced as a composite graft. Split- or full-thickness grafts may be used if only skin and a very small amount of fat are missing from the tip. Grafts may be placed over small areas of bone exposure; however, a sensitive tip may result. Full-thickness grafts are probably more useful and can be taken from the amputated part, if available, or from the hypothenar eminence. The hypothenar area can usually be closed primarily with minimal donor site morbidity. Again, the surgeon must remember that for small defects, healing by secondary intention may incorporate sensate skin and thus be preferable to a small graft. Replacement of amputated parts by a composite graft, ie, skin, fat, and perhaps bone and nail bed, has been somewhat controversial. There is no doubt that the younger the patient, the better composite grafts work. An alternative is replacement of the part as a defatted and deboned composite graft consisting of full-thickness skin and nail bed if present (termed a "cap graft"). Whichever method is used, various techniques have been described to increase the chance of the graft "taking". The most common technique is deepithelialization of a portion of the replaced part and underlapping the deepithelialized skin with the skin of the finger. Others have recommended cooling the fingertip for 3 days.

Flaps

Various flaps have been described for coverage of the fingertip. The most commonly used flaps have been the volar V-Y advancement, the laterally based V-Y advancement, the cross finger, the reverse cross finger (upside down), the thenar crease, and the Moberg flap. These common flaps have been described in many surgery textbooks.

More recent literature has concentrated on various vascularized island flaps based on the same or a neighboring digit. These have been termed the homodigital island flap and the heterodigital island flap, respectively. Several variations of these flaps have been described. All involve taking a portion of the dorsal-lateral skin of the finger and advancing it either as a distally or a proximally based island. The distally based flaps have the disadvantage of transferring denervated skin

to the tip, whereas the proximal islands do not. The donor sites are generally covered with either split- or full-thickness skin grafts. Static 2-point discrimination in proximally based flaps varies, but is usually less than 10 mm. Cold intolerance continues to be a problem with all forms of reconstruction. The etiology of cold intolerance is unknown and treatment is difficult.

The ultimate and penultimate flaps for reconstruction of a traumatized tip are replantation of the part or acute reconstruction with a partial toe transfer. However, most partial toe transfers are delayed because of the crushing nature of the injuries; toe transfers are discussed under nail reconstruction.

Subsequent to the description of the minute arterial anatomy, replantation of the tip, even at the midnail level, has become a reality. A majority of reports of replantation come from the Orient, where loss of even a portion of the fingertip is a social stigma. Replantation from the DIP joint distally is successful in 70% to 80% of the patients. Often, at the nail-bed level, only an artery can be anastomosed and venous drainage obtained through heparin wipes. However, between the level of the DIP and the proximal nail fold, both arterial and venous anastomoses can be achieved with vessels generally under 0.5 mm in diameter. Although technically difficult, replacement of like with like can unequivocally yield the best result, as does replantation in other parts of the body. As with other fingertip reconstructions, cold intolerance and hypersensitivity may be a problem. Sensory return may be excellent, whether or not the digital nerve is repaired.

Nail-Bed Injuries

Following the reporting of the anatomy and physiology of the nail bed in the early 1980s, appropriate repair of nail-bed injuries became common. Since that time many authors have contributed to the various aspects of nail-bed reconstruction. However, in the past 4 or 5 years little new, except for microsurgery, has been reported about nail-bed repair and/or reconstruction.

Acute Injuries

As with fingertip injuries, nail-bed injuries must be assessed accurately. Simple nail-bed injuries, such as transverse lacerations or crush injuries resulting in stellate lacerations may be managed by complete nail removal and suture of the underlying nail bed with 7-0 chromic under loupe magnification. These injuries can be managed in the emergency room using finger tourniquets, and excellent outcomes are expected. The nail plate itself or silastic sheeting may be placed over the nail bed to mold the repair

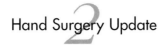
and add protection. The nail plate can also serve to help stabilize small tuft fractures. A dorsal figure-of-8 suture from the hyponychium to about 5 mm proximal to the nail fold offers "tension-band" fixation of small tuft fractures. If sutures are placed in the proximal nail plate to pull it into the nail fold, these sutures must be removed at the first visit to avoid sinus tract formation through the dorsal roof.

Traditional teaching has been that subungual hematomas greater than 25% to 50% require nail-plate removal and suture repair of the nail bed. However, recent reports have noted excellent nail growth and shape following simple evacuation of subungual hematomas, as long as the nail plate itself is still undisturbed. Consequently, nail-plate removal is now recommended only if the nail plate is mostly dislodged.

With loss of soft tissue and nail bed, care must be taken to ensure an adequate base for subsequent nail growth. Without adequate bony support some curving of the nail is expected, and with minimal support a hooked nail results. The combination of local flaps and nail-bed grafts results in a generally esthetic and functional tip, as long as reasonable bony support is present. Full-thickness nail grafts from the amputated part may be placed either on the denuded distal phalanx or the deepithelialized flap used to reconstruct the tip. Grafts and repairs can be done acutely in the emergency room.

Split-thickness nail-bed grafts can be placed acutely when there is avulsion of the nail bed itself. Grafts may be harvested from the same digit, a neighboring finger, or more commonly from the great toe. A template of the defect is made and transferred to the donor nail bed. Generally, if the physician is unable to take a graft from the remaining nail bed of the injured digit, the great toe nail bed is chosen to allow adequate size. The nail is removed and the template placed on the sterile matrix of the great toe. After outlining, the edges of the graft are incised partial thickness using the tip of a 15-blade scalpel. The 15 blade is used to harvest the graft ensuring that the graft is thin enough to visualize the blade at all times. The graft is sutured into place using 7-0 chromic suture. The toe nail plate is placed back onto the toe for comfort and protection.

Full-thickness grafts can also be harvested from any amputated part or digit that will be discarded. Take of both split- and full-thickness grafts is generally excellent, and the grafts can be placed directly on an exposed digital phalanx.

Nail-Bed Reconstruction

Split-Thickness Sterile Matrix Grafts
Split-thickness sterile matrix grafts may be used to reconstruct the sterile matrix when the nail is split or nonadherent. After nail-plate removal, the area of the scar is visualized best by magnification, using either high power loupes or the operating microscope. The scar is excised and a template is made. It is imperative not to invert the template, or the graft will not fit. The graft is harvested and sutured into place. Split sterile matrix graft can only replace sterile and not germinal matrix. Split germinal matrix grafts cannot be used to replace the germinal matrix because the basilar layer must be retained to produce hard nail. Postoperative care is managed using either the old nail plate or 0.020-in reinforced Silastic sheeting.

Germinal Matrix and Composite Grafts
Free grafts of the germinal matrix alone, or in conjunction with the dorsal roof and a portion of the sterile matrix may be used for nail-bed reconstruction when hard-nail production is lacking. However, the outcome from isolated or combined germinal matrix grafting is inconsistent. Composite or germinal matrix grafts were reported to do better in younger patients, but in a recent series of composite grafts no distinct correlation was found between patient age or size of the graft and outcome. It is generally believed that these grafts work better acutely when scarring is not present. Therefore, in delayed reconstruction excision of all scar is important.

When harvesting a composite nail bed graft, depending on the size of the graft needed, it is often easier to harvest the dorsal roof, germinal matrix, and sterile matrix leaving the hard nail plate in place. Such harvesting avoids trauma to delicate structures and stabilizes the graft in its new position. However, enough plate must be removed to facilitate insetting and suturing.

Eponychial Grafts
Composite grafts of the dorsal roof (eponychium) may be used to correct a deformity of an eponychium on a finger. Deformities may occur following excision of a tumor in the eponychium, burns, abrasions, or lacerations. Loss of the dorsal roof often leaves a dull roughened appearance of the nail plate.

First the recipient site is created. In reconstruction the surgeon should cut back to nonscarred tissue. A template is made and the graft harvested from one of the toes. The dorsal roof and the overlying skin are harvested; the roof is sutured with 7-0 chromic and the skin with 5 or 6-0 nylon. The toe is allowed to heal in by secondary intention, which rarely leaves a significant deformity.

Pincer Nail Deformity

The pincer or trumpet nail deformity consists of a marked increase in the side-to-side curvature of the nail, which is more pronounced as the nail progresses distally. The deformity can be so severe as to nearly pinch off the hyponychium. The etiology is unknown, but the deformity has followed trauma and other disease processes.

Most of the reported treatments have included at least partial ablation of the nail bed. Until recently, long-term results of treatment have not been reported. A series of pincer nail deformities corrected by dermal grafting has recently been reported. The nail plate was removed. The radial and ulnar edges of the nail bed, which curves around the lateral aspects of the distal phalanx, were freed from the distal phalanx at the hyponychium and tunnels created under the lateral nail bed to the lateral edges of the germinal matrix. Dermal grafts were pulled through the radial and ulnar tunnels to support and prevent readherence of the nail bed. The abnormal nail plate was discarded and replaced with 0.020-in Silastic sheeting. Pain was relieved, and the appearance of the nail improved.

Hook Nail Deformity

A hook nail deformity primarily results from loss of bony support of the nail bed. Tethering of the nail bed to the hyponychium can also cause some mild hooking. Correction of the established deformity is very difficult. The surgeon must either provide new bony support or shorten the finger so that any remaining nail bed overlies the distal phalanx.

Minor success follows the use of soft-tissue flaps for correction. The technique includes the elevation of the curved portion of the nail bed and a small amount of underlying soft tissue. The gap created is filled in with a cross-finger, thenar, or local flap. The best results have been with partial toe transfers to lengthen the distal phalanx and provide adequate support for the nail bed.

Annotated Bibliography

Anatomy

Strauch B, de Moura W: Arterial system of the fingers. *J Hand Surg* 1990;15A:148–154.

The authors provide a detailed anatomic description of the arterial system of the fingers including the fingertip.

Zook EG, Van Beek AL, Russell RC, Beatty ME: Anatomy and physiology of the perionychium: A review of the literature and anatomic study. *J Hand Surg* 1980;5A:528–536.

This article provides the basic anatomy and physiology of the fingertip.

Fingertip Injuries

Adani R, Busa R, Castagnetti C, Bathia A, Caroli A: Homodigital neurovascular island flaps with "direct flow" vascularization. *Ann Plast Surg* 1997;38:36–40.

The authors illustrate a distally advanced homodigital island flap for fingertip reconstruction. Excellent range of motion and normal to mildly diminished 2-point discrimination usually were achieved.

Bene MD, Petrolati M, Raimondi P, Tremolada C, Muset A: Reverse dorsal digital island flap. *Plast Reconstr Surg* 1994;93:552–557.

A dorsal finger flap based on small subcutaneous arterial and venous branches is rotated distally as an island. Although the blood supply appears somewhat tenuous, the authors report minimal complications in 12 cases.

Bindra RR: Management of nail-bed fracture-lacerations using a tension-band suture. *J Hand Surg* 1996;21A:1111–1113.

A figure-of-8 suture overlying the nail plate is placed from the hyponychium to just proximal to the nail fold as a tension band for distal phalangeal fractures.

Dubert T, Houimli S, Valenti P, Dinh A: Very distal finger amputations: Replantation or "reposition-flap" repair? *J Hand Surg* 1997;22B:353–358.

Fingertip reconstruction using a "reposition-flap" is compared to fingertip replantation. In the reposition-flap technique, the nail unit and the underlying distal phalanx of the amputated part are replaced as nonvascularized grafts; the pulp is reconstructed with a homodigital flap. Results with the reposition flap were less satisfactory than replantation, but the reposition flap provides an alternative when replantation cannot be done.

Germann G, Rutschle S, Kania N, Raff T: The reverse pedicle heterodigital cross-finger island flap. *J Hand Surg* 1997;228 25–29.

The authors describe a reverse heterodigital island flap for cases where a traditional cross-finger or homodigital flap cannot be used. Although the indication for such a flap is uncommon, this paper adds yet another flap to those available for fingertip reconstruction.

Hirase Y: Salvage of fingertip amputated at nail level: New surgical principles and treatments. *Ann Plast Surg* 1997;38:151–157.

The author describes a classification of fingertip amputations that provides a useful guideline for surgical management.

Ishikura N, Tsukada S: An easy method of vascular anastomosis for replantation of fingertips. *J Reconstr Microsurg* 1995;11:141–143.

A vascular stent made from a silicone background is used for anastomosis of tiny vessels during fingertip replantation. The stent facilitates placement of the sutures and can be removed before tying the final suture.

Lee LP, Lau PY, Chan CW: A simple and efficient treatment for fingertip injuries. *J Hand Surg* 1995;20B:63–71.

An occlusive dressing called a fingertip cap is described for healing by secondary intention. Numerous cases are illustrated.

Tsai T-M, Yuen JC: A neurovascular island flap for volar-oblique fingertip amputations: Analysis of long-term results. *J Hand Surg* 1996;218:94–98.

A local advancement flap from the dorsal lateral aspect of the finger just proximal to the nail may be useful in specific cases.

Nail-Bed Injuries

Hirase Y, Kojima T, Matsui M: Aesthetic fingertip reconstruction with a free vascularized nail graft: A review of 60 flaps involving partial toe transfers. *Plast Reconstr Surg* 1997; 99:774–784.

This article provides a useful guideline and several illustrative cases for vascularized nail and fingertip reconstruction.

Koshima I, Moriguchi T, Umeda N, Yamada A: Trimmed second toetip transfer for reconstruction of claw nail deformity of the fingers. *Br J Plast Surg* 1992;45B:591–594.

The authors describe 2 cases of claw or hook nail deformity corrected by a partial toe transfer. The technique represents true reconstruction of the tip and is probably the only way to restore a normal tip from a hook nail deformity.

Kumar VP, Satku K: Treatment and prevention of "hook nail" deformity with anatomic correlation. *J Hand Surg* 1993; 18A:617–620.

The authors describe a technique for correction of a hook nail deformity, first by removal of the nail bed unsupported by the distal phalanx and second by closure with a volar V-Y flap.

Chapter 26
Dupuytren's Disease

Ghazi M. Rayan, MD

Nearly 150 articles related to Dupuytren's disease have been published in the last 6 years. The literature encompasses letters, editorials, case reports, historical accounts and review articles; clinical material, including international epidemiologic studies; and basic science investigations. This plethora of material, especially in the basic science area, reflects the continuing and prodigious interest of clinicians and basic scientists in this enigmatic and elusive disease. Basic information and newly evolved knowledge or lack thereof, will be reviewed in the following sections.

History

Records dating back to the twelfth and thirteenth centuries contain descriptions of a condition resembling Dupuytren's disease. In 1614 Felix Platter, a Swiss physician, described what became known as the stonemason's hand. He believed that the flexion deformity was due to flexor tendon contracture. This error persisted until 1777, coincidentally the year Dupuytren was born, when the British surgeon Henry Cline dissected 2 diseased cadaveric hands and recognized that the true nature of the condition was contracture of the palmar fascia. In 1787, Cline also described palmar fasciotomy and its effect on partial correction of the deformity. Cooper, influenced by Cline, advocated the use of closed fasciotomy in 1822. Elective surgery was rarely performed because anesthesia was not available and fatal sepsis was feared.

The French surgeon Guillaume Dupuytren's 1831 lecture at the Hotel Dieu in Paris established the nature of the permanent retraction of the fingers, and gave the disease its eponym in the late 1800s. Dupuytren likely received the credit because of his thorough description of the condition and his detailed recital of the normal and pathologic palmar fascial anatomy. Unlike Cline and Cooper, who were lecturers, Dupuytren published his findings in 1832 and 1834. Over 250 references to Dupuytren's disease were published between its first description and the turn of the century. In the last 100 years, innumerable clinical and basic science publications have greatly expanded our understanding of Dupuytren's disease.

Epidemiology

Because of a dearth of related epidemiologic research, the true incidence of Dupuytren's disease in the United States is unknown. There is considerable disparity among available international epidemiologic studies regarding its prevalence. Reports of prevalence of Dupuytren's among Japanese males, for example, vary from 3% to 26%. Although the disease is very common in Australia, it is rare among native Australians; similarly the disease is common in the United States yet rare among native Americans. The incidence and prevalence of Dupuytren's disease are influenced by geography, gender, and age. The Nordic theory suggests that the disease originated from one racial group and was distributed in other areas as a result of migration. The Scandinavian invaders were the aboriginals who brought this Viking disease to the modern Europeans. The disease prevalence varies in different parts of the world. Dupuytren's disease is very common in northern Europe, including Scandinavia; common in the United Kingdom, Ireland, Australia, and northern America; uncommon in southern Mediterranean Europe and in South America; and rare in Africa and China. The disease is very common among descendants of the Celts and Caucasians of northern Europe; common among Caucasians of North America; uncommon among native Australians and Asians; rare among native Africans, African Americans, native Americans, and Gypsies.

The male to female ratio has been reported as high as 9:1; however, with advancing age there is an increase in the disease incidence among women, decreasing the ratio to 4:1. The disease is less severe and has later onset in females, and is extremely rare among children below the age of 13 years. Dupuytren reported the first case of a 6-year-old, who had small and ring finger contracture since birth. Congenital or very early onset Dupuytren's disease should raise suspicion of other diagnoses such as camptodactyly. A few pediatric cases were recently reported, but histologic confirmation of fibromatosis was not obtained.

Numerous studies have linked cigarette smoking and alcohol consumption to Dupuytren's disease. Smoking increases the risk of developing Dupuytren's disease and may contribute to its prevalence among alcoholics, who tend to smoke heavily. One study demonstrated that alcoholics have a higher rate of Dupuytren's disease largely due to liver involvement, and nonalcoholic patients with liver disease have a higher incidence than controls. The relationship is probably due to the influence of alcohol on lipid metabolism. In another report, the incidence of Dupuytren's disease was 13% among elderly veterans living in England and Ireland; family history was present in 9%. Drinking, diabetes, and manual occupational demands were not contributing factors. Dupuytren's disease appears to be more prevalent among HIV patients than in the general population.

Recent reports have demonstrated a higher incidence of the disease in diabetic patients, without gender difference; presence of Dupuytren's disease is related to joint stiffness, carpal tunnel syndrome, and flexor tenosynovitis. The patient's age and duration of diabetes are factors predicting the development of a mild form of Dupuytren's disease. Several studies showed an increase incidence of Dupuytren's disease in epileptics linked to the influence of antiepileptic medication. Epileptic patients appear to have more severe Dupuytren's disease than nonepileptic patients. One investigation could not implicate drug therapy (ie, anticonvulsants and phenobarbital) in the etiology of Dupuytren's disease.

Etiologic Factors

Traumatic, neoplastic, and genetic factors may be involved in the etiology of Dupuytren's disease. The controversy regarding traumatic etiology began with Dupuytren's declaration in 1831 that the disease was occupational, due to chronic local trauma. Three years later, Goyrand contested the relationship to manual work citing his hospital manager who had bilateral disease yet did no hard manual labor. He also questioned why bilateral disease would occur in a coachman who whipped with only one hand. Recent occupational medicine studies have demonstrated a relationship between Dupuytren's disease and occupational hand trauma among workers exposed to vibration. An incidence of 19% was reported in patients with vibration white finger compared to 10% among controls. There is insufficient evidence to confirm that manual labor hastens either the onset or progress of the disease. Controlled studies have not linked acute trauma to typical Dupuytren's disease.

Proliferation of fibroblasts in Dupuytren's disease was once suggested to be neoplastic in nature; accordingly, the disease was categorized as a fibromatosis. Modern immunocytochemical techniques have demonstrated a relationship between sarcoma and Dupuytren's disease nodular fibroblasts. One group compared growth characteristics of cultured Dupuytren's disease and fibrosarcoma fibroblasts.

They concluded that the Dupuytren's disease nodule is a benign mesenchymal tumor with high levels of plasminogen activator, and the nodule is a mode of benign tumor progression.

Growth factors present in neoplastic conditions may influence Dupuytren's disease and be involved in its pathogenesis. Basic fibroblast growth factor (BFGF) was identified in Dupuytren's disease tissue. The cellular areas of nodules containing myofibroblasts express high levels of transforming growth factor (TGF)-α and epidermal growth factor. Hurst and Badalamente documented the localization of TGF-β within myofibroblasts, but not in extracellular matrix (ECM), and the effect of TGF-β on myofibroblast proliferation. They also found platelet-derived growth factor (PDGF) to be expressed by Dupuytren's disease tissue, and suggested a role for TGF-β and PDGF in the pathogenesis of Dupuytren's disease. Growth factors are involved in the pathogenesis of neoplasia, Dupuytren's disease, early wound healing, and inflammatory conditions.

Inheritance appears to be an important factor in the etiology of Dupuytren's disease. In one series of 50 patients with Dupuytren's disease, the reported disease incidence among relatives was 16%. When more than 800 relatives of these patients were examined, the true incidence was found to be 68%. The disease has an autosomal dominant mode of transmission with variable penetrance. Heuston described Dupuytren's disease in terms of diathesis, or disease aggressiveness and inherited tendency. Patients with strong diathesis had early onset, severe disease, higher incidence of recurrence, and less favorable outcome.

In a report on identical twins, only one had developed Dupuytren's disease suggesting that genetic background alone is insufficient for development of the disease. Chromosomal abnormalities were detected in karyotyping of cell cultures from Dupuytren's disease. Clones of cells trisomic for chromosome 8 were encountered, along with abnormalities in the Y chromosome. Etiologically, Dupuytren's disease appears to be multifactorial, with genetic factors of primary importance.

Molecular Biology and Pathophysiology

Immunocytochemical and cell culture experiments have provided new insights into the pathophysiology of Dupuytren's disease. Similarities exist between the pathologic changes in Dupuytren's disease nodules and wound healing; in Dupuytren's disease, however, the process is progressive and sporadic. The myofibroblast, the quintessential cell in

Dupuytren's disease, has morphologic characteristics of both fibroblasts and smooth muscle cells (Fig. 1). Although the cell of origin is uncertain, it is likely a modulated contractile fibroblast. The key differences from fibroblasts are its larger size; indented nucleus; cytoplasmic actin microfilaments, ie, stress fibers (alpha smooth muscle type); nonmuscle myosin; and intermediate filament cytoskeletal protein, such as vimentin and desmin. Myofibroblasts can actively contract; their contractile property is influenced by several agents, such as prostaglandins and lysophosphatidic acid. The contractile property is partially responsible for the palmar fascia contracture in Dupuytren's disease. Intracellular actin is a marker for myofibroblasts. A positive correlation has been observed between alpha smooth muscle actin (SMA) expression and the generation of contractile force in Dupuytren's fibroblasts. SMA may be related to a strong diathesis and high postoperative recurrence rate. Macrophages encountered in Dupuytren's tissue are the source of growth factors and free radicals. Increased levels of hypoxanthine and oxygen-free radicals in Dupuytren's disease tissue may contribute to cellular proliferation.

The ECM in Dupuytren's disease is responsible for synthesis and deposition of fibronectin, a protein that connects myofibroblasts to one another (cell-to-cell) and to stromal ECM (cell-to-stroma) by means of integrin. Fibronectin seems to be responsible for transmitting cellular contraction (Fig. 2). Fibronectin is also concentrated around the myofibroblast cell surface. Expression of the extra domain EDA and EDB isoforms of fibronectin is pronounced in Dupuytren's disease tissue, but nominal in normal tissue.

Normal palmar tissue has proteoglycans, type I collagen and a small amount of type III collagen. All 3 components increase in both diseased and normal palmar fascia of patients with Dupuytren's disease. In Dupuytren's disease abundant collagen is produced from both greater synthesis and fibroblast population. There is an increased ratio of type III to type I collagen, especially in the early stages of the disease. Transglutaminase expression is observed in active stages of Dupuytren's disease because of its ability to catalyze cross-linking of collagen molecules.

The myofibroblast is encountered in the active or involutional stage of Dupuytren's disease. However, myofibroblasts have been identified in Dupuytren's disease nodules with variable degrees in all stages (proliferative, involutional, and residual). Types IV and VI collagen, laminin, and fibronectin deposition in ECM are associated with proliferative activity of myofibroblasts and strongly expressed in cellular areas. Type VI collagen is present in normal palmar aponeuroses, but nearly disappears from tissue undergoing fibrotic remodeling.

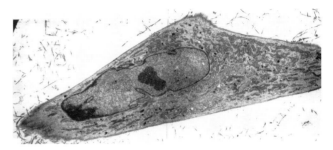

Figure 1

Electron micrograph of a cultured fibroblast, which acquired characteristics of a myofibroblast, in collagen lattice prior to contraction. (Reproduced with permission from Tomasek JJ, Haaksma CJ, Eddy RJ, Vaughan MB: Fibroblast contraction occurs on release of tension in attached collagen lattices: Dependency on an organized actin cytoskeleton and serum. *Anat Rec* 1992;232:359–368.)

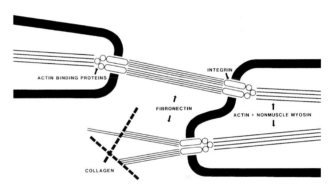

Figure 2

Contractile fibroblasts and extracellular matrix, showing cell-to cell and cell-to-stroma connections. (Reproduced with permission from McFarlane R, McGrouther D, Flint M (eds): *Dupuytren's Disease: Biology and Treatment.* New York, NY, Churchill Livingstone, 1990, p 98.)

There is a possibility that Dupuytren's disease is a T-cell-mediated autoimmune disorder. Whether an autoimmune phenomenon plays a role in the pathogenesis of Dupuytren's disease remains a subject of controversy. HLA-typed Dupuytren's disease patients were found to have HLA-DR3, which was also detected in the peripheral blood of Peyronie's disease patients. Messenger RNAs and cytokines, including interleukin-1, BFGF, and TGF-β, have been identified in Dupuytren's tissue. BFGF and PDGF are mitogenic for normal and diseased fibroblasts. TGF-β is a potent stimulator of collagen deposition and fibroblast proliferation in both cell types. However, Dupuytren's cells are more metabolically active and sensitive to growth factors. Regulation of biochemistry and agents such as SMA and growth factors may one day allow nonoperative control of Dupuytren's disease.

Experiments with continuous traction suggest a role for physical forces in influencing at least temporarily the course of the disease. Continuous elongation applied to diseased and normal fascia causes electron microscopic changes in both tissues. Monofilament stress fibers appear in the endothelial cells of microvessels only in Dupuytren's tissue. The response to mechanical stress probably affects the contractile component of the cytoskeleton. Increased levels of degradative enzymes and loss of tensile strength of the palmar fascia are also observed. One group showed an increase in proliferation of cell cultures subjected to mechanical strain. The increase was highest for Dupuytren's disease-involved tissue, compared to uninvolved fascia from Dupuytren's disease patients and normal fascia. PDGF-β expression was enhanced in diseased palmar fascia, suggesting that it may be the mediator in response to cyclic stress. The response of the diseased tissue to continuous elongation and prolonged splinting contradicts and challenges the popular notion that the disease is progressive and irreversible. Physical forces appear to influence biochemical processes and play a role in the pathogenesis of Dupuytren's disease. Future basic science research will undoubtedly further examine the influence of biomechanical processes on collagen morphology and focus on these physical and chemical interactions. Perhaps nonsurgical control of the disease may one day be attained by mechanical means and pharmacologic agents.

Anatomy

Palmar fascia includes the palmar aponeurosis (PA) and lateral extensions to the thenar and hypothenar areas. The PA has 3-dimensional fiber orientation—longitudinal, transverse, and vertical. The longitudinal fibers are condensed into 5 fascicles or pretendinous bands, one for each digit. Each pretendinous band (PB) divides into 2 slips. Distally, the PB trifurcates into 3 layers. The superficial layer inserts into the dermis. The fibers of the middle layer partly terminate in the proximal digit; the remaining fibers run deep to the neurovascular bundle and natatory ligament as the spiral band, and eventually insert into the lateral digital sheet. The fibers of the deep layer run almost vertically and attach to the extensor mechanism (Fig. 3). The transverse fibers form the natatory ligament and superficial transverse ligament of Albinus, which runs deep to the PBs.

The vertically oriented fibers are of 2 types: multiple minute vertical bands that are superficial to and bind the PA to the dermis; and 8 vertical septa of Legueu and Juvara, which extend from the deep surface of the PA to the interosseous muscle fascia, metacarpals, and deep transverse metacarpal ligaments (Fig. 4). The septa form canals for the

passage of flexor tendons ulnarly and neurovascular bundles and lumbrical muscles radially. The palmodigital fascia consists of transitional tissue between the PA and digital fascia. The web-space fascial coalescence consists of fibers from natatory ligaments, spiral bands, lateral sheets, and vertical

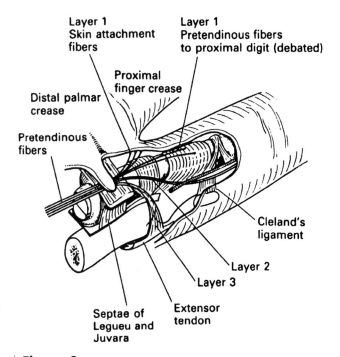

Figure 3

Termination of the pretendinous band into 3 layers. (Adapted with permission from McFarlane R, McGrouther D, Flint M (eds): *Dupuytren's Disease: Biology and Treatment.* New York, NY, Churchill Livingstone, 1990, p 134.)

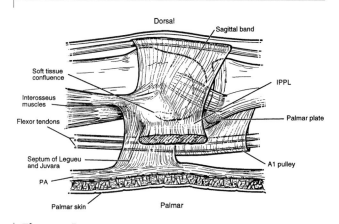

Figure 4

Three-dimensional longitudinal cross-sectional anatomy at the metacarpophalangeal joint level. PA = palmar aponeurosis, IPPL = interpalmar plate ligament (Reproduced with permission from Rayan GM: Palmar fascial complex anatomy and pathology in Dupuytren's disease. *Hand Clin* 1999;15:73–86.)

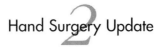
septa. The fibers of the web-space coalescence are bound by digital neurovascular bundles on either side. The digital fascia (Fig. 5) consists of the lateral digital sheet, spiral band, Grayson's ligaments, retrovascular fibers, Cleland's ligaments, and retinacular ligaments. The thumb fascia includes the PB and 2 commissural ligaments, distal (natatory ligament) and proximal (superficial transverse ligament).

Dupuytren's disease is a process of fascial contracture pursued along anatomic pathways, in which normal anatomy becomes distorted in a predictable fashion. The diseased palmar fascia (Fig. 6) includes the pretendinous cord, which originates from the PB and causes metacarpophalangeal (MCP) joint flexion contracture; and the natatory cord, which originates from the natatory ligament, extends dorsally along the lateral side of the digit, and causes web-space contracture. Skin pits are developed by contracture of the superficial layer of the PB. The diseased digital fascia causes proximal interphalangeal joint flexion deformity and includes the central

cord, which may originate from the middle layer of PB or from the fibrofatty tissue, and the lateral cord, which arises from the lateral digital sheet. The retrovascular cord is said to develop from the retrovascular fibers, but some doubt its existence. The spiral cord components are PB, spiral band, lateral digital sheet, and Grayson's ligament. A portion of the web-space coalescence therefore contributes to spiral cord formation. Intraoperatively, it becomes apparent that the nerve is the structure that spirals around the cord. The precursors of the isolated digital cord are the same as the spiral cord without PB contribution. On the ulnar side of the hand, the abductor digiti minimi cord is less defined than other cords. It is adherent to the skin, believed to originate from the muscle fascia, and extends to the ulnar side of the proximal phalanx. The vertical cord develops from the fibers of the PB deep vertical layer, or less frequently the 8 vertical septa. The radial side of the hand is affected less commonly than the ulnar side, and can be a cause of disability. The diseased thumb fascia (Fig.7)

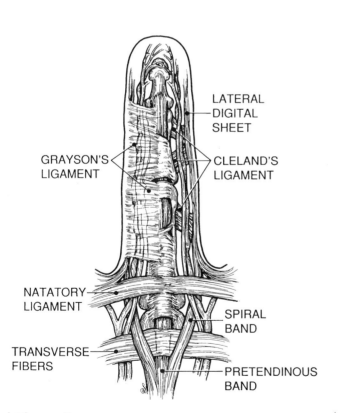

Figure 5

Normal palmar and digital fascial structures, which are precursors of diseased tissue in Dupuytren's disease. (Reproduced with permission from McFarlane RM: Patterns of the diseased fascia in the fingers in Dupuytren's contracture. *Plast Reconstr Surg* 1974;54:31–44.)

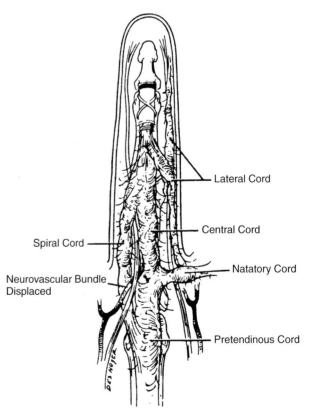

Figure 6

Diseased palmar and digital fascial structures encountered in Dupuytren's disease. (Reproduced with permission from Strickland JW, Basset RL: The isolated digital cord in Dupuytren's contractures: Anatomy and clinical significance. *J Hand Surg* 1985; 10A:118–124.)

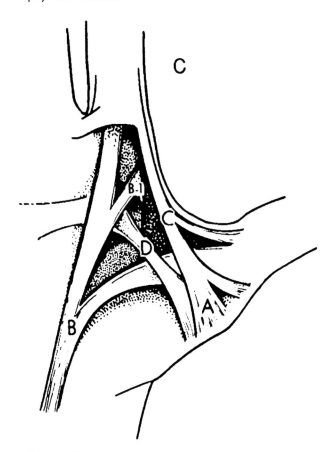

Figure 7
Fascial structure of the radial side of the hand. A = thenar cord insertion, B = pretendinous cord, C = distal commissural cord, D = proximal commissural cord. (Reproduced with permission from Tubiana R: Location of Dupuytren's disease on radial aspect of the hand. *Clin Orthop* 1982;168:222–229.)

disease was described by McFarlane as a white male, northern European, approximately 57 years old, with bilateral disease that may involve more than one digit. Patients with typical disease usually have a family history. In patients with atypical Dupuytren's contracture, race and gender become irrelevant and a family history is not present. The patient may have systemic disease, such as longstanding diabetes, or on occasion rheumatoid arthritis. The condition may develop following hand surgery and a history of trauma, such as wrist or hand fracture, may be present. The disease is confined to the hand, often remains in the palm without digital extension, and usually affects only one hand. The condition is either regressive or nonprogressive. Surgical treatment is rarely indicated in atypical contracture patients. Recurrence of the contracture is uncommon after surgery.

A number of unusual Dupuytren's contracture cases have been reported in the recent literature. These cases include disease among indigenous Africans and African Americans triggered by surgical trauma (eg, carpal tunnel release, trigger-finger releases, and foreign body removal). These unusual cases often share similar clinical backgrounds. Their race and gender vary; family history is absent; and the disease is not severe, is confined to the hand, and rarely bilateral. Surgical treatment is rarely necessary. African Americans are reported to have a less extensive diathesis or severity and predisposition than Caucasians. In a series of patients with distal radius fractures, the incidence of Dupuytren's disease was 9%. The condition developed within 6 months after injury; most patients had nodules or skin pits in the palm in line with the ring finger; digital contracture did not develop; and the disease remained static. These cases are probably atypical Dupuytren's contracture rather than typical. The disparity in reports of the disease prevalence and recurrence rates may be due to lack of distinction between typical and atypical types. Future epidemiologic and outcome studies should take into consideration typical and atypical varieties.

Clinical Findings

The genesis of the typical Dupuytren's disease lesion is ushered by the formation of a nodule and sometimes an associated skin pit. Nodules are located adjacent to the distal palmar crease, often in line with the ring and small fingers, at the base of the thumb and small finger, and near the proximal interphalangeal joint. The nodule gradually regresses, giving way to development of a cord. Nodules and cords have different pathology; some believe they may even have a different tissue of origin. There are 2 schools of thought regarding the origin of nodules in Dupuytren's disease. An

compromises the pretendinous cord, which infrequently causes MCP joint flexion contracture, and the first web commissural cords (the natatory and superficial transverse cords), which both cause first web-space contracture. A less distinct thenar cord can be encountered on the radial side of the thumb; this cord courses along, blends with the thenar muscle fascia, and inserts on the radial aspect of the thumb MCP joint. The thenar cord may be analogous to the abductor digiti minimi cord on the ulnar side of the hand.

Clinical Types

I have observed 2 distinct clinical types of palmar fasial contracture—typical Dupuytren's disease and atypical Dupuytren's contracture. The typical patient with Dupuytren's

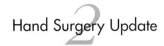
extrinsic theory suggests that the disease originates from fibrofatty tissue outside the palmar aponeurosis; an intrinsic theory proposes that the disease originates from normal palmar fascia. The disease seems to originate in the superficial components of the palmar fascia and its fine extensions into the dermis. The diseased fascia rarely can extend proximal to the wrist crease into the deep layer of the superficial fascia or flexor carpi ulnaris tendon.

Dupuytren's nodules should be differentiated from epithelioid sarcoma. Nodules are painful when associated with stenosing tenosynovitis and trigger finger, which develop either from direct pressure on the flexor tendons and A1 pulley or from a vertical cord. As the disease progresses, palmar and proximal interphalangeal joint nodules transform into pretendinous and digital cords. Digital cords sometimes interconnect with or extend from pretendinous cords. Pretendinous cords should be differentiated from palmar bands or prolapsed flexor tendons due to attenuation of annular pulleys as in rheumatoid arthritis. Ledderhose disease (plantar fibromatosis) and Peyronie's disease (penile fibromatosis) may be encountered in patients with a strong diathesis. Garrod's nodes, or knuckle pads, are fibrosing lesions often associated with bilateral, Ledderhose or Peyronie disease.

One group found a 52% prevalence of spiral nerve intraoperatively; however, 42% had a palpable interdigital soft-tissue mass. The presence of a soft-tissue mass was specific (75%), but not sensitive (59%) for spiral nerve presence. Prolonged proximal interphalangeal joint contracture in Dupuytren's disease may be associated with attenuation of the central slip, especially when the deformity exceeds 60°. After digital fasciectomy, an intraoperative tenodesis test can confirm central slip attenuation. Proximal interphalangeal joint extension splinting after surgery can help restore central slip function.

Dupuytren's disease patients can have significantly higher fasting serum cholesterol and triglyceride levels than controls; elevated serum lipids may play a role in the pathogenesis of the disease. The association of alcohol and phenobarbital with Dupuytren's disease may be through their influence on lipid metabolism. Magnetic resonance imaging, although not practical, can show palmar involvement in Dupuytren's disease. The signal characteristic of the diseased tissue correlates with the cellularity of the lesion as seen histologically.

Treatment

Static painless disease with minimal contracture and without functional compromise merits only observation. Recent basic science research has indicated the potential of certain agents in nonsurgical control of the disease or as an adjunct to surgical treatment. Calcium channel blockers could potentially be used for early stages, and collagenase for late stages of the disease. Steroid injection of nodules has been used in an attempt to suppress the disease. Enzymatic fasciotomy with injection of trypsin, hyaluronidase and lignocaine followed by forcible extension of the digit achieves immediate improvement, but has a high recurrence rate. Intralesional injection of gamma-interferon lessens the symptoms and size of the lesions in both Dupuytren's disease and hypertrophic scars by decreasing alpha SMA expression and collagen production. Radiation therapy was used in early stages to minimize disease progression and avoid surgery. Additional studies on unconventional treatment methods are needed.

MCP joint contracture of greater than 30° and proximal interphalangeal flexion contracture of any degree in the presence of a well-developed cord are indications for surgical treatment. Fasciotomy and limited fasciectomy with local anesthetic are indicated for patients in poor general condition. Partial fasciectomy of only the diseased tissue, rather than total fasciectomy, is the most widely used treatment. Outpatient surgery offers considerable savings and is recommended in an otherwise healthy patient with moderate hand involvement. The outcome of surgical treatment is influenced more by the method of skin closure than the type of surgery. Some surgeons believe that skin grafts fare better than the open palm technique. Dermofasciectomy and skin grafting appear to have better outcomes and lower recurrence rates (especially beneath the graft) than other surgical techniques. Dermatofasciectomy and skin grafting are recommended for recurrent cases and for primary aggressive disease when the nodule-cord unit adheres to the skin. A midterm review of dermofasciectomy results showed a 10% recurrence of nodule formation limited to graft insets (proximal or distal), but no recurrence of cords. Other complications appear to be less common with dermatofasciectomy. A marked increase (from 24% to 79%) in disease extension was noted in one 10-year follow-up of dermofasciectomy patients, but the recurrence rate of the disease remained constant at 47%.

Satisfactory results with the open palm technique continue to be reported. A modified MacCash open palm technique, combining transverse and Bruner incisions and leaving the transverse palmar and digital wounds open, was also used with satisfactory results and a low complication rate. All surgery was done with axillary block on an outpatient basis. Hematoma, skin necrosis, and infection were not encountered; angular correction was 79%. The recurrence rate (41%, 23% of which were severe) was similar to other limited fasciectomy techniques. Early age of onset and involvement of the proximal interphalangeal joint and fifth digit adversely affected results. Segmental aponeurectomy has been proposed as a less extensive procedure for the treatment of Dupuytren's disease. This procedure is done through a series of C-shaped incisions; 1-cm segments of diseased tissue are excised. The procedure limits wound complications and joint stiffness associated with wide dissections. Segmental aponeurectomy was reported to have a similar recurrence rate (38%) to other surgical techniques even though diseased tissue is left behind.

The adjunctive surgical release of proximal interphalangeal flexion after fasciectomy is traditionally indicated for residual deformity greater than 40°, but the recent trend is shifting away from releasing residual proximal interphalangeal joint contracture. Attempts to fully correct severe deformity may lead to scarring or dorsal dislocation of the joint.

Severe contracture of the proximal interphalangeal joint in Dupuytren's disease has been treated by fasciectomy and sequential joint release, followed by 6 months of dynamic extension splints. Improvement in joint contracture was observed at 2 years in 59% of patients who complied with the splinting program; improvement among noncompliant patients was only 25%. Severity of contracture, involved digit, and capsular release did not affect outcome. The authors suggested that soft tissues in Dupuytren's disease respond to continuous dynamic extension and are capable of remolding over time.

Preoperative and postoperative skeletal traction with external fixation devices has been recommended to improve correction of severe proximal interphalangeal joint contractures. In severe cases, continuous elongation prior to fasciectomy has been shown to improve the deformity, facilitate surgery, minimize the need for amputation, and alter the collagen orientation and even the metabolism of the fascia. Although continuous elongation provides additional options for treating difficult cases, it is associated with a high rate of such complications as infection, loosening, recurrence, stiffness, and even amputation. According to one report, residual flexion deformity of the proximal interphalangeal joint after digital fasciectomy can be corrected by gentle passive manipulation without aggressive intervention. Studies comparing the results of fasciectomy with or without capsulotomy showed no advantage to concomitant capsuloligamentous release, but a higher complication rate with release. Rotation flaps from the side of the fourth and fifth digits can be used for treating severe cases of Dupuytren's disease. Distally based dorsal hand flaps can also be useful, especially in recurrent cases, for resurfacing palmar skin defects. Amputation can be avoided by osteotomy, arthrodesis, or arthroplasty of the proximal

interphalangeal joint. Amputation remains an option in management of Dupuytren's disease; it is most commonly indicated for the small finger followed by the ring finger. Amputation is especially useful in severe recurrent cases with digital nerve injury. Because recurrent lack of MCP extension may follow amputations distal to this joint, disarticulation at the MCP joint is preferred by some over more distal amputations. Filleting of the finger and MCP disarticulation allow use of the dorsal skin as a flap for skin shortage. Use of continuous passive motion machine following Dupuytren's disease surgery provides no advantage in rehabilitation.

Complications

Complications related to surgical technique include skin necrosis, peripheral nerve and vascular injury, hematoma, and infection. Complications related to patient physiology include loss of digital flexion, scar contracture, and reflex sympathetic dystrophy. Many complications can be prevented.

Digital stiffness secondary to postoperative hand edema is averted by elevation and early active motion. Skin necrosis secondary to hematoma is averted by tourniquet deflation and adequate hemostasis prior to wound closure. Digital neurovascular injury is often associated with a spiral nerve, and can be avoided by careful dissection using loupe magnification and thorough knowledge of the pathologic anatomy. Digital ischemia following release of the tourniquet in one report was relieved with a cutaneous glyceryl trinitrate patch. The use of perioperative guanethidine in one report did not prevent postoperative reflex dystrophy, a condition that seems to be more common in women.

Continuing disease activity can be in the form of recurrence, extension, or both. True recurrence should be differentiated from scar tissue created by the operation itself. True recurrence is based on the presence of a nodule or a cord, rather than loss of digital extension or proximal interphalangeal flexion contracture. Recurrence should also be differentiated from intrinsic muscle adherence, which can affect the digit operated on as well as adjacent digits. Recurrence and extension of disease appear to be affected by the patient's diathesis. Reports of postoperative recurrence range from 2% to 60% with an average of 33%; the average extension rate is 25%. A greater rate of disease extension has been reported with longer term follow-up. Poor prognostic indicators include proximal interphalangeal joint involvement, small finger disease, the number of digits affected, and the passage of time before surgery and secondary fasciectomy. Surgical treatment is a means of controlling,

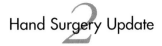

not curing, the disease. Surgical treatment is considered successful when the flexion contracture is fully corrected, full digital flexion is retained, and hand function is restored without complications or recurrence.

Annotated Bibliography

General

Berger A, Delbruck A, Brenner P, Hinzmann R (eds). *Dupuytren's Disease: Pathobiochemistry and Clinical Management.* Berlin, Springer-Verlag, 1994.

This book draws from both basic science and clinical material and includes updated references.

Rayan GM (ed): Dupuytren's disease. *Hand Clin* 1999;15:1–185.

This entire issue is devoted to Dupuytren's disease, and is the most current publication on the subject. The issue contains one of the most comprehensive lists of references available. Over 800 articles related to Dupuytren's disease are cited, including over 200 readings predating 1900.

History

Whaley DC, Elliot D: Dupuytren's disease: A legacy of the north? *J Hand Surg* 1993;18B:363–367.

Conditions resembling Dupuytren's disease were reported in Medieval Scandinavia and Iceland. This article contains a detailed historical account relevant to the origin of the disease.

Etiologic Factors

Badalamente MA, Sampson SP, Hurst LC, Dowd A, Miyasaka K: The role of transforming growth factor beta in Dupuytren's disease. *J Hand Surg* 1996;21A:210–215.

The authors studied the role of TGF-β in stimulation and proliferation of Dupuytren's disease fibroblasts and in the pathobiology of this condition.

Molecular Biology and Pathophysiology

Alioto RJ, Rosier RN, Burton RI, Puzas JE: Comparative effects of growth factors on fibroblasts of Dupuytren's tissue and normal palmar fascia. *J Hand Surg* 1994;19A:442–452.

This article describes an investigation of various growth factors' influence on Dupuytren's disease and normal cell cultures.

Rayan GM, Parizi M, Tomasek JJ: Pharmacologic regulation of Dupuytren's fibroblast contraction in vitro. *J Hand Surg* 1996;21A:1065–1070.

Pharmacologic agents that promote and inhibit Dupuytren's fibroblast contraction are identified. The clinical relevance is the potential for nonsurgical control of the disease.

Terek RM, Jiranek WA, Goldberg MJ, Wolfe HJ, Alman BA: The expression of platelet-derived growth-factor gene in Dupuytren contracture. *J Bone Joint Surg* 1995;77A:1–9.

This immunohistochemical study of PDGF expression in Dupuytren's disease tissue offers a mechanism for its action on fibroblasts.

Tomasek J, Rayan GM: Correlation of alpha-smooth muscle actin expression and contraction in Dupuytren's disease fibroblasts. *J Hand Surg* 1995;20A:450–455.

An immunofluorescence, cell culture, and collagen-lattice model study showed that the expression of alpha smooth muscle actin in Dupuytren's myofibroblasts correlates with their contractility.

Anatomy

Holland AJ, McGrouther DA: Dupuytren's disease and the relationship between the transverse and longitudinal fibers of the palmar fascia: A dissection study. *Clin Anat* 1997;10:97–103.

The authors present an anatomic study of the relationship between the pretendinous band and the transverse fibers of the palmar aponeurosis, and explain the relevance to surgical treatment.

Clinical Types

Chammas M, Bousquet P, Renard E, Poirier JL, Jaffiol C, Allieu Y: Dupuytren's disease, carpal tunnel syndrome, trigger finger, and diabetes mellitus. *J Hand Surg* 1995;20A:109–114.

This comparative prospective study shows the correlation between diabetes, Dupuytren's disease, and other conditions.

McFarlane R: Dupuytren's disease. *J Hand Ther* 1997;10:8–13.

This current review of Dupuytren's disease is from a lecture that contains state-of-the-art information regarding evaluation, treatment, and rehabilitation.

Umlas ME, Bischoff RJ, Gelberman RH: Predictors of neurovascular displacement in hands with Dupuytren's contracture. *J Hand Surg* 1994;19B:664–666.

In this prospective clinical study, the association between interdigital soft-tissue mass, proximal interphalangeal joint flexion contracture, and the presence of Dupuytren's disease spiral nerve was investigated.

Treatment

Brandes G, Messina A, Reale E: The palmar fascia after treatment by the continuous extension technique for Dupuytren's contracture. *J Hand Surg* 1994;19B:528–533.

This group has authored several articles introducing and supporting the concept of continuous elongation in the treatment of Dupuytren's disease.

Breed CM, Smith PJ: A comparison of methods of treatment of PIP joint contractures in Dupuytren's disease. *J Hand Surg* 1996;21B:246–251.

This analysis of different methods of treating residual proximal interphalangeal joint flexion deformity demonstrates that manipulation alone can yield better results and fewer complications than surgical treatment.

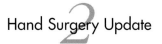

272 Dupuytren's Disease

Brotherston TM, Balakrishnan C, Milner RH, Brown HG: Long term follow-up of dermofasciectomy for Dupuytren's contracture. *Br J Plast Surg* 1994;47:440–443.

This retrospective study of dermofasciectomy and skin grafting for recurrent Dupuytren's disease reported satisfactory outcome with no recurrence beneath the grafts.

Moermans JP: Long-term results after segmental aponeurectomy for Dupuytren's disease. *J Hand Surg* 1996;21B:797–800.

Moermans describes a relatively new conservative approach and its efficiency in the treatment of Dupuytren's disease.

Shaw DL, Wise DI, Holms W: Dupuytren's disease treated by palmar fasciectomy and an open palm technique. *J Hand Surg* 1996;21B:484–485.

This long-term follow-up study demonstrates that the open palm technique yields satisfactory outcomes.

Weinzweig N, Culver JE, Fleegler EJ: Severe contractures of the proximal interphalangeal joint in Dupuytren's disease: Combined fasciectomy with capsuloligamentous release versus fasciectomy alone. *Plast Reconstr Surg* 1996;97:560–567.

In this retrospective comparison of fasciectomy with and without capsulotomy for proximal interphalangeal joint flexion deformity, the authors concluded that there is no advantage to capsuloligamentous release.

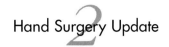
Section VI
Vascular

American Society for Surgery of the Hand

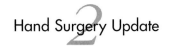

Chapter 27
Ischemia of the Hand

Neil Ford Jones, MD

Ischemia is relatively uncommon in the hand and upper extremity, compared to the lower extremity. The patient's chief complaint is often cold intolerance, or pain in the digit or the entire hand after exposure to cold. Although claudication of the upper extremity is rare, pain in the hand at rest is not. Patients may also present with unilateral or bilateral Raynaud's phenomena, with its characteristic triad of color changes (blanching followed by cyanosis and culminating in hyperemia with associated dysthesia). Splinter hemorrhages in the nail bed may be indicative of microemboli from a proximal source in the upper extremity. The final, catastrophic manifestation of ischemia is gangrene or ulcerations of the distal phalanges and digits.

In their 1961 study of arterial patterns in the hand, Coleman and Anson determined that the superficial arch is complete in only 80% of the population. In the remaining 20%, the superficial arch is incomplete and does not supply all 5 digits; these patients have the highest risk of developing ischemia. If occlusion of the radial or ulnar artery occurs, the collateral circulation may be insufficient to perfuse some or all of the digits. Symptomatic ischemia of a digit will occur if both digital arteries are involved and the collateral dorsal circulation is inadequate.

Examination

Evaluation of the patient should begin with a thorough history and physical examination. All symptoms, including cold intolerance, Raynaud's phenomena, and rest pain, must be documented. Associated risk factors should be considered, such as coronary artery disease, peripheral vascular disease, renal disease, diabetes, connective tissue disorders, smoking, and/or environmental toxins. A rheumatologic and immunologic workup may be necessary to exclude a systemic etiology for the ischemia.

The entire vascular system of the upper extremity needs to be evaluated in order to define the extent of the pathology and the potential for surgical intervention. Proximal occlusion of the subclavian artery may be manifest as a supraclavicular

The author gratefully acknowledges the assistance of Ranjan Gupta, MD in writing this chapter.

fossa bruit or a differential in blood pressure between each arm. Thoracic outlet syndrome may be suggested by Adson's and Wright's provocative maneuvers. Routine Allen testing should be performed in both upper extremities to document the patency of arterial inflow through the radial and ulnar arteries. Areas of pain, pallor, cyanosis, ulceration, and gangrene need to be recorded. If a connective tissue disorder is suspected to be the cause of the ischemia, laboratory tests may be necessary, including a complete blood count, erythrocyte sedimentation rate, rheumatoid factor, antinuclear antibody, anticentromere antibody, serum protein electropheresis, and cryoglobulins. Radiographs of the hand should be obtained to rule out osteomyelitis in patients with gangrene and to delineate the extent of calcification in patients with diabetes and renal vascular disease.

Investigations

The simplest and most informative method of evaluating patients with ischemia of the hand is a pencil Doppler probe. This test can be used to assess the patency of the radial and ulnar arteries, the superficial palmar arch, and the radial and ulnar digital arteries to each digit. The pencil Doppler probe also allows evaluation of pigmented hands or an unconscious patient. Segmental blood pressures can be measured at the elbows and over the radial and ulnar arteries at the wrist. A pressure differential of more than 20 mm Hg between the elbow and wrist or contralateral wrist may indicate stenosis of the distal brachial, radial, or ulnar arteries.

Plethysmography or pulse volume recordings may be used to obtain absolute blood pressures and wave form analysis of each finger. With digital plethysmography, a difference of 15 mm Hg between adjacent fingers or a gradient greater than 30 mm Hg between the wrist and digital pressures is indicative of occlusive disease at the level of the palmar arches or the digital arteries. The ratio between the digital blood pressure and the brachial artery pressure, known as the digital brachial index, normally averages 0.97 (range, 0.78–1.27). Abnormalities in the normal plethysmographic wave forms for each digit may indicate stenosis or occlusion within the digital arteries. The wave forms provide a physiologic profile of blood flow within the hand and fingers.

This technique provides a noninvasive, objective comparison of preoperative and postoperative perfusion in the digits after various treatment modalities.

Isolated cold stress testing can be effective in defining patients with symptomatic vascular insufficiency. Digital temperatures are recorded before and after immersion in cold water. Symptomatic patients will have lower baseline temperatures and abnormal cooling and rewarming curves. Digital plethysmography and laser Doppler flowmetry may be used in association with cold stress testing to evaluate any vasospastic component of arterial insufficiency. Sympathetic vasoconstriction of the digital arteries can be blocked with injection of lidocaine as a local anesthetic. If the decrease in absolute blood pressure and flattening of wave forms can be reversed by this block, these patients may benefit from digital sympathectomy to reverse sympathetic overactivity. Unfortunately, cold stress testing has limited value because cold immersion is extremely painful for many patients with connective tissue disorders or renal vascular disorders.

Bone scintigraphy, with technetium-99m methylene disphosphonate, can be used to investigate a variety of disorders of the hand and wrist. Injection of the conjugate provides an initial angiogram of the upper extremity vasculature, followed by evaluation of the surrounding soft tissues and finally the bone. This technique can define occlusion of the radial or ulnar arteries, and help in evaluation of arteriovenous malformations, Raynaud's phenomena, reflex sympathetic dystrophy, and osteomyelitis.

Color Doppler sonography has been shown to be useful in the identification of small (0.5 to 2 mm) vessel arterial occlusion. Investigators have demonstrated the effectiveness of combining ultrasound imaging, range-gated pulse wave Doppler spectral analysis, and color Doppler imaging to identify arterial occlusion in a rabbit model. This technique has also been effective in evaluating patency rates after single radial and ulnar artery repairs in the forearm. Laser Doppler imaging is a noninvasive technique that can be used to evaluate the spatial distribution and temporal variation of skin blood flow. One group recently used this technique to evaluate patients who had ulnar arteries repaired due to trauma.

The definitive technique for evaluating the vascular anatomy of the upper extremity remains conventional angiography. Emboli, thrombosis, or occlusive disease of the upper extremity can be readily defined with angiography. Angiographic evaluation is recommended for patients with unilateral Raynaud's phenomenon; progressive digital ulceration or gangrene, despite adequate medical management; recurrent digital ulceration; or pencil Doppler evidence of occlusion of the distal radial or ulnar arteries. The entire upper extremity anatomy should be defined from the arch of the aorta to the hand through a femoral puncture. If vasospasm is suspected as a primary cause of the patient's ischemia, angiography should be performed under brachial plexus block anesthesia. Newer contrast agents and refinements in computerized digital subtraction techniques have reduced the amount of contrast medium, thereby reducing the incidence of allergic reactions. Further developments in magnetic resonance angiography may eventually obviate the need for conventional angiography.

Etiology and Pathophysiology

Excluding traumatic transection of the radial, ulnar, or digital arteries, several pathologic processes can produce ischemia of the hand. As with any end-organ, potential mechanisms of ischemia include emboli, increased blood viscosity, thrombosis, occlusive disease, and vasospasm.

Emboli may arise from the heart due to atrial fibrillation or a recent myocardial infarction and lodge at the bifurcation of the brachial artery. The patient will usually have the classic signs and symptoms of pain, pallor, paresthesias, pulselessness, and paralysis. Microemboli may originate from an ulcerated, arteriosclerotic plaque in the subclavian artery or from a mural thrombus in the subclavian artery that has been compressed by the scalene muscles or a cervical rib. These emboli will often lodge in the distal radial or ulnar arteries or may present as splinter hemorrhages or gangrene.

Thrombosis most often affects the distal arteries of the forearm and hand. The most common variant is the "hypothenar hammer syndrome," in which thrombosis of the ulnar artery occurs as it passes through Guyon's canal. Manual laborers such as automobile shop or jackhammer operators have a greater risk of developing this condition because their hands are routinely subjected to repetitive blunt trauma. Patients often present with pain and cold intolerance in the ring and small fingers. Some individuals may also have ulnar nerve symptoms. One recent report described the "corkscrew" sign during angiography, which is suggestive of this condition. It is thought that repetitive trauma to the ulnar artery causes periadventitial scarring, damage to the media and internal elastic lamina, and subintimal hematoma of the vessel. Although less susceptible to spontaneous thrombosis, the radial artery may also be affected secondary to atherosclerosis or repetitive irritation by the extensor pollicis longus tendon. Endothelial damage of the brachial artery secondary to cardiac catheterization, or of the radial artery secondary to arterial pressure monitoring, may also result in localized thrombosis. Other causes of thrombosis include intra-arterial drug injections resulting in a chemical endarteritis or disseminated intravascular coagulation associated with septicemia, both of which result in disastrous gangrene of multiple digits.

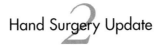
"Sludging" in the distal vessels may occur secondary to increased blood viscosity. This is most often seen in patients with myeloproliferative and immunologic disorders such as polycythemia, leukemia, myeloma, and cryoglobulinemia. Low blood flow states due to vasopressor infusions given to patients in intensive care units can also result in ischemia due to sludging.

Occlusive disease due to intimal proliferation of the arteries in patients with atherosclerosis, connective tissue disorders, and renal vascular disease may result in progressive narrowing of the internal lumen of the common and proper digital arteries. This narrowing eventually results in focal stenoses and segmental occlusions of the vessels. Two recent articles have described the neurologic and ischemic complications in patients with hemodialysis access grafts. In one series of 13 patients with hemodialysis grafts who underwent angiography for investigation of hand ischemia, obstructive arterial disease was responsible for the ischemia in 7 cases and graft "steal" in 3 cases. Patients with arterial stenosis were treated with angioplasty; 80% had improvement or resolution of symptoms. Another study described 22 patients with chronic renal failure who had neurologic and ischemic symptoms distal to the arteriovenous fistula created for hemodialysis. One subset of patients developed symptoms immediately after construction of the fistula. The other group developed progressive ischemic symptoms such as nonhealing ulcers and gangrene. Patients whose fistulas were removed as soon as ischemic symptoms occurred fared the best.

Vasospasm or vasoconstriction of the digital arteries may also result in ischemia of the hand and digits. Vasoconstriction may be the result of sympathetic overactivity leading to Raynaud's phenomena, especially in patients with connective tissue disorders. (Raynaud's symptoms without an underlying disorder is referred to as Raynaud's disease; Raynaud's symptoms with an underlying disorder is called Raynaud's phenomena.) Raynaud's disease is usually seen in young women (aged 11 to 30 years), and is a diagnosis of exclusion after 2 years without developing an underlying disorder. Recent studies have shown that smoking increases the vascular resistance in digital vessels. Ultrasonic Doppler velocimetry was used as a noninvasive, quantitative method of assessing blood flow in digital arteries after smoking for only 3 minutes. After smoke inhalation there was a decrease in peak blood flow velocity, mean volumetric flow, and average luminal area in a specific digital artery.

Treatment

Ischemia of the hand may be acute or chronic. Acute ischemia is most often caused by trauma, emboli, acute thrombosis, intra-arterial drug injections, and low-flow states in acutely ill patients. With any acute ischemic event, immediate diagnosis is critical. The pencil Doppler probe can be used as the initial investigative technique, but angiography will provide the definitive diagnosis. In patients with emboli in the brachial, distal radial, or ulnar arteries, surgical embolectomy or intra-arterial infusion of streptokinase is indicated. Investigation of patients in intensive care units often reveals patent vasculature with sludging being responsible for the distal ischemia. Although heparin, dextran-40, stellate ganglion blocks, and axillary blocks have all been tried, this problem remains unsolved. For thrombosis of the distal radial or ulnar arteries, interventional angiography with a Fogarty catheter can be used to remove the thrombus. Alternatively, resection of the thrombosed segment and interposition vein grafting may be performed.

One recent study reported the use of intra-arterial urokinase in the management of ischemia secondary to palmar and digital arterial occlusion in 9 patients with unilateral upper extremity ischemia. The 3 patients with thromboemboli demonstrated clinical and angiographic improvement. Three of the 4 patients with traumatic arterial occlusion showed clinical improvement but only 1 of the 4 had documented angiographic improvement. This form of treatment was ineffective for patients with organized thrombi or atheroemboli. Although more expensive than streptokinase, urokinase is a direct plasminogen activator and can lyse clots more rapidly with less fibrinogenolytic effect. This results in shorter infusion times and fewer hemorrhagic complications. Because urokinase is a human protein, allergic reactions are rare. Further study is needed, however, before this agent can be used routinely.

Patients with chronic ischemia of the upper extremity often present to the hand surgeon with Raynaud's phenomena, cold intolerance, nonhealing ulcers, or gangrene. Initial treatment of these patients should include recommendations to avoid cold exposure and to stop smoking. Various pharmacologic agents (including intra-arterial reserpine, intravenous guanethidine and phenoxybenzamine, low molecular weight dextran-40, calcium channel blockers, and topical nitroglycerin) have been used with mixed results. Areas of ulceration or dry gangrene are routinely allowed to autoamputate to maintain finger length. If the gangrene has advanced to the level of the distal interphalangeal joint, or if the patient is in significant pain, then formal surgical debridement or amputation is recommended. Bone must be shortened to allow loose approximation of the skin without any tension. Digital sympathectomy and microsurgical revascularization are advocated in selected patients to promote ulcer healing, alleviate symptoms, and prevent progression of the gangrene. Long-term follow-up data supporting these forms of treatment are still not available.

Annotated Bibliography

Investigations

Bornmyr S, Arner M, Svensson H: Laser Doppler imaging of finger skin blood flow in patients after microvascular repair of the ulnar artery at the wrist. *J Hand Surg* 1994;19B:295–300.

Laser Doppler imaging was used to evaluate the spatial distribution and temporal variation of skin blood flow. Sixteen patients who underwent ulnar artery repair after trauma were evaluated and compared to 14 control subjects. A slower recovery of blood flow values occurred after cold provocation in 4 of the 16 subjects.

Holder LE, Merine DS, Yang A: Nuclear medicine, contrast angiography, and magnetic resonance imaging for evaluating vascular problems in the hand. *Hand Clin* 1993;9:85–113.

Koudsi B, Petti CA, Halpern DE, Backus A, Nichter L: Assessment of acute microcirculatory changes by color Doppler sonography. *J Hand Surg* 1994;19A:488–494.

Color Doppler sonography was used for the transcutaneous assessment of acute changes in microvascular flow in a rabbit model. A strong linear correlation existed between Doppler identification of arterial occlusion, but not venous occlusion.

Koman LA, Nunley JA, Goldner JL, Seaber AV, Urbaniak JR: Isolated cold stress testing in the assessment of symptoms in the upper extremity: Preliminary communication. *J Hand Surg* 1984; 9A:305–313.

This classic article is the original description of the technique of cold stress testing and its potential diagnostic role.

Rothkopf DM, Chu B, Gonzalez F, Borah G, Ashmead D IV, Dunn R: Radial and ulnar artery repairs: Assessing patency rates with color Doppler ultrasonographic imaging. *J Hand Surg* 1993;18A:626–628.

Color Doppler ultrasonographic imaging was used to evaluate the patency and graphically display vascular flow in 31 forearm artery repairs. This study confirmed a high patency rate of arterial repairs, especially those without vein grafting.

Sumner DS: Noninvasive assessment of upper extremity and hand ischemia. *J Vasc Surg* 1986;3:560–564.

The author describes the technique of digital plethysmography, or pulse volume recordings, for the diagnosis of vascular problems of the upper extremity.

Etiology and Pathophysiology

Hammond DC, Matloub HS, Yousif NJ, Sanger JR: The corkscrew sign in hypothenar hammer syndrome. *J Hand Surg* 1993;18B:767–769.

Angiography of a manual laborer presenting with numbness and cold intolerance of the middle and ring fingers demonstrated filling defects in the digital arteries of these 2 fingers together with a "corkscrew-like" configuration of the ulnar artery in Guyon's canal.

Lee KL, Miller JG, Laitung G: Hand ischaemia following radial artery cannulation. *J Hand Surg* 1995;20B:493–495.

Digital ischemia following radial artery cannulation is uncommon, and usually the result of thrombotic occlusion of a dominant radial artery. This article reviews the possible mechanisms of digital ischemia following radial artery cannulation and discusses the therapeutic options available.

Morecraft R, Blair WF, Brown TD, Gable RH: Acute effects of smoking on digital artery blood flow in humans. *J Hand Surg* 1994;19A:1–7.

A 20 MHz-pulsed ultrasonic Doppler velocimeter was used to assess hemodynamic parameters in digital arteries before and after smoke inhalation. The authors reported an increased vascular resistance in the fingers and a decrease in volumetric blood flow through the arteries and in tissue perfusion.

Redfern AB, Zimmerman NB: Neurologic and ischemic complications of upper extremity vascular access for dialysis. *J Hand Surg* 1995;20A:199–204.

This study reviews the clinical course of 22 patients with chronic renal failure on hemodialysis with ischemic or neurologic problems in the upper extremity distal to an A–V fistula.

Valji K, Hye RJ, Roberts AC, Oglevie SB, Ziegler T, Bookstein JJ: Hand ischemia in patients with hemodialysis access grafts: Angiographic diagnosis and treatment. *Radiol* 1995;196:697–701.

Thirteen patients with hemodialysis grafts who developed ischemia of the hand underwent angiography. The authors discuss their findings and the effectiveness of transcatheter angioplasty in those patients with arterial stenoses.

Treatment

Jones NF: Acute and chronic ischemia of the hand: Pathophysiology, treatment, and prognosis. *J Hand Surg* 1991; 16A:1074–1083.

Pathophysiologic mechanisms producing ischemia in the hand are emphasized to provide a logical rationale for surgical treatment. Techniques of extended digital sympathectomy and microsurgical revascularization are described.

Wheatley MJ, Marx MV: The use of intra-arterial urokinase in the management of hand ischemia secondary to palmar and digital arterial occlusion. *Ann Plast Surg* 1996;37:356–363.

This article presents a retrospective review of 9 patients treated with intra-arterial infusion of urokinase for severe, unilateral ischemia of the upper extremity. This treatment was most effective for patients with thromboemboli, and was clinically effective in 3 of 4 patients with traumatic arterial occlusions. There was no clinical or angiographic improvement in patients with organized or atherosclerotic lesions.

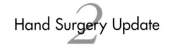

Chapter 28
Replantation Surgery

Steven J. McCabe, MD

Contemporary Developments

Advances in replantation research and techniques continue to improve management of patients with amputations in the upper extremity. However, replantation decisions today are influenced by several global trends that rival the impact of traditional research.

The value of replantation, compared to revision amputation, has come under the scrutiny of a cynical public. Cost containment in a managed care environment most certainly influences replantation decisions, particularly for more distal amputations and less clear indications. Finally, patients have assumed an increasingly proactive role in the decision-making process, and their perspective is the major focus in measuring outcome.

Indications and Contraindications for Replantation

Indications for replantation have historically been related to expected recovery of function based on the anatomic level. However, other patient and injury characteristics complicate the decision to proceed with replantation.

Level of Injury
The level of injury remains the most important factor in replantation recommendations. Anatomic indications for replantation have been derived from observation of functional results.

Amputation of the thumb is a strong indication because of the importance of the thumb, the good function that can be achieved with replantation, and the inferiority of other forms of reconstruction. Multiple digit amputations, and amputations through the palm, wrist, and distal forearm are also strong indications for replantation. Replantation of the single digit, however, is a subject of some controversy. Replantation is generally indicated for amputation distal to the level of the insertion of the superficialis tendon. Amputations through the proximal third of the forearm, the elbow, and arm require cautious consideration. The morbidity of these proximal procedures is much higher than more distal replantation, and the result is less predictable.

Age
Replantation is generally recommended in healthy children. Increasing age is a negative factor that must be balanced against the potential value of the replantation. Advanced age increases the risk of morbidity from the procedure. The higher probability of significant chronic medical illness in older patients reduces the quality of the recovery. These patients also have a shorter time horizon to enjoy benefits from replantation. The surgeon must consider the age of the patient, weighing its importance against other patient and injury characteristics. The more distal the level of amputation, however, the less important is patient age.

General Medical Condition
The presence of conditions such as heart disease or diabetes can make the procedure more dangerous, reduce the probability of success, and lessen the quality of the functional result. Existence of significant medical problems is a negative factor in the decision for replantation.

Ischemic Time
Although ischemic time is an important consideration in replantation, there are no strict criteria for maximum ischemic time in replantation. Cold protects against ischemic injury and is widely used in the transportation of severed parts. Digits have survived after prolonged ischemia up to 42 hours. In major replantation of parts containing skeletal muscle, the ischemic time is more important than in replantation of digits. Eight hours of warm ischemia and up to 16 hours of cold ischemia are considered the upper limits in proximal amputations.

Injury Mechanism
Avulsion injuries and broad crush injuries are negative factors that can influence the choice of procedure. However, these injuries are not clear contraindications. A broad crush injury can be debrided sharply to noninjured tissue, and there are many reports of successful replantation after

avulsion injuries. Nonetheless, these injuries increase the difficulty of surgery, reduce the possibility of success, and lessen the quality of functional recovery.

Digital Replantation

Multiple digital amputations or amputation of the thumb are strong indications for replantation. The technical aspects of the procedure and the postoperative care have changed very little over the past decade. The surgery requires debridement and bone shortening; fixation of the skeleton; repair of arteries, veins, nerves, and tendons; and skin cover. Postoperative care focuses on prevention and early detection of thrombosis and functional rehabilitation of the part.

Because the functional results will reflect the severity of the injury to multiple digits and structures, it is difficult to define and measure the improvement that could be provided by replantation compared to revision amputation. Recent articles reviewing patients with replantation tend to focus on the cost of the procedure and the hospital stay required. One group compared 24 patients who had at least one digit survive in a multiple digit or thumb amputation to 6 patients with no surviving digits. The primary purpose of the study was to define the costs of treatment. The largest single cost was for sick leave, and the second highest cost was the operation. Ward costs were next, with an average length of stay of 11.6 days. There were no dramatic differences in patient responses to 23 questions about activities of daily living. Replantation patients had significantly better mobility, power, and performance measured by a standardized strength test.

The authors included several key findings from clinical research on replantation of the digits. Severe injuries to the digits are complex, involving multiple digits and multiple structures. An individual patient may concurrently be a replantation and amputation patient, and also have other digits that are severely injured and repaired yet do not require replantation or amputation. Measuring the benefit of replantation in the context of such complicated injury is a difficult problem.

Although the replantation patients did not score any higher when questioned on function, cosmesis, and quality of life, 92% would still prefer to have replantation. This important point requires further evaluation with outcome instruments.

Thumb Replantation

Amputation of the thumb is still considered a strong indication for replantation. The survival rate for thumb replanta-

tion can serve as a good marker of the success of a replantation center, because of the reduced influence of patient selection on the results. The survival rate in thumb replantation is strongly influenced by the mechanism of injury. In a large series from Louisville, 88% of the thumbs survived when minimally damaged; however, the survival rate was reduced to 58% in avulsion injuries, and 12% in crushing avulsions or severe crush injuries. In minimally damaged thumb amputations, the survival rate was 94% when replantation surgery was done within 8 hours after injury but decreased to 74% for surgery more than 8 hours after injury.

Initial ischemic time contributed to the success of reexploration of failing replants. Although 45% of 20 failing thumb replants survived, those patients with an interval between injury and initial replantation of less than 8 hours had a 75% success rate at reexploration; uniform failure occurred when the interval exceeded 8 hours. The time interval between injury and replantation may be an important predictor of salvage of the failing replant.

In another review of patients with isolated thumb replantation or revascularization, the mechanism of injury and the level of the amputation were the key factors influencing functional results. Of 46 patients, 85% resumed their preinjury employment; 100% returned to work.

Distal Replantation

Local or regional anesthetic can be used in fingertip replantation. After sharp debridement, one successful method is to fix the bone with two Kirschner wires and repair the nail bed. Two small triangular flaps of dermis are raised from the adjacent margins of the pulp. The distal part is not dissected. The arteries of the proximal part are located, and their position is used to find the arteries in the distal pulp. Any tubular structure in the distal part can be used for inflow if the surgeon is uncertain that an artery can be found. After anastomosis, the tourniquet is deflated and blood is allowed into the amputated part in order to identify palmar veins. A corresponding vein can be located in the proximal stump and repaired. A second artery can be repaired for inflow or outflow, whichever is needed. The nerves are then repaired and the skin flaps sutured. Should vein grafts be needed, the small crossing veins at the flexor side of the distal forearm are a good size match. The skin is then repaired. If no veins can be located, the part can be allowed to bleed or leeches can be used. With careful management of the degree of bleeding, blood transfusion can be avoided. The patient is usually admitted for 3 to 4 days and treated with low molecular weight dextran and heparin.

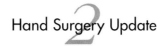
The value of replantation of distal parts continues to be a focus of research. Common indications for replantation of a single digit include those amputations distal to the insertion of the flexor digitorum superficialis, but replantation in the distal phalanx is a subject of some controversy. Differing terminology used to describe the level of amputation and replantation in the distal phalanx further confuses the issue. Papers published since 1993 may refer to any of 4 different zone descriptions proposed by various authors, or use "replantation distal to the insertion of the flexor digitorum superficialis" as a general description.

There is no question that distal replantation is possible; several recent studies have demonstrated the feasibility and evaluated specific aspects of the procedure. The concern today is that the procedure has not received uniform support, and is not widely performed except at specialized replantation centers. The magnitude of the replantation procedure and postoperative care may be perceived as much more involved than revision amputation; however, the difficulty of small vessel repair is more than compensated for by the ease of bone work and the absence of the need for tendon repair.

Mechanism of injury plays an important role in the survival rate of distal replantation. As with more proximal levels and amputations of the thumb, sharp cutting injuries fare better. However, a growing body of evidence indicates that avulsion injury and crush injuries do not preclude successful replantation.

Nail growth following distal replantation depends on the level of amputation: those distal to the lunula are more likely to result in normal nail appearance whereas those in the germinal matrix will have more problems of nail growth.

Because opportunities to perform distal replantation are uncommon, randomized trials of replantation and revision amputation are difficult to conduct. When comparison of the 2 procedures has been attempted, however, the results have favored replantation.

Transmetacarpal Amputation

The transmetacarpal amputation is an interesting injury that is widely considered a strong indication for replantation due to the magnitude of the injury itself; however, results of treatment to date have not supported such an enthusiastic endorsement. During the procedure the debridement should include the distal interosseous and lumbrical muscles, allowing the distal tendon position to be controlled by splinting. Depending on the level of the injury

and debridement, the redundant vascular supply of the hand may provide perfusion of multiple digits with each arterial repair. This redundancy, however, can cause hematoma at the site of replantation unless care is taken to identify and ligate multiple deep and superficial arteries.

Further improvements in the management of these injuries have been described in 2 recent reports of replantations at the transmetacarpal level. These articles include reviews of other studies evaluating the results of replantation for transmetacarpal amputations. Using Chen's criteria to score postoperative results, the proportion of grade 1 and 2 results was low, with the exception of one series of 4 patients who had results approaching those expected for wrist and distal forearm replantation.

Noting the sparse literature on this injury, one group reviewed a series of patients with amputations and devascularizations. Secondary surgery was common not only in this series but also in other reported series. Only 1 supervisor resumed his preinjury occupation; no manual workers returned to their preinjury livelihood. The discouraging results were attributed to intrinsic muscle ischemia and "creation of a common wound."

Further refinement in the postoperative care of these injuries was evident in the results reported by Scheker and associates. They attributed good results to resection of the distal intrinsic muscles and a carefully controlled postoperative regimen, including a specific splinting protocol and early motion. An ingenious splint allows gentle active motion and controls the position of the scarring intrinsic tendons. Two of the 4 patients in this study had repeat surgery. The results of this splinting program show promise for replantations of the forearm and wrist as well as the transmetacarpal level.

Hand and Distal Forearm Amputation

Large power saws are the predominant injury mechanism for reported amputations through the wrist and distal forearm. This type of injury is an excellent indication for replantation, requiring relatively straightforward microsurgery and offering good potential for functional recovery.

Extensive debridement is required, followed by bone shortening and stable bone fixation using plates if possible. Arthrodesis or proximal row carpectomy can be used to stabilize the skeleton in amputations through the carpus. Although all structures are typically repaired in one procedure, many patients with replantation at this level have secondary surgery for revisions and other corrections.

Scheker's description of a postoperative regimen with the crane outrigger splint offers precise suggestions for controlled early mobilization. The regimen provided good results in his patients, who were very satisfied with replantation at this level. Return to useful employment is a realistic goal after this injury and procedure.

Replantation in Children

Indications for replantation are much broader for amputations in children. If the part is available and surgery can be safely performed, an attempt to replant is almost always warranted. Children have a better (and sometimes unpredictably high) potential for excellent functional recovery compared to adults. Nerve recovery, for example, is superior in children following repair.

The technical aspects of the surgery and postoperative care in children are similar to adults. In a review of a large number of replantations and revascularizations in children performed at Duke University Medical Center, the mechanism of injury was the most important predictor of survival of the revascularized or replanted part. The survival rate was 72% after laceration injury, and dropped to 53% when the amputation resulted from a crush or avulsion injury. Survival in replanted digits was lower for children older than 9 years. Return to the operating room for a failing digit rarely reversed the problem.

The functional results revealed that fingers with injuries distal to the flexor digitorum superficialis insertion recovered better proximal interphalangeal (PIP) joint motion than fingers with injuries proximal to the PIP joint. The average 2-point discrimination was 8 mm in patients who had replantation. In children younger than 9 years, 12 of 17 replanted parts had 2-point discrimination less than 5 mm. Functional recovery after replantation in children is difficult to measure. At present it is impossible to determine whether the more inclusive criteria for replantation in adults can be applied to pediatric patients.

Growth Disturbance

Severe injuries and subsequent replantation or revascularization can lead to premature closure of growth plates. The use of distraction to elongate replanted parts has been reported in 2 recent articles. Two cases of forearm lengthening and 1 instance of thumb lengthening have been described; bone grafting of the gap was required in 2 of the cases. In a rat model, growth deficiency was related to the ischemic insult, suggesting the importance of rapid revascularization of amputations in children.

Postoperative Monitoring

Numerous methods can be used to monitor the replanted digit after surgery. The objective of monitoring is to detect and reoperate on a digit that has suffered thrombosis of the anastomosis. Many reexplored cases have been salvaged. One group evaluated the use of thermometry and laser Doppler flowmetry, 2 common methods of postoperative monitoring of the replanted digit. Thermometry is probably the easiest method (other than an experienced examiner). Heat is delivered to the digit with blood flow via the intact anastomosis and is lost to the atmosphere. Thermometry is particularly applicable to replantation because of the large surface area of the digit compared to the area of its contact to the hand. In the event of thrombosis, heat cannot reach the fingertip by conduction through its small area of contact with the body. Because of direct conduction of heat, however, thermometry may not be well-suited for a thin free flap with a large area of contact. If the surgeon uses direct warming of the replanted part postoperatively, thermometry may not be sensitive; alternative methods should be used to detect thrombosis. Laser Doppler has received a lot of interest. Hovius and associates created ROC (receiver operator characteristics) curves for laser Doppler flowmetry and thermometry, confirming that both can be useful. Their methodology may not be comparable to that used in a clinical setting, however. Longitudinal evaluation of temperature provides useful information and is a highly sensitive test; this evaluation will alert the surgeon to a need for personal evaluation before committing to repeat surgery.

Thrombolysis

Intermittent case reports have described use of thrombolytic therapy for salvage of failing replantation when surgical options have been exhausted. One group used recombinant tissue plasminogen activator for salvage of a forearm replantation with venous occlusion. This approach shows promise and should be a topic of continuing research.

Cold Sensitivity

Sensitivity to cold is nearly universal after digital replantation. Despite the prevalence and morbidity of this problem,

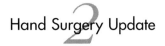

there is no clear description of its physiology or any widely used treatment. Cold-induced vasospasm has been implicated as one cause of cold sensitivity. It develops in the first year and does not seem to improve with time; however, patient complaints of this symptom diminish over time, suggesting that the 2 are not perfectly linked. In one 12-year study, investigators found that patients with moderate symptoms improved over time; however, there was no plethysmographic improvement. Another group used local and systemic cooling to evaluate cold-induced vasospasm for 3 years after digital replantation. They noted that cold-induced vasospasm is not present in the first few weeks after replantation, but develops in the first year. Although not all patients had cold-induced vasospasm, once acquired it seemed unlikely to improve.

Microvascular Research

Microvascular anastomosis is an area of microsurgery that would benefit from improved ease and efficiency. Unlike most free-tissue transfers, the long-term success of replantation usually requires long-term patency of the microanastomosis. This puts special demands on nonsuture methods of repair. Various anastomotic coupling devices have been used in clinical settings with success. In one report, surgeons from France and Australia used a ring device to perform 17 microvascular anastomoses in digital replantation. Seven of the anastomoses were considered critical for survival of the part. All 15 anastomoses available for evaluation were patent after 6 months. This is a fascinating area for further research.

Another group reported the use of fibrin glue for microsurgical anastomosis. This glue was used as an adjunct to suture anastomosis. The authors believed the surgical time was reduced in 21 cases of finger replantation. Thirty-two of 36 digits survived. Although the methodology used does not allow definition of any benefit from the use of the glue, its use does not seem to be harmful to patency.

Information Technology

One interesting application of information technology is the suggested use of electronic mail to transmit digital images of injuries and radiographs for evaluation at a replantation center. This may obviate the expensive transfer of patients to a microsurgery center if replantation is clearly not feasible. The practicality and benefit is not clear-cut, however; the same replantation center could be the best location to deal with the extensive nonmicrosurgical aspects of the injury. The Internet provides great potential in other aspects of microsurgery, such as patient education, teaching, and dissemination of research findings.

Annotated Bibliography

Digital Replantation

Holmberg J, Lindgren B, Jutemark R: Replantation-revascularization and primary amputation in major hand injuries. Resources spent on treatment and the indirect costs of sick leave in Sweden. *J Hand Surg* 1996;21B:576–580.

This interesting paper reviews 30 patients whose severe injuries made them candidates for replantation. Replantation or revascularization was successful in 24 patients; there were 3 failed attempts and 3 primary revisions. The highest costs were sick leave, followed by the operation, and then ward costs. The successful patients did not self-evaluate their hands to be any more functional than the failures or amputations did. A standardized strength test demonstrated better results in the replantation patients.

Thumb Replantation

Arakaki A, Tsai TM: Thumb replantation: Survival factors and reexploration in 122 cases. *J Hand Surg* 1993;18B:152–156.

A large group of replanted thumbs was used in this analysis of the factors leading to failure of replantation. The mechanism of injury was the most important factor, with survival of 88% in minimally damaged thumbs, 58% in avulsion injuries, and 12% in crush avulsions. The time lapse between injury and replantation was important for survival in the minimally damaged group; those patients returned to the operating room for reexploration.

Janezic TF, Arnez ZM, Solinc M, Zaletel-Kragelj L: Functional results of 46 thumb replantations and revascularisations. *Microsurgery* 1996;17:264–267.

In this contribution from Slovenian surgeons, 46 patients with successful thumb replantation or revascularization were evaluated. Functional recovery was related to the mechanism of injury and the level of injury. All patients returned to some type of work; 67% returned to the same occupation.

Distal Replantation

Dubert T, Houimli S, Valenti P, Dinh A: Very distal finger amputations: Replantation or "reposition-flap" repair? *J Hand Surg* 1997;22B:353–358.

The results of distal replantation in 10 patients were compared to "reposition flap repair" in 6 patients. The results of replantation were superior, but with longer hospital stays (average 8 days). Interestingly, the replantation patients returned to work more quickly. The focus of the article is a general review of the techniques, technical problems, and solutions of distal replantation.

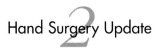

Elliot D, Sood MK, Flemming AFS, Swain B: A comparison of replantation and terminalization after distal finger amputation. *J Hand Surg* 1997;22B:523–529.

In this interesting article, the authors compare the results of replantation of a single finger in 11 patients with amputations distal to the flexor digitorum superficialis insertion to revision amputation in 19 patients who failed replantation or had primary revision. Perhaps because of the small group size, no statistical analysis is provided. The authors emphasize the discouraging results of terminalization, and include some cost information.

Nishi G, Shibata Y, Tago K, Kubota M, Suzuki M: Nail regeneration in digits replanted after amputation through the distal phalanx. *J Hand Surg* 1996;21A:229–233.

Nail regeneration was evaluated after replantation of 48 digits amputated through the distal phalanx. Replantations distal to the lunula showed near normal nail regeneration, whereas more proximal injuries may cause problems with nail growth. Four cases are reported in more detail with photographs.

Yamano Y: Replantation of fingertips. *J Hand Surg* 1993; 18B:157–162.

This review of 207 fingertip replantations also details several specific cases. Survival in zone 1, distal to the base of the nail, was related to the mechanism of injury. The article includes some interesting information about average hospital stay, cost of treatment, and time off work.

Transmetacarpal, Hand, and Distal Forearm Amputation

Scheker LR, Chesher SP, Netscher DT, Julliard KN, O'Neill WL: Functional results of dynamic splinting after transmetacarpal, wrist, and distal forearm replantation. *J Hand Surg* 1995;20B:584–590.

The authors introduce a precise postoperative protocol for management of replantations at the forearm, wrist, and transmetacarpal levels. At the heart of the program is a crane outrigger splint, which is described and illustrated. The results in this small patient group are especially good for transmetacarpal and wrist-level replantations.

Vanstraelen P, Papini RP, Sykes PJ, Milling MA: The functional results of hand replantation; The Chepstow experience. *J Hand Surg* 1993;18B:556–564.

The injuries, surgery, postoperative care, and results of 8 wrist and distal forearm level replantations are thoroughly described. Late functional assessment of 6 patients included a questionnaire on activities of daily living. This article provides concise documentation of the current state of this surgery and postoperative evaluation.

Weinzweig N, Sharzer LA, Starker I: Replantation and revascularization at the transmetacarpal level: Long-term functional results. *J Hand Surg* 1996;21A:877–883.

This review of 13 consecutive transmetacarpal replantations and revascularizations revealed good success regarding survival, but discouraging functional results. Eleven of the 13 hands required secondary surgery, with an average of 4.5 procedures per hand. Range of motion averaged 109° per digit; pinch and grip strength was weak or absent. Using Chen's criteria, 31% were grade 2, 31% were grade 3, and 38% were grade 4. Only one supervisor resumed his preinjury occupation; however all patients were satisfied with the surgery. This is an excellent review of the literature on replantation at this level.

Replantation in Children

Graf P, Biemer E: Treatment of post-replantation retardation of bone growth by callus distraction: A report of two cases. *J Hand Surg* 1993;18B:147–151.

Postreplantation discrepancy forearm bone length was corrected in 2 patients. In one case, a radius adequately reossified after distraction. The second case required ulnar grafting.

Saies AD, Urbaniak JR, Nunley JA, Taras JS, Goldner RD, Fitch RD: Results after replantation and revascularization in the upper extremity in children. *J Bone Joint Surg* 1994;76A:1766–1776.

The authors present a 14-year review of revascularization and replantation in the hand of pediatric patients from Duke University Medical Center. Injuries of 123 children were divided between amputations and devascularizations and separated into 3 anatomic zones of injury. The major predictor for survival of amputated parts following microsurgery was the mechanism of injury. The recovery was measured using range of motion and sensibility. The authors note the difficulty of measuring functional use of the hand, especially in children. This important article reviews the procedure and its results in a population in which replantation is rarely discouraged.

Postoperative Monitoring

Hovius SE, van Adrichem LN, Mulder HD, van Strik R, van der Meulen JC: Comparison of laser Doppler flowmetry and thermometry in the postoperative monitoring of replantations. *J Hand Surg* 1995;20A:88–93.

The authors measured the perfusion units with a laser Doppler, and compared the results to temperature measurement of the replanted digits. They used the lowest temperature and perfusion units as the index score, and looked at the status of the digit at that time. ROC curves were generated, and the authors concluded that laser Doppler flowmetry is more sensitive and specific (a better diagnostic test for thrombosis). Although this is an interesting study, the use of the lowest score favors the laser Doppler because this is not the way thermometry would be used in clinical practice. In addition, revascularizations may be different than replantation. Both methods demonstrated high sensitivities and specificities.

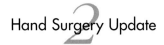
Cold Sensitivity

Backman C, Nystrom A, Backman C, Bjerle P: Arterial spasticity and cold intolerance in relation to time after digital replantation. *J Hand Surg* 1993;18B:551–555.

Cold intolerance may be the most disabling problem after digital amputation. These authors measured digital blood pressures during local cooling and systemic cooling to examine arterial spasticity. Not all patients developed this problem, but it persisted for the 3 years of the study in the patients who did develop it.

Povlsen B, Nylander G, Nylander E: Cold-induced vasospasm after digital replantation does not improve with time: A 12 year prospective study. *J Hand Surg* 1995;20B:237–239.

This long-term follow-up demonstrates that cold-induced vasospasm does not improve with time. Those patients with moderate symptoms of cold sensitivity showed improvement in symptoms, whereas patients with severe symptoms showed no improvement.

Microvascular Research

Isogai N, Cooley BG, Kamiishi H: Clinical outcome of digital replantation using the fibrin glue-assisted microvascular anastomosis technique. *J Hand Surg* 1996;21B:573–575.

Thirty-two of 36 digits survived when anastomosis was performed with 4–6 sutures and fibrin glue. The average operative time was 3.2 hours per digit. The authors believe the operative time was less because the glue allowed them to use less sutures.

Lanzetta M: Use of the 3M precise microvascular anastomotic system in hand surgery. *J Hand Surg* 1995;20A:725–730.

Lanzetta details the experience with the 3M ring device in microsurgery of the hand. Seventeen anastomoses were performed (7 critical for survival of tissue) in replantations and revascularizations. All 15 of the available anastomoses were open more than 6 months after surgery when evaluated by Doppler. The longest follow-up was 15 months. The time required to perform the anastomosis with the ring device was 6 minutes.

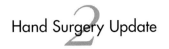
Chapter 29
Free-Tissue Reconstruction

Randy Sherman, MD

Introduction

Phenomenal progress has been made in the treatment of a vast spectrum of upper-extremity acquired ailments and congenital differences. While advances in all of the subspecialties within hand surgery have been quite notable, none have been as spectacular as those in the field of free-tissue reconstruction. With enhanced instrumentation, magnification systems, and microsuture, dedicated upper extremity reconstructive microsurgeons have revolutionized the treatment of previously uncorrectable sequelae of trauma, cancer, infection, and anomalies of development. The objective of free-tissue reconstruction is the replacement of absent, impaired, or destroyed tissues with heterotrophic analogs that most closely mirror normal appearance and function. The classic precept of restoring tissue in kind has supplanted osteoplastic thumb reconstruction with toe-to-thumb transfers, currently the mainstay for all the free-tissue reconstructive procedures. Over the last 5 years, significant progress has been made in the technical refinements, maturation of indications, selection of techniques, and understanding of long-term outcomes. The wide range of available free-tissue transfers can now be applied in more specific and appropriate circumstances.

History

Through the twentieth century, surgeons have been fascinated with the concept of anastamosis of blood vessels. The triangulation technique, currently the most commonly used option in microvacular anastomosis, was first described in 1906. Gibson discussed the concepts of tissue transfer on vascular pedicles, while Murray accomplished the first successful kidney transplantation in 1955. Littler described the neurovascular island pedicle flap in 1956, further refining composite tissue transfer. With the successful reports of arm replantations in the US and China in 1962, the corresponding fields of replantation and microvascular reconstruction took flight. Second toe-to-thumb transfers were reported in 1966, and great toe-to-thumb transfers in 1969. Millesi described his work in peripheral microneurosurgery in 1969. After Ack-

land pioneered the fabrication of new instrumentation and suture in 1972, successful transfer of vascularized bone, nerve, and muscle were reported. Further refinements in the application of free-tissue transfers to the hand and upper extremity were reported in 1980 with the temporoparietal fascial free flap and the partial toe transfer, in 1982 with the radial forearm flap, and in 1984 with the lateral arm flap. Studies on ever larger series of toe-to-finger transplants, as well as motorized muscle transfers, have continued to raise the standards of functionalized microvascular reconstruction.

Indications

Trauma

The most prevalent indication for free-tissue reconstruction is posttraumatic deformity. Nonreplantable digital amputation is the most common indication for toe-to-finger transfer. Thumb reconstruction can be accomplished using the great toe, the second toe, the wraparound procedure, the twisted two-toe procedure, or bipolar lengthening. Single or multiple finger amputations are best managed by second toe transfer. When preservation of length is required, neurovascular island flaps from the toe web space can be used for distal pulp surfaces; this transfer allows the reconstruction of glabrous skin involved in basic pinch and grasp functions and can restore highly discriminatory 2-point sensation. Loss of full-thickness skin on either the dorsal or palmar surface of the hand with exposure of tendons and/or other underlying surfaces may be amenable to reconstruction using one of several highly vascularized free-tissue transfers, including the radial forearm, dorsal pedis, lateral arm, proximal forearm, and temporoparietal fascial flaps. Composite defects of the dorsal hand, including skin and tendon involvement, can be addressed with tendonocutaneous flaps or bilaminar fascial flaps and nonvascularized tendon grafts (ie, temporoparietal fascial with deep temporal fascia). Increasingly complex defects that involve skin, tendon, and bone, as well as loss of metacarpal diaphyseal length, are appropriately addressed with osteocutaneous flaps from the lateral arm, radial forearm, and dorsalis pedis (Figs. 1–4). Larger cosmetic defects of the forearm, elbow,

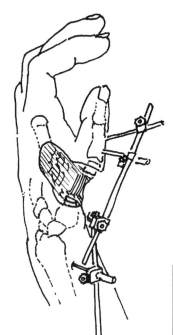

Figure 1

Composite defect of the thumb metacarpal diaphysis, including loss of extensor pollicis longus, digital nerves, subcutaneous tissue, and skin.

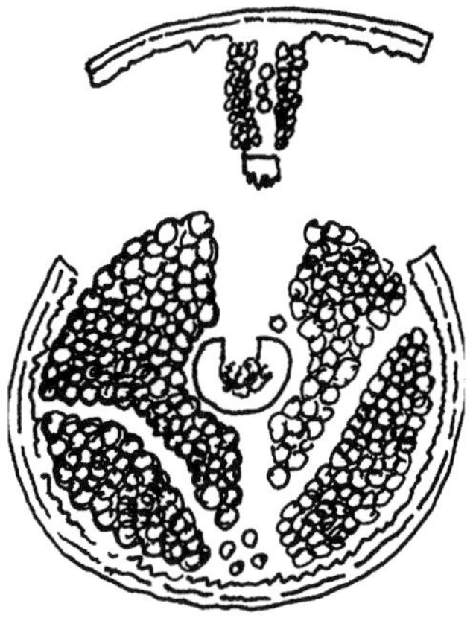

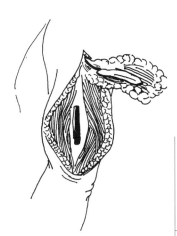

Figure 2

Lateral arm osteocutaneous flap raised with cortical segment of humerus, including posterior radial collateral artery and vein and posterior cutaneous nerve to the arm and forearm.

Figure 3

Cross-sectional view of lateral arm osteocutaneous flap, showing obligatory cuff of triceps.

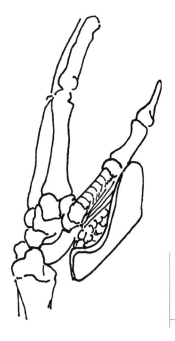

Figure 4

Schematic view of transposed lateral arm osteocutaneous flap, with humeral segment replacing lost metacarpal shaft.

and brachium are usually covered with free muscle transfers followed by split-thickness skin grafts. Common donor muscles include the latissimus dorsi, serratus anterior, rectus abdominus, and gracilis. Long-bone defects can be managed most effectively with fibular transfer, either as a vascularized bone only or osteocutaneous flap. In certain circumstances, motorized muscle transfers can be used to restore extrinsic finger flexion or extension, as well as biceps function; the gracilis muscle is selected most frequently, followed by the latissimus dorsi.

Tumor

Complex postablative defects may be created by limb salvage tumor resection. These defects are best reconstructed with free-tissue transfer. Digital restoration with toe transfers may be required, usually after resection secondary to melanoma. Long bone defects, which are often secondary to resections of osteosarcomas, chondrosarcomas, or malignant fibrous histocytomas, can be successfully reconstructed using the vascularized fibula to replace the resected bone segment. If endoprostheses are chosen as the

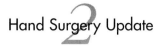
reconstructive alternative for skeletal restoration, muscle transfers are frequently used to obtain secure wound closure. In rare instances, when a proximal humeral neoplasm is treated with amputation, distal free-tissue transfers from the amputated arm can be used to close the residual brachial defects. A filleted, extended radial forearm-osteocutaneous flap has been used to provide coverage of the thorax and brachial plexus after resection of a proximal humeral desmoid tumor.

Infection

Wounds resulting from major infection include those that are secondary to necrotizing and/or clostridial infections. These massive wounds often occur in immunocompromised patients, such as severe diabetics or those suffering from advanced stages of cancer. Tissues lost most often include skin and subcutaneous tissue, with compromise of muscle compartments. Reconstruction usually focuses on wound coverage and closure; again, this is best accomplished with large surface area muscle transfers. The latissimus dorsi muscle is most suitable for these circumstances, and is easily covered by split-thickness skin grafts. Fortunately, osteomyelitis is infrequent in the upper extremity; when present, it rarely requires massive debridement to an extent that would necessitate free-tissue transfer reconstruction. The resultant wounds should be approached similarly to posttraumatic or postablative deformities.

Congenital

Significant progress has been made in the last 5 years to further define indications for free-tissue reconstruction in the congenitally different hand. Second toe-to-hand transfer—either taken unilaterally or bilaterally—had been used in the reconstruction of symbrachydactyly, constriction band syndrome, complex syndactyly, transverse deficits, acrosyndactyly, and adactylous hands. There is now general agreement that when multiple digits are transferred, they are best done during a single stage. Three-jointed second toe transplants, including the metatarsal phalangeal joint, with meticulous intrinsic muscle repair has been proven superior. Minimizing ischemic time with multiple nerve microneurorrhaphy has also improved outcomes.

Long-bone transfer with vascularized epiphyseal transplantation in radial club hands has been reported, but not adequately followed to assess long-term growth and functional outcome. Vascularized joint transfer has also been attempted in several centers with modest improvement in joint function.

Burn

Free-tissue reconstruction is rarely indicated in the acute management of burn patients. Free skin flaps have been used after release of severe contractures of the axilla, elbow, and wrist. The parascapular fascia cutaneous flap or, more recently, the extended lateral arm/proximal forearm fascia cutaneous flaps have served well to allow full restoration of flexion extension arcs after complete release of burn contractures. Digital web space contractures are most often amenable to split-thickness skin grafting. In those unusual cases in which underlying structures are exposed, small segmental free muscle flaps or free toe web space transfers can be transferred. The radial forearm or temporoparietal fascia flaps are best reserved for moderate resurfacing in dorsal hand injuries involving skin, with exposure or destruction of tendons or other underlying structures.

Reconstruction by Location

Thumb

Transfer options for thumb reconstruction include the total great toe, second toe, great toe wraparound, trimmed great toe, and twisted two toes. There are 5 considerations for selection of one of these options—the level of the thumb amputation, associated injuries or other deformities of the hand, the size match and appearance of the opposite intact thumb in relation to the donor great toe and second toe, functional requirements of the patient, and patient's choice. The total great toe is indicated for amputation at or proximal to the metacarpophalangeal (MCP) joint, with good size match to the opposite (normal) side, and a need for optimal thumb function; the second toe, for patients with a significant size discrepancy, who are intolerant to loss of great toe, need less than optimal function, or for children; great toe wraparound, for amputation distal to the interphalangeal (IP) joint, skin and nail avulsion distal to the MCP joint with intact IP joint function; and trimmed great toe transfer is indicated for large size discrepancy and IP joint motion equal in importance to thumb appearance (Fig. 5).

In several large series in which patients had completed occupational therapy, including sensory reeducation, the average 2-point discrimination varied between 13 and 15 mm. Grip strength ranged from 60% to 75% of the opposite normal side. Range of motion of the transferred joint was best in the total great toe (followed by the second toe), with no IP motion possible after wraparound procedures.

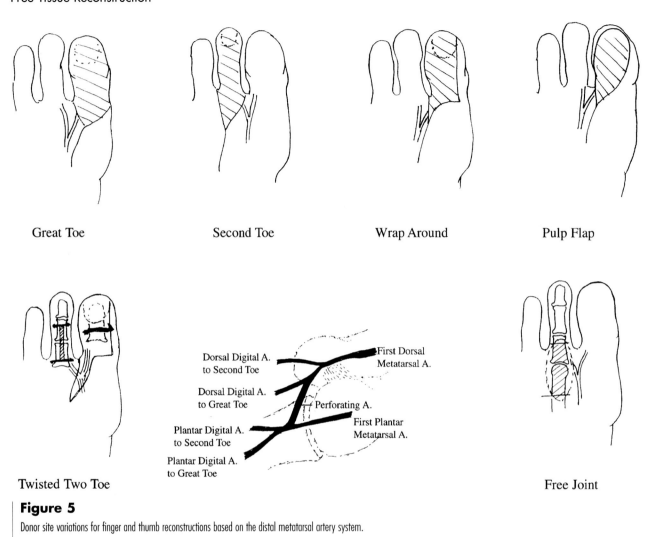

Great Toe

Second Toe

Wrap Around

Pulp Flap

Twisted Two Toe

Dorsal Digital A.
to Second Toe

Dorsal Digital A.
to Great Toe

Plantar Digital A.
to Second Toe

Plantar Digital A.
to Great Toe

First Dorsal
Metatarsal A.

Perforating A.

First Plantar
Metatarsal A.

Free Joint

Figure 5

Donor site variations for finger and thumb reconstructions based on the distal metatarsal artery system.

Maximal functional restoration in thumb reconstruction requires an intact metacarpophalangeal joint, and a normal, stable, functioning carpometacarpal joint.

Fingers

Loss of an individual finger is rarely an indication for digital reconstruction. Multiple digital loss, compromising basic key and chuck grasp as well as pinch functions, remains the primary indication for toe-to-finger transfers. Reconstructive options have been limited to second toe transfers from one or both feet. Reports of en bloc multiple toe transfers have been discouraging in regard to both hand function and donor site morbidity. Some centers have used partial toe transfers for distal digital reconstruction; however, the indications for this procedure remain controversial. Wei and associates classified these metacarpal hand injuries, with

determinants for reconstructive options based on subtype components (Table 1).

Full-thickness skin deformities, whether on the palmar or dorsal surface of the digits, may occasionally require coverage with free-tissue reconstruction; first web-space flaps are best suited for this coverage. A neurovascular island flap can be constructed using the first dorsal metatarsal artery with accompanying cutaneous nerves. Recent advances in both proximally and distally based homodigital and heterodigital neurovascular island flaps have reduced the need for web-space neurovascular free-tissue reconstructions.

Palm

Free-tissue reconstruction plays a limited role in palmar wound coverage. Temporoparietal fascia with overlying skin graft or proximal forearm flaps allow for wound closure with

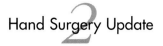

Table 1

Metacarpal hand injury classification and toe-transfer guidelines

Type		Definition	Reconstruction Options
I		Loss of all fingers proximal to midproximal phalanx, with normal thumb or thumb tip amputation only	
	A	Amputations distal to MCP joint	Bilateral second toes (amputations distal to web) Combined second and third toes (amputations proximal to web)
	B	Amputations through MCP joint with normal articular surface	Combined second and third toes (composite joint transfer)
	C	Amputations through or proximal to MCP joint with compromised articular surface	Combined second and third toes (transmetatarsal transfer)
II		Loss of all fingers proximal to midproximal phalanx, with amputated thumb proximal to interphalangeal joint	
	A	Thumb amputation distal to metacarpal neck	Whole or trimmed great toe transfer with transproximal phalangeal transfers
	B	Thumb amputation proximal to metacarpal neck with intact thenar function	Interposition bone graft with trimmed great toe or transmetatarsal second toe
	C	Thumb amputation at any level without thenar function	Thumb reconstruction following finger reconstruction and tendon transfer for restoration of opposition
	D	Thumb amputation at any level with damage to the carpometacarpal joint	Same options as IIA and IIB, with reconstruction of immobile thumb post

(Adapted with permission from Wei FC, el-Gammal TA, Lin CH, Chuang CC, Chen HC, Chen SH et al: Metacarpal hand: Classification and guidelines for microsurgical reconstruction with toe transfers. *Plast Reconstr Surg* 1997;99:122–128.)

minimal palmar bulk. One recent report described use of a free pronator quadratus muscle flap based on the anterior interosseous vessels. This technique is limited to reconstruction of small defects, primarily in the region of the MCP joints, because of the limited size of the muscle as well as the short vascular pedicle.

Dorsal Hand

Because of the extremely thin, relatively fragile nature of the skin on the dorsum of the hand, full-thickness loss with tendon exposure or segmental tendon loss is typically encountered more often than palmar skin loss. Occasionally, composite defects of skin, tendon, and bone are seen, most often in urban environments from gunshot wounds. Full-thickness skin loss alone can be reconstructed with a variety of thin fascial or fasciocutaneous flaps, including TPF, lateral arm, proximal forearm, opposite radial forearm, or in some cases reversed pedicle radial ipsilateral forearm.

When tendons are lost, tendonocutaneous flaps can be used—including the dorsalis pedis artery with the long toe extensors, the radial forearm with brachioradialis and palmaris longus, the lateral arm with vascularized tricep tendon, and/or the bilateral temporoparietal flap with interposition tendon grafts. Although the dorsalis pedis flap is the closest analog for tendonocutaneous reconstruction, it requires meticulous dissection and frequently results in donor site morbidity. The lateral arm vascularized triceps tendon transfer has been reported, but without any long-term functional evaluation. Radial forearm flap, incorporating the brachioradialis and palmaris longus muscles, has resulted in reasonable function but has been rarely employed.

Composite defects resulting in loss of diaphyseal metacarpal segments along with tendon and/or skin are best reconstructed using either the lateral arm osteocutaneous flap or the radial forearm osteocutaneous flap. Both flaps have the advantage of combining vascularized cortical bone with a thin skin covering and a reasonably long vascular pedicle. Both carry vascularized nerve that can be used for interposition nerve reconstruction. The radial forearm flap should be reserved for larger cutaneous defects with larger bone defects. The lateral arm osteocutaneous flap can yield a skin paddle up to one third the circumference of the humeral skin, with a bone transfer measuring no greater than 4 cm long by 1 cm wide. A cuff of triceps muscle must be harvested with the bone segment to ensure adequate vascularity. Stabilization of these osseous segments is accomplished with miniplates and/or K-wires. External fixators can be used to further protect the reconstruction in the early phase.

Forearm
Full-thickness skin and subcutaneous loss with exposure of nerves, vessels, and/or bone can best be covered using large, ample muscle transfers. The latissimus dorsi free flap is the first choice for this type of reconstruction. A myocutaneous construct is rarely used; split-thickness skin grafts placed over the latissimus muscle at the time of transfer is the norm. The rectus abdominis has been described for coverage of small to moderate lesions in the forearm and antebrachium. When skin flaps are desired, either parascapular or scapular/cutaneous flaps or lateral arm/proximal forearm flaps can usually accommodate the particular reconstructive needs. Long-bone deficiencies are usually diaphyseal, and are best reconstructed using a vascularized fibular transfer. Based on the peroneal vessels, up to 20 cm of fibula can routinely be harvested. The proximal fibula must be protected to avoid injury to the peroneal nerve, while the distal 6 to 8 cm of fibula is left untouched to protect the ankle mortise and syndesmotic region of the tibia and fibula. When the fibula is harvested, a longitudinally oriented distal skin paddle over the posterior intercrural septum can be reliably carried on the septal perforators from the peroneal vessels as they pass the fibular periosteum. While fibular osteoarticular reconstructions have been reported after resection of giant cell tumors of the distal radius, no long-term follow-up has proven their superiority over nonvascularized techniques. Motorized muscle transfer for extrinsic finger flexion and/or extension is primarily accomplished using the gracilis muscle. This expendable thigh adductor has a dominant neurovascular pedicle including the medial circumflex femoral vessels and anterior branch of the obturator nerve. In the case of flexor digitorum profundus reconstruction, the most common procedure is vascular anastamosis to the radial or ulnar arteries, with the microneurorrhaphy targeting the anterior interosseous nerve. Finger extension is accomplished with free muscle gracilis anastamosed to the radial artery as well as microneurorrhaphy to the posterior

interosseous nerve. Muscle resting tension must be marked by suture ligature every 5 cm on the donor muscle prior to harvest. Tendons are woven through the distal musculotendinous unit using Pulvertaft weaves. Maximal finger flexion is accomplished prior to tensioning of the muscle transfer. Long-term occupational therapy and strong patient motivation are key to successful functional outcome.

Elbow and Brachium
Large traumatic and postablative defects about the elbow and brachium are best covered by large muscle transfers. In most cases, the latissimus dorsi muscle can be transferred with its thoracodorsal pedicle intact. The vascularized fibula serves nicely for reconstruction of the humeral segmental diaphyseal loss. Muscle transfer to improve elbow flexion can be accomplished using either the gracilis muscle as a free-tissue transfer, or the latissimus and/or pectoralis muscles as islandized, rotational transfers. Both the origin and insertion for each muscle must be reestablished.

Various techniques have been tried for restoration of function after brachial plexus injuries. Attempts to provide active shoulder abduction with motorized free muscle transfer have failed to provide enough power and stabilization to improve joint function. Optimal results have come from motorized gracilis transfers for elbow flexion. Successful renervation has been described using 2 or 3 intercostal nerves. Distal flexor and/or extensor reconstruction using free muscle transfers innervated by nerve grafts extending from the intercostals have failed to yield any functional improvement.

Recent Technical Advances

Procedures
In the area of digital reconstruction, procedures such as partial toe transfers, free nail transfers, and extended modified twisted toe transfers have added a series of technically difficult but rewarding surgical options to improve the aesthetic outcome of proven functional reconstructions. Aggressive, delayed sensory reeducation can significantly improve all parameters of sensory nerve function in transferred toes. Free skin and fasciocutaneous flap transfers have been advanced by the introduction of the extended lateral arm flap or proximal forearm flap, which is based on superficial plexus extending out from the posterior radial collateral vessels. This provides a source of thin, pliable, sensate skin for hand and wrist coverage.

Prefabrication of free flaps has provided interesting theoretical options, but few have been practically employed. Vein grafts have been used for some time to bridge the gap between

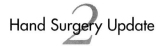
tissue deficit and usable recipient vasculature. Although reported sporadically, complication rates were significantly greater. The increased experience with these venous adjuncts has led to patency rates consistent with primary anastomosis in free-tissue transfer of the upper extremity. Several authors have reported variations in recipient vascular extension by using distally based recipient arteries to provide inflow to free-tissue reconstructions. An axiomatic prerequisite is patency of the palmar arches. These options would allow use of the radial artery that is divided proximal to the wrist to be brought antegrade, and used for anastamosis and coverage of the antebrachium and humeral regions; the digital vessels could be used to vascularize small reconstructions and toe-to-thumb or finger transfers with intact pulp collaterals. Randomly designed venous flaps have been further refined by modification to include multiple venous outflow channels with only a single high-pressure inflow route via end-to-side arterial venous loop formation. These flaps, which are usually constructed in the proximal volar forearm region, have yet to find their way into the mainstream of free-tissue transfer options.

In those rare cases of massive longitudinal injuries that are deemed salvageable, sequential anastomosis of multiple free flaps has been reported. One case described incorporated the use of the fibula osteocutaneous flap for distal radius reconstruction with radial carpal fusion, coupled with the lateral arm fasciocutaneous flap anastomosed to the distal peroneal vessels. Other potential combinations would require the primary flap to contain flow-through vessels (eg, the peroneal vessels of the fibula, or the radial artery and vein of the radial forearm free flap).

Prosthetics

Microanastomotic coupling devices have been used frequently in hand and upper extremity free-tissue reconstruction and replantation. Patency rates are equivalent to or greater than comparably-sized hand-sewn anastamosis. Few problems have been reported, other than 2 cases of discomfort secondary to transcutaneous perception of the coupling device on the dorsal surface of the digits.

Polytetrafluoroethlyene (PTFE) grafts of less than 3 mm in diameter have been used for microarterial reconstruction in the palmar arches. Prostheses as small as 1.5 mm in diameter have been reported. 3M microanastomotic couplers can be used for anastomosis between the PTFE grafts and the native vasculature.

Performance

Success of free-tissue reconstruction using loupe magnification alone is well documented. Patency rates in one series of over 250 procedures were equivalent to others using standard opposable microscopic magnification. Recommended magnification is 5.5 × loupes, with anastomotic repair being done either in interrupted or running fashions. If appropriately selected for larger diameter vessels (2 mm and above), free-tissue reconstruction should be technically equivalent to procedures performed under loupe magnification by cardiac and vascular surgeons. Assuming equivalent patency, clear advantages include cost savings, portability, and operator freedom.

Protocols

Major areas of research in the field of free-tissue reconstruction involve microsurgery, or the anastomosis of vessels smaller than 0.5 mm; prefabrication and tissue engineering of free flaps prior to transfer; and tolerable long-term immunosuppression for limb allotransplantation. The ability to reliably anastomose vessels between 0.2 and 0.5 mm could open a new level of tissue transfer and/or tissue salvage; current limitations include magnification, suture material, and technical competency. Laser-welding anastomosis remains controversial in routine microvascular surgery because of pseudoaneurysmal formation, but may play an increasing role for coaptation of extremely small-diameter vessels.

A better working knowledge of tissue growth factors, as well as the coupling of porous implants allowing in-growth and compatible hydrogels, may allow prefabrication of free-tissue transfers that meet multiple recipient needs. Finally, limb allotransplantation is the focus of many reconstructive microsurgical laboratories, with most research effort now concentrated on the evolution of minimally toxic long-term immunosupression. Pharmacologic immunosupression has evolved away from steroid immunosuppression to more selective agents such as cyclosporin, antilymphycocyte globulins, and FK 506. Significant issues with respect to patient tolerance and long-term toxicities have yet to be resolved, and have spurred recent investigators to continue the search for more tolerable immunosuppressive agents.

Annotated Bibliography

History

Buncke HJ: Forty years of microsurgery: What's next? *J Hand Surg* 1995;20A:S34–S45.

This is an excellent historical review of reconstructive microsurgery over the last 40 years, by the undisputed father of the discipline. The bibliography is comprehensive. Historic firsts both in replantation and free-tissue transfer are neatly tabulated for quick reference. This should be required reading for all students and practitioners of free-tissue reconstruction.

Technique

Dzwierzynski WW, Sanger JR, Yousif NJ, Matloub HS: Case report: Sequential vascular connection of free flaps in the upper extremity. *Ann Plast Surg* 1997;39:303–307.

In this case study, 2 free flaps were joined in series during a delayed reconstruction of a previously revascularized forearm after a mutilating crush injury. A lateral arm flap was anastomosed to the distal peroneal vessels of a transferred fibula flap in an attempt to simultaneously reconstruct bone, skin, and gliding surfaces for further tendon reconstruction. The authors propose that simultaneously transferred free flaps hooked in series allow composite reconstruction, better monitoring of buried osseous free flaps, and optimal position of the 2 free flaps.

Ge XZ, Huang GK: Use of distal arteries for microvascular reconstruction in forearm and hand surgery. *Microsurgery* 1996;17:180–183.

Nine patients underwent a variety of upper extremity microvascular reconstruction procedures in which a distal artery, usually the radial artery, provided vascular inflow after proximal ligation and recipient artery reorientation. Procedures included toe-to-hand transfers, replantation, cutaneous transfers, and brachial artery reconstruction. Advantages were reported to include elimination of vein grafts, single anastomosis, and minimization of size discrepancies. Adequate collateral circulation is an absolute prerequisite.

Germann G, Steinau HU: The clinical reliability of vein grafts in free-flap transfer. *J Reconstr Microsurg* 1996;12:11–17.

Ninety-three interpositional vein grafts in 55 patients were studied for patency. Subgroups examined included arterioarterial venovenous and arteriovenous loop interpositions. A 15% revision rate was noted. Flaps revascularized with the aid of vein grafts had a success rate (96%) equivalent to a similar large series without vein grafts. The authors conclude that the well-planned use of interpositional vein grafts does not result in an increased rate of flap loss.

Kind GM, Buncke GM, Buncke HJ: Foreign-body sensation following 3M coupler use in the hand. *Ann Plast Surg* 1996;37:418–421.

Two symptomatic patients are presented after replantation in which the 3M microanastomotic coupler was used. Eleven patients underwent various microsurgical procedures to the hand employing the 3M coupler; no intraoperative problems or postoperative thromboses were reported. The 2 symptomatic patients complained of tender subcutaneous masses over the area of the coupling device, which was located in the dorsum of the hand. Although the authors strongly support use of the 3M device, they caution against its use in the dorsum, where subcutaneous tissue is sparse.

Lanzetta M: Use of the 3M precise microvascular anastomotic system in hand surgery. *J Hand Surg* 1995;20A:725–730.

The 3M microanastomotic coupler was used in 17 patients requiring replantation and/or revascularization after trauma. Nearly all of the vessel repairs were at or distal to the superficial palmar arch; many were in distal digital arteries. Sixteen of 17 coupled anastomoses were arterial, with diameters averaging 1 to 2 mm. Five anastomoses were at the distal interphalangeal joint. Neither early thromboses nor late aneurysmal formation were noted.

Shenaq SM, Klebuc MJ, Vargo D: Free-tissue transfer with the aid of loupe magnification: Experience with 251 procedures. *Plast Reconstr Surg* 1995;95:261–269.

A large series of free-tissue transfers is described, using loupe magnification instead of the operating microscope to perform anastomoses. Magnification of 5.5 × loupes, coupled with overhead lighting in microvascular anastomoses averaging 1.5 mm in diameter, resulted in an overall success rate of 97%; this compares favorably with many large series using the operating microscope. This alternative is advocated on the basis of cost-effectiveness, portability, and operator freedom.

Toe Transfers

el-Gammal TA, Wei FC: Microvascular reconstruction of the distal digits by partial toe transfer. *Clin Plast Surg* 1997;24:49–55.

The distal digit is defined as that part of the finger distal to the sublimis insertion or (in the thumb) the interphalangeal joint. Ideal reconstruction maintains length, nail function, soft-tissue padding, near normal sensation, and aesthetics. Most donor free-tissue transfers are based on the first dorsal metatarsal artery axis. Options detailed include pulp flaps of the great and second toes, great or second toe nails, wraparound flaps, distal trimmed great toe, and partial lesser toes.

Iglesias M, Butron P, Serrano A: Thumb reconstruction with extended twisted toe flap. *J Hand Surg* 1995;20A:731–736.

A series of 12 patients undergoing thumb reconstruction with the twisted toe flap is described. The donor site was a complex combination of a neurovascular-cutaneous flap from the great toe plus an osteotendinous flap from the second toe, harvested together on the first dorsal metatarsal artery. One of the 12 transfers failed, with an overall 17% major complication rate reported. Results at both donor and recipient sites were described as adequate. This procedure is advocated for patients who refuse classic great toe transfer because of cosmetic, cultural, or work considerations.

Kay SP, Wiberg M: Toe to hand transfer in children: Part 1. Technical aspects. *J Hand Surg* 1996;21B:723–734.

In this large series of microvascular toe transfers, 14 children underwent single toe transfers, while 26 children had 2 toe transfers. Congenital differences, the reason the majority being symbrachydactyly, were the impetus for 85% of the procedures. All transfers survived. Many underwent subsequent tenolysis or tendon transfer. Of the 66 toes transferred, only 2 were complete great toe donors, and 2 wraparound free flaps. The only monobloc second and third toe combination that was transferred was from a highly abnormal foot that was subsequently amputated.

Kay SP, Wiberg M, Bellew M, Webb F: Toe to hand transfer in children: Part 2. Functional and psychological aspects. *J Hand Surg* 1996;21B:735–745.

All 40 children in the report annotated above were followed and tested independently for motor and sensory functional restoration as well as psychosocial effect. The older the child at the time transfer, the better the end range of motion (ROM). Passive ROM exceeded active ROM by an average of 60%, despite tenolyses and transfers. All recovered protective sensation, with most achieving good levels of 2-point discrimination. All transfers were incorporated into naturally occurring use patterns, with most reporting a very positive psychosocial effect.

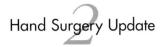
Wei FC, Chen HC, Chuang CC, Chen SH: Microsurgical thumb reconstruction with toe transfer: Selection of various techniques. *Plast Reconstr Surg* 1994;93:345–357.

In this study, 103 toe-to-thumb transfers are reviewed over a 9-year period, in an attempt to provide guidelines for optimal selection of donor site alternatives. Alternatives include second toe, total great toe, great toe wraparound and trimmed great toe. Second toes are best for nontolerance of great toe as donor, sizable second toe, and children. Total great toe is best for those who need maximal function, and for amputations at MCP joint with matching donor and opposite thumb. Wraparound is best for amputations distal to IP joint, or distal skin avulsion with normal IP joint function. Trimmed toe is best for large size discrepancy between donor and opposite thumb, and where IP joint motion and appearance are equally important.

Congenital

Vilkki SK: Advances in microsurgical reconstruction of the congenitally adactylous hand. *Clin Orthop* 1995;314:45–58.

In this study of 18 second toe transplants for reconstruction of congenital adactyly, results, while mostly favorable, varied as a function of the number of joints transferred per toe (3 better than 2); inclusion of intrinsic muscle repair at time of transfer; and repair of as many nerves as possible, including dorsal sensory nerves. Reconstruction of pinch and growth of epiphyses was noted in an overwhelming majority of patients.

Wei FC, el-Gammal TA, Lin CH, Chuang CC, Chen HC, Chen SH: Metacarpal hand: Classification and guidelines for microsurgical reconstruction with toe transfers. *Plast Reconstr Surg* 1997;99:122–128.

This article proposes a classification for the metacarpal hand using the presence of a functioning thumb (Type I) or absence of a functioning thumb (Type II) as the main differentiator. Subclassification is based on the level of the finger amputations in Type I, and level of the thumb amputation in Type II. Different toe transfer procedures are recommended based on this classification.

Flap Harvest

Adani R, Castagnini L, Balsam M, Caroli A: First web space reconstruction by a free flap from the contralateral paralysed hand. *Microsurgery* 1995;16:827–829.

This case report involves the use of a dorsal hand skin flap harvested from a useless, insensate hand prior to amputation, used to reconstruct the first web space of the opposite injured hand. The tenet "spare parts whenever possible" is nicely demonstrated in this article. While the opportunities for such donor sites are rare in hand and upper extremity, they should be seized whenever feasible.

Brandt KE, Khouri RK: The lateral arm/proximal forearm flap. *Plast Reconstr Surg* 1993;92:1137–1143.

Fifteen patients underwent harvesting of the posterolateral forearm skin as an extension of the lateral arm flap, with the pedicle remaining as the posterior radial collateral artery and vein. Advantages include a larger flap, thinner skin, a longer vascular pedicle, and more reliable sensory recovery in the transferred tissue based on the posterior cutaneous nerve to the forearm. The longest flap was 35 cm, while the largest in volume 476 cm².

Brown DM, Upton J, Khouri RK: Free flap coverage of the hand. *Clin Plast Surg* 1997;24:57–62.

This article is a limited review of the use of skin and fascial free flaps for full-thickness dorsal and palmar defects of the hand. The lateral arm flap, proximal forearm flap (or extended lateral arm flap), contralateral radial forearm flap, dorsalis pedis flap, and temporoparietal fascia flap are considered. Scapular, groin, deltoid, and lateral thigh flaps are discouraged because of their bulkiness.

Chuang DC: Functioning free muscle transplantation for brachial plexus injury. *Clin Orthop* 1995;314:104–111.

In this series, 64 patients underwent some form of functioning free muscle transplantation and nerve transfer after brachial plexus injury. The most successful outcomes were in those who had biceps restoration using a gracilis muscle motored by 2 or 3 intercostal nerves. Other free muscle donors used included latissimus, rectus femoris, and gastrocnemius. Muscle transplants designed to restore shoulder abduction were unsuccessful. The results of transplants motorized by either cranial nerve XI or contralateral spinal nerves were highly variable.

Dautel G, Merle M: Pronator quadratus free muscle flap for treatment of palmar defects. *J Hand Surg* 1993;18B:576–578.

The pronator quadratus muscle, previously described by different authors as both a proximally based and distally based pedicle flap, is used as a free-tissue transfer to free the muscle from its short arc of rotation. The anterior interosseous pedicle is used, and is described as extremely short with very small diameter vessels, ie, venae comitantes 0.6 mm. The average muscle belly measured 4 × 5 cm, and could only be used for small defects. No deficit in pronation was noted during posttransfer muscle testing.

Desai SS, Chuang DC, Levin LS: Microsurgical reconstruction of the extensor system. *Hand Clin* 1995;11:471–482.

Various options for microvascular reconstruction of the dorsal hand extensor system are described. The authors detail use of the radial forearm flap harvested with a portion of the brachioradialis and palmaris longus as tendon donors in addition to the dorsalis pedis flap with the short extensors to the lesser toes. Functioning muscle transferred for extensor defects includes gracilis, latissimus, tensor fascia lata, or soleus harvested with fibula for composite defects. One-stage reconstruction with early institution of therapy is strongly advocated.

Friedman JD, Sherman R: Options for vascularized bone transfer in the upper extremity. *Problems in Plastic and Reconstructive Surgery* 1993;3:312–326.

The history, potential donor sites, indications, and operative techniques are described for use of the fibula, iliac crest, lateral arm/humerus, and parascapular flaps as alternatives for vascularized bone transfers in reconstruction of composite osseous defects of the upper extremity. Case reports are provided for further illustration.

Jeng SF, Wei FC, Noordhoff MS: The composite groin fascial free flap. *Ann Plast Surg* 1995;35:595–600.

Seven patients with composite loss of dorsal hand skin, subcutaneous tissue, and tendons underwent reconstruction with a classically described groin flap using the superficial circumflex iliac artery and vein, then extended by including well-vascularized external oblique aponeurotic fascia. All transfers were successful, with the vascularized

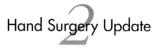
fascia employed to provide a gliding surface for tendon reconstruction. Tendon reconstruction was done by simultaneous grafting or tendon transfer. The authors note excellent cosmesis, minimal donor site morbidity, and one-stage reconstruction as the distinct advantages.

Krimmer H, Hahn P, Lanz U: Free gracilis muscle transplantation for hand reconstruction. *Clin Orthop* 1995;314:13–18.

Fifteen patients received motorized gracilis transfer to restore either finger flexion or extension. A majority of patients had developed Volkman's ischemic contracture after trauma. The survival rate was 87%, with all viable transfers demonstrating some functional return. Secondary procedures were required in half of the transfers to achieve optimal outcomes. Wrist fusion significantly improved finger flexion power in 2 cases.

Reynoso R, Espinosa A, Mendoza M, Clifton J: The arterialized antebrachial skin flap for hand reconstruction. *J Reconstr Microsurg* 1997;13:267–275.

In this study, 20 patients underwent arterialized venous skin free flaps. Distal forearm antebrachial skin was the preferred donor site. Afferent, controlled arterial venous inflow with multiple efferent venovenous anastomoses yielded better results than uncontrolled inflow and single vessel outflow. All flaps suffered some degree of congestion. Excellent coverage was achieved in 75% of patients. The main advantage of these flaps is that they do not sacrifice important donor vessels.

Yajima H, Tamai S, Fukui A, Ono H, Inada Y: Free and island flap transfer for soft tissue defects in the hand and forearm. *Microsurgery* 1996;17:150–154.

This 20-year retrospective review described 226 flaps used in upper extremity reconstruction. Seventy-nine patients underwent 82 free flaps, with a 94% survival rate. Four of the 5 flap failures involved a dorsalis pedis donor site. Island pedicle flaps and free flaps are compared. Indications for the primary use of free flaps include thumb, multiple finger, and large composite tissue defects.

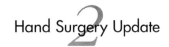

Chapter 30
Congenital and Pediatric Vascular Malformations

David Netscher, MD

Saleh M. Shenaq, MD

Incidence and Classification

Hemangiomas are the most common vascular tumors of infancy and childhood, occurring in 4 to 5 of every 100 newborns, and because 40% to 60% of lesions are evident at birth, hemangiomas are also the most frequent congenital anomaly. After ganglions, giant cell tumors, and inclusion cysts, vascular lesions are the fourth most common hand tumor.

Overall, the nomenclature for the classification of vascular malformations has changed with better understanding of the pathogenesis. The unifying classification system is helpful in predicting behavior of a given lesion and then recommending rational treatment. The authors of a classic study published in 1982 concluded that the involuting hemangiomas could be distinguished from the noninvoluting growths (or vascular malformations) by histologic and radiologic evaluation, and by careful history taking and clinical examination. In fact, most lesions can be categorized by clinical evaluation of appearance, location, and flow characteristics (palpable thrill and audible auscultatory bruit) without having to resort to special investigations such as angiography, magnetic resonance imaging (MRI), or color Doppler imaging (CDI).

Old terms, such as strawberry nevus and port wine stain, have given way to hemangioma and capillary malformation, respectively; while cavernous lesions are now classified either as hemangiomas or venous malformations, depending on their characteristics. Likewise, the terms lymphangioma and cystic hygroma have been substituted by lymphatic malformation. Thus, there are now considered to be 2 distinct subclasses of pediatric vascular lesions, hemangiomas and vascular malformations. Only 30% of hemangiomas are visible at birth, but almost all appear during the neonatal period. Rapid growth then occurs followed by proportionate growth, and finally a slow process of involution. Three times as many females as males are affected by hemangiomas. In contrast, malformations are all present at birth (but may not

be seen until later years), and they tend to enlarge in proportion to the child unless accelerated growth is stimulated by trauma, hormonal changes, infection, or surgical intervention. Other differences between hemangiomas and vascular malformations are noted in Table 1.

Vascular malformations are, in turn, subclassified based on the vessel size and flow characteristics of the lesion. Thus, there are capillary, venous, lymphatic, and arteriovenous malformations. The first 3 are low-flow lesions and the latter is a high-flow lesion. There also are various combinations such as lymphaticovenous malformations and capillary venous malformations. Certain syndromal conditions may be associated with limb hypertrophy. These include Klippel-Trénaunay syndrome, a capillary-venous-lymphatic malformation that may diffusely affect an extremity and is associated with the blush of an overlying port wine stain (Fig. 1) and Parkes-Weber syndrome, which is an association of port wine stain, multiple arteriovenous malformations, and limb overgrowth. In both these syndromes, the vascular malformations are restricted to the cutaneous and subcutaneous tissues. They usually do not involve muscles and joints. In contrast, pure venous malformations of extremities also involve muscles and other tissues. Maffucci's syndrome is characterized by the coexistence of vascular malformations and dyschondroplasia (Ollier's disease).

Evaluation of Vascular Lesions

History and Physical Examination

Hemangiomas grow very rapidly during the proliferative phase, they begin to involute slowly before 1 year of age, and they are generally quiescent by 5 years of age. The characteristic growth and regression distinguishes hemangiomas from vascular malformations. The beginning of involution can be seen by graying of the surface of the lesion. Spontaneous ulceration may occur during the proliferative phase.

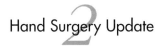

Table 1

Characteristics of pediatric vascular lesions

	Hemangioma	**Malformation**
Clinical	Forty percent present at birth; rapid growth, slow involution; female:male ratio 3:1	All present at birth; growth commensurate with child; no resolution; female:male ratio 1:1
Cell biology	Endothelial proliferation; increased mast cells; multilaminated basement membrane	Flat endothelium, slow turnover; normal mast cell count; normal basement membrane
Hematologic	Platelet trapping thrombocytopenia (Kasabach-Merritt)	Primary venous stasis with consumptive coagulopathy
Radiographic	Seldom a "mass effect" on adjacent bone	Phleboliths seen in low-flow lesions
	On angiography they appear as organized, gland-like neoplasms with "lobular-parenchymal staining"	Venous malformations show rarefaction of bone and hypoplasia; mixed capillary-venous and capillary-arteriovenous lesions may have bone hypertrophy
		Angiography shows a collection of tortuous vessels without a "parenchymal" mass, and there may be arteriovenous shunting

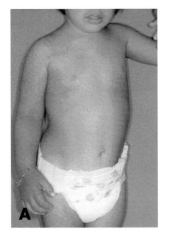 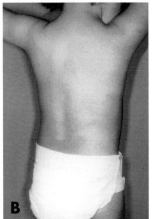 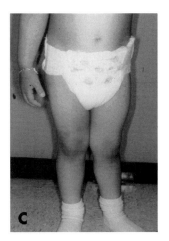 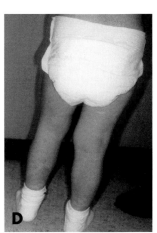

Figure 1

Child with capillary venous malformations showing hypertrophy of right upper extremity and capillary port wine skin staining of upper extremity **(A)**, trunk **(B)**, and legs **(C** and **D)**.

Healing by epithelialization of the ulceration leaves a pale central scar (Fig. 2). Involution is progressive, although skin redundancy or a residual fibrofatty mass may remain once it is completed; in the upper extremity, this is rarely problematic (6%). Fifty percent of these anomalies are regressed by age 5 years and 70% by age 7 years.

Vascular malformations, in contrast, grow commensurately with the child. Expansion can occur with the pubertal growth spurt, during pregnancy, following trauma, while taking birth control medications, or after subtotal excision. Although malformations are said to be present at birth, many are inconspicuous and do not appear until late childhood.

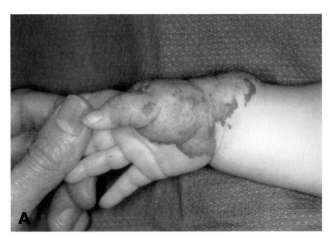
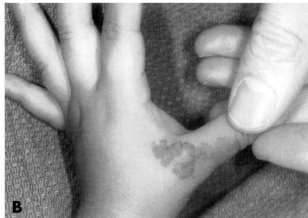

Figure 2

A and **B,** Two patients showing hemangiomas of the hand with classic involutional phase appearance.

Port wine stains (capillary malformations) may be present at birth, but only in later life may it become obvious that they are associated with a deeper, low-flow venous or lymphatic anomaly or, less frequently, with a high-flow arteriovenous malformation. The extent of a port wine stain (also called naevus flammeus in the pink stage early in life) usually does not change with growth, and in the extremities there is no tendency for a particular dermatomal distribution as there is with trigeminal involvement on the face. With time the stain assumes a purple hue, and the skin develops a cobblestone appearance.

Venous and lymphatic malformations may coexist and may be insidious in their development, but are usually obvious by 4 or 5 years of age. Venous malformations are distinguished clinically by enlargement when the limb is lowered, and they decompress when the limb is elevated. Phleboliths may be palpable and indicate the presence of a venous malformation. Epidermal vesicle formation of clear serous fluid is pathognomonic of a lymphatic lesion (especially when it occurs in an incisional scar), but this dermal involvement may not always occur with lymphatic malformations, especially when they are deeply located.

By contrast, arteriovenous malformations have features of increased blood flow, such as increased warmth, subcutaneous pulsations, a thrill, and a bruit. A large lesion proximal to the wrist may demonstrate a positive Branham's sign, which is a reduction in heart rate when a proximal occluding tourniquet is applied.

Complications

Hemangiomas and vascular malformations may have local or systemic complications.

Hemangiomas About 30% of upper limb hemangiomas ulcerate. Maceration and infection may develop. Fingertip hemangiomas may be accompanied by acute or chronic paronychial infections, especially among children who suck their fingers.

Extensive upper extremity hemangiomas usually do not cause compressive symptoms, nerve palsies, or significant compromise of major muscle-tendon units. Very occasionally, local distortion and tissue destruction may occur. These larger lesions may cause high output congestive failure in neonates.

Kasabach-Merritt syndrome is a coagulation disorder that occurs with hemangiomas in infancy; usually these are very large or multiple systemic hemangiomas. There is a profound thrombocytopenia and consumptive coagulopathy. This is a self-limited condition, and the platelet level returns to normal once the hemangioma regresses.

Venous Malformations Pain may occur with venous vascular malformations. The pain may be related to muscle involvement, with vascular engorgement, or to episodes of thrombosis or intralesional hemorrhage. Painful subcutaneous thrombi and calcified phleboliths are less symptomatic on nonpercussive surfaces. Intermittent joint pain and swelling may be caused by joint effusions or hemarthroses. The latter may be caused by malformations that are intra-articular in location or secondary to consumptive coagulopathy. With time, increased weight and bulk of venous lesions are bothersome. Larger lesions are better tolerated in the proximal extremity than in the hand and wrist where dependency increases the weight and size, and functional disturbances of the mobile hand structures are more likely to ensue. In areas where extensive skin involvement occurs, pruritus is likely during summer months, and there is an increased need for skin lubrication.

Skeletal hypertrophy occurs with the syndromal vascular malformations. However, with pure venous malformations, demineralization and hypoplasia of underlying skeletal structures are common. Pathologic fractures may occur.

Patients with large low-flow venous malformations have a somewhat different coagulopathy than those with the Kasabach-Merritt syndrome of hemangiomas. A chronic localized intravascular coagulation results in a very low plasma fibrinogen level, elevation of fibrin split products, and a moderately low platelet count. This chronic consumptive coagulopathy causes episodes of thrombosis, which lead to intralesional phlebolith formation, or bleeding (hemarthroses, hematomas, or intraoperative bleeding) (Fig. 3). Elastic stockings that compress the malformation and reduce blood stagnation also reduce the chronic localized coagulopathy. The condition worsens after cessation of use of elastic stockings, therapeutic intervention (embolization or surgical procedure), spontaneous bone fracture, or during pregnancy or menses in women. When a surgical procedure is considered, treatment with low-molecular-weight heparin minimizes risk of excessive hemorrhage.

Lymphatic Malformations These malformations are seldom painful. Compressive neuropathies do not occur. However, chronic lymphedema may result, and function may be restricted by the bulk of the lesion. Compressive garments are not very effective in the more distal extremity, probably because the cystic channels in the hand and digits are small, unlike those in the more proximal extremity.

When skin is involved, there may be persistent fluid leakage and recurrent infections. Skin incisions made in these areas will often break down and discharge fluid from deep cystic pockets. Beta-hemolytic streptococcus is the cause of most cellulitic episodes.

Children with massive lymphatic malformations of more than 1 extremity may have diffuse involvement of the pulmonary system, liver, and gastrointestinal tract. Malabsorption and protein-losing enteropathy may become life-threatening.

Arteriovenous Malformations As with other vascular lesions, complications of arteriovenous malformations may be localized or systemic. There is proximal arterial collateral enlargement with "parasitic" reversed flow in the artery distal to the arteriovenous connection. Additionally, increased pressure in the veins causes varicosity and pericapillary fibrin cuffing. The latter, together with reduced distal arterial flow, results in distal tissue ischemia and necrosis (Fig. 4). Increased blood volume returning to the heart ultimately results in increased cardiac output from both tachycardia and increased cardiac stroke volume. High output cardiac failure may ensue.

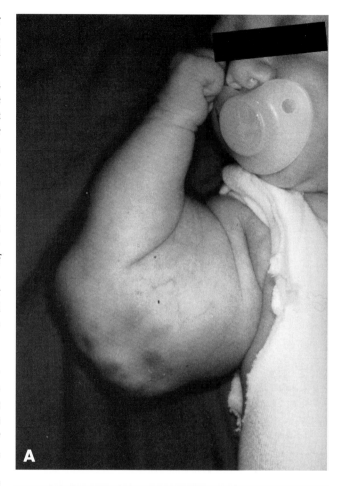

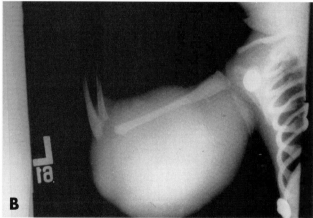

Figure 3

A, This neonate had a very large venous malformation affecting the axilla and upper arm. **B,** Intralesional phleboliths are seen on the plain radiograph. This child had a chronic consumptive coagulopathy and had both hemarthroses and gastrointestinal bleeding that required blood transfusions. She died suddenly at age 10 months from acute disseminated intravascular coagulopathy after developing a relatively minor respiratory infection.

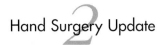

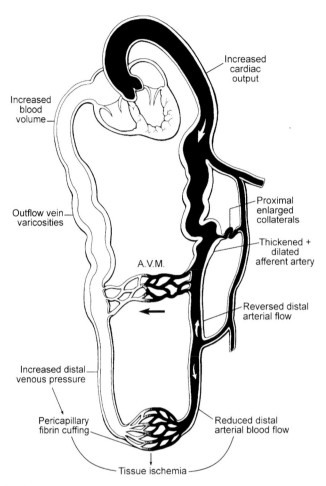

Figure 4

Circulatory pathophysiologic changes that develop with arteriovenous malformations and result in distal extremity ischemia.

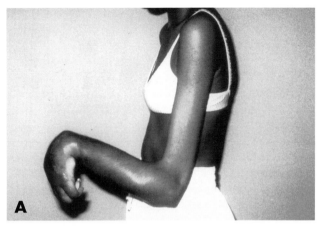

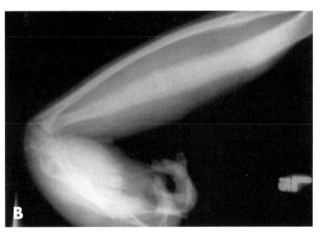

Figure 5

A, Patient with a pure venous malformation and Volkman's-like contracture (at age 17 years). **B,** Radiograph showing the contracted wrist and finger position and the skeletal changes.

Venous and arteriovenous malformations may sometimes develop the sequelae of Volkman's-like ischemic contracture (Fig. 5).

Atypical Vascular Lesions

Hemangiomas and vascular malformations may have synovial involvement. In a joint, this involvement may result in acute painful hemarthrosis; whereas, in the flexor tendon sheath, it may mimic that of tenosynovitis. MRI will help confirm the suspected diagnosis, and treatment involves resection of the lesion and synovectomy.

Perineural vascular malformations are uncommon. Frequently the diagnosis is not suspected before surgical exploration and the appearance is often that of a painful extremity mass. Nerve involvement is of three types: type 1 is an intraneural extrafascicular malformation that is easily removed

with magnification; type 2 is an intrafascicular encompassing malformation that is unresectable because of potential serious nerve damage; and type 3 has both intraneural and extraneural components.

Some question the diagnosis of "blue rubber bleb nevus syndrome" (BRBNS) and believe that it is simply a variety of venous malformation characterized by distinctive vascular lesions of the skin and gastrointestinal tract. The skin vascular malformations are superficially located and are red to blue in color. The lesions are soft and easily compressible, leaving an empty, wrinkled sack that refills slowly. They can be macular, papular, or nodular. Overlying skin may show increased sweating. Unlike the cutaneous lesions, the gastrointestinal lesions bleed readily, and often produce anemia that requires transfusion. Skeletal abnormalities are often associated.

Vascular malformations have been described in conjunction with other lesions. A case of multiple painful glomus tumors associated with arteriovenous shunting and finger joint nodular lesions has been described. Congenital transverse limb defects have also been associated in familial patterns with vascular malformations covering over the end of the extremity stump.

Finally, other lesions may masquerade as congenital vascular lesions. This is highlighted by a recent report of 2 cases of congenital fibrosarcoma that were initially thought to be hemangiomas. In both of the reported cases there was a soft compressible mass associated with the presence of moderate thrombocytopenia. Differentiation was finally made on the suspicion that the diagnostic criteria of hemangioma were not fully met. These vascular tumors had ectatic superficial veins. The lesions did not feel quite as spongy as hemangiomas, and the modest thrombocytopenia was that of a tumor-related disseminated intravascular coagulopathy (DIC) rather than a true depiction of the profound thrombocytopenia that would be expected with Kasabach-Merritt syndrome. The MRI showed an inhomogeneous mass caused by intralesional bleeding, whereas hemangiomas are homogeneous and may show flow voids on MRI T2-weighted images. Angiography showed classic tumor vessels. The differentiation between hemangioma and fibrosarcoma is, of course, essential so that timely management of the latter may be instituted.

Diagnostic Imaging

Routine Radiographs Bone thinning and osteolytic changes occur with pure venous malformations, whereas skeletal hypertrophy may be associated with syndromal lesions such as those in Klippel-Trénaunay syndrome. Calcified phleboliths may also be seen in the slow-flowing venous lesions. A skeletal survey will provide accurate measurement of bone girth and length and will help in deciding management of and providing follow-up for associated bone hypertrophy.

Technetium Nuclear Medicine Scanning Technetium labeled red blood cell (Tc-RBC) scans are helpful in a number of ways. They differentiate vascular from nonvascular lesions. Thus, lymphangiomas or, for example, the lipodystrophy associated with Klippel-Trénaunay syndrome may be distinguished from vascular malformations. Furthermore

Tc-RBC scanning routinely images the entire body, thereby allowing for evaluation of multiple masses in different parts of the body and for the diagnosis of occult vascular lesions.

Some deep soft-tissue masses not only are difficult to diagnose as vascular lesions, but also may be difficult to distinguish from one another (eg, a deeply located hemangioma and a vascular malformation). This is especially the case for an infant in whom time has not made the character of the lesion evident. Parents often are asked to wait and let the nature of the lesion demonstrate the diagnosis. The Tc-RBC scan allows definitive diagnosis at an earlier age, permitting the physician to give accurate diagnostic prognostic information to the parents. The scan is reported to have diagnostic accuracy of 97%. Hemangiomas show intense focal uptake, but are homogeneous throughout the lesion; in contrast, the malformations show abnormal vessels or diffusely increased activity.

Doppler Imaging CDI is very helpful in the diagnostic workup of vascular malformations. Both high-flow and low-flow lesions can be accurately diagnosed. Follow-up CDI can document the increased inflow arterial rates in treated arteriovenous malformations and aid evaluation for persistent thrombosis of low-flow malformations.

Magnetic Resonance Imaging MRI can be used to determine the anatomic relationship of the malformation to the adjacent nerves and muscles, information that has significant therapeutic considerations (Fig. 6). MRI easily distinguishes between high-flow and low-flow malformations and, therefore, is also an excellent tool for specific diagnosis of the type of vascular malformation to be treated. In

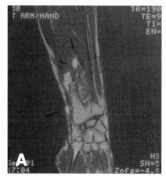
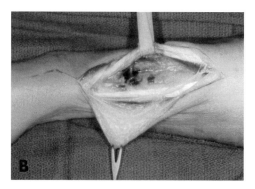

Figure 6

A, A patient who had distal arm pain was seen by magnetic resonance imaging to have a localized venous malformation. **B,** The patient's pain responded to total excision of this lesion.

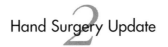

addition to the typical T1 and T2 signal intensities, flow sensitive spin-echo (SE) techniques of scanning are now used. Areas of signal void on SE sequences are not specific for flow, but are confirmed to be flow related by high signal intensity with gradient-echo sequences. Hemangiomas and venous malformations may on occasion be difficult to distinguish clinically. However, unlike venous malformations on MRI, hemangiomas consistently have high-flow signal voids within the lesion.

Magnetic resonance angiography (MRA), at least in 1 institution, has replaced arteriography in the management of vascular malformations of the hand. The technique provides detailed imaging of arterial and venous components of the lesion without requiring contrasting enhancement or an invasive procedure. MRA combined with the various MRI sequences enables resectability to be assessed based on the extent of involvement and flow characteristics.

Arteriography Although arteriography was for a long time the "gold standard" diagnostic evaluation, it is now reserved for use as a preliminary to surgical treatment for arteriovenous malformations. A recommended algorithm for diagnosis has been suggested (Fig. 7). Most patients may be adequately evaluated by clinical examination alone. Following clinical evaluation, MRI would be the next step in the diagnostic ladder. It will reveal either a diffuse or localized low-flow lesion, or a high-flow lesion. Diffuse

low-flow vascular malformations will then generally be treated by nonsurgical measures and observation, while discrete low-flow lesions will be excised for specific indications. Symptomatic high-flow vascular lesions will then require selective angiography to more clearly identify the "feeding" vessels for surgical excision or to enable superselective embolization before surgical removal.

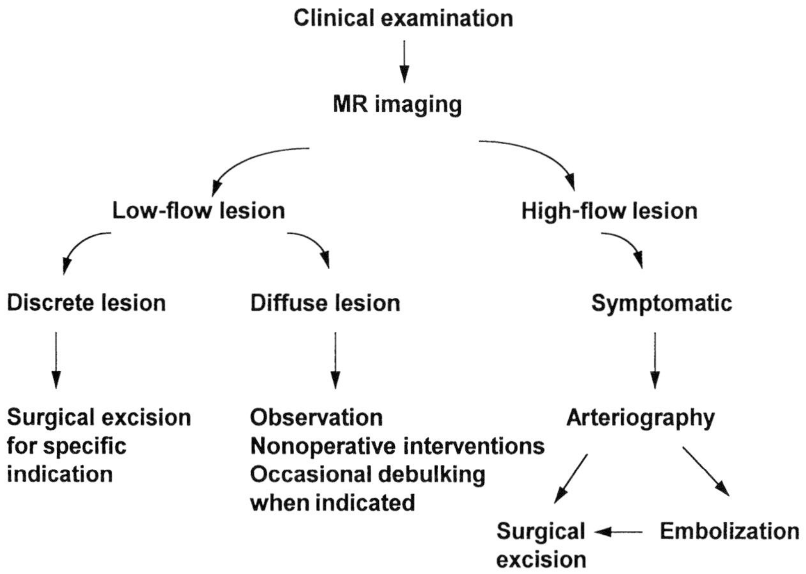

Treatment of Vascular Anomalies

Hemangiomas

Small localized hemangiomas may be excised; this treatment will reduce parental anxiety and annoyances with ulcerations. However, as a general rule, parents must be convinced that watchful waiting is always the best course of treatment for hemangiomas. In the upper extremity, redundant fibro-fatty tissue after involution is seldom a problem that requires surgical contouring (in contrast, perhaps, to facial areas).

Local wound care is all that is needed for an ulcerated hemangioma. Hand splints may be needed to separate digits when there are interdigital ulcerations. Active children and those who suck their fingers should have them immobilized with special rigid elbow splints (similar to those used in the postoperative period with cleft palate patients) that will keep the elbow extended and fingers away from the mouth.

Specific systemic treatment is indicated for complications such as high output cardiac failure and Kasabach-Merritt syndrome. The recommended dosage of steroids is 2 to 3 mg of prednisolone per kg/day, administered orally for 2 to 3 weeks. If the lesion is sensitive, a response is usually noted in this time. Dosage can then be lowered to 1 mg/kg/day. Intralesional injection of methylprednisolone or a triamcinolone/betamethasone combination using 2 injections per week has also been successfully used to treat hemangiomas. Interferon alpha-2a as daily subcutaneous injections (up to 3 million units/m^2 of body surface area) has been used to treat life-threatening hemangiomas in infancy, usually in those who have failed steroid therapy.

Capillary Malformations

Argon laser and tunable dye laser are the most publicized treatments for port wine stains. High-energy light is converted to heat, causing thrombosis or

Clinical examination

↓

MR imaging

Low-flow lesion   **High-flow lesion**

Discrete lesion   **Diffuse lesion**   **Symptomatic**

↓   ↓   ↓

Surgical excision for specific indication   **Observation Nonoperative interventions Occasional debulking when indicated**   **Arteriography**

Surgical ← **Embolization**
excision

Figure 7

Algorithm for diagnostic evaluation of pediatric vascular anomalies.

perivascular narrowing that diminishes the size of the capillary malformation, hopefully, with minimal dermal scarring. Appropriate light wave length in the observed spectrum of oxyhemoglobin results in selective vascular injury. Repeated treatments may be required until the desired degree of lesion lightening has been achieved. Excision and resurfacing with split-thickness skin grafts may be considered for the hypertrophic cobblestoned port wine stains in older patients in whom laser treatments are unlikely to be effective or when oozing and vesicles are present.

Venous Malformations

Treatment of upper extremity venous lesions is initially conservative. Arteriography is generally not indicated. Localized malformations, especially those involving only subcutaneous tissues (as seen on MRI scans) can be readily excised. However, caution must be exercised when considering surgical treatment of diffuse venous malformations. Curative resection is unlikely and complications (such as flap necrosis and poor wound healing) are common, particularly when prior radiation therapy may have been performed. (Irradiation, incidentally, is generally not recommended for treatment of either venous malformations or hemangiomas. It is an outdated therapy because of inconclusive treatment results and serious complications, such as permanent skin changes, induction of future cancers, and potential postsurgical problems.)

Localized pain from venous malformations often occurs. The cause of this pain is often unclear. It may be caused by localized phlebothrombosis. Aspirin or acetaminophen, elevation, and elastic support are the initial treatment for pain. Chronic pain in small, localized malformations on percussive surfaces can be helped by excision and linear closure.

For functional and aesthetic reasons, subtotal excision can be contemplated occasionally for extensive lesions (Fig. 8). Staged resections should begin distally and progress proximally. Preoperative clotting must be assessed, and meticulous intraoperative hemostasis must be achieved. Circumferential flaps should not be raised. Incisions must be planned so that cutaneous vascularity is not compromised and scarred areas of previously operated-on regions are not reentered. There also must be avoidance of intraneural dissection, although external median and ulnar nerve decompressions may be indicated.

Potential complications of these debulking excisions include ischemic flap necrosis, distal digital necrosis, adverse hypertrophic cutaneous scarring, cicatricial tendon adhesions, cicatricial adhesive neuropathy and nerve palsy or chronic pain, and precipitation of DIC.

Lymphatic Malformations

Treatment is required for episodic infections and involves elevation, immobilization, and systemic antibiotics. When repeated cellulitis is problematic, long-term prophylactic antibiotics may be required. Individuals with these malformations must take meticulous care of the skin and nails to prevent entry portals for infection.

Compressive garments control swelling, but are not as effective in reducing bulk as they are with venous malformations. Home compression pumps are also helpful when there is extensive extremity involvement. Coban (a self-adherent tape) wrapping to the digits and hand at night are also effective for helping swelling.

Occasionally, staged surgical debulking may be indicated. Principles of excision are similar to those for the larger venous malformations—mainly avoidance of reentering previously operated-on scarred regions, preservation of cutaneous nerves and dorsal veins, and avoidance of extension of dissections more than 180° circumferentially around the limb. The Charles procedure (ie, complete excision of affected skin and subcutaneous tissue with skin graft replacement) is generally not appropriate for the upper extremity because it leaves unaesthetic results with recurrent skin breakdown and contractures. Lymphatic malformations in the upper arm are often contiguous with chest wall malformations, and single-stage chest wall and axillary dissection may be required. However, dissection within the brachial plexus region should be performed with great caution; it seldom is indicated in order to minimize perineurial scarring and subsequent intractable pain. Massive, diffuse lesions in a functionless limb may best be treated by amputation.

Combined Lymphatic Venous Malformations

Usually nonsurgical interventions are favored; although, occasionally, staged debulking procedures may be required with the already alluded to precautions, such as preoperative coagulation evaluation and careful planning of incisions with preservation of uninvolved neurovascular elements. Upper limb skeletal overgrowth usually is not a functional problem (in contradistinction to the lower limb). Epiphysiodesis is seldom indicated in upper limb hypertrophy. Very rarely, if there is differential overgrowth of either the radius or the ulna, the relevant bone may require shortening to avoid deviation and instability of the carpus and hand.

Arteriovenous Malformations

There are 3 types of arteriovenous malformations. The truncal type has connections between major arteries and veins. Diffuse arteriovenous malformations have multiple small connections between arterial and venous systems. The

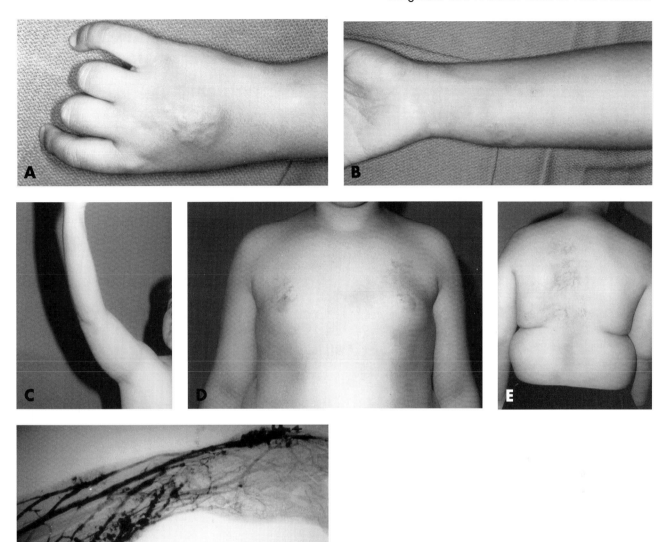

Figure 8

This child is affected by a diffuse venous vascular malformation that clinically affects the dorsum of the hand (**A**), the ulnar aspect of the distal forearm (**B**), the inner upper arm (**C**), and the anterior (**D**) and posterior (**E**) trunk. **F,** Arteriogram shows diffuse venous lakes in the venous phase of the study.

third type is localized, is hemodynamically quieter than the first 2 types, and is more amenable to surgical ablation.

One investigator believed that early treatment of arteriovenous malformations was required to minimize chances of enlargement. However, others have recommended initial conservative treatment and reserve intervention for complications, such as spontaneous projectile bleeds, pain, and increasing size that interferes with function.

Selective transcatheter embolization usually is not recommended as the sole treatment because there is a high recurrence rate. However, staged treatment with initial embolization followed by surgical excision in 24 to 48 hours may reduce the hazards of excision alone. In the distal extremity, embolization poses a particular problem because the endarterial vessels distally have no collaterals. Occlusion of these vessels may result in significant tissue loss. Highly selective embolization into 1-mm diameter vessels is possible and minimizes distal complications.

Intraosseous arteriovenous malformations of extremities are rare and difficult to treat successfully. Usually preliminary

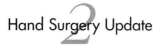
306   Congenital and Pediatric Vascular Malformations

selective embolization is performed. Cortical windows are subsequently surgically opened into the affected bone, the angiomatous tissue is scooped out, and the resulting cavities are filled with bone cement or autogenous bone.

Partial excisions and deafferentation should not be attempted. Instead, a complete dissection of the affected region should be planned. The surgeon must be prepared to use microvascular techniques to reestablish distal circulation. Judicious use of a tourniquet controls blood loss. Complete excision of the anomalous soft tissue with preservation of nerves, skeletal structures, and joints is required. Involved muscle-tendon units, skin, and subcutaneous tissue may be reconstructed or replaced. Split-thickness skin grafts and even free-flap coverage may be required.

Use of total circulatory arrest may be entertained as an adjunct to facilitate excisions of large lesions, especially when located more proximally where tourniquet control is not possible.

Amputation may be the only way to cure a patient with a nonfunctional limb, intractable pain, or where multiple previous surgeries have failed (Fig. 9). Amputations may be lifesaving where extensive malformations result in high-output cardiac failure or consumptive coagulopathy.

There is said to be a complication rate as high as 50% after surgical resection of extremity arteriovenous malformations. Complications include wound breakdown, flap necrosis, distal tissue necrosis, intractable pain, and tendon adherence. Incomplete excision invariably results in proximal expansion of the lesion.

Annotated Bibliography

Incidence and Classification

Mulliken JB, Glowacki J: Hemangiomas and vascular malformations in infants and children: A classification based on endothelial characteristics. *Plast Reconstr Surg* 1982;69: 412–422.

The authors attempt to unify the classification of hemangiomas and vascular malformations. Suggested classifications fall into 6 broad categories: embryology, histology, clinical features, dynamics of growth, hemodynamic pattern, and cell biology. A classification is useful only if it has diagnostic applicability and aids in planning therapy and in understanding of the pathogenesis.

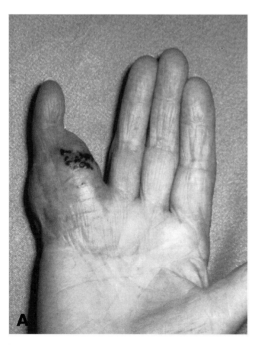
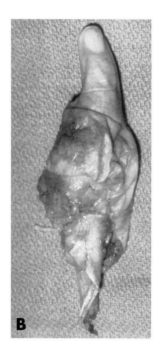
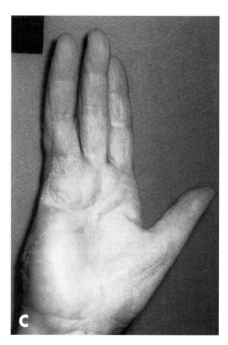

Figure 9

A, Patient with arteriovenous malformation of the little finger was able to be treated by total resection of the lesion by performing (**B** and **C**) a ray amputation of that digit.

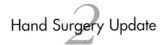
Palmieri TJ: Vascular tumors of the hand and forearm. *Hand Clin* 1987;3:225–240.

This provides a compilation of a large review of vascular upper extremity tumors. The overall incidence of these tumors is described.

Evaluation of Vascular Lesions

Chan P, Lee CP, Lee YH: High output cardiac failure caused by multiple giant cutaneous hemangiomas. *Jpn Heart J* 1992; 33:493–497.

This is a case description of a patient who developed high-output cardiac failure secondary to multiple right upper limb giant hemangiomas.

Enjolras O, Ciabrini D, Mazoyer E, Laurian C, Herbreteau D: Extensive pure venous malformations in the upper or lower limb: A review of 27 cases. *J Am Acad Dermatol* 1997;36:219–225.

This review of pure venous malformations draws the distinction between isolated venous malformations and mixed lesions. Coagulation profiles frequently demonstrated localized intravascular coagulation problems. Most patients had conservative management (elastic stockings), and use of compressive garments had a beneficial effect on the intravascular coagulopathy.

McClinton MA: Tumors and aneurysms of the upper extremity. *Hand Clin* 1993;9:151–169.

This descriptive article on vascular tumors of the upper extremity includes a thorough discussion of the congenital and pediatric vascular disorders. It places the classification system and distinction between hemangiomas and vascular malformations in perspective. It also subdivides the capillary, venous, and arteriovenous malformations by diagnostic and treatment categories.

Nakada K, Kawada T, Fujioka T, et al: Hemangioma of the upper arm associated with massive hemorrhage in a neonate. *Surg Today* 1993;23:273–276.

This case report of young child who had a large axillary hemangioma that required resection because of massive hemorrhage and progressive cardiac failure is used to illustrate the point that rapid surgical intervention may on occasion be required to prevent clinical deterioration in such cases. After resection of that hemangioma, extensive defects of the skin and subcutaneous tissue required closure by a skin flap technique.

Upton J: Vascular malformations of the upper limb, in Mulliken JB, Young AE (eds): *Vascular Birthmarks: Hemangiomas and Malformations.* Philadelphia, PA, WB Saunders, 1988, pp 343–380.

This book chapter, which antedates the value of MRI, is nonetheless an excellent review of vascular anomalies in the upper extremity and their treatment.

Complications and Atypical Vascular Lesions

Boon LM, Fishman SJ, Lund DP, Mulliken JB: Congenital fibrosarcoma masquerading as congenital hemangioma: Report of two cases. *J Pediatr Surg* 1995;30:1378–1381.

The authors report on 2 infants who had large congenital fibrosarcomas that initially were believed to be hemangiomas. They review anatomic findings, hematologic differences, and radiologic clues that can help to differentiate congenital fibrosarcoma from congenital hemangioma.

Filling-Katz MR, Levin SW, Patronas NJ, Katz NN: Terminal transverse limb defects associated with familial cavernous angiomatosis. *Am J Med Genet* 1992;42:346–351.

Although transverse terminal limb defects are rarely reported as familial, this report is that of a patient known to have familial angiomatosis in which 2 relatives had similar terminal transverse defects of the midforearm. The vascular malformation was located at the apex of the distal amputation. The supposition is that familial cavernous angiomatosis may be a new cause of vascular disruption, resulting in terminal transverse limb defects.

Hall BD: Vascular abnormalities at the site of limb deficiency. *Am J Med Genet* 1992;43:619–620.

This is a case report of a child with a transverse limb deficiency and an angiomatous lesion over the tip of the forearm at the site of the deficiency. Again, potential associations of vascular abnormalities and limb deficiencies are discussed.

Louis DS, Fortin PT: Perineural hemangiomas of the upper extremity: Report of four cases. *J Hand Surg* 1992;17A:308–311.

This report reviews 4 cases in which there were neurologic symptoms associated with vascular malformations. The authors found only 8 other previously reported cases in the literature. The greater the extent of intrafascicular involvement, the more difficult is total eradication of the hemangioma. The surgeon should avoid intraneural dissection of these lesions.

Moodley M, Ramdial P: Blue rubber bleb nevus syndrome: Case report and review of the literature. *Pediatrics* 1993;92:160–162.

This article describes a case with the classical cutaneous features of compressible vascular bleb-like lesions of the skin associated with gastrointestinal vascular lesions. This blue rubber bleb nevus syndrome may represent a variant of venous vascular malformation.

Nakamura K: Multiple glomus tumors associated with arteriovenous fistulas and with nodular lesions of the finger joints. *Plast Reconstr Surg* 1992;90:675–683.

This case report associates multiple glomus tumors with arteriovenous fistulas.

Rico AA, Holguin PH, Gonzalez IG, Coba JM: Flexor tendon synovial sheath haemangioma mimicking subacute tenosynovitis. *J Hand Surg* 1994;19B:704–705.

A case of hemangioma arising from the synovial sheath of the flexor tendons is described. The initial symptoms are those of subacute tenosynovitis. The tumor did not affect the flexor tendons and could be completely resected with functional recovery.

Diagnostic Imaging

Barton DJ, Miller JH, Allwright SJ, Sloan GM: Distinguishing soft-tissue hemangiomas from vascular malformations using technetium-labeled red blood cell scintigraphy. *Plast Reconstr Surg* 1992;89:46–55.

The authors describe an accuracy of 97% in distinguishing hemangiomas and vascular malformations in children from each other using Tc-RBC. This technique is particularly useful when the clinical diagnosis of the lesion is not evident, such as with deeper lesions. Not only can biopsy be avoided but parents can be reassured when the child is at an earlier age and given accurate information regarding prognosis.

Disa JJ, Chung KC, Gellad FE, Bickel KD, Wilgis EF: Efficacy of magnetic resonance angiography in the evaluation of vascular malformations of the hand. *Plast Reconstr Surg* 1997;99:136–147.

In this series, MRA was efficacious in the management of vascular malformations of the hand. This technique provided detailed images of both arterial and venous components of the lesion without contrast enhancement or an invasive procedure. Resectability could be determined based on the extent of involvement of surrounding tissues and the flow characteristics.

Pearce WH, Rutherford RB, Whitehill TA, Davis K: Nuclear magnetic resonance imaging: Its diagnostic value in patients with congenital vascular malformations of the limbs. *J Vasc Surg* 1988;8:64–70.

This article describes the fact that diagnosis of vascular lesions can frequently be made on clinical evaluation. The first-line diagnostic test when there is clinical uncertainty is MRI scan, which will, in turn, differentiate diffuse from discrete lesions and high-flow from low-flow lesions. An algorithm then follows for further diagnostic evaluation and treatment of patients with peripheral congenital vascular malformations.

Rak KM, Yakes WF, Ray RL, et al: MR imaging of symptomatic peripheral vascular malformations. *Am J Roentgenol* 1992;159:107–112.

Low-flow venous malformations can be distinguished from high-flow arteriovenous malformations and fistulas on the basis of spin-echo MRI signal characteristics.

Yakes WFJ, Dake MD: Angiographic and interventional procedures in the hand, in Gilula LA, Yin Y (eds): *Imaging of the Wrist and Hand*. Philadelphia, PA, WB Saunders, 1996, pp 499–522.

The role of noninvasive vascular studies, such as color flow Doppler imaging and MRI, is evaluated. These diagnostic imaging modalities are recommended as a first line investigation for pediatric vascular malformations. Arteriography is specifically used for arteriovenous malformations when surgery is anticipated and can be done as a preliminary embolization procedure before surgical excision of these lesions.

Treatment of Vascular Anomalies

Hemangiomas

Castello MA, Ragni G, Antimi A, et al: Successful management with interferon alpha-2a after prednisone therapy failure in an infant with a giant cavernous hemangioma. *Med Pediatr Oncol* 1997;28:213–215.

A giant cavernous hemangioma of the left arm with severe thrombocytopenia and consumptive coagulopathy was described. Prednisone and transfusions had failed to control the bleeding. The child was then treated with daily subcutaneous infusions of Interferon alpha-2a. The hemangioma regressed progressively and disappeared after 4 months of treatment, and the coagulopathy rapidly improved and transfusions were reduced.

Ezekowitz RA, Mulliken JB, Folkman J: Interferon alfa-2a therapy for life-threatening hemangiomas of infancy. *N Engl J Med* 1992;326:1456–1463.

Interferon alpha-2a appears to induce early regression of life-threatening corticosteroid resistant hemangiomas of infancy. In 18 of 20 patients who had failed to respond to corticosteroid therapy, the hemangiomas regressed by 50% or more after an average of 7.8 months of treatment.

Capillary Malformations

Geronemus RG: Pulsed dye laser treatment of vascular lesions in children. *J Dermatol Surg Oncol* 1993;19:303–310.

Superficial vascular lesions such as port wine stains respond effectively to treatment with the pulse dye laser while a more variable response is noted with deeper vascular lesions, early proliferative lesions, and ulcerated hemangiomas. The procedure was found to be safe with a low incidence of adverse scarring, depigmentation, and ulceration.

Venous Malformations

Hill RA, Pho RW, Kumar VP: Resection of vascular malformations. *J Hand Surg* 1993;18B:17–21.

In this retrospective review of 15 cases of congenital vascular malformations of the upper extremity, malformations are classified on the basis of tissue involvement into local and diffuse types, and the outcome of radical surgical approach is assessed. There were 7 cases of recurrence (47%). Recurrences were more frequent in the diffuse type and when excision was considered incomplete. Prior irradiation added significantly to the postoperative complication rate.

Upton J, Mulliken JB, Murray JE. Classification and rationale for management of vascular anomalies in the upper extremity. *J Hand Surg* 1985;10A:970–975.

A rationale for classification and treatment is described. The trend is toward conservativism with the more diffuse venous, lymphaticovenous, and arteriovenous malformations. However, where indicated, guidelines for surgical treatment are outlined. Pitfalls and avoidance of complications are highlighted.

Arteriovenous Malformations

Dickey KW, Pollak JS, Meier GH III, Denny DF, White RI Jr: Management of large high-flow arteriovenous malformations of the shoulder and upper extremity with transcatheter embolotherapy. *J Vasc Interv Radiol* 1995;6:765–773.

Large high-flow arteriovenous malformations are refractory to intravascular treatment because of the diffuse involvement of soft tissues by the lesion. Transcatheter embolotherapy in these lesions should be reserved for patients undergoing resection to help decrease intraoperative bleeding.

Koshima I, Soeda S, Murashita T: Extended wrap-around flap for reconstruction of the finger with recurrent arteriovenous malformation. *Plast Reconstr Surg* 1993;91:1140–1144.

Treatment of arteriovenous malformations of the finger is difficult because complete resection of malformations by ligation or en bloc resection is impossible. This is a case report of a patient who had

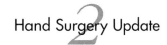
previous resections to the index finger. Following complete resection, the finger was resurfaced with a wrap-around flap.

Loose DA: Combined treatment of congenital vascular defects: Indications and tactics. *Semin Vasc Surg* 1993;6:260–265.

This author describes combined therapy that may be required for high-flow lesions, including embolization and surgical endeavors. Additionally, the author tries to define the role of nonsurgical techniques such as laser, cortisone, and sclerotherapy for low-flow vascular lesions.

McCarthy RE, Lytle JO, Van Devanter S: The use of total circulatory arrest in the surgery of giant hemangioma and Klippel-Trenaunay syndrome in neonates. *Clin Orthop* 1993;289:237–242.

This article describes 2 neonates who required deep hypothermia and circulatory arrest to provide central control of blood loss for the resection of giant vascular peripheral lesions. The surgery in both cases was done as a life-saving measure because the infants were suffering from high-output cardiac failure. In both cases, because of the small total blood volumes, circulatory arrest was critical in excision of these hypervascular tumors.

Perrelli L, Cina G, Cotroneo AR, Falappa P, Nanni L: Treatment of intraosseous arteriovenous fistulas of the extremities. *J Pediatr Surg* 1994;29:1380–1383.

The authors describe successful treatment of 3 patients with intraosseous arteriovenous fistulas of the upper extremities. Embolization was performed followed by an operation at which cortical windows were opened over the affected bone, the angiomatous material curetted, and the cavities filled with bone cement.

Polsen C, Anous M, Netscher D, Shenaq S, Safi HJ: Hypothermia and cardiopulmonary bypass during resection of extensive arteriovenous malformation followed by microvascular reconstruction. *Ann Plast Surg* 1995;34:642–649.

The authors describe the use of hypothermic hypoperfusion to facilitate excision of an intraosseous mandibular arteriovenous malformation. This method may be implemented for resection of large proximal upper limb hypervascular lesions when tourniquet control is not possible. The method of hypoperfusion, while providing effective hemostasis, gives some margin of safety compared with complete cardiac arrest.

Yamamoto Y, Ohura T, Minakawa H, et al: Experience with arteriovenous malformations treated with flap coverage. *Plast Reconstr Surg* 1994;94:476–482.

Twelve patients requiring free-tissue transfer and 2 in whom pedicle-flap transfer was performed following arteriovenous malformation resection are described. Wide resections must be performed, and soft-tissue coverage by means of complex reconstructions help ensure total resection of arteriovenous malformations.

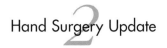

Section VII
Arthritis

Chapter 31
Rheumatoid Arthritis

Chapter 32
Osteoarthritis of the Hand

Chapter 33
Other Arthritides

American Society for Surgery of the Hand

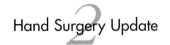

Chapter 31
Rheumatoid Arthritis

Robert Lee Wilson, MD

Rheumatoid arthritis is a systemic autoimmune disorder characterized by chronic symmetric erosive synovitis involving the peripheral joints. The wrist and small joints of the hand are the articulations most frequently involved. Rheumatoid disease is a more appropriate term than arthritis because it acknowledges the nonarticular aspects—vasculitis, pericarditis, pulmonary nodules and fibrosis, episcleritis, and subcutaneous nodules. From 1% to 2% of the world's population is affected. The prevalence increases with age; women predominate in a ratio of 2.5 to 1. Genetics plays a role (HLA-DR4/DR1). Research is focused on bacteria and viruses as possible etiologic agents.

Pathologically, the initial event is thought to be an injury to the synovial microvascular endothelial cells. The vessel lumens are blocked with platelets, leukocytes, and fibrin thrombi. The synovium proliferates and becomes thickened. Polymorphonucleocytes (PMNs) are the predominant cell in the joint effusions and mononuclear cells surround the vessels. The PMNs are attracted to the synovial fluid by chemotactic factors, releasing proteinases, prostaglandins, and leukotrienes as well as activating the complement cascade. Endothelial cells play a role in recruitment of inflammatory cells. Macrophages are the major component of the infiltrating cell population in rheumatoid synovium. They produce an extensive list of inflammation mediators and have a phagocytic function themselves. Bone is eroded by immature, highly active fibroblast-like cells; osteoclasts proliferate and are responsible for subchondral osteopenia. The cartilage surface is destroyed by enzymes in the inflammatory milieu. In restricted areas, such as the carpal tunnel, a mass of hypertrophic synovium may produce ischemic tendon changes. The surgeon must understand the natural course of the disease, the stage of involvement, and the patient's functional limitations before initiating a treatment program.

When first evaluating a rheumatoid patient, the examiner must obtain a detailed history and initiate a regional examination starting proximally at the shoulder. A systemic evaluation should include observation of the skin for atrophy or nodules; the joints for synovitis, stiffness, and pain; the tendons for tenosynovitis and triggering; and muscle and nerve function. The surgeon must understand the effects of a drug program and the basics of medical management. Nonsteroidal anti-inflammatory drugs (NSAIDs) may decrease inflammation and pain, but will not inhibit synovial proliferation. The effectiveness of NSAIDs is related to prevention of prostaglandin synthesis. Low-dose corticosteroids are often beneficial in treating symptoms of inflammatory joints. One recent study demonstrated that steroids may halt progression of the disease. Remittive agents include antimalarial drugs, sulfasalazine, methotrexate, gold, D-Penicillamine, immunosuppressive agents (azathioprine and cyclophosphamide), and cyclosporine. Nonsurgical treatment must also include rest, controlled exercise, splinting, and patient education.

Surgical Indications and Principles of Treatment

When managing patients with rheumatoid disease involving the upper extremity, the priorities are pain relief, restoration or improvement of function, prevention of deformities, and the appearance of the hand. The presence of a deformity is not of itself an indication for surgery. The patient with metacarpophalangeal (MCP) ulnar drift and flexion contractures, but good grip strength and no pain, may not be a candidate for MCP joint arthroplasty. If similar deformities exist in both hands and present a functional problem, one hand should be corrected to facilitate large object grasp. However, the contralateral hand might be left undisturbed to provide small object grasp and possibly more power than the operated hand. For the patient with multiple deformities, the surgeon's concern should be whether an operative procedure will provide sufficient improvement. A functional evaluation by a knowledgeable hand therapist will often define the troublesome areas, allowing the surgery to address the problems of greatest concern.

The surgeon needs to understand the natural history of the disease itself and the specific deformity. With a progressive course, an operation will provide only temporary benefit.

The author is grateful to Peter J. Campbell, MD for his assistance with this chapter.

The examiner may decide that a patient has progressed past the point where a preventive procedure such as a synovectomy can be performed successfully, yet reconstructive joint surgery is premature. The critical questions are where the patient is in the course of the disease, what impact we can make now, and what further progression will occur.

Each rheumatoid hand deformity has defined stages and progresses in a distinct manner. When evaluating a swan neck, the multiple causes need to be recognized. The significance of patient progression from stage II (flexible) to stage III (limited motion) must be understood. In general, surgery conducted before the development of fixed joint contractures yields much better results. Postoperative motion at the MCP and proximal interphalangeal (PIP) joints is directly related to tendon function. The patient who has had fixed swan-neck deformities for a number of years is unlikely to regain sustained motion after joint releases or implant arthroplasties because the extensor and flexor tendon function cannot be revived. Before technically difficult procedures such as MCP arthroplasty are performed, treatment of a painful wrist with an ulnar head resection is recommended. This straightforward procedure requires no patient compliance, will gain the individual's confidence, and will give the surgeon valuable insight into the patient's condition.

When planning upper extremity operations, proximal joints (shoulder and elbow) should generally be operated on before more distal ones (hand and wrist). In the hand, surgery at the MCP joints is recommended before approaching the PIP joints. Realignment of the proximal joints and restoration of motion will significantly improve hand function.

Mobilizing procedures and stabilizing operations should be carried out at different times. Arthrodesis of the wrist and thumb MCP joint can be accomplished simultaneously; however, combining these with MCP implant arthroplasties that require prompt remobilization may compromise the end result. Lower extremity procedures are usually performed before upper extremity operations. Careful coordination is required. The ambulatory aides that are required after lower extremity surgery can be detrimental to recently performed hand procedures.

Disease involvement in one joint will affect adjacent joints and overlying structures. A zig-zag deformity may occur in multiple planes. This is best seen in the coronal plane with the wrist in radial deviation and the fingers in ulnar deviation. However, it can also occur in the sagittal plane with a swan-neck deformity. A swan neck is usually associated with an intrinsic contracture (intrinsic-plus). One author demonstrated that a swan neck can result from an extrinsic-minus condition. Carpal collapse results in extrinsic extensor tendon lengthening, which produces weakness that allows the intrinsic muscles to overpower the hand. This problem can be treated by restoring carpal height.

Extensor Tendons

Extensor tenosynovitis often presents as a painless dorsal wrist mass distal to the retinaculum. The mass consists of synovium filled with fluid. Adhesions can occur and infiltration of the extensor tendons can result in erosion and rupture. A more frequent cause of extensor tendon rupture is from an eroded distal ulna (Vaughn-Jackson lesion). A tenosynovectomy is indicated for persistent tenosynovitis unresponsive to medical treatment, a tenosynovial mass increasing in size, or rupture of an extensor tendon.

A tenosynovectomy begins with careful evaluation of all the tendons (Fig. 1). A nodule present within the substance

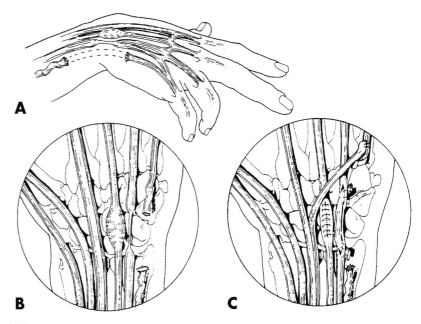

Figure 1

A and **B,** Tendon damage from rheumatoid disease can include infiltration with nodule formation (middle finger), attenuation with pseudotendon interposition (ring), or tendon rupture (little). **C,** Tendon nodules are excised and the tendon repaired (middle finger). Attenuated tendons can be treated with a graft (ring). Ruptured tendons can be reconstructed with a transfer (EIP to little finger EDC, or EDM). (Reproduced with permission from Wilson RL, DeVito MC: Extensor tendon problems in rheumatoid arthritis. *Hand Clin* 1996;12:551–559.)

of a tendon should be excised. If the tendon is weakened by the disease or the procedure, suturing is necessary. A tendon that is markedly frayed but not ruptured should be protected with an overlay graft. When pseudotendon is encountered, it should be treated like a ruptured tendon with a transfer or graft. The extensor retinaculum can be returned to its normal position if the bed on which the extensors are gliding is normal. Returning the retinaculum to its anatomic position above the tendons is contraindicated if the extensors are frayed or if tendon grafts or transfers have been carried out. Complications that can occur after a tenosynovectomy include skin slough, tendon adhesions, and further tendon rupture.

The most serious complication of untreated dorsal tenosynovitis is tendon rupture. When the patient presents with a sudden loss of finger extension, the surgeon should locate the possible rupture site by palpation. Other causes for loss of finger extension include ulnar extensor tendon subluxation, MCP joint dislocation, posterior interosseous nerve compression at the elbow, and tendon nodules in both the flexors and extensors. Extensor tendon reconstruction is indicated after a tendon rupture. Before performing an operative procedure, the wrist and MCP joints are carefully evaluated. At surgery, traction to the distal end of the extensor tendon will determine if simultaneous extensor centering at the MCP joint will need to be performed while reconstructing the extensor tendon proximally. Extensor tendon grafts (Fig. 2) and tendon transfers have both proven effective.

The patient with a single extensor tendon rupture usually has loss of little finger extension. Recommended treatment is transfer of the ruptured little finger extensor tendon to the ring finger extensor digitorum communis (EDC); alternatives are extensor indicis proprius (EIP) transfer or a tendon graft. Double extensor ruptures frequently involve the ring and little fingers. The customary management is suturing the ruptured ring finger extensor to the middle finger EDC. The EIP is then transferred to the little finger or a tendon graft can be used. On occasion, the middle and ring finger communis tendons are ruptured. In this situation, the middle finger tendon can be transferred to the index EDC and the ring finger tendon to the little finger. Another possibility is rupture of all 4 EDC tendons leaving the EIP and

extensor digiti minimi (EDM) intact. The preferred treatment for this case is a tendon graft for the middle and ring finger extensors. A triple extensor rupture usually involves the ulnar 3 finger tendons. The recommended treatment is transfer of the ruptured middle finger tendon to the index communis and the EIP to both the ring and little finger extensors. Alternatives include a tendon graft for all 3 EDC tendons, or use of the flexor digitorum superficialis (FDS) for the ring and little finger ruptures and an adjacent transfer for the middle to the index finger. Fortunately, rupture of all the extensor tendons to 4 fingers (communis as well as the proprius tendons) is rare. The recommended treatment is to use both the middle and ring finger flexor superficialis tendons placed either through the interosseous membrane or around the radial aspect of the hand into the 4 communis tendons. The patient presenting with a single or double rupture has the best prognosis. If the patient's distal joints are satisfactory, nearly complete motion can be expected.

Rupture of the extensor pollicis longus (EPL) can occur as an isolated incident or in association with digital extensor ruptures. Several treatment possibilities exist. An EIP to EPL

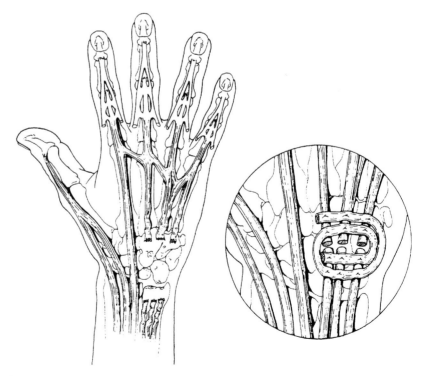

Figure 2

Extensor reconstruction with a tendon graft looped through the proximal and distal ends to bridge the gap. (Reproduced with permission from Wilson RL, DeVito MC: Extensor tendon problems in rheumatoid arthritis. *Hand Clin* 1996;12:551–559.)

transfer can be performed, or an extensor graft and transfer of the extensor pollicis brevis (EPB) to the EPL at the MCP joint level. When rupture of wrist tendons includes both radial wrist extensors, an arthrodesis will be required.

Flexor Tendons

Flexor tenosynovitis can contribute to a rheumatoid patient's complaints of weak grip, morning stiffness, volar wrist swelling, and median nerve compression. The tenosynovitis may be diffuse or create discrete nodules that can limit tendon excursion.

At the wrist, a tenosynovectomy is indicated for median nerve compression, a painful tenosynovial mass, or a tendon rupture. During surgery, any bony spicules in the carpal canal should be removed and the capsule closed over the denuded bone. The most common flexor rupture (Mannerfelt syndrome) involves the flexor pollicis longus (FPL). When the thumb interphalangeal joint is damaged, fusion or tenodesis is indicated. If the patient has satisfactory interphalangeal joint function, a tendon bridge graft, a 2-staged flexor graft, or a superficialis transfer can be performed. A profundus rupture within the carpal canal may be masked by an intact superficialis. Treatment of a ruptured profundus is suture to an adjacent intact tendon. Flexors other than the FPL can be damaged; the presence of 1 tendon rupture is an indication to promptly perform surgery to prevent further tendon damage.

The palm is the most common location of flexor tenosynovitis. Indications for a flexor tenosynovectomy in the palm include pain with use, triggering, tendon rupture, and passive flexion of the fingers that is greater than active flexion. Secondary interphalangeal joint stiffness can result from prolonged tenosynovitis. With digital flexor tenosynovitis, the problem is the bulk of the tenosynovial mass compared to the annular pulleys. When the nodularity is present in the distal palm, the finger is usually locked in flexion. However, with a profundus tendon nodule distally at the A2 pulley, the finger will be locked in extension. Treatment of digital flexor tenosynovitis includes removal of the abnormal tissue, nodule excision, and tendon repair. If profundus excursion remains limited, the sheath contents are debulked by excising one half or possibly the entire FDS. The A1 pulley should be preserved, as division will compound volar MCP subluxation, bowstringing, and ulnar deviation. One group demonstrated good or excellent results (67%), but experienced a clinical recurrence of 31% requiring reoperation in 15%. The best results occur when tenosynovitis is limited to the wrist and palm.

When treating flexor tendon ruptures in the palm and digits, a single tendon rupture may pass unnoticed or be confused with a nodule within the tendon. With a profundus rupture, a tenosynovectomy will protect the remaining superficialis. For rupture within the digit, a profundus tenodesis or distal interphalangeal (DIP) fusion should be considered. Profundus grafts through an intact superficialis are contraindicated. When both tendons are ruptured in the palm, the profundus may be sutured to an adjacent profundus, or a superficialis from an adjacent finger can be transferred to the profundus. When both tendons are ruptured in a digit, consideration should be given to a staged tendon graft; however, this should be done only in a younger patient with good interphalangeal joint motion. Another option is to fuse both the PIP and DIP joints.

Wrist

Synovitis in the wrist characteristically starts on the ulnar aspect. It initially involves the distal radioulnar and radiocarpal joints and spares the midcarpal joint. Radiographs demonstrate erosive changes involving the ulnar styloid, the sigmoid notch of the radius, the insertion of the radioscapholunate ligament, and the scaphoid waist. With damage to the extrinsic and intrinsic ligaments compounding these bony changes, the wrist is shortened, the metacarpals angulate radially, and a series of carpal abnormalities (supination, palmar dislocation, and ulnar translocation) occur. Radial rotation will produce relative ulnar prominence and facilitate the progression of deformities distally (MCP ulnar drift). A dorsal wrist synovectomy is indicated for painful poorly controlled synovitis and minimal articular damage. Contraindications include translocation of the lunate, marked erosion, subluxation, or instability. Recurrence of synovitis and the necessity for further wrist surgery are minimized if the operation is performed before erosive changes occur. Following a synovectomy, the dorsal retinaculum can be placed beneath the extensor tendons to reinforce the capsule and relocate the extensor communis ulnaris (ECU) dorsally. If the wrist is positioned in radial deviation and passively can be moved ulnarward, transfer of the extensor carpi radialis longus to the ECU will remove the radially deviating force and may augment ulnar deviation.

A partial arthrodesis, either radiolunate or radioscapholunate, is recommended for wrists with significant erosive changes or instability following a synovectomy. Contraindications include midcarpal ankylosis or resorption of the scaphoid and lunate. One author recommended inserting an implant in the capitate head to maintain motion at this level. Another team observed that a radial-lunate arthrodesis would prevent dislocation of an unstable wrist, but that the operation could not repress further degeneration. Those

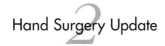
patients with advanced erosion and excessive bone loss were more likely to deteriorate. Complete radiocarpal arthrodesis is indicated for severe wrist pain, a significant deformity, poor bone stock, and ruptured wrist extensor tendons. The best position for wrist fusion is neutral or slight flexion. If both wrists need to be fused, one should be in neutral and the other in 10° to 15° of flexion. The wrist joint is stabilized with one or more longitudinal Steinmann pins, with further oblique pins or staples as needed. Results have demonstrated 95% good or excellent function.

To preserve wrist motion, numerous arthroplasty procedures have been described. These include a synovectomy with stabilization, temporarily pinning the wrist, and the creation of a fibrous ankylosis between the radius and the proximal row. A palmar shelf arthroplasty will not provide sustained pain relief, and a proximal row carpectomy is contraindicated.

A number of wrist implants have been devised. The most commonly used—the silicone implant—is indicated in the low-demand patient with satisfactory wrist extensor tendons, no deformity, good bone stock, and a stable wrist. The technique is more demanding than a wrist fusion, requiring preservation of the capsule to stabilize the wrist implant and careful preparation of both the radius and the carpus. Although one recent study noted satisfactory results, the implant fracture rate was 22%. Previous stud-

ies demonstrated failure rates over 40% at 10 years. A total replacement is limited to patients with advanced disease and satisfactory bone stock. A recent series of 57 cases followed at least 5 years indicated 24% failures, often involving loosening of the distal implant. Several authors have used an uncemented wrist implant. Complication rates following total wrist replacement vary from 16% to 40%; the biggest problems are bone resorption and component loosening, radial-ulnar imbalance, and attrition tendon ruptures.

Pain and dysfunction at the distal radioulnar joint is a frequent problem in rheumatoid patients. A synovectomy of the joint is appropriate for early localized disease with associated pain. An ulnar head excision is indicated for marked tenderness localized to the joint, pain that increases with pronosupination, or extensor tendon ruptures. The remaining ulna stump is stabilized using either local tissue including triangular fibrocartilage complex remnants, a flap of volar capsule placed dorsally, or a retinacular flap with an ulnar base attached to the radius (Fig. 3). A Sauvè-Kapandji procedure may prove helpful in the young patient with a sufficient ulnar head. One group reported that the palmar and ulnar translocation of the carpus was prevented with such a procedure. Others have found that wrist dislocation is due more to the disease process than either resection or preservation of the ulnar head. An ulnar head implant,

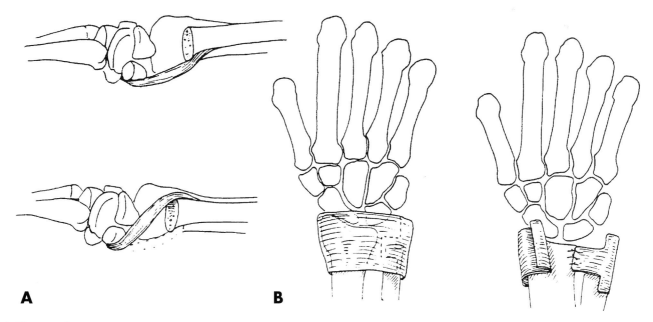

A   **B**

Figure 3

A, A distally based flap of capsule and periosteum is sutured to the dorsum of the ulna, depressing it. **B,** An ulnar-based retinacular flap is attached to the radius, covering the resected ulna. (Reproduced with permission from Wilson RL: Rheumatoid arthritis of the hand. *Orthop Clin North Am* 1986;17:313–343.)

which covers the end of the ulna but will not buttress the carpus or prevent a shift of the carpus in an ulnar direction, is rarely indicated.

Metacarpophalangeal Joints

The most frequent deformities at the MCP joint are palmar dislocation of the proximal phalanx and ulnar deviation of the fingers. The MCP joint has multiplanar motion with flexion and extension as well as abduction, adduction, and rotation. The collateral ligaments are the major restraints to radial and ulnar deviation and are asymmetrical, as is the metacarpal head. The transverse metacarpal ligament is attached to the volar plate that also suspends the A1 pulley. The extensor tendon is centered over the MCP joint by the sagittal bands that insert on the volar plate. The sagittal bands stabilize and centralize the extensor tendon. The ulnar band is stronger than the radial band. The static forces (volar plate, collateral ligaments, and sagittal bands) and the dynamic ones (extensor, flexor, and intrinsic tendons) intersect at a point Zancolli termed the force nucleus. As the inflammatory process disrupts the static stabilizers, the dynamic forces propel the nucleus away from the weakened side (Fig. 4).

The wrist, PIP, and DIP joints proximal and distal to the MCP joint should be evaluated to fully understand their impact on MCP deformities. Radiographs of the hand should be graded for arthritic joint involvement and evaluated for erosion of the proximal phalanx base. The joint should be examined for subluxation or complete dislocation. A tangential view of the metacarpal head (Brewerton view) will show cortical erosions at the collateral ligament insertions.

MCP synovectomy is indicated for painful persistent MCP joint synovitis that has not responded to medical treatment and demonstrates minimal cartilage damage radiographically (Fig. 5). The patient with subluxation that cannot be relocated (disruption of the force nucleus) is not a candidate for MCP synovectomy. The technique includes release of the ulnar intrinsics and the abductor digiti minimi, reefing or recessing of the radial collateral ligaments, crossed intrinsic tendon transfers, and centralization of the extensor tendon. Postoperatively, the patient must be promptly remobilized with a program similar to that used after implant arthroplasties. Although an expected result is overall improvement with decreased pain and correction of ulnar drift, decreased motion at the MCP joint may occur. If the disease itself is not overly aggressive, correction will be maintained.

Implant arthroplasty is indicated in patients with a decreased arc of motion (40° or less), marked flexion contractures with a poor functional position, MCP joint pain with associated radiographic abnormalities, and severe ulnar

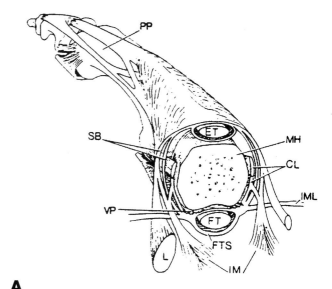

A

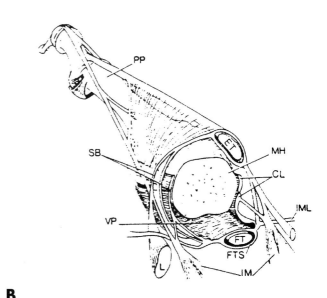

B

Figure 4

A, Normal anatomy of the metacarpophalangeal joint. **B,** Rheumatoid MCP deformities. CL = collateral ligament, ET = extensor tendon, FT = flexor tendon, FTS = flexor tendon sheath, IM = interosseous muscle or tendon, IML = intermetacarpal ligament, MH = metacarpal head, PP = proximal phalanx, VP = volar plate, SB = sagittal bands, L = lumbrical. (Reproduced with permission from Wilson RL, Carlblom ER: The rheumatoid metacarpophalangeal joint. *Hand Clin* 1989;5:223–227.)

drift with loss of function. Contraindications include poor bone stock, presence of vasculitis (lupus), or poor skin condition (scleroderma). The operative technique includes complete soft-tissue release after sufficient joint exposure, adequate bone resection, preparation of the medullary

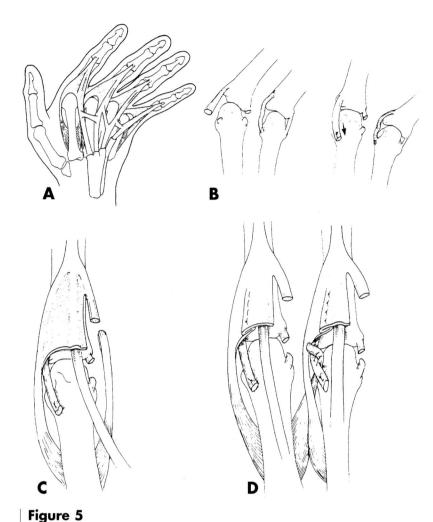

Figure 5

A, Metacarpophalangeal joint synovectomy. Synovectomy of the MCP joints is indicated when the subluxation can be reduced manually and no significant cartilage damage is present. **B,** After a complete joint synovectomy, the joint is reduced and the radial collateral ligament plicated or recessed (arrow). **C,** The ulnar intrinsic is released and transferred to the radial capsule of the adjacent ulnar digit. **D,** The extensor tendons are recentered by either plicating the radial hood or looping a portion of the extensor tendon through the dorsal capsule. (Reproduced with permission from Wilson RL, Carlblom ER: The rheumatoid metacarpophalangeal joint. *Hand Clin* 1989;5:223–227.)

a shift in the arc of motion into extension for the patient presenting with flexion contractures. Some studies have shown a mild loss of motion over time. Recurrent deformity can occur in patients whose disease course is progressive.

Interphalangeal Joints

Two characteristic PIP deformities occur in the rheumatoid hand. The attitude that the digit manifests is determined by the imbalance that occurs in the flexor/ extensor system. A thorough understanding of the complex, dynamic relationship between the intrinsic and extrinsic components is necessary to properly evaluate these patients.

The swan-neck deformity is characterized by hyperextension at the PIP joint and flexion at the DIP joint. The causes are numerous, and can be attributed to pathology focused at the wrist, MCP, PIP, or DIP joints (Fig. 6). Carpal collapse and migration effectively lengthen the extrinsic system, causing increased mechanical advantage in the lumbrical/interosseous complex that accentuates the swan-neck posture. Palmar MCP joint subluxation increases the extensor force at the base of the middle phalanx. This mechanism is accentuated by progressive contracture of the intrinsic tendons. PIP joint synovitis can attenuate the volar structures (volar plate, collateral ligaments, FDS insertion), allowing a position of hyperextension. Synovitis at the DIP joint can disrupt the terminal extensor tendon (mallet), causing DIP joint flexion and contributing to a swan-neck posture.

Swan-neck deformities have been classified by the severity of the deformity. Type I is mild with minimal functional loss, and is characterized by full passive motion at the PIP joint. Conservative treatment includes joint injections and figure-of-eight splints to prevent hyperextension. Surgical intervention is directed at the involved joint. DIP joint arthrodesis or tenodermodesis corrects a mallet deformity. Soft-tissue procedures at the PIP joint, such as FDS tenodesis or oblique retinacular ligament reconstruction, are designed to prevent hyperextension.

canals, and correct implant selection. Reconstruction is completed with collateral ligament reattachment on the radial side, centralization of the extensor tendon, and possibly use of crossed intrinsic transfers. Problems can occur from marked bony erosion, particularly with dorsal bone loss on the proximal phalanx, and release of the little finger flexor, producing insufficient little finger MCP flexion. Implant fracture is not infrequent (at least 15%), but revision surgery is relatively rare. The patient needs to be involved in a prolonged splinting and exercise program, with subsequent instruction in joint protection to avoid abuse of the operated hand. Expected results are decreased pain, and

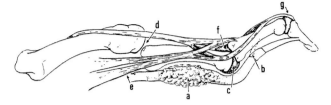

Figure 6

Swan-neck deformity. Flexor tenosynovitis (a), superficialis rupture (b), volar plate laxity (c), MCP joint subluxation/dislocation (d), intrinsic contracture (e), PIP joint synovitis (f), DIP joint synovitis (g). (Reproduced with permission from Wilson RL: Rheumatoid arthritis of the hand. *Orthop Clin North Am* 1986;17:313–343.)

Type II deformities are associated with MCP joint disease. The passive motion at the PIP joint is dependent on MCP position. Extension at the MCP joint limits passive PIP flexion (positive intrinsic test). Treatment involves intrinsic release with or without MCP joint reconstruction, depending on the severity of MCP involvement.

Type III swan-neck deformity is characterized by loss of PIP motion regardless of MCP position, but with preservation of PIP joint space on radiographic images. MCP joint dislocation is addressed with an implant arthroplasty followed by PIP joint manipulation. If this manipulation fails to recover sufficient motion, an open lateral band mobilization will be necessary to allow volar migration of the intrinsic component. If full passive flexion is not attained, a collateral ligament release and even a central slip lengthening may be necessary. Motion must be checked by applying traction to the flexor tendons. A dorsal skin release distal to the PIP joint and Kirscher-wire fixation are often necessary.

In type IV deformities, limited PIP motion is correlated with radiographs confirming joint destruction. Surgical options include arthrodesis or implant arthroplasty. Arthrodesis should be considered for index and middle digits if pinch is required. Implant arthroplasty is recommended only for the ring and little fingers, if the collateral ligaments and both flexor and extensor tendon function is intact. One recent study evaluating silicone implant arthroplasty in 40 PIP joints showed fair or poor results in 28 of 40 fingers. Digits with swan-neck deformities showed an 86% recurrence rate and lost a significantly greater amount of motion than did fingers with boutonnière deformities.

Boutonnière deformities are common in rheumatoid arthritis. Unlike a swan-neck deformity, which can evolve from numerous joints, a boutonnière deformity is specific to disease at the PIP joint. Synovitis at the PIP joint attenuates the extensor mechanism, elongates the central slip, and stretches the triangular ligament, allowing volar migration of the lateral bands and producing DIP joint hyperextension. Compensatory hyperextension of the MCP joint occurs. Initially these deformities are passively correctable but later become fixed deformities. Classification and treatment of a PIP boutonnière is based upon the severity of the deformity.

Stage I, or preboutonnière deformity, presents with proliferative PIP joint synovitis. PIP range of motion is preserved but DIP flexion may be decreased. Treatment at this stage includes splinting, joint injection, or synovectomy. A distal extensor tenotomy can gain DIP joint flexion. In stage II, a PIP joint flexion deformity (30° to 40°) remains passively correctable. Radiographs indicate maintenance of joint space. Restoration of PIP joint function involves synovectomy and either central slip repair following resection of the attenuated tendon or reconstruction using the lateral bands. Stage III disease is characterized by a fixed contracture with the inability to passively extend the PIP joint. Function may be satisfactory and treatment should be individualized. Surgical indications are pain, a progressive flexion contracture, or inability to grasp large objects. Attempted restoration of extensor function by itself will be unsuccessful. Treatment options include arthrodesis or arthroplasty. A recent study of implant arthroplasty in patients with a boutonnière deformity showed no overall improvement in motion; however, the arc of motion was placed in a more functional range. Those fingers with a prior or concurrent MCP arthroplasty gained motion, while those without MCP arthroplasty lost motion. Stage IV boutonnières present with contractures greater than 70°. Fusion is indicated for joint pain, instability, and deformity associated with functional loss.

Thumb Deformities

The thumb of rheumatoid patients is frequently involved (two thirds of the time) and can include all 3 joints. The boutonnière deformity (type I) is the most common thumb abnormality (70%). Synovitis of the MCP joint attenuates the dorsal capsule and EPB tendon, permitting ulnar displacement of the EPL and eventually allowing palmar subluxation of the proximal phalanx. Interphalangeal joint hyperextension occurs from increased tension on the thumb intrinsics; with EPL displacement, the thumb becomes adducted.

Recommended early treatment includes MCP joint synovectomy and reconstruction of the extensor mechanism. One recent study evaluating EPL rerouting and EPB reattachment showed excellent subjective results in 11 cases with a 38-month follow-up. Good extensor strength was preserved, but range of motion of the MCP and interphalangeal joints was variable. Previous studies have shown a high

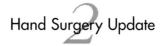

recurrence rate requiring additional surgery. With an advancing boutonnière deformity, the MCP flexion deformity becomes fixed with a passively correctable interphalangeal joint. The goal of treatment should be to preserve motion in at least one of these joints. MCP arthrodesis is the recommended procedure if motion can be maintained at the trapeziometacarpal (TMC) and interphalangeal joints. In the advanced boutonnière deformity, the MCP and interphalangeal joints are destroyed. Surgical reconstruction includes interphalangeal joint fusion with MCP joint fusion or arthroplasty. The latter should only be considered if the TMC joint is mobile and pain free.

The swan-neck deformity (type III) is the second most common rheumatoid thumb deformity pattern. Synovitis at the TMC joint leads to dorsal lateral metacarpal subluxation, which is accentuated by the pull of the abductor pollicis longus and pinch forces. With persistent TMC joint pain, an arthroplasty is indicated, removing sufficient bone (a portion of the trapezium and the metacarpal if necessary) to allow soft-tissue interposition. If the MCP joint is passively correctable without erosive changes on radiographs, a soft-tissue procedure (volar capsulodesis or flexor tenodesis) can be considered. Otherwise, an MCP joint fusion is indicated.

A gamekeeper's deformity (type IV) has a presentation similar to the laxity found with MCP ligament trauma. Synovitis at the TMC joint is associated with a metacarpal adduction contracture. MCP joint synovitis produces attenuation of the ulnar collateral ligament with instability on stress radialward. If treated early, a synovectomy and ligament reconstruction is possible. When articular destruction occurs, an MCP joint arthrodesis is necessary. With an advanced deformity, a supplemental adductor tenotomy and first web release with a Z-plasty will be required.

The type V deformity describes MCP joint hyperextension with resultant interphalangeal flexion due to tension on the FPL. This needs to be differentiated from the type III deformity, as there is neither TMC involvement nor first web space contracture. Treatment consists of stabilizing the MCP joint by capsulodesis or arthrodesis.

Type VI deformity is characterized by skeletal collapse and loss of bony substance, such as seen in arthritis mutilans, a psoriatic variant. Treatment includes arthrodesis of the distal joints if adequate bone stock remains.

Complex Rheumatoid Wrist and Hand Problems

Patients with rheumatoid deformities can rarely be approached in a straightforward fashion. The deformities rarely occur alone and are usually compounded by multiple joint involvement. Correction of one problem requires a thorough understanding of the adjacent joint and tendon difficulties. After complete assessment of all problem areas, plans are made to perform sequential procedures, first directing attention to those that cause the patient the most pain and impairment. Multiple concurrent operations may be carried out. While this approach will decrease the patient's surgical morbidity, it requires that the surgeon be experienced in all of the operations, have clear indications for performing each, and be able to coordinate the postoperative rehabilitation.

The patient with a degenerated painful wrist and marked MCP joint deformities can be treated with a simultaneous partial or complete wrist fusion while performing MCP joint arthroplasty. However, a logical and safe choice is elimination of wrist pain and creation of a stable wrist without deformity as the first procedure, and MCP implant arthroplasty as the second. The patient with wrist pain, ruptured digital extensor tendons, and MCP problems is even more difficult to manage, no matter which strategy is selected. If planning sequential procedures, the patient should first undergo MCP implant arthroplasties, maintaining passive MCP motion with an exercise program, followed by a wrist arthrodesis and lastly extensor tendon reconstruction. To carry out all 3 of these simultaneously requires experience, thorough knowledge of each procedure, cautious selection of surgical incisions, and the availability of an experienced hand therapist. Patients with deformities of both MCP and PIP joints also require careful planning. The preference is to retain motion at the MCP joints while gaining stability and optimal position at the PIP level. Implant arthroplasties of both MCP and PIP joints are rarely indicated; trying to regain PIP motion in such situations is rarely satisfying, nor does it add to the functional improvement of the patient. A preferred approach is to perform MCP implant arthroplasties and correct the PIP joint problems with releases and joint pinning. On occasion, it may be necessary to correct the PIP problems before performing MCP surgery; most frequently, however, these can be performed at a later stage.

When faced with a complex situation including tendons and joints, the recommended treatment is reconstruction of the flexor tendons, then the MCP joints, and lastly the extensors. Should one repair extensor ruptures but not have satisfactory MCP motion, the reconstructed extensors will fail to function and will not respond to a later tenolysis after MCP reconstruction. Overall, the sequential approach of staged reconstruction is more predictable than multiple concurrent procedures.

Annotated Bibliography

Nonsurgical Treatment

Massarotti EM: Medical aspects of rheumatoid arthritis: Diagnosis and treatment. *Hand Clin* 1996;12:463–475.

The author discusses the medical management, differential diagnosis, and nonsurgical treatment of rheumatoid arthritis, with special emphasis on the hand.

Tendons

de Jager LT, Jaffe R, Learmonth ID, Heywood AW: The A1 pulley in rheumatoid flexor tenosynovectomy: To retain or divide? *J Hand Surg* 1994;19B:202–204.

This study compares 55 digits in which the A1 pulley was divided during flexor tenosynovectomy to 45 digits in which the A1 pulley was retained. Volar subluxation occurred in 49% when the A1 pulley was divided, compared to 11% when the pulley was preserved. Ulnar deviation increased by 7° when the A1 pulley was divided. The authors suggest that palmar subluxation and ulnar deviation is increased when the A1 pulley is sacrificed.

Wheen DJ, Tonkin MA, Green J, Bronkhorst M: Long-term results following digital flexor tenosynovectomy in rheumatoid arthritis. *J Hand Surg* 1995;20A:790–794.

In this retrospective review of 15 patients (61 digits) who underwent digital flexor tenosynovectomy, follow-up averaged 4 years. Active flexion improved an average of 2.2 cm. Clinical recurrence rate was 31%. The subset of patients that required excision of a slip of FDS had a statistically significant reduction in recurrence and reoperation rates.

Williamson SC, Feldon P: Extensor tendon ruptures in rheumatoid arthritis. *Hand Clin* 1995;11:449–459.

This article is a discussion of the tendon reconstruction options available in the rheumatoid patient who presents with extensor tendon disruption.

Wilson RL, DeVito MC: Extensor tendon problems in rheumatoid arthritis. *Hand Clin* 1996;12:551–559.

This review of the common presentations of rheumatoid extensor tendon disease at the wrist places emphasis on surgical treatment options and technique.

Wrist

Adolfsson L, Nylander G: Arthroscopic synovectomy of the rheumatoid wrist. *J Hand Surg* 1993;18B:92–96.

The authors describe the technique and results of arthroscopic synovectomy of the wrist in 16 patients. They demonstrated good pain relief with increased grip strength and no postoperative stiffness. The arthroscopic technique may minimize the disadvantages of conventional surgical synovectomy.

Bosco JA III, Bynum DK, Bowers WH: Long-term outcome of Volz total wrist arthroplasties. *J Arthroplasty* 1994;9:25–31.

Eighteen Volz total wrist arthroplasties (14 rheumatoid arthritis, 4 degenerative joint disease) were evaluated with an average follow-up of 8.6 years. A 24% loss in carpal height was noted during the study period. Four metacarpal components (22%) were loose and 1 radial component (6%) loosened. Fifteen of 18 wrists (83%) had little or no pain. The 3 wrists with moderate to severe pain, and 3 of the 5 loose components, were in patients with degenerative joint disease.

Cobb TK, Beckenbaugh RD: Biaxial long-stemmed multipronged distal components for revision/bone deficit total-wrist arthroplasty. *J Hand Surg* 1996;21A:764–770.

The authors describe results of 10 revision arthroplasties using a multipronged distal component. Follow-up averaged 3.8 years. Two patients required arthrodesis. Six of the 8 remaining patients had no pain; the other 2 reported mild pain. These results imply greater longevity for the custom component when treating patients with deficient bone stock.

Cobb TK, Beckenbaugh RD: Biaxial total-wrist arthroplasty. *J Hand Surg* 1996;21A:1011–1021.

In a follow-up study (average 6.5 years) of 57 biaxial total wrist arthroplasties, pain was reported as nonexistent in 75%, mild in 19%, and severe in 3%. Range of motion averaged 36° extension, 29° flexion, 10° radial deviation, and 20° ulnar deviation. Grip strength improved from 4.1 kgf to 5.9 kgf. Failure occurred in 20%.

Della Santa D, Chamay A: Radiological evolution of the rheumatoid wrist after radio-lunate arthrodesis. *J Hand Surg* 1995; 20B:146–154.

The authors evaluated 26 wrists treated surgically and 20 wrists treated nonsurgically with a 5-year follow-up. Radiolunate arthrodesis can prevent dislocation of an unstable wrist but deterioration around it can still occur. The operation selected (partial or complete arthrodesis or total arthroplasty) depends on the stage and type of the disease.

Lundborg G, Branemark PI: Anchorage of wrist joint prostheses to bone using the osseointegration principle. *J Hand Surg* 1997;22B:84–89.

Results of 5 patients who underwent total wrist arthroplasty using titanium screw fixation, proximally in both the radius and ulna and distally in the metacarpals, are described. No bone resorption or screw loosening at the interface occurred.

Shapiro JS: The wrist in rheumatoid arthritis. *Hand Clin* 1996; 12:477–498.

This is an excellent review of the rheumatoid wrist, including the natural history, biomechanics, and operative intervention.

Stanley JK, Tolat AR: Long-term results of Swanson silastic arthroplasty in the rheumatoid wrist. *J Hand Surg* 1993; 18B:381–388.

The authors present results of a long-term follow-up of 50 Swanson wrist arthroplasties. Range of motion averaged 25° extension and 31° flexion. Implant fracture rate was 22%; 14% were symptomatic and required reoperation. There was no symptomatic synovitis from particular debris. Previous studies have not produced comparable results.

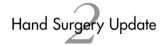

Terrono AL, Feldon PG, Millender LH, Nalebuff EA: Evaluation and treatment of the rheumatoid wrist. *J Bone Joint Surg* 1995; 77A:1116–1128.

A comprehensive review of the evaluation, treatment, and operative technique of the wrist pathology found in rheumatoid arthritis is presented.

Distal Radioulnar Joint

Blank JE, Cassidy C: The distal radioulnar joint in rheumatoid arthritis. *Hand Clin* 1996;12:499–513.

This review article looks at the etiology and surgical options for treating deformities at the distal radioulnar joint. The authors' preferred techniques are presented in detail, and an extensive list of reference is provided.

Van Gemert AM, Spauwen PH: Radiological evaluation of the long-term effects of resection of the distal ulna in rheumatoid arthritis. *J Hand Surg* 1994;19B:330–333.

The authors studied carpal translation in 28 patients, comparing unilateral distal ulnar resection with the nonoperated hand radiographically (before surgery, and 4 to 8 years postoperative). They concluded that ulnar carpal translation results from the disease process itself and is not accelerated by the distal ulnar resection.

Vincent KA, Szabo RM, Agee JM: The Suave-Kapandji procedure for reconstruction of the rheumatoid distal radioulnar joint. *J Hand Surg* 1993;18A:978–983.

Twenty-one wrists in 17 patients were followed an average of 39 months following a Suavè-Kapandji procedure. There was high patient satisfaction with regard to pain relief, stability, and range of motion. Ulnar and palmar translocation was prevented in wrists with normal geometry at the time of surgery. With preexisting carpal translocation, further progression will occur.

Weiler PJ, Bogoch ER: Kinematics of the distal radioulnar joint in rheumatoid arthritis: An in vivo study using centrode analysis. *J Hand Surg* 1995;20A:937–943.

The distal radioulnar joint was evaluated in 10 wrists by computed tomography, studying varying degrees of pronosupination. Normal subjects as well as rheumatoids prior to bone erosion showed the center of rotation to lie within a well defined area. With erosion at the dorsal border of the sigmoid notch, the ulna becomes dorsally positioned relative to the radius. Significant kinematic alterations occur.

Interphalangeal Joints

Adamson GJ, Gellman H, Brumfield RH Jr, Kuscher SH, Lawler JW: Flexible implant resection arthroplasty of the proximal interphalangeal joint in patients with systemic inflammatory arthritis. *J Hand Surg* 1994;19A:378–384.

In a long-term follow-up of silicone implant arthroplasties in 40 proximal interphalangeal joints, overall results were 12 good, 18 fair, and 10 poor. PIP implant arthroplasty in digits with a swan-neck deformity or joints ankylosed prior to surgery was not recommended. Performing an MCP arthroplasty prior to or concurrently with an implant arthroplasty for a boutonnière deformity will provide an improved functional range of motion.

Rizio L, Belsky MR: Finger deformities in rheumatoid arthritis. *Hand Clin* 1996;12:531–540.

In this review of the anatomy, pathology, and treatment of rheumatoid interphalangeal joint deformities, swan-neck and boutonnière deformities are discussed at length.

Ruther W, Verhestraeten B, Fink B, Tillmann K: Resection arthroplasty of the metacarpophalangeal joints in rheumatoid arthritis: Results after more than 15 years. *J Hand Surg* 1995; 20B:707–715.

In this long-term (15 to 22 years) retrospective study of 128 MCP joints treated with resection arthroplasty without interpositional material, overall patient satisfaction was high. Average active motion arc measured 35°. Ulnar deviation greater than 15° occurred in 30%. One third of the patients were rated as good, one third fair, and one third poor.

Thumb Deformities

Manueddu CA, Bogoch ER, Hastings DE: Restoration of metacarpophalangeal extension of the thumb in inflammatory arthritis. *J Hand Surg* 1996;21B:633–639.

Eleven patients with early boutonnière deformities were treated by EPL rerouting. Follow-up ranged from 1 to 5 years (average, 3.2 years). Early results showed preservation of good extensor strength with variable postoperative interphalangeal joint motion. Longer follow-up is necessary to evaluate recurrence.

Stein AB, Terrono AL: The rheumatoid thumb. *Hand Clin* 1996; 12:541–550.

In this review of the common deformities found in the rheumatoid thumb, the authors discuss etiology, classification, and surgical treatment.

Complex Deformities

Blair WF: An approach to complex rheumatoid hand and wrist problems. *Hand Clin* 1996;12:615–628.

This comprehensive article presents a strategy for treatment of the rheumatoid hand and wrist. A series of complex cases illustrates treatment for patients with multiple deformities.

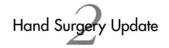

Chapter 32
Osteoarthritis of the Hand

Edward Diao, MD

Introduction

Osteoarthritis (OA) is a degenerative condition in which a hyaline cartilage disorder develops in diarthrodial joints. It is distinct from inflammatory arthropathies, such as rheumatoid arthritis, in which the primary component is an inflammatory/systemic pathophysiology. Although the term OA can be used to refer to all the degenerative conditions of articular cartilage, other than those caused by rheumatoid arthritis and seronegative spondyloarthropathies, idiopathic OA, or "primary idiopathic OA," is reserved to describe situations in which articular cartilage degeneration occurs without clear etiology. Idiopathic OA excludes posttraumatic arthritis or arthritic conditions resulting from crystalline deposition disease, obvious infection, or other known causes.

Epidemiology of Hand Osteoarthritis

The prevalence of OA of the hand increases with age; it is more common in men than women until women reach menopause. In individuals older than 65 years of age, the prevalence of radiographic OA of the hand has been estimated to be as high as 78% in men and 99% in women. The most affected joints are the distal interphalangeal (DIP) joint, the proximal interphalangeal (PIP) joint, and the base of the thumb. In a recent study, the cumulative incidence of radiographic hand OA was evaluated in 751 men and women (mean age, 55 ± 5.58 years). Baseline right-hand radiographs were taken between 1967 and 1969, and follow-up radiographs were taken 24 years later. Among patients without baseline OA, the incidence of developing OA in almost all hand joints was greater in women than in men. In both men and women, the joints most frequently affected were the DIP joint, followed by the base of the thumb, PIP joint, and metacarpophalangeal (MCP) joint. However, only the MCP joint had a similar incidence of OA development in both men and women.

Significant OA in 1 or more joints in a row, for example the PIP joints, markedly increased the risk of subsequent OA in all other joints in the same row. Also, significant OA in 1 joint in a finger increased the risk of subsequent OA in other joints in that finger. The presence of interphalangeal (IP) joint OA at baseline appeared to be associated with subsequent OA in all hand joints. However, baseline OA in the thumb was not as strong a predictor of subsequent progressive disease.

Patterns of OA also vary among different geographic and racial populations. For example, trapeziometacarpal (TMC) disease is much more prevalent among Caucasian populations. In one anatomic study, severe disease with eburnation of joint surfaces occurred in 50% of the Caucasian specimens, chondromalacia in 25%, and normal hyaline cartilage in 25%. In the Asian specimens, eburnation of joint surfaces was seen in only 8%, chondromalacia in 48%, and normal joint surfaces in 44%.

Pathophysiology and Pathobiology of Osteoarthritis

Recent studies have identified the interaction between biomechanical and biochemical factors in clinical OA. The TMC joint is the joint most frequently operated on in the osteoarthritic upper extremity and provides a unique isolated model for examination of pathobiology and biomechanics. One study analyzed 12 fresh postmortem specimens and 7 postsurgical specimens. The specimens were grouped into 6 surgically harvested specimens from patients with symptomatic joint disease, 6 fresh postmortem specimens with grossly normal articular surface, and 5 fresh postmortem specimens with significant eburnation, resembling that of the surgical group in both extent and topographic distribution. Regional biochemical analysis was performed on specimens from 4 compartments of the TMC joint surface. Glycosaminoglycan (GAG) analysis and proteoglycan extraction and analysis were conducted. The highest levels of total GAG and hydroxyproline (Hyp) corroborated the localization of severe osteoarthritic lesions to the palmar region of the TMC joint. Loss of GAG consistently preceded and exceeded that of Hyp, which suggests a selective, initial biochemical decomposition of diseased articular cartilage rather than simple mechanical wear of otherwise normal surface material.

Specific GAG analysis demonstrated a declining ratio of chondroitin sulfate (CS) to keratan sulfate (KS), which follows the normal skeletal aging process. However, in surgical specimens and cadaver specimens with OA, this pattern was reversed, implying that stimulation of the chondrocyte in osteoarthritic articular cartilage accounts for increased synthetic activity and increase in the CS to KS ratio.

In cases of severe OA, functional incompetence of the palmar beak ligament was found, resulting in pathologic laxity, abnormal translation of the metacarpal and the trapezium, and presumably generation of increased sheer forces between the joint surfaces. The resulting sharply demarcated zones of eburnation refutes an arthritic etiology based on the presence of a degraded enzyme in the synovial fluids, which would bathe the entirety of the joint surfaces. Mechanical instability resulting from beak ligament insufficiency is therefore assumed to modulate the geographic biochemical breakdown of the articular cartilage.

In another study, surface ultrastructure in the TMC joint was evaluated by scanning electronic microscopy. Materials from a variety of surgically harvested specimens in 3 stages of articular disease (normal cartilage, intermediate disease, and end-stage disease with eburnation) were compared. Intermediate disease was most commonly found in the palmar contact areas of TMC surface removed during basal joint arthroplasty. Ultrastructural changes were paralleled by an increase, then a decrease in the cellular elements. This pattern occurred in a geographic distribution that related to joint contact areas. The areas with early signs of disruption of normal surface ultrastructure and progressively the most severe areas of destruction were concentrated in the contact zones of the palmar compartment of the joint. These findings suggest an interdependence of biochemical and biomechanical events in the pathogenesis of OA.

To evaluate contact patterns in the TMC joint, 3 cadaver specimens were mounted on a base and their muscles loaded to simulate lateral pinch. Pressure-sensitive film was used to evaluate joint contact pressures in various functional positions. The palmar compartment of the TMC joint was found to be the primary contact area during flexion adduction of the thumb ray in lateral pinch. Simulation of dynamic pinch and release resulted in enlargement of the contact pattern, suggesting physiologic translation of the metacarpal on the trapezium. Detachment of the palmar beak ligament resulted in dorsal translation of the contact area, which produced a pattern similar to that of cartilage degeneration in osteoarthritic joints. This study validated the primary role of the palmar beak ligament that had been proposed earlier.

The primary importance of the beak ligament or anterior oblique ligament was reiterated in a study in which 30 hand specimens were dissected and 5 ligamentous structures were identified. The anterior oblique ligament was the primary stabilizer of the TMC joint; it was noted to be taut in abduction, extension, and pronation when the specimens were stress tested (Fig. 1).

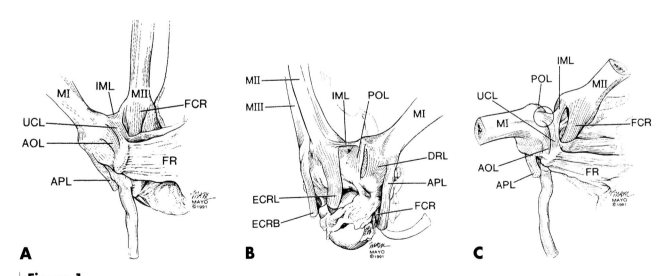

Figure 1

Left trapezoimetacarpal joint. **A,** Palmar view. **B,** Dorsal view. **C,** Distal view. AOL = anterior oblique ligament, UCL = ulnar collateral ligament, IML = first intermetacarpal ligament, APL = abductor pollicis longus tendon, FCR = flexor carpi radialis tendon, FR = flexor retinaculum, MI = first metacarpal, MII = second metacarpal, MIII = third metacarpal, POL = posterior oblique ligament, DRL = dorsoradial ligament, ECRL = extensor carpi radialis longus tendon, ECRB = extensor carpi radialis brevis tendon. (Reproduced with permission from the Mayo Foundation, Rochester, MN.)

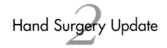

Nonsurgical Treatment

Initial treatment of OA in the hand and wrist is directed at the mechanical and biologic aspects of the disease. To decrease mechanical stresses in the affected joints, a period of activity modification, rest, and judicious splinting is appropriate. For the IP joints, finger splints for night use and selective day use can be considered. For the basilar thumb joint, an opponens splint, either hand-based or across the wrist, can be beneficial. Similarly, a wrist cock-up splint can be used for intercarpal and radiocarpal OA.

To counteract biologic aspects of OA, anti-inflammatory medication can be used. Systemic oral nonsteroidal anti-inflammatory drugs (NSAIDs) are the mainstay of early management of symptomatic OA. A myriad of NSAIDs are available. No single compound has been found to be singularly effective in the treatment of OA. Responses vary among patient populations. Any and all may alleviate the inflammatory response to OA to some degree. Agents are selected for efficacy, convenience of dosing intervals, and minimal incidence of gastrointestinal upset and renal and liver side effects. When these treatments fail, surgical therapy is indicated.

Diagnosis and Treatment of Specific Joints

Distal Interphalangeal Joint

OA of the DIP joint is characterized by primary enlargement of the distal joint with formation of so-called Heberden's nodes. It often is painless, and is noticeable primarily because of the deformity of the joint. After loss of joint space and formation of Heberden's nodes, angulatory and rotational deformities of the terminal phalanx can develop.

Nodular involvement of the joint combined with bone spurs can lead to the formation of ganglion cysts in conjunction with the OA. These cysts are called mucous cysts. With or without mucous cyst formation, OA of the DIP can cause secondary deformity of the nail plate, with loss of its normal sheen; in more severe cases, grooving or even splitting of the nail plate can result. These lesions must not be treated as primary skin or dermatologic lesions because shaving of the mass or drainage or cautery of the lesion can lead to formation of a draining sinus or even to septic arthritis of the DIP joint.

The indications for treatment may be purely cosmetic, as in the painless OA of the DIP joint with Heberden's node formation, or to resolve a mucous cyst situation (either a cyst that remains intact, or a mucous cyst with an associated draining sinus or skin lesion). The main surgical treatments have consisted of debridement of the Heberden's nodes and/or removal of the mucous cyst if it occurs. In rare circumstances, when joint destruction is severe and maintenance of a DIP joint in acceptable alignment is difficult to achieve by any other means, arthrodesis is considered.

Most cases of DIP joint OA are successfully treated with limited surgical excision. The concept of surgical excision of mucous cysts and marginal osteophytes was described in 1973. A recent review of 178 patients (average age, 57 years) treated for mucous cysts between 1973 and 1992 confirmed the efficacy of these procedures. The mucous cyst was carefully dissected and the cyst walls were traced down to the point of origin on the dorsal ulnar or the dorsal aspect of the DIP joint. After excision of the cyst, osteophytes were removed with rongeur and curettes. There were only 2 recurrences and 2 postoperative infections in the series. Associated nail-bed deformities were resolved in 46 cases. This treatment is significantly more successful than simple excision of the cysts, which has a recurrence rate of 25%, or cryosurgery, with recurrence rates of 11% to 14%. Moreover, this study confirms that skin grafting is unnecessary for successful treatment of these lesions.

In some instances, DIP joint arthrodesis may be indicated, particularly to correct severe angulatory or rotational deformity that is cosmetically or functionally unacceptable to the patient. A study of 30 cadaveric DIP joints compared DIP arthrodesis by tension band wiring versus that using a Herbert screw. These are alternatives to simple Kirscher wire (K-wire) fixation, which can be associated with failure of the arthrodesis. The results indicated that the mean minimum width of the distal phalanx (3.55 mm) is less than the diameter of the screw (3.90 mm). Fracture or thread penetration at the tip of the distal phalanx occurred in 25 of the specimens during screw placement. However, the Herbert screw had significantly greater anterior-posterior bending strength and greater torsional rigidity when compared with tension band wiring techniques. Some of the benefits of Herbert screw fixation may be obtained with fewer complications with use of the Herbert miniscrew (Zimmer, Inc, Warsaw, IN), an implant with a smaller trailing thread diameter (3.2 mm) that can be more easily accommodated in a terminal phalanx, particularly in smaller patients and females.

In certain circumstances of DIP arthritis, silicone implant arthroplasty may be an alternative to arthrodesis. An 11-year experience with 23 patients (average age, 58.3 years) with a total of 38 silicone interpositional arthroplasties of the DIP joint was reported in 1997. This procedure was undertaken as an alternative to DIP joint arthrodesis, and the implants were in place for an average of 10 years. Fewer than 10% of the implants required removal. A dorsal T-shaped incision was used with division of extensor tendon, bone contouring, placement of silicone implant, and then extensor tendon repair. The mean extension lag was 12.7° (range, 0° to 45°). The active range of motion ranged from 10° to 50° with a mean of 33.2°. In 10 of 23 patients (43%), the joints were stable to lateral stress; 12 patients (52%) showed some degree of lateral mobility, but with a stable end point. There was only 1 case of gross instability. Three patients had complications with this procedure. Silicone interpositional arthroplasty can be performed at the DIP joint, and may have some limited applications to DIP joint OA treatment.

Proximal Interphalangeal Joint

The PIP joint is less commonly involved with OA than the DIP joint. The main indications for surgery are pain refractory to medical management, deformity that interferes with function, and contracture secondary to osteophyte formation and soft-tissue fibrosis. Because PIP joint motion is so critical to normal hand function, surgery should be avoided when an acceptable arc of motion is present. Infrequently, significant instability associated with joint destruction is an indication for surgical reconstruction via arthrodesis or arthroplasty, especially if the joint deformity is associated with pain or limitation of function.

When the amount of OA is relatively modest, but effects of trauma or idiopathic arthritis lead to fibrosis of the soft tissues, total collateral ligament excision for treatment of contracted PIP joints has been demonstrated to be effective. Although traditional belief is that the collateral ligament complex could not be totally removed without a major compromise to joint stability, total excision of thickened, fibrosed collateral ligaments was proposed to achieve significant improvement in motion (Fig. 2). In a 1993 review of 16 patients with PIP joint contractures treated by this method, the average range of motion increased from 38° preoperatively to 78° postoperatively. There was no evidence of late instability of the PIP joints on manual lateral stress testing and stressed radiographic examination. The surgery did not improve range of motion in 2 patients with a preoperative total arc of motion of 70° to 80°; therefore, this surgery is recommended only when the total arc of motion is 70° or less.

A follow-up study performed on these patients with late magnetic resonance imaging (MRI) revealed that after total collateral ligament excision, scar formation and scar remodeling under the stimulus of active motion allow the soft tissues to remodel into a structure that resembles normal collateral ligament, in terms of function in restoring stability and in MRI appearance. Total collateral ligament excision can be coupled with flexor sheath release, with volar plate

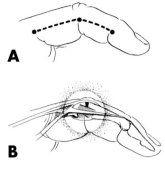
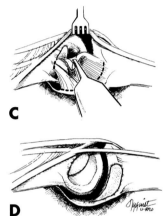

Figure 2
A, Midaxial incision. **B,** Relationship of extensor mechanism to collateral ligament. **C,** Dorsal mobilization of extensor mechanism allows total collateral ligament excision along dotted lines at condyle of proximal phalanx and insertion at base of middle phalanx and on palmar plate. **D,** Appearance of proximal interphalangeal joint after total collateral ligament excision. (Reproduced with permission from Diao E, Eaton RG: Total collateral ligament excision for contractures of the proximal interphalangeal joint. J Hand Surg 1993;18A:395–402.)

contracture release in selected patients, and with modest marginal osteophyte excision.

For joints that have more severe OA with significant bone destruction and loss of alignment, treatment alternatives include both arthrodesis and arthroplasty. The traditional means of achieving arthrodesis is by temporary K-wire fixation. Although relatively simple to perform from a technical standpoint, pin complications and lack of compression can lead to failure of arthrodesis. In one review of 203 patients (average age, 47 years), 290 small joint arthrodeses of MCP and PIP joints were performed using tension band technique. K-wire pins (0.028- or 0.035-in) were used to create bone tunnels, and 25- or 26-gauge stainless steel wires were threaded through holes. Tension band techniques were then used with the stainless steel wires over the K-wires. Arthrodesis was favored over arthroplasty because of gross instability, prior history of sepsis, deficient bone stock, inadequate soft-tissue coverage or support, or a combination thereof. The PIP joints were approached through a dorsal longitudinal incision. A 3% nonunion rate was reported, and the incidence of hardware removal was 9%. Four patients had painless pseudarthrosis. Tension band wiring should be considered as an excellent option

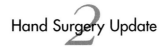
for PIP joint arthrodesis. Its reliability, ability to provide stable fixation with some compression, and ability to dispense with external splinting in compliant patients make this treatment an attractive alternative to conventional temporary K-wire arthrodesis techniques.

In a recent comparison of various arthrodesis techniques, 37 patients had Herbert screw fixation, 100 had conventional K-wire fixation, 69 patients had tension band wiring, and 11 had plate fixation. None of the patients who had arthrodesis for OA had nonunions. For other conditions, however, nonunions did occur. K-wires were associated with the highest nonunion rate; tension band wiring had an intermediate nonunion rate, and Herbert screws had the lowest nonunion rate.

Silicone implant arthroplasty remains a viable and appropriate treatment for severe OA of the PIP joint, particularly in nonborder digits. Silicone implants, such as Swanson's original design or variations thereof, are well suited to the PIP joint. Smaller sized implants than those for the more common MCP joint replacements are usually necessary. Traditionally, a dorsal approach is used with a longitudinal extensor tendon-splitting approach and detachment of the central slip. Joint surfaces are prepared and the implant placed, followed by extensor tendon repair and skin closure. Judicious protection of the extensor mechanism for 4 to 6 weeks is necessary to prevent failure of the extensor mechanism at the PIP joint and subsequent boutonnière deformity.

In the palmar approach, Eaton's volar plate arthroplasty approach is followed to expose the PIP joint. Reflection of flexor sheath between A2 and A4 pulleys, retraction of the flexor tendons, detachment of the volar plate, and excision of collateral ligaments can then be followed by preparation of joint surfaces and placement of the implant. A retrospective review of 47 patients (average age, 52 years) with 87 PIP joint silicone replacement arthroplasties performed through a palmar approach revealed excellent clinical results. Eleven patients were excluded; of the remaining 36 patients, 18 were undergoing reconstruction for OA. Average preoperative extension deficit of the PIP (17°) improved 8° postoperatively. Average preoperative total active motion at the PIP joint was 44°; after surgery it was 46°. Sixty-seven digits were relieved of pain immediately postoperatively and all had improved function. The benefits in terms of protection of the extensor mechanism warrant this approach as a preferred alternative to dorsal placement of the implant.

Trapeziometacarpal Joint

The TMC joint is the most common upper extremity site of surgical reconstruction for OA. Indications for surgery are primarily pain and secondarily deformity that interferes with activities of daily living. The main elements of TMC anatomy have been confirmed and amplified by recent studies. The basal joint is semiconstrained and incongruous and has been likened to 2 saddles with the axes of the opposing saddles perpendicular to each other, one essentially upside down and rotated at 90°. This anatomy permits flexion-extension, abduction-adduction, and rotation to allow thumb opposition and circumduction. The critical ligament is the palmar ligament, anterior oblique ligament, or beak ligament. The diagnosis of basal joint arthritis is suspected when there is a history of pain with thumb use and movement, particularly with gripping across the thumb joint. The loading of the joint causes subluxation and increases contact joint forces. The pain is a diffuse aching localized to the thumb abductor muscles and the thenar muscles. The diagnosis is confirmed at physical examination when the examiner reproduces the pain by exerting digital pressure over the capsule of the TMC joint volarly, radially, and dorsally. It is important to differentiate TMC joint arthritis pain from that associated with other etiologies of radial-sided wrist pain, such as thumb MCP joint arthritis or instability, de Quervain's tenosynovitis, second dorsal compartment tendinitis affecting wrist flexors, tendinitis in the other dorsal wrist compartments, and intercarpal or radiocarpal arthritis. In the early stages of basal joint arthritis, significant deformity or crepitus may not be evident. In later stages, these findings should be discernible.

Eaton and Littler described 4 radiographic stages of basal joint disease. In stage 1, the articular contours are normal, and there is no subluxation or joint debris. The joint space may be widened if an effusion is present. In stage 2, there is slight narrowing of the thumb TMC joint, but the joint space and articular contours are preserved. Joint debris less than 2 mm in size may be present. In stage 3, there is significant TMC joint disruption, with sclerotic or cystic changes in subchondral bone and osteophytes greater than 2 mm in size. Stage 4 disease is pantrapezial arthritis, in which both TMC and scaphotrapezial joints are affected, and these articular surfaces show radiographic signs of severe degeneration.

The palmar oblique or beak ligament is the most important one in preventing carpometacarpal joint thumb subluxation and migration, and insufficiency of this ligament is implicated in the pathomechanics of the development of basal joint arthritis. It therefore stands to reason that reconstruction or reconstitution of the stabilizing function of such a ligament would be a cornerstone of successful surgical treatment for basal joint disease.

The decision to treat basal joint disease and ultimately to perform surgery on it should be independent of radiographic staging. Patients with stage 1 OA could be symptomatic enough to require surgical reconstruction and be candidates for a successful outcome. Some patients with significant stage 3 or 4 OA, on the other hand, might be relatively asymptomatic and thus should not be encouraged to have surgical reconstruction. Nonsurgical treatment includes the use of NSAIDs, cortisone injections, and judicious splinting. Unfortunately, these measures are not enough in a significant percentage of clinical cases, which go on to require surgical reconstruction.

Stage 1 disease that requires surgical treatment is relatively rare. The only candidates are patients who have enough symptoms to require surgical reconstruction, yet have joint surfaces that are completely free of eburnation and demonstrate only the slightest, if any, changes of chondromalacia in the contact areas of the palmar aspect of the joint. Because the pathomechanics of the joint are such that mechanical instability and subluxation lead to arthrosis, the ligamentous restraints to the thumb metacarpal should be reconstructed and augmented with a slip of flexor carpi radialis tendon. For such a reconstruction to be successful, assessment of the articular surfaces must confirm that they are, at most, minimally involved. Exposure for this assessment is provided by the Wagner approach, in which the thenar musculature is reflected from the base of the metacarpal and the slip of the abductor pollicis longus that attaches to the thenar muscles is divided. With good preservation of the joint surfaces and the bulk of the cartilage, reconstruction with the flexor carpi radialis tendon is highly successful. Ligament reconstruction to render the symptomatic hypermobile joint more stable may retard the progression of the degenerative articular process, as well as resolve the immediate symptoms of joint arthrosis.

In stages 2, 3, and 4, joint surfaces are no longer normal. Therefore, reconstructive efforts must be directed at elimination of painful arthritic joints about the trapezium, with salvage techniques used to decrease pain while preserving function. TMC joint arthrodesis is 1 of several possible treatments for stage 2 or 3 basal joint arthritis. It is not appropriate for stage 4 OA, in which the scaphotrapezial joint is also involved. An advantage of this procedure is the prevention of thumb ray shortening, and good results have been achieved in laborers. One disadvantage is that the scaphotrapezial joint, which bears all the thumb ray motion after surgery, has increased wear and the reconstruction can fail when arthrosis of the scaphotrapezial joint becomes significant. Another downside is that the success rate of the arthrodesis itself varies from 50% to 100%, and postoperative immobilization may be required for several months.

Four methods of fixation of the TMC joint—crossed K-wire, cup-and-cone osteotomy with single K-wire fixation, cerclage wiring, and tension band wiring with a single longitudinal K-wire—have been compared. The tension band wiring and cerclage techniques were superior in terms of stiffness of construct and minimal toggle displacement. The major limitation of this technique relates not only to successful bony healing, but also to subsequent loss of motion and inability to manipulate the hand so that the thumb can abduct to allow the palm to flatten against a flat surface such as a table or floor.

Another technique for basal joint reconstruction is simple excisional arthroplasty. Weakness and instability have been reported as drawbacks of this surgery. Proximal migration of the metacarpal with shortening of the thumb ray may present functional problems and can compromise long-term results. Another approach involves excision of the trapezium and placement of interposition material. The flexor carpi radialis "anchovy spacer" is one of these. Other tendons, fascia, tissue bank fascia, and gelfoam have also been proposed as interpositional materials after trapeziectomy.

A stemmed silicone trapezial implant has been used for TMC joint arthritis, but failed to seat satisfactorily in the trapezium fossa in over 25% of cases. A modified cannulated silicone trapezial implant, which allows insertion of a slip of abductor pollicis longus into the base of the index metacarpal as a portion of the overall arthroplasty procedure, has been used clinically on a limited basis. In a recent review of the Niebauer TMC arthroplasty prostheses, the authors found that 88% of patients were pleased and would have undergone the operation again. Postoperative subluxation occurred in 83% of the patients. However, in 24 of 27 patients pain was relieved and satisfactory motion and stability were achieved.

Eaton and Littler's original flexor carpi radialis technique and variations such as Burton's ligament reconstruction tendon interposition (LRTI) have withstood the test of time (Fig. 3). A recent report indicates that at 9-year follow-up, LRTI reconstructions are durable and continue to have good performance clinically. Average grip strength increased 10 kg, a 93% improvement over preoperative values, and has steadily improved over time. In 92% of patients, the tip of the thumb could be brought to the MCP joint base of the little finger, and average web angle was 40°. Stress radiographs showed metacarpal base subluxation of 11% at 9 years; average loss of height was 13% at 9 years. The authors concluded that these ligament reconstructions have excellent long-term durability with pain relief and even late increases in strength.

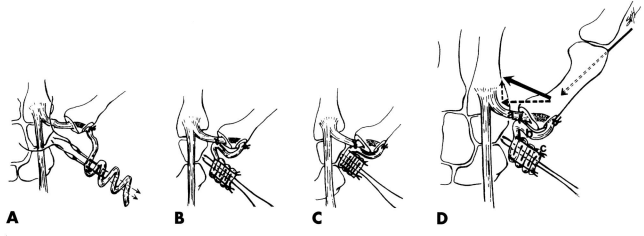

Figure 3

Schematic representation of the ligament reconstruction-tendon interposition arthroplasty. **A,** Flexor carpi radialis (FCR) slip has been passed through the bone tunnel in the thumb metacarpal. **B,** FCR is stabilized at bone tunnel by suturing the tail to itself. **C,** FCR interposition is delivered into the trapezial space. The forces in function producing proximal migration and radial subluxation of the metacarpal are neutralized by the ligament reconstruction, as indicated in the vector diagram (**D**). a = ligament reconstruction, b = metacarpal resurfacing, c = tendon arthroplasty spacer. (Reproduced with permission from Tomaino MM, Pellegrini VD Jr, Burton RI: Arthroplasty of the basal joint of the thumb: Long-term follow-up after ligament reconstruction with tendon interposition. *J Bone Joint Surg* 1995;77A:346–355.)

In another report of the LRTI reconstruction, outcome studies of 27 patients revealed that 24 (89%) were satisfied with their pain relief; 23 (87%) would undergo the same procedure again. Eighteen patients noted improvement in their ability to perform activities of daily living. Postsurgical improvements were noted in web space measurements and grip and pinch strength determinations. The trapezial space ratio decreased 51% following arthroplasty when compared to normal values in the literature, and 33% compared to preoperative values in the study.

When the flexor carpi radialis is used as the source of LRTI arthroplasty, the suspension point is determined by the insertion of the flexor carpi radialis. If this tendon is not split all the way to its osseous insertion, the consequence is an even more proximal suspension point with potential for developing laxity. One surgeon described a technique using a slip of abductor pollicis longus, maintained with its bony insertion on the dorsal base of the thumb metacarpal and detached at the musculotendinous junction proximally. Bone tunnels are then created obliquely from the dorsal metaphysis of the thumb metacarpal to exit the center of the articular surface of the metacarpal. Thereafter, the tendon is passed obliquely through the radial facet of the index metacarpal and out through the dorsum to be woven up to the extensor carpi radialis longus tendon. Originally designed as the salvage for failed Swanson interposition arthroplasties, this technique has been effective as an index

procedure for basal joint OA in stages 2, 3, and 4. The ability to control the location of the suspension point bone tunnel with use of the abductor pollicis longus is one advantage. It also is possible to set the tension of the ligament reconstruction more directly by pulling the abductor pollicis longus taut through the tunnel while suturing, thus more closely simulating the anterior oblique ligament in both direction and function.

A variation of this reconstruction has been used clinically for the last 10 years, and its performance has been excellent. Patients have been returned to heavy labor, repetitive hand use, and high-demand occupations, such as orthopaedic and neurologic surgery. In addition to determining patient outcomes, biomechanical testing has been conducted to ascertain thumb metacarpal base stability after basal joint reconstruction. In this study, the relative migration of the base of the thumb metacarpal in the proximal, dorsal, and radial directions was tested in a cadaver model, with standardized force generated by loading the digital flexor tendons with weights. Trapezial excision was performed on 15 fresh, frozen cadaver hands randomized into 3 groups—LRTI, Thompson's suspensionplasty with abductor pollicis longus, and a modification thereof. Specimens were fixed with an index metacarpal-radius intramedullary rod, and a pinch force of 5 kg/cm^2 was generated by hanging weights on tendons and measured with a miniature pressure transducer. Postreconstruction migration of the thumb metacarpal base was measured using a sonic digitizer tracking system. The modified suspensionplasty with the more distal abductor pollicis longus suspension point was superior to the other 2 techniques. It provided the best stability and minimized proximal migration of the thumb metacarpal (Figs. 4–6).

In the future, arthroscopic surgery may be used to treat TMC joint arthritis of the thumb. In a 1996 report, 33 patients were evaluated after arthroscopic partial resection of the trapezium and interpositional arthroplasty. A 2.7-mm arthroscope was used to view the TMC joint, and a 2.9-mm round burr was used to perform trapezial resection. Intrapositional material, palmaris longus, autogenous tendon graft, Gore-Tex®, or fascia lata allograft was then inserted. There was satisfactory pain relief and no complications in 87.8% of patients. The author claimed that preservation of joint capsule and ligaments was an advantage of this technique. Adequate interposition is assumed to cause the beak ligament to become taut and functional again, but this has not been confirmed biomechanically and clinically.

Scaphoid-Trapezium-Trapezoid Osteoarthritis

Ideal treatment of symptomatic scaphoid-trapezium-trapezoid (STT) OA is by STT arthrodesis. This procedure was originally described as the triscaphe arthrodesis. It effectively eliminates the affected arthritic joint. STT arthrodesis remains the prototype for other intercarpal arthrodeses, which are effective treatments for intercarpal ligament insufficiencies, either acute or chronic, as well as focal OA or post-traumatic arthritis. These arthrodeses are effective methods of maintaining overall carpal height in situations where a carpal bone or bones must be removed, for example in fracture nonunion or severe osteonecrosis.

The disadvantage of intercarpal arthrodesis is that with alteration of normal wrist kinematics, neighboring joints are subjected to increased stress. A recent review of STT arthrodesis pointed to significant complications in 14 patients with a 62-month average follow-up. Eight had significant residual symptoms; 9 returned to presurgery occupations. Overall motion was reduced by 30% to 60%. Eleven patients had complications; 3 had nonunions, and 6 required subsequent surgery. The most frequent complication was progressive TMC or radioscaphoid arthrosis.

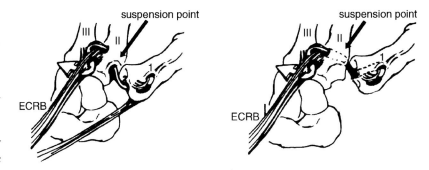

Figure 4

Schematics of abductor pollicis longus tendon suspensionplasty procedures with weave into the extensor carpi radialis brevis (ECRB). **A,** Suspension point at the proximal index metacarpal facet in Thompson's original description. **B,** The more distal metaphyseal suspension point in Diao's modification.

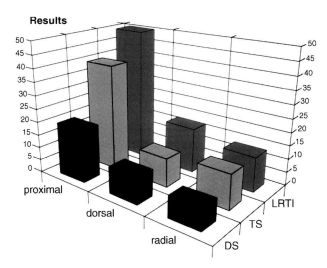

Figure 5

Comparison of migration in proximal, dorsal, and radial directions in cadaver study of ligament reconstruction with tendon interposition (LRTI), Thompson suspensionplasty (TS), and Diao suspensionplasty (DS). DS demonstrated the least migration of the thumb metacarpal

Although some of the poor results were attributed to technical problems, initial excellent results in some patients deteriorated over time. The overall rate of progressive radiocarpal arthrosis was 33%.

Complications of intercarpal arthrodesis were reviewed in another recent study of 50 patients; 3 patients were excluded for inadequate follow-up data. Operations reviewed included STT fusion (25 patients) and lunotriquetral fusion (14 patients). At 34-month follow-up, there were 18 good, 16 fair, and 13 poor results. Of the 50 patients, 36 had complications; 25 underwent further surgery, 16 for nonunion.

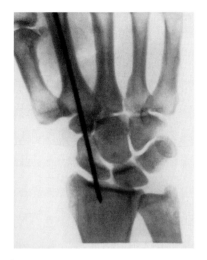

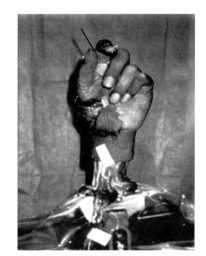

Figure 6

Experimental protocol for basal joint cadaver study.

Alternatives to STT arthrodesis are trapezium excision and ligament reconstruction-interposition arthroplasty, supplemented by trapezial-trapezoid joint interposition by tendon as well. This prevents subsequent thumb metacarpotrapezial arthritis, which may lead to failure of the original treatment and necessitate further surgery.

Intercarpal-Radiocarpal Osteoarthritis

Radiocarpal arthritis is most commonly the sequela of trauma (distal radius fracture, scaphoid fracture, or intercarpal-radiocarpal dislocation). It can also occur in a pattern described as scapholunate advanced collapse, or SLAC wrist, a progressive condition that can be idiopathic or induced by trauma to the intercarpal and radiocarpal wrist ligaments. SLAC wrist is characterized by scapholunate ligament insufficiency, which leads to progressive arthritis at the radioscaphoid joint and, subsequently, the capitolunate joint. Motion-sparing reconstruction can take advantage of the normal radiolunate joint, which tends to be spared of disease. Scaphoid excision followed by capitolunate arthrodesis or, more commonly, 4-corner fusion (capitate-lunate-hamate-triquetrum) addresses the radioscaphoid and capitolunate arthritis and the carpal instability and collapse, relying on the radiolunate joint to preserve wrist motion.

The natural history of SLAC wrist includes a pattern of progressive radiocarpal and intercarpal arthritis. However, early or mild forms of this deformity may progress slowly and may not necessitate surgical treatment. Two years after initial incidental SLAC wrist diagnosis, 20 of 30 wrists were found symptom-free in one recent study. The authors concluded that in some patients, especially older and low-demand patients, surgery may not be warranted, because the natural history of SLAC wrist does not always lead to rapidly worsening symptoms and radiographs.

One group of authors reported results of 100 scaphoid excisions and 4-corner fusions with 44-month average follow-up. Most patients had good to excellent results, with 72° arc of flexion-extension, radioulnar deviation of 37°, and 80% of the grip strength of the opposite side. Only 2 patients had progressive radioulnar arthritis, and only 3 had nonunions. Twelve percent had dorsal impingement of the capitate and radius, which was believed to be related to malalignment at the time of surgery.

Salvage procedures for symptomatic SLAC wrists and other osteoarthritic conditions that affect radiocarpal and intercarpal joints include proximal row carpectomy (PRC) and total wrist fusion. In PRC, the scaphoid, lunate, and triquetrum are excised, and a pseudarthrosis or pseudoarticulation is formed between the distal carpal row (trapezium, trapezoid, capitate, and hamate) and the distal radius. In the original description of this procedure, a normal proximal capitate was necessary to have a functional articulation to the lunate fossa of the distal radius. However, a modified technique for PRC involves resecting the proximal capitate to create a broader interface to distribute radiocarpal compressive forces more evenly. In a recent review of 12 patients treated with this technique, all had radiocarpal degenerative disease, including SLAC wrist with radiolunate or capitolunate involvement. Range of motion improved from 80° to 94° of flexion-extension. Flexion improved from 38° to 46° ($p < 0.01$). In the last 4 patients, in whom a dorsal wrist capsule was also interposed between the radius and carpus, the final arc of flexion-extension averaged 111°. Strength improved from 19 kg to 26 kg on average ($p < 0.01$ by paired t-test). These results compared quite favorably with those of other reported treatments.

Outcomes were reviewed for 23 wrists treated by PRC using conventional techniques, with an average 6-year follow-up. Carpectomies were performed for scapholunate dissociation, scaphoid nonunions, and Kienböck's disease. Twenty patients were satisfied with their outcomes. The flexion-extension arc averaged 74°, or 61% of the opposite wrist. Grip strength, corrected for dominance, averaged 79% of the opposite side, with an average improvement of 15 kg of force. Three patients subsequently developed radiocarpal arthritis, but only 1 required revision to arthrodesis. Similar results were obtained in a multicenter study of PRC in 1993. A retrospective review of the 20 patients 3.5 years after surgery showed a 15% decrease in motion but a 22% improvement in grip strength. Eighty-two percent were satisfied and stated that they would repeat the procedures.

A variety of different techniques for SLAC wrist have been compared. A recent review evaluated the outcomes of 6 different reconstructive procedures for stages 2 and 3 SLAC wrist in 55 patients with an average follow-up of 50 months. Treatments compared included scaphoid excision and intercarpal arthrodesis, 4-corner fusion, capitolunate fusion, PRC, radioscapholunate arthrodesis, radioscaphoid arthrodesis, and primary total wrist arthrodesis. In general, patients had less wrist pain postoperatively. There were 4 capitolunate nonunions, and 2 4-corner fusion nonunions. Six of 51 motion-preserving procedures required subsequent conversion to total arthrodesis. With scaphoid excision and 4-corner fusion, a 54° flexion-extension arc was obtained. Of all procedures, PRC preserved the best wrist mobility, with a flexion-extension arc of 71°.

Two studies looked specifically at whether PRC or limited intercarpal arthrodesis was superior for SLAC reconstruction. In one study, 24 wrists treated with either of the 2 procedures between 1980 and 1990 were retrospectively reviewed 5.5 years postoperatively. The authors concluded that both treatment groups had satisfactory results, except for 3 patients with PRC. Both groups showed improvements in grip strength and range of motion, which were sustained for at least 1 year postoperatively. Incorrect capitolunate alignment, which would result in diminished wrist extension, was noted with limited wrist arthrodesis. In another study of 28 patients, 4-corner arthrodesis patients had 95° motion compared to 115° for the PRC group. Grip strength averaged 74% of the opposite wrist in the arthrodesis group and 94% in the PRC group. There were 3 failures in the intercarpal arthrodesis group, and none in the PRC group. Both studies concluded that in wrists without capitolunate arthritis, PRC is superior. These authors did not perform the modified PRC with capitate excision, and they recommended limited wrist arthrodesis when capitolunate arthritis is significant.

The ultimate salvage for wrist OA (radiocarpal, intercarpal, or combined) is wrist arthrodesis. It can be used as a primary treatment for severe radiocarpal or intercarpal arthritis, has the great advantages of excellent reliability in terms of pain relief and durability, and can offer the patient an upper extremity that can be used for repetitive activities and heavy labor. The disadvantages are that wrist flexion-extension and radioulnar deviation motions are eliminated, and the only wrist motion that remains is forearm pronation-supination. Historically, wrist arthrodesis could be performed a multitude of ways. Iliac crest allografts with cast immobilization have been described, as well as intramedullary transfixing pin techniques. More recently, dorsally applied osteosynthesis compression plates with compression screws have been highly effective for wrist arthrodesis.

The iliac crest and pin technique was recently reviewed. The treatment was used for patients with connective tissue disorders, congenital wrist disorders, and some acquired wrist disorders. In the acquired wrist disorder group, average time of fusion was 12 weeks. In 2 patients, there was failure of arthrodesis. The disadvantage of this technique is the required cast and splint immobilization for a prolonged time until satisfactory wrist arthrodesis has been achieved.

Modern designs of osteosynthesis plates have improved the predictability of wrist arthrodesis. One review looked at wrist arthrodesis in 28 consecutive patients (average age, 34 years) with a combination of dorsal plate and local bone graft at an average follow-up of 2 years. All patients had a solid wrist arthrodesis. Grip strength, pronation, supination, and digital motion did not change from preoperative status. There were no instances of postoperative wrist pain or instability. Extensive tendinitis in 4 patients necessitated plate removal. One patient had carpal tunnel syndrome that required subsequent decompression, and one had distal radioulnar joint pain requiring corticosteroid injection therapy. Rigid plating imparts immediate stability in OA when bone stock is adequate to accept screws, and it decreases the amount of bone graft required, allowing local bone graft to suffice without need to resort to iliac crest graft. After surgery, these patients can be treated using removable wrist splints, without rigid, full-time cast or splint application; usually splints can be discontinued at 6 to 8 weeks. The main disadvantage of wrist arthrodesis with a plate is the need for a second operation for hardware removal. However, use of the plate has diminished the incidence of nonunions and pin-fixation-related complications, including pin tract infections and loss of positioning of the wrist.

One concern regarding wrist arthrodesis is how well the upper extremity functions afterward. In one 54-month follow-up of patients, a clinical questionnaire, Jebsen Hand Function Test, and Buck-Gramcko-Lohmann Functional Grading Scale were used. Fifteen of 23 patients returned to their original jobs, and all patients noted that although they could do most of the tests, they had to do them in a modified fashion. Perineal care and hand manipulation in tight spaces remained the 2 most difficult daily tasks. The Jebsen Test had a 64% completion rate with the fused wrist

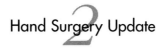
compared to a 78% completion rate for normal wrists. The Buck-Gramcko-Lohmann evaluations had an average score of 8.3 out of a possible 10. The conclusion is that patients who have had wrist arthrodesis can accomplish most activities of daily living, with some modifications.

The final treatment category that bears discussion is total wrist arthroplasty. Unfortunately, the overall success of total joint arthroplasty in the hip and knee, and increasingly in the shoulder and elbow, has not readily been transferred to the wrist. Complication rates of wrist arthroplasty have been as high as 50% in some series. For significant wrist arthritis, wrist arthrodesis remains the treatment of choice. However, some alternatives still exist in terms of use of total wrist arthroplasty. Between 1986 and 1991, 50 revised Meuli total wrist prostheses were implanted in 45 patients, 33 with rheumatoid arthritis and 12 with traumatic arthritis. The prosthesis is designed to be inserted through a longitudinal dorsal approach with distal radius and proximal carpal row resection. The anchoring stems are placed in an intramedullary position in the radius and in the second and third metacarpals distally. The proximal radial component contains the titanium ball head, and the distal cup is polyethylene. This unconstrained ball-and-socket joint allows motion in all planes as well as slight distraction with the theoretical limits of 50° flexion, 80° extension, and 70° of radioulnar deviation. There was an average 4.5-year follow-up. Results were excellent in 24 wrists, good in 12, fair in 5, and poor in 8; 1 patient died during the follow-up period. Overall average range of motion of those who still had their index arthroplasty procedure was 30° flexion, 40° extension, 10° radial deviation, and 10° ulnar deviation; pronation and supination were each 85°. Of the 12 posttraumatic OA patients, 10 showed improvement in grip strength postoperatively. This modified implant, used in uncemented fashion, demonstrated acceptably good results, with most complications ascribed to technical errors in placement of the carpal component; most failures related to this problem occurred within the first year. The authors believe this is an acceptable treatment and certainly compares favorably with some of the other reports of total wrist arthroplasty.

Since 1983, a biaxial total wrist prosthesis has been used at the Mayo Clinic because of an unacceptable loosening rate with the original Meuli and ball-and-socket designs. The biaxial implant has an ellipsoidal concave-shaped device within the proximal radial component and the distal carpal component with a single intramedullary stem containing a convex metal component. Fifty-seven patients with rheumatoid arthritis were followed-up for a minimum of 5 years or until failure. The mean follow was 6.5 years, and average patient age was 58 years. Follow-up pain was reported absent in 75% of patients, mild in 19%, moderate in 3%, and severe in 3%. The range of motion averaged 35° extension, 29° flexion, 10° radial deviation, and 20° ulnar deviation. There were 11 failures—8 distal loosenings, 1 infection, 1 dislocation, and 1 progressive soft-tissue imbalance.

Other prostheses currently in early clinical trials have been designed to improve methods of fixation and decrease the incidence of loosening, particularly of the carpal components. It remains to be seen whether these will offer improvements over existing prostheses. The notion of a salvage wrist operation for severe joint destruction that still retains motion is attractive, but the primary application at present is for patients with rheumatoid arthritis and only selected patients with OA. Revision of failed prostheses is particularly challenging, with subsequent loss of bone stock that generally requires either a custom prosthesis or an arthrodesis with significant supplemental bone grafting. Total wrist arthroplasty remains a therapy with very limited applications, compared to PRC, intercarpal arthrodesis, and total wrist arthrodesis, which remain the appropriate treatment for most osteoarthritic conditions in the wrist.

Annotated Bibliography

Epidemiology of Hand Osteoarthritis

Chaisson CE, Zhang Y, McAlindon TE, et al: Radiographic hand osteoarthritis: Incidence, patterns, and influence of pre-existing disease in a population based sample. *J Rheumatol* 1997;24:1337–1343.

Seven hundred fifty-one members of the Framingham cohort for cardiac disease had baseline right-hand radiographs taken in 1967 to 1969, with follow-up radiographs 24 years later. Patterns of OA were evaluated, including comparisons of the likelihood of progressive OA in different joints and relative risks of occurrence in men and women.

Pathophysiology and Pathobiology of Osteoarthritis

Ateshian GA, Ark JW, Rosenwasser MP, Pawluk RJ, Soslowsky LJ, Mow VC: Contact areas in the thumb carpometacarpal joint. *J Orthop Res* 1995;13:450–458.

Eight cadaver hands were tested with the thumb in the lateral pinch position. Small muscle loads were attached to simulate thumb flexion, extension, abduction, and adduction in neutral positions. A stereophotogrammetric technique was used to determine contact areas of the articular surfaces. Maps of cartilage thickness were determined for 9 specimens. The volar-ulnar, ulnar, and dorsal radial regions of the trapezium were the most common sites of thin cartilage and corresponded to the loading patterns in the lateral pinch position. The authors hypothesized that mechanical stresses lead to OA in this joint.

Imaeda T, An KN, Cooney WP III, Linscheid R: Anatomy of trapeziometacarpal ligaments. *J Hand Surg* 1993;18A:226–231.

Stabilizing ligaments of the thumb TMC joint were identified and studied with 30 anatomic cadaver dissections. Five ligamentous structures were identified—the anterior oblique ligament, the ulnar collateral ligament, the first intermetacarpal ligament, the posterior oblique ligament, and the dorsal ligament.

Imaeda T, Niebur G, An KN, Cooney WP III: Kinematics of the trapeziometacarpal joint after sectioning of ligaments. *J Orthop Res* 1994;12:205–210.

In this selective cutting experiment in 12 cadavers, a magnetic tracking system was used to note loading patterns after sectioning of ligaments. The combination of the anterior oblique and ulnar collateral ligaments was determined to be the most important in providing constraint of the TMC joint during simulated thumb circumduction.

Pellegrini VD Jr, Olcott CW, Hollenberg G: Contact patterns in the trapeziometacarpal joint: The role of the palmar beak ligament. *J Hand Surg* 1993;18A:238–244.

K-wires were used to mount 23 cadaver forearm specimens with the wrist at 30° extension and the thumb MCP joint in 20° of flexion. Extrinsic and intrinsic muscles were loaded with hanging weights, resulting in reproducible contact between the thumb pulp and index finger for pinch.

Pellegrini VD Jr, Smith RL, Ku CW: Pathobiology of articular cartilage in trapeziometacarpal osteoarthritis: I. Regional biochemical analysis. *J Hand Surg* 1994;19A:70–78.

Seven surgical specimens and 12 fresh postmortem specimens were evaluated; 6 postmortem specimens had no gross joint disease and 5 contained large well-defined areas of eburnation. Biomechanical analysis was performed on the hyaline cartilage from 4 quadrants in surgically harvested specimens. Chondromalacic surfaces were noted in the palmar contact areas and characterized by preferential loss of GAG, retention of collagen, and increasing CS/KS ratio, which is consistent with known biochemical changes in osteoarthritic joints.

Pellegrini VD Jr, Smith RL, Ku CW: Pathobiology of articular cartilage in trapeziometacarpal osteoarthritis: II. Surface ultrastructure by scanning electron microscopy. *J Hand Surg* 1994;19A:79–85.

Scanning electron microscopy was used to characterize the surface ultrastructure of TMC hyaline cartilage in osteoarthritic specimens and to grade the specimens into normal, intermediate OA, and severe OA categories. Osteoarthritic changes occurred in a geographic pattern relating to joint contact areas, with the highest incidence of changes occurring on the palmar contact areas of the TMC surfaces.

Distal Interphalangeal Joint

Kasdan ML, Stallings SP, Leis VM, Wolens D: Outcome of surgically treated mucous cysts of the hand. *J Hand Surg* 1994;19A:504–507.

The authors studied 190 mucous cysts from 178 patients (average age, 57 years) treated from 1973 to 1992. The long finger most frequently resolved. There were only 2 recurrences and 2 postoperative infections. Associated nail deformities were corrected in 46 cases. Surgical excision of marginal osteophytes proved to be an extremely effective treatment.

Wilgis EF: Distal interphalangeal joint silicone interpositional arthroplasty of the hand. *Clin Orthop* 1997;342:38–41.

This is a review of 38 digits with DIP joint silicone, interpositional arthroplasty. Average patient age was 58 years at surgery, and mean follow-up was 10-years. Fewer than 10% of the implants were removed, and an average of 33° of motion was obtained.

Wyrsch B, Dawson J, Aufranc S, Weikert D, Milek M: Distal interphalangeal joint arthrodesis comparing tension-band wire and Herbert screw: A biomechanical and dimensional analysis. *J Hand Surg* 1996;21A:438–443.

In 30 cadaveric DIP joints, Herbert screw or tension band wire technique was used to stimulate arthrodesis. Three-point lateral bending, anterior-posterior bending, and axial torsion were studied. The Herbert screw had greater anteroposterior bending strength and torsional rigidity despite fracture or thread penetration of the tip of the distal phalanx during screw placement in 25 of 30 specimens.

Proximal Interphalangeal Joint

Diao E, Eaton RG: Total collateral ligament excision for contractures of the proximal interphalangeal joint. *J Hand Surg* 1993;18A:395–402.

The complete excision of scarred PIP collateral ligaments as the cornerstone of surgical treatment for PIP joint contractures was evaluated. Sixteen patients had preoperative range of motion of 38°; at follow-up, postoperative range of motion of 78° with no instances of instability. The only surgical failures were in patients with a preoperative range of motion of ≥ 70°.

Leibovic SJ, Strickland JW: Arthrodesis of the proximal interphalangeal joint of the finger: Comparison of the use of the Herbert screw with other fixation methods. *J Hand Surg* 1994;19A:181–188.

This is a review of 224 PIP joint arthrodeses with a variety of techniques: Herbert screw (37); K-wires (100); tension band wiring (69); plates (11); and miscellaneous techniques (7). Clinical union was achieved in an average of 7 weeks, and radiographic union in 10 weeks. There were 31 cases of nonunion in 24 digits. The lowest nonunion rate was with Herbert screws.

Lin HH, Wyrick JD, Stern PJ: Proximal interphalangeal joint silicone replacement arthroplasty: Clinical results using an anterior approach. *J Hand Surg* 1995;20A:123–132.

The authors reviewed 69 PIP joint silicone arthroplasties using a palmar zigzag approach in 36 patients. The interval between A2 and A4 pulleys was used for implantation. Follow-up was 3.4 years. Extension deficit improved from 17° preoperatively to 8° postoperatively, with no significant increase in total active motion. Pain relief was maintained in 67 digits. The anterior approach allows presentation of the central slip insertion and initiation of immediate active and passive joint motion.

Stern PJ, Gates NT, Jones TB: Tension band arthrodesis of small joints in the hand. *J Hand Surg* 1993;18A:194–197.

Two hundred ninety tension band arthrodeses of the MCP joint and PIP joints of the hand in 203 patients (average age, 47 years) were studied. Nine patients failed to achieve bony union, 4 had painless

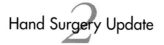
pseudoarthrosis, and 1 had a small finger amputation. Twenty-five fusions (9%) required hardware removal. There were 10 superficial infections and 3 malrotated fusions.

Trapeziometacarpal Joint

Diao E, Iida H, Lotz JC: Thumb metacarpal base stability after basal joint reconstruction: A biomechanical study. *Orthop Trans* 1997;21:316.

Fifteen fresh frozen cadaver hands had trapezial excision and 1 of 3 types of reconstruction—LRTI as described by Burton, adductor pollicis longus (APL) suspensionplasty as described by Thompson, or Diao's modification of the suspensionplasty with the APL suspended more distally on the index metacarpal base.

Lins RE, Gelberman RH, McKeown L, Katz JN, Kadiyala RK: Basal joint arthritis: Trapeziectomy with ligament reconstruction and tendon interposition arthroplasty. *J Hand Surg* 1996; 21A:202–209.

Twenty-seven consecutive patients who had basal joint arthritis were treated with LRTI. Most patients were satisfied with the pain relief and said they would undergo surgery again.

Menon J: Arthroscopic management of trapeziometacarpal joint arthritis of the thumb. *Arthroscopy* 1996;12:581–587.

Thirty-three patients had trapezial partial resection using 2.7-mm arthroscope imaging and 2.9-mm burr resection followed by intraposition arthroplasty with either autogenous tendon graft, Gore-Tex®, or fascia lata allograft. Twenty-nine patients (88%) had satisfactory pain relief. No complications were associated with the other 4 patients who had persistent pain and required a second operation. Preoperative pin strength improved from 6 lbs to 11 lbs postoperatively.

Sotereanos DG, Taras J, Urbaniak JR: Niebauer trapeziometacarpal arthroplasty: A long-term follow-up. *J Hand Surg* 1993;18A:560–564.

Thirty Niebauer TMC prostheses in 27 patients were reviewed with average follow-up of 9 years (minimum, 4 years). Most prostheses were placed for OA. Of the patients, 88% said they would undergo the procedure again, despite postoperative subluxation that occurred in 83%; these subluxations were not painful. One case of silicone synovitis was encountered. The authors recommend Niebauer arthroplasty as a satisfactory treatment for TMC joint arthritis.

Stokel EA, Tencer AF, Driscoll HL, Trumble TE. A biomechanical comparison of four methods of fixation of the trapeziometacarpal joint. *J Hand Surg* 1994;19A:86–92.

Twenty thumb TMC specimens were fixed with tension band wiring, crossed K-wire technique, cup and cone joint preparation with a single K-wire, or cerclage interosseous wiring technique. Biomechanical stability was tested under axial compression, torsion, and cantilever bending. The tension band technique had superior fixation in torsion, the cerclage technique in flexion-extension, and both in axial loading.

Thompson JS: Complications and salvage of trapeziometacarpal arthroplasties, in Barr JS Jr (ed): *Instructional Course Lectures XXXVIII*. Park Ridge, IL, American Academy of Orthopaedic Surgeons, 1989, pp 3–13.

Treatment of TMC arthritis, particularly after failed silicone implantation, is reviewed. The abductor pollicis longus suspensionplasty surgical technique is reviewed.

Tomaino MM, Pellegrini VD Jr, Burton RI: Arthroplasty of the basal joint of the thumb: Long-term follow-up after ligament reconstruction with tendon interposition. *J Bone Joint Surg* 1995;77A:346–355.

Twenty-four thumbs of 22 patients who underwent LRTI with average 9-year follow-up were evaluated. Twenty-one patients (95%) had excellent relief of pain and were satisfied with the outcome.

Scaphoid-Trapezium-Trapezoid Osteoarthritis

Fortin PT, Louis DS: Long-term follow-up of scaphoid-trapezium-trapezoid arthrodesis. *J Hand Surg* 1993;18A:675–681.

Nineteen consecutive patients with STT arthrodesis for chronic scapholunate instability or isolated arthrosis were reviewed. Eight of the 14 patients available for follow-up had significant residual symptoms or limitations, and there were 11 complications. STT arthrodesis was not predictable in this series.

Intercarpal-Radiocarpal Osteoarthritis

Ashmead D IV, Watson HK, Damon C, Herber S, Paly W: Scapholunate advanced collapse wrist salvage. *J Hand Surg* 1994;19A:741–750.

One hundred wrists with scaphoid excision and limited 4-corner wrist arthrodesis were reviewed for SLAC wrist. An average 44-month follow-up revealed excellent functional status. Extension-flexion averaged 72° (53% of the normal opposite wrist), radioulnar deviation 37° (59%), and grip strength 80% of the opposite side.

Cobb TK, Beckenbaugh RD: Biaxial total-wrist arthroplasty. *J Hand Surg* 1996;21A:1011–1021.

Sixty-four consecutive biaxial total wrist arthroplasties for rheumatoid arthritis in 62 patients between 1983 and 1988 were reviewed. Forty-six intact surviving implants were followed for 6.5 years. The average patient age was 58 years. There were 11 failures. Pain was absent in 75%, mild in 19%, moderate in 3%, and severe in 3%.

Culp RW, McGuigan FX, Turner MA, Lichtman DM, Osterman AL, McCarroll HR: Proximal row carpectomy: A multicenter study. *J Hand Surg* 1993;18A:19–25.

Twenty patients were reviewed retrospectively at 3.5 years. For non-rheumatoid patients, motion decreased 15% after surgery but mean grip strength improved 22%.

Fassler PR, Stern PJ, Kiefhaber TR: Asymptomatic SLAC wrist: Does it exist? *J Hand Surg* 1993;18A:682–686.

Twenty-five patients (30 wrists) had asymptomatic SLAC wrist discovered incidentally on comparison radiographs when evaluated for other problems. All patients were evaluated an average of 2 years later. At that time, 20 wrists were completely symptom-free and 10 had occasional pain related to heavy activity. No patients had SLAC wrist.

Krakauer JD, Bishop AT, Cooney WP: Surgical treatment of scapholunate advanced collapse. *J Hand Surg* 1994;19A:751–759.

Six different reconstructive procedures for SLAC wrist were reviewed, including scaphoid excision and intercarpal arthrodesis, PRC, radioscapholunate arthrodesis, radioscaphoid arthrodesis, and primary total wrist arthrodesis. Proximal row carpectomy best preserved wrist stability, with flexion and extension arc of 71°.

Lee DH, Carroll RE: Wrist arthrodesis: A combined intramedullary pin and autogenous iliac crest bone graft technique. *J Hand Surg* 1994;19A:733–740.

Forty-six wrist arthrodeses, using intramedullary Steinmann pin and autogenous iliac crest dorsal bone grafting in 36 patients for a variety of disorders, were reviewed. For osteoarthritic patients, an average of 12 weeks was required until satisfactory fusion.

McAuliffe JA, Dell PC, Jaffe R: Complications of intercarpal arthrodesis. *J Hand Surg* 1993;18A:1121–1128.

This review of 50 patients at 34-month follow-up revealed 18 patients with good, 16 with fair, and 13 with poor results; 3 patients had inadequate follow-up data. Thirty-six patients had complications, and 25 patients underwent further surgery. The most common indication for reoperation was nonunion (16 patients).

Meuli HC, Fernandez DL: Uncemented total wrist arthroplasty. *J Hand Surg* 1995;20A:115–122.

The modified Meuli prosthesis, developed in 1986, is reviewed in 50 wrists (12 with traumatic arthritis). After an average of 4.5 years, results were excellent in 24 wrists, good in 12, fair in 5, and poor in 8. One patient died during the follow-up period.

Salomon GD, Eaton RG: Proximal row carpectomy with partial capitate resection. *J Hand Surg* 1996;21A:2–8.

Twelve patients underwent PRC with a modification of partial resection of the proximal capitate. Ten patients had SLAC wrist or chronic scaphoid nonunion with secondary arthritis; 7 had capitolunate disease. At mean follow-up of 55 months, 7 patients had no pain and 4 patients had only occasional pain.

Tomaino MM, Delsignore J, Burton RI: Long-term results following proximal row carpectomy. *J Hand Surg* 1994;19A:694–703.

Twenty-three wrists were examined 6 years after PRC. The patients were satisfied with functional performance and pain relief.

Tomaino MM, Miller RJ, Cole I, Burton RI: Scapholunate advanced collapse wrist: Proximal row carpectomy or limited wrist arthrodesis with scaphoid excision? *J Hand Surg* 1994;19A:134–142.

Twenty-four wrists were treated for SLAC wrist between 1980 and 1990 with either PRC or limited wrist arthrodesis with scaphoid excision. Retrospective review at an average of 5.5 years noted satisfactory results of both procedures. These results were similar in subjective and objective results, which included range of motion and grip strength.

Weiss AP, Hastings H II: Wrist arthrodesis for traumatic conditions: A study of plate and local bone graft application. *J Hand Surg* 1995;20A:50–56.

Twenty-eight consecutive patients (average age, 34 years) underwent wrist arthrodesis by dorsal osteosynthesis compression plate fixation technique. Average duration of symptoms was 2.1 years, and average follow-up was 2 years. With the use of more rigid fixation techniques, local bone graft was acceptable; iliac crest bone grafts were not required in any patients.

Weiss AC, Wiedeman G Jr, Quenzer D, Hanington KR, Hastings H II, Strickland JW: Upper extremity function after wrist arthrodesis. *J Hand Surg* 1995;20A:813–817.

The authors undertook comprehensive functional evaluation of 23 patients who had undergone wrist arthrodesis. The clinical questionnaire, Jebsen hand functional test, and functional rating by Buck-Gramcko-Lohmann were administered at an average of 54 months postoperatively. The patients did well with all evaluations. Activities of daily living can be done after wrist arthrodesis, although some adaptation is required for these tasks.

Wyrick JD, Stern PJ, Kiefhaber TR: Motion-preserving procedures in the treatment of scapholunate advanced collapse wrist: Proximal row carpectomy versus four-corner arthrodesis. *J Hand Surg* 1995;20A:965–970.

Of 28 SLAC wrists, 17 had scaphoid excision and 4-corner arthrodesis, and 11 had PRC. Total motion averaged 95° in patients after 4-corner arthrodesis and 115° after PRC.

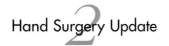

Chapter 33
Other Arthritides

Edward Akelman, MD

Juvenile Rheumatoid Arthritis

Juvenile rheumatoid arthritis (JRA) is a chronic systemic idiopathic inflammatory disorder affecting children and adolescents prior to puberty. Its major manifestation is inflammatory arthritis of synovial joints. JRA is the most common connective tissue disease in children, affecting as many as many as 250,000 children in the United States alone.

General diagnostic criteria for JRA classification include age younger than 16 years at onset; arthritis in 1 or more joints, defined by swelling and effusion; limited range of motion; tenderness or pain on motion and increased heat; duration of disease of 6 weeks to 3 months; and exclusion of other rheumatoid diseases. Although laboratory data in JRA are helpful in classifying patients into different subgroups, they are not in and of themelves diagnostic. Diagnostic criteria are shown in Table 1. JRA is characterized by chronic

Table 1
Modes of onset of juvenile rheumatoid arthritis

	Systemic	Polyarticular		Pauciarticular	
Presentation	Extra-articular manifestations (fever, rash, organomegaly serositis, myalgia, hematologic changes) and arthritis	Symmetric arthritis involving large and small joints Five or more joints affected		Asymmetric arthritis involving few joints, usually large Less than five joints affected, frequently only one joint	
		RF negative	RF positive	Type I	Type II
Percent of patients	20%	25% to 30%	10%	25%	15% to 20%
Age at onset (median)	5 years	3 years	> 8 years	2 years	10 years
Sex distribution	M = F	F > M	F > M	F > M	M > F
Rheumatoid factor	Generally negative	Negative	Positive	Generally negative	Generally negative
Antinuclear antibodies	Generally negative	Positive in 25%	Positive in 75%	Positive in 50%	Generally negative
Course	Systemic manifestations are self-limited; arthritis may become chronic, with 25% of patients developing severe destructive arthritis	Majority do well, 10% develop severe sequelae, particularly hip and temporomandibular joint problems	Resembles adult rheumatoid disease, severe destructive arthritis in 50% of cases	Arthritis mild; morbidity associated with ocular problems (eg, iridocyclitis)	Course variable; patients may develop ankylosing spondylitis pattern

(Reproduced with permission from Jay S, Helm S, Wray BB: Juvenile rheumatoid arthritis. *Am Fam Physician* 1982;26:139–147.)

synovial inflammation and hyperplasia. Diagnosis can only be confirmed by pathologic biopsy, although this is not generally necessary. Pathologic findings include synovial vascular hyperplasia with infiltration by lymphocytes and plasma cells. Although the pathogenesis of JRA is not entirely clear, some have suggested that etiologic factors include infection, autoimmune phenomenon or a stress response.

Three major subgroups of JRA are recognized by history and clinical findings, laboratory analysis, and patient presentation: (1) systemic JRA, or Still's disease; (2) polyarticular JRA; and (3) pauciarticular JRA (Table 1).

Young children may present with different symptoms than adolescents. Patients may experience stiffness in the morning and have difficulty with ambulation. Parents may report that their children complain of fatigue and low-grade fever, as well as general malaise. Findings in the upper extremity are loss of wrist motion, specifically extension, and ulnar deviation of the carpus and metacarpals. Lack of digital flexion as well as radial deviation at the metacarpophalangeal (MCP) joint are noted. Radiographs may show closed epiphyses and diminished osseous growth (Fig. 1).

Medical treatment is directed to diminish the inflammatory process. Salicylates are the initial treatment of choice. If an adolescent does not show appropriate response to salicylate therapy, nonsteroidal anti-inflammatory medications have been shown to be useful. At later stages of disease, the use of Gold salts has yielded excellent results. Hydroxychloroquinine has been used in older children unresponsive to treatment with aspirin or nonsteroidal anti-inflammatory agents. Methotrexate has been reported to have the greatest potential for treating JRA and inducing disease remission. Corticosteroids have been used in severe cases of systemic JRA.

Surgical Management

The indications for surgery in young patients with JRA are the same as those for patients with adult rheumatoid arthritis. Surgery is only carried out after nonsurgical methods of treatment have failed. The goals of surgery in a patient with JRA are to alleviate pain, limit progression of disease, improve patient function, and occasionally to improve cosmetic appearance.

Thumb and Fingers

JRA involving the thumb carpometacarpal (CMC), MCP, and interphalangeal (IP) joints is best treated with splints. If indicated, thumb IP and MCP joint arthrodesis improves pinch strength and reduces joint pain.

Patients with JRA have significant involvement with the MCP and proximal interphalangeal (PIP) joints approximately 50% of the time. As in adults, some patients may have radial deviation of the hand, ulnar deviation of the PIP joints, and MCP joint flexion deformities. Older children may present with radial deviation of nondeformed fingers at the MCP joint; they often have limited MCP joint flexion. After physes are closed, Silastic arthroplasties may have a role in treatment of severe erosive deformity of the finger MCP joints.

The joints of fingers in children younger than 4 years of age are most commonly seen to have MCP and IP joint flexion deformities. These may evolve into boutonnière deformities more frequently than into swan-neck deformities. Flexor tenosynovitis is very common in patients with JRA. This can manifest as flexor tendon nodules, swelling, fullness, and difficulty with grip. Triggering may be seen in some patients. Occupational therapy can generate significant improvement in maintaining full active and passive range of motion during active flexor tenosynovitis. Anti-inflammatory medication

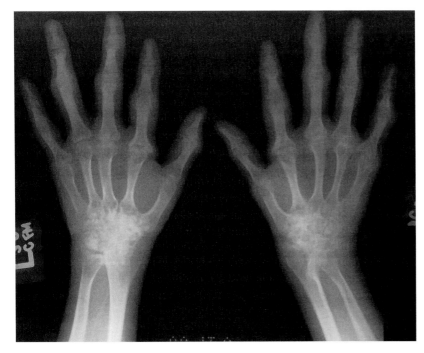

Figure 1

A 13-year-old patient with juvenile rheumatoid arthritis with closed epiphysis.

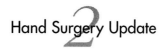

and splinting may improve digital motion. Some authors have recommended general anesthesia and steroid injection in young patients. Tenosynovectomy has been described in severe cases, especially when passive flexion is greater than active flexion.

Thumb Conservative management of the thumb includes the use of an opponens splint, with emphasis on maintaining thumb and index web space. Severe involvement of the IP and MCP joint requires arthrodesis. Carpometacarpal arthroplasty is recommended for joint involvement at the CMC level.

Fingers Well-positioned intrinsic-plus splints will help control digital pain and deformity. Flexor tenosynovitis is a significant problem for most patients with JRA. Tenosynovectomy may be required for both digits and thumb in patients with diminished active motion but better passive motion. At the MCP joint, synovectomies and MCP joint Silastic arthroplasties seem to provide excellent pain relief; motion is improved with MCP joint arthroplasty. Finger IP joints may develop into boutonnière deformities, and less commonly into swan-neck deformities. Surgical reconstruction is indicated in patients with diminished function and pain in their digits.

Radiocarpal and Intercarpal Joints

The wrist is involved in large numbers of patients with JRA. Patients generally present with synovitis at the distal radioulnar joint. In patients with intercarpal, CMC joint, and radiocarpal disease, limited motion is often seen at the radiocarpal joint, even in patients without pan-carpal wrist arthrodeses. Splinting in a neutral wrist position provides excellent relief of pain and will maintain an optimal functional wrist position. Intra-articular corticosteroid injections can reduce pain, decrease synovitis, and increase the ability to judiciously begin motion at the wrist. As in patients with adult rheumatoid arthritis, dorsal tenosynovectomies may be performed with or without wrist synovectomy. If there is distal radioulnar joint pain and lack of congruity, a distal ulnar arthroplasty may be performed.

Psoriatic Arthritis

The diagnosis of psoriatic arthritis is made when a patient presents with inflammatory hand arthritis with corresponding skin and nail changes. The classic patient presenting with psoriasis has a scaly, erythematous skin rash. Although it has been estimated that only 5% to 7% of patients with psoriasis develop arthritis, 95% of those patients may have involvement of peripheral joints (Fig. 2). Five percent of patients have involvement of the spine alone, while 20% to 40% have both peripheral and axial involvement. The association with HLA-B27 occurs only when there is spinal involvement. HLA-ADR7 and HLA-ADR4 studies have been reported as being positive. Other patients present with a more classic spondyloarthropathy, with oligoarticular findings in the legs and swollen digits. Psoriatic arthritis may assume a rheumatoid arthritis-like pattern. Laboratory findings reflect an inflammatory arthritis, with findings of an inflammatory joint fluid and elevated sedimentation rate.

Moll and Wright initially classified psoriatic arthritis into 5 broad clinical groups: patients with distal interphalangeal (DIP) involvement, patients with widespread effusions, patients with symptoms indistinguishable from rheumatoid arthritis except for the absence of rheumatoid arthritis, patients with monoarticular arthritis, and patients with ankylosing spondylitis. Nalebuff modified this classification based on radiographic and clinical changes seen in the hand, identifying 3 distinct types. In type I (spontaneous ankylosis), ankylosis is common at the DIP and PIP joints but not at the MCP joint level. Functional loss is less severe with this subgroup. In type II (osteolysis), bone loss is common and is not restricted only to the DIP joint level. Arthritis mutilans is the worst example of osteolysis. Many patients have significant functional loss and deformities. In type III, rheumatoid arthritis-like deformities with stiffness, patient symptoms superficially resemble rheumatoid arthritis but have significant differences.

When nail involvement is noted, the most common nail finding is pitting, representing the involvement of the proximal nail matrix. Characteristic radiographic findings of osteolysis include bony destruction and widening of joint spaces.

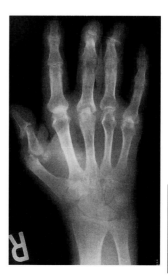

Figure 2

A 27-year-old man with psoriatic arthritis. Note the destruction and subluxation of the MCP joint of the thumb and osteolysis of the PIP and MCP joints.

At the joint level, the proximal bone tapers with greater involvement, creating a "pencil and cup" appearance at the joint. As multiple digits begin telescoping, the condition may be described as an "opera glass" hand. There is a lower incidence of tenosynovitis and tendon ruptures in psoriatic arthritis compared to rheumatoid arthritis. Patients may have an asymmetric involvement in both hands.

Nonsurgical Treatment
Medical treatment of psoriatic arthritis begins with non-steroidal anti-inflammatory agents, which are often the only medications required. Methotrexate, Gold, antimalarials, sulfasalazine, and cyclosporine may be used in an attempt to control more resistant arthritis. In severe cases of psoriatic arthritis, which have been described as "explosive," physicians should consider the possibility of HIV infection.

Thumb
Hand-based or forearm-based spica splints help control pain and discomfort at the IP, MCP, and CMC joint levels. If there is no improvement, surgery should include IP and MCP fusions with CMC arthroplasty.

Fingers
Intrinsic-plus splints will help control pain, discomfort, and swelling in patients with psoriatic arthritis. In recalcitrant cases, surgery should be based on the type of psoriatic arthritis. In the Nalebuff type I group, spontaneous DIP joint fusions require no treatment. PIP joint fusions in poor position may be treated by osteotomy and arthrodesis of the index and middle finger, with revision arthroplasties performed at the ring and small finger PIP joint. PIP joint fusions are required in patients who need MCP joint arthroplasty.

In Nalebuff type II digits, fusion is required at every joint level. Firm fixation is required. Occasionally, a bone graft is required to provide adequate bony contact.

In Nalebuff type III joints, MCP arthroplasty can be performed in patients with limited extension. In patients with MCP joint hyperextension, manipulation and/or soft-tissue releases may be required. Based on the digit involved, IP joint deformities are treated with either corrective osteotomies, arthrodesis, or arthroplasties.

Surgical Treatment: Thumb and Fingers
Resection arthroplasty has been employed to treat basal joint disease in psoriatic arthritis. Nalebuff suggested that the appropriate treatment of spontaneous ankylosis of the digits with PIP joints in poor position is arthroplasty or osteotomy, depending on which individual digit is involved. The index and long finger are generally fused, while the ring and small finger are treated with arthroplasty.

In patients with bone loss, fusion is the only surgical procedure that preserves bone length and stops further shortening. Supplemental bone grafts may be needed to allow these joints to fuse.

In patients with rheumatoid arthritis-like joints with stiffness and deformity, MCP arthroplasties provide excellent relief of MCP joint pain and improve motion. Joint manipulation can be used in some patients with MCP joints fixed in hyperextension.

Wrist
Nonsurgical therapy at the wrist level is directed at maintaining joint motion and muscle strength. Neutral resting wrist splints may help control wrist discomfort and pain. Skin rashes can be treated with ultraviolet light and medication. Increased positive bacterial cultures have been found in psoriatic skin. Skin problems may need to be treated before considering any surgical procedure.

The procedure of choice at the level of the wrist is radio-carpal and intercarpal arthrodesis with or without ulnar arthroplasty.

Surgery at the wrist is indicated when pain does not improve with conservative, medical, or occupational therapy. Synovectomy has been noted to provide pain relief without improvement in range of motion. Treatment of distal radio-ulnar joint involvement may include distal ulnar arthroplasty as well as distal radioulnar joint synovectomy. Most radio-carpal and intercarpal involvement progresses to spontaneous arthrodeses. Reconstructive surgery may include corrective extension osteotomies. Standard dorsal extensor compartment tenosynovectomies may be required.

Involvement of the radiocarpal joint is common in psoriatic arthritis. Most wrists with psoriatic arthritis fuse spontaneously; a significant number become stiff in a functionally adequate position. Surgery is limited to resection of the distal ulna and/or ulna arthroplasty in patients with limited supination and pronation and pain in the ulnar side of the wrist.

Gout

Gouty arthropathy is caused by the rapid increase or decrease in uric acid concentration in the body. Ninety percent of individuals with hyperuricemia have impaired or relatively impaired excretion of uric acid rather than over-production. Patients present with symptoms of gouty arthropathy when high uric acid levels result in the deposition of monosodium urate crystals in soft tissues and joints. Lower temperature has an effect on the solubility of uric acid, and the peripheral joints of the hands and feet are

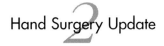
involved initially because of lower distal temperatures. The diagnosis of gout depends on the demonstration of monosodium urate monohydrate (MSU) crystals when a joint is aspirated. MSU crystals are long, thin needle-shaped structures with a strong negative biorefringency. Serum uric acid levels may be normal in the face of an acute gouty attack.

Patients with gout may give a history of being awakened in the middle of the night, without previous pain, by pain in the affected toe or hand and wrist (Fig. 3). Joint pain is severe. Patients have quick onset of joints that are warm, erythematous, and swollen. In the hand, the small joints are more frequently involved than the wrist. The olecranon bursa is commonly involved.

The medical treatment of acute gouty arthropathy is challenging. Colchicine is best used in the initial 24 hours of a gouty attack. However, colchicine requires both intact kidneys and liver for its metabolism and excretion. Colchicine has been associated with granulocytopenia, with overwhelming infection and death. Nonsteroidal anti-inflammatory medications are also used in acute attacks. In a patient with more frequent attacks, medications that increase renal excretion of uric acid and xanthine oxidase inhibitors are the medications of choice; these include probenecid, sulfinpyrazone, and allopurinol.

Conservative and Surgical Treatment

In its early stages, acute gout should be treated with medications as described above and wrist and digital splints supporting radiocarpal, thumb, and digital joints. As pain subsides, joint mobilization techniques are helpful in preserving function. The most common treatment of gout is medical and conservative. However, gouty tenosynovitis can cause rupture of extensor and flexor tendons, cause acute or chronic carpal tunnel syndrome, and may increase in size such that bulk destroys soft-tissue coverage. Surgery in this situation consists of debridement of gouty tophi, tenosynovectomy, occasional tendon transfer, and soft-tissue coverage procedures. When tophaceous deposits are removed, tendon gliding may be improved, joint range of motion increases, and pain from nerve compression is reduced. At later stages, because of the destruction of distal or proximal IP joints, arthrodesis is generally recommended (Fig. 4).

Pseudogout (Calcium Pyrophosphate Deposition Disease)

Calcium pyrophosphate crystalline deposition disease (CPPD) was first named pseudogout because this disease process was felt to mimic clinical gout. However, recent advances in understanding of this disease render CPPD disease a more appropriate name. The etiology of CPPD is not clearly understood. It is thought to develop initially in areas about articular cartilage, more commonly at the chondrocyte level. Most scientists believe an increase in either calcium or inorganic pyrophosphate in cartilage leads to crystal formation within cartilage and the clinical syndrome of CPPD. CPPD can be classified as hereditary or idiopathic and may be associated with trauma and other metabolic diseases. Some patients present with low-grade inflammation lasting weeks or months. Patients may present with morning stiffness, digital flexion contractures, and a high

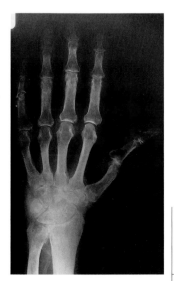

Figure 3

A 60-year-old man with a history of gout, presenting with severe ulnar-sided wrist pain. Note the erosion of the distal ulnar.

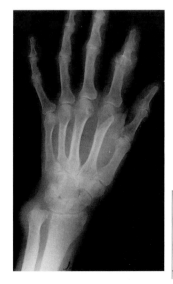

Figure 4

A 31-year-old patient with end-stage gouty arthropathy of the proximal interphalangeal joint of the index finger. Arthrodesis is indicated.

sedimentation rate. Diagnosis is confirmed by joint aspiration. In contradistinction to monosodium urate crystals, CPPD crystals have a negative or weak positive biorefringency. Pathognomonic radiographs include involvement of knee menisci and the triangular fibrocartilage complex at the level of the wrist (Fig. 5). CPPD is occasionally seen between bones of the carpus.

Patients generally present with symptoms of acute inflammation that may improve rapidly. Symptoms of pain are not as severe as in gouty arthropathy. MCP joints and wrist joints may be involved in chronic arthrosis and occasionally bear clinical resemblance to rheumatoid arthritis.

As in all patients with acute inflammation, resting individual joints is helpful in the acute inflammatory stage; joint mobilization and range of motion techniques are initiated as acute inflammatory symptoms subside. Intra-articular steroids as well as nonsteroidal anti-inflammatory medications have been used to reduce inflammation. However, no regimen currently exists to remove CPPD crystals from joints. Colchicine has been used for frequent recurrent attacks. Surgery is rare; crystal-induced tendon ruptures are believed to occur because of chronic inflammatory changes about the tendon.

Systemic Lupus Erythematosus

Systemic lupus erythematosus (SLE) is an autoimmune disease that may affect all bodily organ systems. Each patient may present with an individually specific disease course. Females are much more commonly affected than males with this condition, with a reported incidence ratio of 5:1. There appears to be a genetic predisposition; family members are known to share an inherent tendency towards an autoimmune disease in general rather than to SLE. Criteria for lupus classification have been developed by the American College of Rheumatology. Joint involvement is common in SLE; up to 90% of patients develop hand and wrist problems. Patients present with multiple symptoms. The diagnosis of SLE is suspected specifically if a patient has a facial butterfly or malar rash. Most patients present with laboratory abnormalities of autoantibodies such as antinuclear antibodies, antidoublestranded DNA antibodies, antiSmith antibodies, and antiRNP antibodies.

In the hand, patients have been noted to have Raynaud's phenomenon, synovitis, skin rashes, and ligamentous laxity. Joint involvement includes swelling, erythema, and pain at the MCP and PIP joints. Articular cartilage is not commonly involved, and may appear radiographically normal despite severe deformities. At the level of the wrist, dorsal subluxation of the distal radioulnar joint is common, and radiographs may demonstrate mild translocation of the carpus (Fig. 6). The most common finding relating to fingers is ulnar subluxation of extensor tendons during digital flexion.

SLE arthritis is controlled with the same therapy directed for SLE in general. Aspirin and nonsteroidal anti-inflammatories are used as first medical treatments, with the addition of hydroxychloroquinine if these medications do not have an effect. Low-dose oral steroids have been used in more significant cases of multiorgan involvement. Therapy is directed towards passively correctable deformities, using exercises and occupational therapy splints. Resting splints at the level of the thumb, digits, or wrist may be useful to keep MCP joints straight.

Because dorsal subluxation of the distal ulna is common, with occasional extensor tendon rupture, distal ulnar arthroplasty with extensor tendon reconstruction is sometimes required. At the intercarpal joints, occasionally intercarpal or radiocarpal arthrodesis is required.

At the MCP joints, Nalebuff has attempted to restore MCP alignment and function with soft-tissue surgery. Long-term results of this surgery have not been described. Fixed MCP deformities require the addition of MCP joint arthroplasty, which appears to perform well. At the IP joint

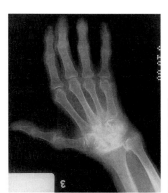

Figure 5

A 70-year-old woman with longstanding calcium pyrophosphate deposition disease. Note the calcification of the triangular fibrocartilage complex and at the radioulnar joint.

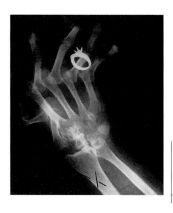

Figure 6

A 46-year-old woman with longstanding lupus. Note the carpal translocation.

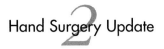
level, arthrodesis remains the treatment of choice. In the thumb, IP joint fusion is required. At the MCP joint level, soft-tissue reconstruction may be undertaken if the joint is passively correctable. If passive correction is not possible, the MCP joint must be fused. At the CMC joint level, soft-tissue arthroplasty is required if the MCP and IP joints are fused.

Surgery

Unlike rheumatoid arthritis, soft-tissue procedures to correct MCP joint deformities in SLE have not been uniformly successful. Despite multiple surgical techniques, failure rates of 70% have been reported prior to fixed deformity.

PIP joint deformities, particularly swan-neck deformities, are corrected at the MCP joint level. Volar plate laxity secondary to swan-neck deformity requires soft-tissue reconstruction, including superficialis tenodesis and/or volar plate advancement.

Patients with thumb involvement in SLE generally have a correctable MCP joint flexion deformity and hyperextension of the IP joint. These may be addressed with IP and MCP joint fusions. CMC joint involvement may require treatment with CMC joint arthroplasty.

Scleroderma

Systemic sclerosis, or scleroderma, is a multiorgan disease process that also affects the hand and wrist. Patients generally have thickened, tight skin, and present with kidney, esophageal, and lung involvement. Arthritis and joint pain occur in up to 70% of patients in the early phases of disease. Raynaud's phenomenon and digital tip ulcerations are common (Fig. 7). Laboratory studies show a positive ANA in a large percentage of cases. An anticentromere antibody is present in over half the patients with limited disease.

The clinical presentation of scleroderma includes swollen hand and digits associated with an inflammatory arthritis. Disease may occur in a disseminated cutaneous form or limited cutaneous form. In the crest form of disease (calcinosis, Raynaud's phenomenon, esophageal dysfunction, sclerodactyly, telangiectasias), 80% of patients test positive for the anticentromeric antibody. Raynaud's phenomenon in scleroderma is commonly associated with painful fingertip ulcers leading to pits and scars. Because of the pain associated with Raynaud's phenomenon, conservative measures such as warm or heated gloves or calcium channel blockers have been reported to be effective. Digital sympathectomy has been recommended in severe cases.

The most common digital deformities occur at the MCP and PIP joints, with progressive PIP joint flexion contractures and hyperextension of the MCP joints. At the thumb, adduction contractures are common; as the PIP joint flexes, soft-tissue involvement of the skin over the PIP joint level is compromised. Nonsurgical measures include physical and occupational therapy to improve active and passive range of motion and prevent contracture and subluxation.

PIP contractures may be unmanageable by nonsurgical treatment. Arthrodesis is required to control established PIP joint contractures in scleroderma. Occasionally, calcific deposits must be removed if they start to necrose or erode through skin.

Nonsurgical methods may be useful in early stages of disease. Physical therapy, including active range of motion exercises, massage, and paraffin baths, has been noted to be beneficial.

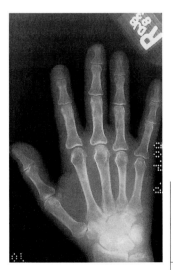

Figure 7

A 62-year-old patient with longstanding scleroderma. Note the index finger shortening and distal phalanx loss secondary to digital tip ulceration.

Annotated Bibliography

Adamson GJ, Gellman H, Brumfield RH Jr., Kuschner SH, Waller JW: Flexible implant resection arthroplasty of the proximal interphalangeal joint in patients with systemic inflammatory arthritis. J Hand Surg 1994;19A:378–384.

The authors review long-term results of surgical treatment of PIP joint deformities using silicone elastomer flexible implants. Nineteen patients were followed for an average of 94 months. Three patients had JRA, 2 had SLE, and one had mixed connective tissue disease. The authors showed that digits with boutonnière deformities with previous or concurrent MCP joint silicone arthroplasties had a much more successful outcome than those that did not. They suggested that MCP joint arthroplasty should be performed before or concurrently with PIP joint arthroplasty to restore extrinsic and intrinsic function. They also noted that in joints that were ankylosed prior to surgery or in digits with swan neck deformities, flexible implants did not perform very well.

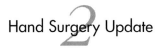
346   Other Arthritides

Evans DM, Ansell BM, Hall MA: The wrist in juvenile arthritis. *J Hand Surg* 1991;16B:293–304.

This is an excellent review article of the natural history of disease of the radiocarpal and intercarpal joints.

Naidu SH, Ostrov BE, Pellegrini VD Jr: Isolated digital swelling at the initial presentation of juvenile rheumatoid arthritis. *J Hand Surg* 1997;22A:653–657.

Seven patients with JRA presented with isolated finger swelling as the initial manifestation of their disease. This presentation of JRA should be recognized so the appropriate management can be instituted promptly.

Nalebuff EA: Surgery of psoriatic arthritis of the hand. *Hand Clin* 1996;12:603–614.

This unique review article describes a senior hand surgeon's experience with psoriatic arthritis. The author stresses the unique aspects of this particular entity. Physicians and surgeons treating these patients should be aware of the differences from other arthritides in order to properly advise or treat.

Nalebuff EA: Surgery of systemic lupus erythematosus arthritis of the hand. *Hand Clin* 1996;12:591–602.

Systemic lupus erythematosus is described by this senior author as a disease that superficially resembles rheumatoid arthritis. SLE involves the hand and wrist and is significant to hand surgeons. The author shows what specific characteristics differentiate SLE from psoriatic arthritis and scleroderma.

O'Brien BM, Kumar PA, Mellow CG, Oliver CG: Radical microarteriolysis in the treatment of vasospastic disorders of the hand, especially scleroderma. *J Hand Surg* 1992;17B:447–452.

This report describes a favorable outcome in a lengthy microscopic surgical procedure for scleroderma. Although the authors give short follow-up, patients are reported to have improvement from their severe pain and ulceration.

Ruperto N, Ravelli A, Levinson JE, et al: Long-term health outcomes and quality of life in American and Italian inception cohorts of patients with juvenile rheumatoid arthritis: II. Early predictors of outcome. *J Rheumatol* 1997;24:952–958.

In this excellent article, the authors use clinical and immunogenetic variables that are measurable within 6 months of onset of JRA to predict future disability, pain, and well being. The quality of life appears more difficult to forecast, perhaps due to the multiple domains that make up this outcome. The best predictor of higher disability was the articular severity score, while a positive antinuclear antibody test foretold less disability. Early hand involvement was the strongest predictor of poor overall well being.

Simmons BP, Nutting JT, Bernstein RA: Juvenile rheumatoid arthritis. *Hand Clin* 1996;12:573–589.

JRA should be suspected in a child with arthralgias and systemic signs of sepsis. Serologic methods of diagnosis show great promise for improved classification, and randomized trials are providing better information on pharmacologic treatment. Surgery—reserved for cases that do not improve with medical and occupational therapy—addresses delay or prevention of joint destruction and epiphyseal closure deformity, pain, and maintenance of growth and joint motion.

Wigley FM, Wise RA, Miller R, Needleman BW, Spence RJ: Anticentromere antibody as a predictor of digital ischemic loss in patients with systemic sclerosis. *Arthritis Rheum* 1992;35:688–693.

Anticentromere antibody (ACA) has been typically used to differentiate primary Raynaud's phenomenon from secondary Raynaud's phenomenon, limited scleroderma from diffuse scleroderma, and scleroderma from other connective tissue diseases. In this intriguing study, clinical and serologic risk factors for digital ischemia were evaluated. In patients with scleroderma, the presence of ACA predicted an increased risk of losing one or more digits secondary to ischemia. Age, race, smoking status, duration of Raynaud's phenomenon, and length of disease were not predictive of digital loss.

Section VIII
Tumors

Chapter 34
Multidisciplinary Treatment of Tumors of the Hand

Chapter 35
Cutaneous Tumors of the Hand

Chapter 36
Management Principles of Aggressive Tumors of the Hand and Forearm

Chapter 37
Benign, Aggressive, and Malignant Neoplasms

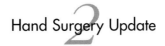

Chapter 34
Multidisciplinary Treatment of Tumors of the Hand

William G. Kraybill, MD

Soft-Tissue Tumors

Clinical and Radiographic Evaluation

The evaluation of soft-tissue sarcoma (STS) masses should include a careful history and physical examination, with a focus on potential sites of metastasis. Some STSs (eg, epithelioid sarcomas, synovial sarcomas, and rhabdomyosarcomas [RMS]) have a propensity for lymph node metastasis. Although STSs are frequently differentiated from benign tumors by their large size (≥ 5 cm) and depth, as many as one third of all sarcomas are in a subcutaneous location and are frequently small. The possibility that a benign-appearing, small, unexplained mass is malignant should always be considered, particularly when small tumors of the hand are being evaluated. Because of the propensity for STSs to metastasize to the lung, patients with potentially malignant hand tumors should have a chest radiograph.

Following a complete history and physical examination with routine blood work and a chest radiograph, consideration should be given to imaging the primary tumor. If there is even a remote possibility that a soft-tissue tumor may be malignant, it should be imaged before biopsy. Plain films, while important in evaluating bone tumors, are of less value in soft-tissue tumors. Although ultrasound by experienced personnel may offer a low-cost method of identifying or delineating some benign lesions, magnetic resonance imaging (MRI) is the gold standard for evaluation of soft-tissue tumors. Scintigraphy, while useful in identifying skip lesions in bone tumors, is less helpful with soft-tissue tumors. Computed tomography (CT) is less valuable in evaluating soft-tissue masses compared to bone tumors. Following full clinical evaluation, biopsy is required. The biopsy should be directed or carried out by the surgeon who will be doing the definitive resection.

The biopsy should be planned to avoid disruption to the surrounding tissue planes and compartments. In any tumor suspected of being malignant, the biopsy should be an incisional, core needle, or aspiration biopsy. In tumors for which there is a very low index of suspicion for malignancy, excisional biopsy is an option. Although diagnoses by aspiration cytology have been reported, the accuracy of cytologic diagnoses in soft-tissue tumors is not uniform. Nevertheless, aspiration cytology may be extremely useful in the evaluation of suspected recurrent soft-tissue tumors. Technological advancements in MRI will soon allow MRI-directed needle biopsy. MRI-directed small-core needle biopsies should cause less disruption and facilitate more accurate diagnoses. Needle biopsies are less disruptive than open biopsies.

For patients with STSs known to have an increased propensity to metastasize to lymph nodes, performing sentinel lymph node biopsy to assess the status of lymph nodes is an intriguing concept. However, data are insufficient to support routine recommendation of this procedure at the present time.

Multidisciplinary Considerations

Once assessment has been completed—including evaluation for comorbidities, physical examination, imaging, and biopsy—the total management of these complex cases should be considered in a multidisciplinary forum. Input should be sought from the surgical oncologist, radiation oncologist, medical oncologist, hand surgeon, and physical or occupational therapist. The therapeutic plan should consider pre- and postoperative adjuvant regional and systemic therapies, reconstruction, and rehabilitation.

Management Considerations

The exact management of a given STS depends on histopathologic diagnosis, tumor grade, and extent of disease. There are over 100 different types of STSs. Groups of STSs that behave in similar ways will be reviewed in this chapter.

The histologic distribution of STSs in the wrist and hand is somewhat different than in other areas. A series of 23 STSs of the hand and wrist reported from Memorial Sloan-Kettering Cancer Center included 8 synovial sarcomas, 2 epithelioid sarcomas, 1 clear cell sarcoma, 1 peripheral neuroectodermal tumor, 1 angiosarcoma, and 3 RMS. Other series have reported similar distributions of histologies.

Chemotherapy plays an important role in patients with neuroectodermal tumors, Ewing's sarcoma, and RMS. Clear cell sarcomas, epithelioid sarcomas, and synovial sarcomas have a propensity to metastasize to lymph nodes. These characteristics must be considered when evaluating and managing these patients. Of the 23 patients in the Memorial Sloan-Kettering series, 20 were high grade and 15 were considered deep tumors. Survival data on 16 patients who presented without metastatic disease were compared to that of 152 patients who had sarcomas smaller than 5 cm in other sites. Survival was less for hand sarcoma patients, compared to patients with sarcomas in other extremities ($p = 0.0008$). Subset analysis demonstrated that this difference existed only for patients with positive margins ($p = 0.01$). Among patients with negative margins, survival was equivalent in both groups. Patients with deep STS of the hand also had much worse survival than those with deep STS in other extremities. On this basis, the authors of the Memorial Sloan-Kettering Study have emphasized the importance of negative margins in the management of STS of the hand. If negative margins cannot be obtained, amputation should be considered. Although radiation was used in selected patients in this series, its use was not emphasized and did not improve survival.

Another group reported results in 25 patients with STS of the forearm and hand; however, only 9 had tumors of the hand or wrist. Radiation was used in 20 patients, usually preoperatively. There were only 3 local recurrences, all in patients with deep STS of the forearm. Patients with close margins were treated with a boost of 16 Gy following preoperative radiation and resection. This group also noted the importance of negative surgical margins, but emphasized their experience with surgery combined with radiation therapy.

In a series of hand STSs in 16 patients at Massachusetts General Hospital, all gross tumor was removed, but negative microscopic margins were not necessarily obtained. These patients were then treated with an aggressive external beam radiation program. Local control was achieved in 13 of 16 patients. The authors emphasized the importance of close communication between the oncologic surgeon and the radiation oncologist, and advocated the use of preoperative radiation in patients with larger tumors and in patients who had an incisional biopsy.

A different spectrum of histologic diagnoses was the subject of a National Cancer Institute (NCI) report that emphasized the combination of chemotherapy, radiation, and surgery. The patients in the NCI report were almost exclusively children and young adults; median age was 18 years. Of 28 patients with sarcomas of the hand and foot, 15 cases were of the Ewing's sarcoma family (ESF) of tumors (classic and atypical Ewing's sarcoma and primitive neuroectodermal tumors); 7 were alveolar RMS; and 6 cases were nonrhabdomyosarcoma soft-tissue sarcomas (NRMS). Of the 15 patients with ESF tumors, 14 were only biopsied and then treated with chemotherapy and radiation therapy; 1 patient underwent a ray amputation. There were only 2 local failures, and 7 of the 15 patients died of systemic tumor. In 6 patients with alveolar RMS, the primary tumor was only biopsied; gross residual disease remained. The patients were then treated with radiation and aggressive multi-agent chemotherapy. There were no local recurrences, but 4 of 6 patients with systemic disease died. One patient underwent a ray amputation. In 5 patients with NRMS, 1 patient died of distant disease and the remainder were free of disease. This study emphasizes the importance of diagnosis in the management of soft-tissue tumors. For ESF tumors and alveolar RMS, local control can be secured easily in most circumstances with chemotherapy and radiation therapy.

Another group recently reviewed their experience with RMS and NRMS of the hand in children. Surgery for RMS of the hand consisted of biopsy only in 5 cases; local excision in 3; and 1 case each of wide local excision, above-elbow amputation, and ray amputation. All patients received multi-agent chemotherapy; radiation therapy was used selectively. All 7 patients who presented with metastatic disease died of their disease. Radiation was successful in 3 patients with microscopically positive margins. In the remainder, radiation was the primary therapeutic modality for control of metastatic sites. Of 7 patients with NRMS, 2 received radiation for microscopic positive margins; neither had recurrence. Four patients treated with wide local excision or ray amputation were also free of recurrence. One child with a malignant hemangiopericytoma was treated with multi-agent chemotherapy and radiation therapy for metastatic disease; this child died. The authors emphasized the importance of conservative surgery and selective use of radiation and multi-agent chemotherapy in patients with RMS of the hand. In pediatric patients with NRMS, conservative surgery or limited (ray) amputation were recommended, with selective use of radiation therapy.

These reports underscore the importance of careful diagnosis and multidisciplinary management of STS of the hand. A cautious combination of radiation and surgery is appropriate in the management of STS of the hand in adults. Chemotherapy plays an important role in management of hand sarcomas in children and selected adults.

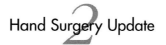
Innovative Treatments

Two additional local therapies, brachytherapy and hyperthermic isolated limb perfusion, have been used in other clinical situations; however, very little has been published specific to their use in STS of the hand. Brachytherapy is routinely employed in treatment of STS at Memorial Sloan-Kettering Cancer Center and at other cancer centers, but the use of brachytherapy in hand sarcomas has not been addressed in the literature. Hyperthermic isolated limb perfusion with tumor-necrosing factor and melphalan has also been used to achieve limb salvage in patients with unresectable STS in extremities; however, there are no reports of its use in the hand. This therapy would need to be combined with surgery and possibly other modalities with consideration of the morbidities of each. In extremity STS, the combination of radiation and hyperthermic isolated limb perfusion with tumor-necrosing factor and melphalan has been associated with significant morbidity. Combination of these two modalities should be approached with extreme caution.

Cutaneous Tumors

Clinical and Radiologic Evaluation

Cutaneous neoplasms of the hand and wrist are evaluated in a similar manner to cutaneous neoplasms in other locations. Physical examination should include a complete skin examination to search for other skin tumors. Many skin tumors have some propensity for lymph node metastasis. This propensity varies in degree by tumor type. All lymph node stations should be carefully inspected. Routine laboratory work should include a complete blood count and liver function tests. It may be difficult to differentiate advanced cutaneous neoplasms that have ulcerated from locally aggressive soft-tissue tumors that have also ulcerated. Any tumor with evidence of invasion of the subdermal tissues should be thoroughly imaged by MRI to assess the relations of the tumor to deep structures. Imaging in search of distant metastasis is more frequently indicated with soft-tissue tumors than cutaneous tumors. For most skin tumors (eg, melanoma, squamous cell cancer, and adenexal tumors), a chest radiograph will suffice. Even in patients with melanoma, chest CT scans are not routinely indicated. In one report, chest CT in patients with cervical lymphadenopathy had the highest likelihood of positive findings (20%); pelvic CT in patients with groin lymphadenopathy was positive in only 7.4% of 94 patients in the series. Although selective use of chest CT in patients with cervical adenopathy or pelvic CT in the presence of bulky groin disease may be useful, the yield will be low.

Once clinical examination has been completed, a biopsy must be done. The method of biopsy of cutaneous neoplasms is different for pigmented lesions than other skin lesions. Pigmented lesions should be excisionally biopsied, but this may not be possible in a confined area like the hand. In such cases, an incisional or punch biopsy of the thickest component of the pigmented lesion is recommended. Shave biopsies should never be done for pigmented lesions. Pigmented lesions beneath the nail require removal of the nail plate for biopsy. The nail plate should be submitted for pathologic evaluation, because tumor may be identified on the nail plate.

The prognosis with cutaneous melanoma is closely related to thickness of the tumor. Sentinel lymph node biopsy has been demonstrated to be effective in accurately assessing the presence or absence of positive lymph nodes in clinically negative lymph node stations. Sentinel lymph node biopsy should be performed in all patients with primary melanomas that are thicker than 1.0 mm at the time of surgical management of the primary tumor. Formal resection of primary melanoma prior to sentinel lymph node biopsy disrupts the lymphatics and may alter the results of sentinel lymph node biopsy.

Sentinel lymph node biopsy should be considered in other cutaneous tumors known to have a propensity for lymph node metastasis. One group recently reported early results of sentinel lymph node mapping for Merkel cell tumors. Although the long-term implications of these findings remain unclear, a finding of a positive lymph node could provide more accurate staging and better prognostic information, resulting in more aggressive regional therapy. Patients with negative sentinel lymph nodes still require careful follow-up, including assessment of lymph node stations.

Multidisciplinary Considerations

Once the clinical evaluation and biopsy have been completed, this information should be considered in a multidisciplinary forum. Although the format for this interaction will vary from institution to institution, individuals who are familiar with the natural history of the specific type of cutaneous neoplasm involved should participate. This group should include a surgical oncologist, radiation oncologist, medical oncologist, hand surgeon familiar with reconstructive techniques, and a dermatopathologist. With the tumor information and relevant comorbidities as a base, a plan of treatment and rehabilitation should be outlined.

Malignant Melanoma

Cancer statistics include one estimate that there were over 41,000 melanomas in 1998. Melanoma is the most rapidly increasing tumor in the United States. Of all cutaneous melanomas, approximately 2% occur on the hand. The most important prognostic factor in cutaneous melanoma is tumor thickness.

The preferred excision margin for tumors 1 to 4 mm in thickness is 2 cm. In confined areas like the hand, however, most surgeons accept margins of 1 to 2 cm for tumors under 2 mm in thickness. For tumors deeper than 2 mm, 2-cm margins should be sought (Table 1). This may require partial or even complete hand amputation in some situations.

In one recent series of 116 patients with melanomas of hands and feet (26 were melanomas of hands), tumors no greater than 1.5 mm in thickness had a low incidence of nodal metastases and were effectively treated with a 1-cm margin. Thicker melanomas were associated with a rate of regional or systemic failure exceeding 50%. In the absence of metastatic disease, these patients should undergo local excision with a 2-cm margin and sentinel lymph node biopsy followed by lymphadenectomy if the sentinel node is positive. Although acral lentiginous melanomas are more common and were thought to carry a higher risk than other melanomas of corresponding thickness, tumor thickness was found to be the predominant prognostic indicator. Resection of the distal phalanx has been found to be sufficient treatment of subungual tumors in most patients.

Sentinel lymph node biopsy allows the assessment of lymph node stations without submitting patients to radical prophylactic lymph node dissection. At Roswell Park Cancer Institute, patients first go to nuclear medicine for lymphoscintigraphy. About 2 hours later, they proceed to the operating room where isosulfan blue is injected around the primary tumor. Lymphoscintigraphy, a gamma counter, and isosulfan blue all aid in the search for the sentinel node. This technique is indicated in all patients with primary melanomas over 1 mm thick. Some high-risk melanomas less than 1 mm in thickness, when combined with other poor prognostic factors, may also benefit from this method. This technique requires skill and coordination of surgical oncology, nuclear medicine, and pathology. A breakdown in any one of these services can result in failure. Patients with positive sentinel lymph nodes or biopsied clinically positive lymph nodes should undergo regional lymphadenectomy.

Some patients will present with locally advanced malignant melanoma of the hand; they often have clinically apparent regional lymph node metastasis. These patients should also be evaluated for distant metastasis and managed with more aggressive surgical resection. In patients with more advanced primary melanoma of the hand, recurrent tumor of the hand, or satellitosis, hyperthermic isolated limb perfusion with melphalan (or with melphalan and tumor necrosis factor) may be helpful in obtaining control of the primary or recurrent tumor without amputation. Another alternative is a combination of radiation and surgery; however, data concerning use of this combination in melanomas of the hand are sparse. Some patients may still require amputation. Patients with advanced lymph node metastasis will usually benefit from radical surgical lymphadenectomy. In these patients with bulky regional disease that is confirmed after surgery, radiation therapy may be instituted to help control regional disease.

Nonpigmented Cutaneous Tumors of the Hand and Wrist

Ultraviolet radiation, skin type, carcinogens, ionizing radiation, and chronic irritation play major roles in skin cancers. Human papillomavirus and heredity may also be factors. Over 100 benign and malignant tumors are listed for the skin and subcutis. Only the more common tumors and categories of tumors will be covered in this chapter.

Keratoacanthomas are benign cutaneous tumors characterized by initial rapid growth, followed by a leveling off of growth and then regression. The incidence is unknown, but in one large retrospective review the relative incidence of keratoacanthoma to squamous cell cancer (SCC) was reported to range from 1:2 to 1:17. Keratoacanthomas frequently occur in sun-exposed areas, such as the dorsum of the hand. Diagnosis of keratoacanthoma can be difficult because of its similarity to SCC. Local excision is usually recommended, and local recurrence of keratoacanthoma is uncommon. Should local recurrence occur, the possibility of SCC should be reconsidered.

Table 1

Margins for melanoma excision

Tumor thickness (mm)	Excision margin (cm)
In situ	0.5–1.0
0–1	1.0
1–2	1 or 2*
2–4	2
> 4	≥ 4

*2-cm margin is preferable, but 1 cm is appropriate in anatomically restricted areas. (Reproduced with permission from Ross MI, Balch CM: Surgical treatment of primary melanoma, in Balch CM, Houghton AN, Sober AJ, Soong S (eds): *Cutaneous Melanoma*. St. Louis, MO, Quality Medical Publishing, 1998, pp 141–153.)

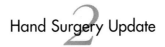
Sweat gland tumors of the hand are uncommon. Although the hand does not have apocrine sweat glands, it has a large number of eccrine sweat glands. The most common eccrine tumor is eccrine poroma, an entity that may be confused with a basal cell cancer. Eccrine tumors should be treated by excision and primary closure. Malignant eccrine poromas can arise from existing benign eccrine poromas. Other cutaneous malignant tumors of eccrine origin may be very malignant, with capability for lymph node and hematogenous metastasis. Cutaneous tumor biopsy specimens should be evaluated by an experienced dermatopathologist; the expected behavior of the neoplasm should be carefully assessed.

Pilosebaceous tumors occur on the dorsum of the hand because of an absence of pilosebaceous organs on the palm. Tumors with hair differentiation include trichoepithelioma, trichoadenoma, pilomatrixoma, tricholemmona, and folliculoma; although all of these lesions are benign, they may occasionally require excision for diagnosis or aesthetics.

Premalignant Lesions

A number of premalignant lesions of the skin can develop on the hand. Most that occur on the dorsum result from ultraviolet radiation. Cutaneous horns are benign protrusions of conical hyperkeratosis from the epidermis. SCC can be found in up to 15% of horns; treatment is excision with a base of 2 to 3 mm.

Actinic keratosis is a premalignant condition appearing in sun-exposed areas of the body, typically in the head and neck as well as on the dorsum of the hands and forearms. Multiple discrete dry, rough, and scaly areas are frequently present and can remain for years without progressing. The conversion to SCC has been estimated to be 1 in 100 actinic keratoses per year. Most can be treated with 5% fluorouracil. Nodular lesions may require excision.

Arsenic keratoses are caused by prolonged sublethal ingestion of arsenic. Arsenic keratosis may progress to Bowen's disease or invasive SCC. Treatment is surgical excision.

Malignant Nonmelanotic Tumors

Dermatofibrosarcoma is a locally aggressive soft-tissue neoplasm; histologically, it is a low-grade fibrosarcoma. Dermatofibrosarcoma rarely involves the hand. Treatment of these lesions is a wide (2.5 to 3 cm) excision. In confined areas such as the hand, Mohs surgery (resection with continuous frozen section microscopic assessment) has promise. If surgical treatment of dermatofibrosarcoma is not feasible or requires a radical procedure, consideration

should be given to radiation therapy in combination with conservative surgery, or to radiation therapy alone in special circumstances.

Basal cell carcinoma (BCC) is a malignant epithelial neoplasm arising from either basal cells or pluripotential appendageal cells of the epidermis. The most common etiology is sun exposure; the vast majority of these tumors occur on the face. Only 3% to 12% of hand malignancies are BCC, usually on the sun-exposed dorsum of the hand. Other risk factors include radiation exposure, immunosuppression, Gorlin's syndrome, and arsenic exposure. Metastases from BCC are rare. A 1- or 2-mm margin is adequate for BCC; however, morphea tumors usually advance well beyond their apparent margin. In confined areas such as the hand, Moh's surgery allows concurrent mapping of the histologic margins as the dissection proceeds. BCC may also be responsive to radiation therapy.

Squamous cell carcinoma is a tumor of epidermal keratinocytes and accounts for 75% to 90% of all hand malignancies. It affects men more than women, and is the most common malignancy of the nail bed. Sun exposure is the most commonly implicated etiology, but etiologic factors similar to those found in BCC are also important in squamous cell carcinoma. Patients receiving immunosuppression experience a 4-fold increase in incidence of skin cancer; they also have greater recurrence and metastasis rates. Tumors smaller than 1.5 cm in diameter that are not ulcerated, not fixed, and have no evidence of regional lymphadenopathy have a high cure rate; most of these tumors can be treated with simple excision. A small percentage are considerably more aggressive and capable of infiltration of surrounding tissues, lymph node metastasis, and hematogenous metastasis; these are usually treated by local excision with a 1-cm margin. All margins that are indurated should be removed, and margins should be checked histologically. The tumor should be excised one tissue plane below the tumor. Squamous cell carcinoma of the nail bed will usually require amputation of at least the distal phalanx. MRI can be very useful in assessing the extent of tumor prior to resection. Principles of reconstruction should be adhered to when amputation is necessary.

On rare occasions, squamous cell carcinoma of the hand may become quite extensive prior to treatment, requiring more extensive surgery. Every effort should be made to preserve function, but not at the risk of increased local recurrence. Surgical resection combined with radiation is one approach. Responses to isolated hyperthermic limb perfusion with melphalan and tumor necrosis factor have also been reported. This may be a consideration when hand or arm amputation is the only alternative. However, there is relatively little experience employing this treatment in the management of advanced squamous cell carcinomas.

Patients with regional metastasis to the epitrochlear and axillary lymph nodes may benefit from lymph node dissection and adjuvant radiation of the node station if the primary tumor has been controlled. In one large series (685 patients with squamous cell carcinoma of the trunk and limbs), the metastatic rate was 4.9% and the overall mortality rate was 3.4%. The mortality rate was 70.6% in patients with metastasis; correspondingly, 30% of patients with operable metastasis were salvaged.

Cutaneous malignancies have also been associated with organ transplantation secondary to immunosuppressive drugs. In one series of 1,300 kidney transplants, there were 176 skin malignancies; many of these occurred on the back of the hand. Because of the propensity for field cancerization, these patients were treated with resection of the dorsal surface skin with good results.

Merkel cell cancer is a rare and highly aggressive cutaneous malignancy that usually occurs in the head, neck, and upper extremities. Nodal disease occurs in over half of these patients at some time during their course. Wide excision with local radiation and regional node dissection or regional radiation therapy have been recommended for these lesions. Sentinel node biopsy was recently suggested for these tumors and good results have also been reported with isolated hyperthermic limb perfusion.

As with STS, cutaneous neoplasms have widely differing behaviors. Management of these varied tumors depends on their expected behavior and the knowledge base for therapy decisions. Accurate diagnosis and multidisciplinary consultation are critical to successful management of these tumors.

Annotated Bibliography

Soft-Tissue Tumors

Bray PW, Bell RS, Bowen CV, Davis A, O'Sullivan B: Limb salvage surgery and adjuvant radiotherapy for soft tissue sarcomas of the forearm and hand. *J Hand Surg* 1997;22A:495–503.

This study of 25 patients with soft-tissue sarcomas of the hand and forearm focused on a combination of radiation and surgery in the management of these difficult cases. Eighty-eight percent of patients surviving did not require amputation.

Brien EW, Terek RM, Geer RJ, Caldwell G, Brennan MF, Healey JH: Treatment of soft-tissue sarcomas of the hand. *J Bone Joint Surg* 1995;77A:564–571.

Management of 23 patients with soft-tissue sarcomas of the hand is reviewed. Patients were treated at Memorial Sloan-Kettering Cancer Center.

Eggermont AM, Schraffordt Koops H, Klausner JM, et al: Isolated limb perfusion with tumor necrosis factor and melphalan for limb salvage in 186 patients with locally advanced soft tissue extremity sarcomas: The cumulative multicenter European experience. *Ann Surg* 1996;224:756–765.

In this series, 186 patients were managed with hyperthermic isolation limb perfusion with melphalan and tumor necrosis factor over a period of almost 4.5 years in a number of institutions. Excellent limb salvage is reported.

Enzinger FM, Weiss SW (eds): *Soft Tissue Tumors,* ed 3. St. Louis, MO, Mosby, 1995.

This is an authoritative text on the pathology of soft-tissue tumors.

Fong Y, Coit DG, Woodruff JM, Brennan MF: Lymph node metastasis from soft tissue sarcoma in adults: Analysis of data from a prospective database of 1,772 sarcoma patients. *Ann Surg* 1993;217:72–77.

This study reviews the incidence of lymph node metastasis from Memorial Sloan-Kettering Cancer Center's sarcoma database.

Gross E, Rao BN, Pappo AS, et al: Soft tissue sarcoma of the hand in children: Clinical outcome and management. *J Pediatr Surg* 1997;32:698–702.

Seventeen patients treated for soft-tissue sarcomas of the hand at St. Jude Children's Research hospital are reviewed. This study emphasizes the management of histologies more typical of this young age group.

Hoglund M: Ultrasound diagnosis of soft-tissue tumours in the hand and forearm: A prospective study. *Acta Radiol* 1997;38:508–513.

Fifty soft-tissue tumors were diagnosed by ultrasonography or histopathology as belonging to 1 of 5 soft-tissue tumor groups. The reported ultrasound diagnoses and the histopathologic results were compared, and their sensitivity was calculated.

Johnstone PA, Wexler LH, Venzon DJ, et al: Sarcomas of the hand and foot: Analysis of local control and functional result with combined modality therapy in extremity preservation. *Int J Radiat Oncol Biol Phys* 1994;29:735–745.

This article describes the management of young adults and children with soft-tissue tumors of the hand and foot. Ewing's sarcoma and rhabdomyosarcomas are emphasized.

Lufkin RB, Gronemeyer DH, Seibel RM: Interventional MRI: Update. *Eur Radiol* 1997;7(suppl 5):187–200.

The development of interventional MRI capability is described.

Okunieff P, Suit HD, Proppe KH: Extremity preservation by combined modality treatment of sarcomas of the hand and wrist. *Int J Radiat Oncol Biol Phys* 1986;12:1923–1929.

This review of 17 patients with soft-tissue sarcomas of the hand and wrist managed with surgical resection and radiation therapy emphasizes limb salvage.

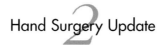
Peh WC, Truong NP, Totty WG, Gilula LA: Pictorial review: Magnetic resonance imaging of benign soft tissue masses of the hand and wrist. *Clin Radiol* 1995;50:519–525.

In this review of the use of MRI in evaluation of soft-tissue masses of the hand, the authors describe certain conditions under which the diagnosis may be made or strongly suspected from characteristic MRI features.

Pisters PW, Harrison LB, Leung DH, Woodruff JM, Casper ES, Brennan MF: Long-term results of a prospective randomized trial of adjuvant brachytherapy in soft tissue sarcoma. *J Clin Oncol* 1996;14:859–868.

Long-term results of a randomized prospective trial in soft-tissue sarcomas treated with resection and brachytherapy or resection alone are reported.

Rydholm A, Gustafson P, Rooser B, Willen H, Berg NO: Subcutaneous sarcoma: A population-based study of 129 patients. *J Bone Joint Surg* 1991;73B:662–667.

This is one of the few population-based studies of soft-tissue sarcomas-an important resource for those interested in these uncommon tumors.

Simon MA, Finn HA: Diagnostic strategy for bone and soft-tissue tumors. *J Bone Joint Surg* 1993;75A:622–631.

This is a review of diagnostic strategies in the evaluation of bone and soft-tissue tumors.

Terek RM, Brien EW: Soft-tissue sarcomas of the hand and wrist. *Hand Clin* 1995;11:287–305.

This review article on the multidisciplinary management of sarcomas of the hand lists 52 references.

Vrouenraets BC, Keus RB, Nieweg OE, Kroon BB: Complications of combined radiotherapy and isolated limb perfusion with tumor necrosis factor alpha +/− interferon gamma and melphalan in patients with irresectable soft tissue tumors. *J Surg Oncol* 1997;65:88–94.

This study describes complications associated with sequential treatment of patients with radiation and isolation perfusion.

Cutaneous Tumors

Ho VC, Sober AJ, Balch CM: Biopsy techniques, in Balch CM, Houghton AN, Sober AJ, Soong S (eds): *Cutaneous Melanoma*, ed 3. St. Louis, MO, Quality Medical Publishing, 1998, pp 135–140.

This chapter of a text devoted to melanoma reviews biopsy techniques of pigmented lesions. The book is a superb resource for those interested in malignant melanoma.

Kuvshinoff BW, Kurtz C, Coit DG: Computed tomography in evaluation of patients with stage III melanoma. *Ann Surg Oncol* 1997;4:252–258.

These authors reviewed CT evaluation of patients with positive lymph nodes. Routine CT in patients with clinical stage III melanoma infrequently identified metastatic disease. Selective use of chest CT in patients with cervical adenopathy or use of pelvic CT in the presence of groin disease may be useful.

Morton DL, Wen DR, Cochran AJ: Management of early-stage melanoma by intraoperative lymphatic mapping and selective lymphadenectomy. *Surg Oncol Clin North Am* 1992;1:247–259.

This is an early review of sentinel lymph node biopsy by the group that developed and popularized this technique.

Pfeifer T, Weinberg H, Brady MS: Lymphatic mapping for Merkel cell carcinoma. *J Am Acad Dermatol* 1997;37:650–651.

The authors describe early results and the rationale for lymphatic mapping in Merkel cell carcinoma.

Reintgen DS, Rapaport DP, Tanabe KK, Ross MI: Lymphatic mapping and sentinel lymphadenectomy, in Balch CM, Houghton AN, Sober AJ, Soong S (eds): *Cutaneous Melanoma*, ed 3. St. Louis, MO, Quality Medical Publishing, 1998, pp 227–244.

Another chapter in the melanoma text reviews the indications and techniques for sentinel lymph node biopsy in patients with malignant melanoma.

Malignant Melanoma

Albertini JJ, Cruse CW, Rapaport D, et al: Intraoperative radio-lympho-scintigraphy improves sentinel lymph node identification for patients with melanoma. *Ann Surg* 1996;223:217–224.

The authors emphasize the benefits of blue dye labeling used in combination with radiolabeling for sentinel node biopsy.

Ang KK, Peters LJ, Weber RS, et al: Postoperative radiotherapy for cutaneous melanoma of the head and neck region. *Int J Radiat Oncol Biol Phys* 1994;30:795–798.

This is one of the more extensive reviews of the role of radiation in melanoma of the head and neck.

Balch CM, Urist MM, Karakousis CP, et al: Efficacy of 2-cm surgical margins for intermediate-thickness melanomas (1–4 mm): Results of a multi-institutional randomized surgical trial. *Ann Surg* 1993;218:262–269.

Balch and associates compared 2-cm and 4-cm margins in melanomas thicker than those in Veronesi's trial. There was no significant difference in local recurrence and survival.

Fraker DL: Hyperthermic regional perfusion for melanoma of the limbs, in Balch CM, Houghton AN, Sober AJ, Soong S (eds): *Cutaneous Melanoma*, ed 3. St. Louis, MO, Quality Medical Publishing,1998, pp 281–300.

This chapter describes the role of hyperthermic regional perfusion in management of patients with melanoma.

Landis SH, Murray T, Bolden S, Wingo PA: Cancer statistics, 1998. *CA Cancer J Clin* 1998;48:6–29.

This is a statistical report on tumors per year in the United States.

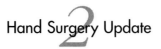

Stadelmann WK, Rapaport DP, Soong SJ, Reintgen DS, Buzaid AC, Balch CM: Prognostic clinical and pathologic features, in Balch CM, Houghton AN, Sober AJ, Soong S (eds): *Cutaneous Melanoma*, ed 3. St. Louis, MO, Quality Medical Publishing, 1998, pp 11–35.

This chapter focuses on relevant prognostic clinical and pathologic features of malignant melanomas.

Tseng JF, Tanabe KK, Gadd MA, et al: Surgical management of primary cutaneous melanomas of the hands and feet. *Ann Surg* 1997;225:544–553.

This review of 116 patients with melanoma of the hand and feet provides a useful overview of this difficult problem.

Veronesi U, Cascinelli N: Narrow excision (1-cm margin): A safe procedure for thin cutaneous melanoma. *Arch Surg* 1991; 126:438–441.

This follow-up report further confirms the value of the smaller margin for thin melanomas.

Veronesi U, Cascinelli N, Adamus J, et al: Thin stage I primary cutaneous malignant melanoma: Comparison of excision with margins of 1 or 3 cm. *N Engl J Med* 1988;318: 1159–1162.

In a European trial, 1- and 3-cm excisions for melanomas were compared. This study demonstrates the value of 1-cm margins in patients with thin melanomas.

Warso M, Gray T, Gonzalez M: Melanoma of the Hand. *J Hand Surg* 1997;22A:354–360.

This article presents a review of 39 patients with melanoma of the hand.

Nonpigmented Cutaneous Tumors of the Hand and Wrist

Fink JA, Akelman E: Nonmelanotic malignant skin tumors of the hand. *Hand Clin* 1995;11:255–264.

An extensive review emphasizing the importance of careful histopathologic diagnosis, this article covers 87 references.

Hashimoto K, Lever WF: Tumors of skin appendages, in Fitzpatrick TB, Eisen AZ, Wolff K, Freedberg IM, Austen KF (eds): *Dermatology in General Medicine*. New York, NY, McGraw-Hill, 1993, pp 873–898.

Skin appendage tumors are described in this chapter.

Haws MJ, Neumeister MW, Kenneaster DG, Russell RC: Management of nonmelanoma skin tumors of the hand. *Clin Plast Surg* 1997;24:779–795.

This extensive and thorough review article on the management of nonmelanoma skin tumors of the hand mentions 72 references.

Lever WF, Schaumburg-Lever G (eds): *Histopathology of the Skin*, ed 6. Philadelphia, PA, JB Lippincott, 1983.

This book outlines pathologic histology of skin diseases and tumors.

Rook A, Whimster I: Keratoacanthoma: A thirty year retrospect. *Br J Dermatol* 1979;100:41–47.

This is a large clinical review of keratoacanthoma.

Safai B: Cancers of the skin, in DeVita VT, Rosenberg SA, Hellman S (eds): *Cancer: Principles & Practice of Oncology*, ed 4. Philadelphia, PA, JB Lippincott, 1993, vol 2, pp 1567–1611.

This exhaustive text on cancer includes a chapter describing the multidisciplinary management of skin cancers.

Premalignant Lesions

Fleegler EJ: Skin tumors, in Green DP, Hotchkiss RN (eds): *Operative Hand Surgery*, ed 3. New York, NY, Churchill Livingtstone, 1993, vol 2, pp 2173–2196.

A chapter of this comprehensive text of operative hand surgery is devoted to skin tumors.

Klein E, Stoll HL Jr, Milgrom H, Helm F, Walker MJ: Tumors of the skin: XII. Topical 5-Fluorouracil for epidermal neoplasms. *J Surg Oncol* 1971;3:331–349.

Results of an early trial of the use of 5-fluorouracil in skin tumors are described.

Malignant Nonmelanotic Tumors

Ames SE, Krag DN, Brady MS: Radiolocalization of the sentinel lymph node in Merkel cell carcinoma: A clinical analysis of seven cases. *J Surg Oncol* 1998;67:251–254.

The sentinel node was identified and removed successfully in 7 patients using radiolocalization. This technique is useful in the staging and therapy of patients with Merkel cell carcinoma.

Ariyan S: Benign and malignant soft tissue tumors of the hand, in McCarthy JG, May JW Jr, Littler JW (eds): *Plastic Surgery: The Hand, Part 2*. Philadelphia, PA, WB Saunders, 1990, vol 8, pp 5483–5509.

This chapter describes management of soft-tissue tumors of the hand.

Dawson R, Williams OM, Mansel RE: Isolated hyperthermic limb perfusion chemotherapy in Merkel cell tumour: A case report. *J R Coll Surg Edinb* 1996;41:255–256.

This is a case report on isolated limb perfusion in a patient with a Merkel cell tumor.

Fenig E, Brenner B, Katz A, Rakovsky E, Hana MB, Sulkes A: The role of radiation therapy and chemotherapy in the treatment of Merkel cell carcinoma. *Cancer* 1997;80:881–885.

In a report of 40 patients with Merkel cell carcinoma, the authors conclude that data support the use of chemotherapy followed by radiation therapy for patients with advanced locoregional Merkel cell carcinoma.

Fitzpatrick TB, Johnson RA, Polano MK, Suurmond D, Wolff K (eds): *Color Atlas and Synopsis of Clinical Dermatology: Common and Serious Diseases*, ed 2. New York, NY, McGraw-Hill Health Professions Division, 1992.

This is an atlas of clinical dermatology.

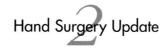
Haas RL, Keus RB, Loftus BM, Rutgers EJ, van Coevorden F, Bartelink H: The role of radiotherapy in the local management of dermatofibrosarcoma protuberans: Soft Tissue Tumours Working Group. *Eur J Cancer* 1997;33:1055–1060.

This European article describes the use of combined radiation and surgery in 17 patients. Local control was achieved in 82%.

Joseph MG, Zulueta QP, Kennedy PJ: Squamous cell carcinoma of the skin of the trunk and limbs: The incidence of metastases and their outcome. *Aust N Z J Surg* 1992;62:697–701.

This is an excellent review of the implications of nodal metastasis from squamous cell cancer.

Lejeune F, Lienard D, Eggermont A, et al: Efficacy of the tumor necrosis factor-alpha (rTNF-alpha) associated with interferon-gamma and chemotherapy in extracorporeal circulation in the limb in inoperable malignant melanoma, soft tissue sarcoma and epidermoid carcinoma: A 4-year experience. *Bull Cancer* 1995;82:561–567.

In addition to reporting treatment of sarcomas and melanomas with isolated limb perfusion, the authors describe management of some squamous cell cancers with perfusion.

Marks ME, Kim RY, Salter MM: Radiotherapy as an adjunct in the management of Merkel cell carcinoma. *Cancer* 1990;65:60–64.

Four patients diagnosed with Merkel cell carcinoma were treated with surgery followed by radiation therapy. The authors recommend radiation and surgery in the management of Merkel cell carcinoma.

Ratner D, Thomas CO, Johnson TM, et al: Mohs micrographic surgery for the treatment of dermatofibrosarcoma protuberans: Results of a multi-institutional series with an analysis of the extent of microscopic spread. *J Am Acad Dermatol* 1997;37:600–613.

This updated article on the role of Moh's surgery in the management of patients with dermatofibrosarcoma protuberans reviews the records of 58 patients. The importance of negative microscopic margins is emphasized.

Ross MI, Balch CM: Surgical treatment of primary melanoma, in Balch CM, Houghton AN, Sober AJ, Soong S (eds): *Cutaneous Melanoma*, ed 3. St. Louis, MO, Quality Medical Publishing, 1998, pp 141–153.

This chapter describes the surgical treatment of primary melanoma.

Schiavon M, Mazzoleni F, Chiarelli A, Matano P: Squamous cell carcinoma of the hand: Fifty-five case reports. *J Hand Surg* 1988;13A:401–404.

In a report of 55 patients with squamous cell carcinoma of the hand, the authors emphasize an aggressive surgical approach.

Scholtens RE, van Zuuren EJ, Posma AN: Treatment of recurrent squamous cell carcinoma of the hand in immunosuppressed patients. *J Hand Surg* 1995;20A:73–76.

Fourteen patients with kidney transplants were treated by total skin resection for recurrent squamous cell carcinoma of the skin on the dorsum of the hand.

Yiengpruksawan A, Coit DG, Thaler HT, Urmacher C, Knapper WK: Merkel cell carcinoma: Prognosis and management. *Arch Surg* 1991;126:1514–1519.

Seventy patients with Merkel cell carcinoma were treated at Memorial Sloan-Kettering Cancer Center between 1969 and 1989. Recommended treatment includes wide excision of the primary tumor and either elective or early therapeutic regional node dissection. The role of adjuvant radiotherapy or chemotherapy remains unclear.

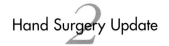

Chapter 35
Cutaneous Tumors of the Hand

L. Scott Levin, MD

The history of skin tumors in the hand is linked closely with predisposing factors that have contributed to skin cancers. For example, exposure to arsenic has been incriminated in the development of arsenic keratoses and basal cell carcinomas (BCCs). Excess exposure to ionizing radiation has been recognized to result in skin cancer since the early 1900s.

Before the advent of aggressive treatment for osteomyelitis, burns, and chronic wounds, fistulae from sinus tracts were common. Those chronic inflammatory conditions led to Marjolin ulcers, aggressive squamous cell carcinomas (SCCs); these are much rarer today than many years ago.

Finally, the recreational history of the United States population has changed. There is more emphasis on outdoor activity, tanning, and sun exposure, leading subsequently to a higher incidence of melanoma and other cutaneous malignancies.

The Normal Skin

The skin is the organ system that serves as the barrier between the relatively closed systems of the human body and the external environment. It is strong, elastic, waterproof, protective, and self-repairing, and serves both as a sensory and an excretory organ. It regulates heat loss by sweat glands and, in some places, by hair.

The skin also has important immunologic functions, with 3 major cell types present in the epidermis. These are keratinocytes (from ectoderm), melanocytes (from neuroectoderm), and Langerhans cells (derived from mesenchyme). Langerhans cells express immunoglobulin A (IgA) antibody antigens and have receptor sites for the Fc portion of the IgG antibody and complement components (C3). These cells assist in the cutaneous immunologic response. Ultraviolet (UV) light adversely affects the function of Langerhans cells, impairing their ability to process antigens.

Skin color in humans is due largely to the content of melanin within keratinocytes. The number of melanocytes is the same for a specific region of skin. Melanin inhibits transmission of radiation through the skin; for example, an up to tenfold decrease in UV light passes through the epidermis of dark skinned persons. Moreover, exposure to UV light is thought to be a principal etiologic factor in the development of human malignant melanoma and other malignancies that will be discussed.

Principles and Goals of Treatment

The principles of treatment of skin tumors of the hand are (1) to recognize pathology early; (2) to have a high index of suspicion for any skin lesion that has appeared recently or for a preexisting lesion that has undergone changes in consistency, texture, or size; (3) to consider any such lesion a neoplasm until proved otherwise; (4) to perform appropriate biopsy with proper surgical technique; (5) to provide appropriate treatment that includes adequate margins when surgery is used for treatment; (6) to establish regular post-treatment surveillance of the primary lesion; and (7) to consider adjunctive therapy, depending on the tumor and its extent.

If surgical management is chosen, the goal should be eradication of the tumor without regard to hand function unless completion and adequate tumor resection can be assured while preserving function. Inadequate margins of resection obtained to preserve function lead to high local recurrence rates and ultimate higher morbidity after subsequent ablative surgery. Certain tumors, based on their size, location, and biologic behavior, require less aggressive resection, and in these cases hand function can be preserved.

Basic Science

Biologic behavior of hand skin tumors is variable; some follow a relatively benign course while others progress to cause local morbidity, later metastasis, and even death. Biologic aggressiveness in different tumors is related to the epithelial growth factor receptor concentration found in the peripheral palisade layer of the skin. This layer contains the most actively dividing cells in the skin.

Cell-mediated immunity is the host-defense mechanism that guards against invasion by BCC and SCC. Natural killer (NK) cells and T cells prevent tumor growth progression. T cells that produce interferon and interleukin 2 stimulate NK cells that play a significant role in tumor rejection. Reports of decreased NK-cell activity in mice receiving long-term UV radiation suggest impaired immunity and susceptibility to tumor induction by UV-light exposure. Immunosuppressive agents such as those used in renal transplant patients have been linked to the development of spontaneous malignancies. Approximately 30% of the skin tumors arising in immunosuppressed patients are very aggressive.

Predisposing Factors for Skin Cancers

UV radiation plays a role in skin cancer pathogenesis. The only clinically significant wavelengths are in the UV spectrum. The sun is the natural source of UV radiation, but the long-term effects of using sun lamps and tanning beds cannot be ignored. Solar radiation that penetrates to the surface of the earth is almost void of the UVC wave band. The ozone layer of the stratosphere absorbs UV wavelengths below 290 nm so that only UVB and UVA reach Earth's crust. Over 95% of solar UV radiation is in the UVA wave band; however, the UVB wave band is responsible for acute sunburn as well as chronic sun damage and malignant degeneration that occur in human skin. The UVB rays are the most carcinogenic.

Actinic damage is the only recognized risk factor for development of skin cancer. Geographic distribution of skin cancer is related to a person's susceptibility to UV light, which is inversely proportional to the melanocyte content of the skin. Individuals of Celtic ancestry do not tan well and tend to sunburn with solar exposure; they have a predilection for development of skin cancers.

Surgical Management

Biopsy Methods

Tumors on the hand that are suspected of being malignant should be biopsied either with a punch, shave, or excisional biopsy. Excisional biopsy using a scalpel should be done with the intent to close the defect primarily, assuming that margins are adequate. Frozen section can be obtained in BCCs or SCCs, but Mohs' micrographic surgery is a better choice if surrounding tissue is to be preserved. Frozen section is not performed in cases of malignant melanoma. Shave excision is best suited for pedunculated, papular, or exophytic lesions. Nevertheless, the procedure can be used as a deep shave for macular or indurated lesions, permitting sampling into the papillary dermis. It should not be used for biopsying melanomas or inflammatory lesions.

Cryotherapy is a versatile procedure that is technically easy to perform, does not require the injection of local anesthetic, and can be used for both benign and for some malignant lesions. Liquid nitrogen is the most commonly used cryogen. The mechanism of tissue injury is related to rapid crystal formation, recrystallization patterns during thaw, and ischemia secondary to vascular stasis and endothelial damage. The "ice ball" formed in the tissue during therapy must reach appropriate horizontal and vertical dimensions to effect adequate treatment. The amount of tissue damage in cryosurgery is increased by rapid freezing followed by slow thaw and repeated freeze-thaw cycles.

Actinic keratoses are frozen until white for 10 to 15 seconds. Cure rates up to 95% have been reported for both BCCs and SCCs. It is only the small well-defined lesions, however, that are best suited for this treatment.

The skin curette is a useful tool for the removal of a variety of lesions. It is best suited for use on soft or friable tumors, such as actinic keratoses or selected BCCs and SCCs. Growths on concave surfaces (as compared to convex surfaces) are more suited for removal by curettage.

In the treatment of benign or premalignant lesions, bleeding is often controlled by light electrodesiccation. However, curettage must be followed by vigorous electrodesiccation when treating nonmelanoma skin cancers by this method. Both the wound bed and a small (< 1 mm) rim of normal tissue beyond that removed by the curette should be seared. Three sequential cycles of curettage and electrodesiccation are generally recommended for an individual malignant lesion.

Mohs' Micrographic Surgery

In most cases of invasive skin cancer, surgical excision is the standard goal. Mohs described micrographic surgery in 1932. He called it chemosurgery because it combines zinc chloride as a fixative (chemo) and microscopic control with excision of margins created with a knife (surgery). The technique involves excision of all visible tumor in saucer-like layers while mapping the exact size and shape of the lesion. Horizontal frozen sections taken from the undersurface of the excised tissue are examined microscopically; wherever tumor is found, it is localized on the map and the area is marked for further resection. This progress is repeated until all tumor is removed.

The indications for Mohs' micrographic surgery in the treatment of malignant skin tumors of the hand follow. Tumors should be recurrent BCCs and SCCs, and primary lesions should meet one or more of the following criteria: (1) tumors are in sites reported to have a relatively high recurrence rate, (2) tumors have poorly delineated borders arising from scar tissue, (3) lesions are over 2 cm or tumors

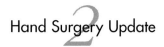
have aggressive malignant features, (4) they are morpheaform or sclerosing BCCs, (5) tumors are in critical locations where it is desirable to preserve as much uninvolved tissue as possible (eg, the hand), and (6) there are SSCs with perineural invasion. Microcystic adenexal carcinomas, dermatofibrosarcoma protuberans, and malignant melanoma may also be considered for Mohs' surgery.

Actinic Keratoses

Actinic keratoses are the most frequent epidermal tumors, with most arising on sun-exposed skin. The term solar keratosis is more specific because it refers to a variety of rays. Actinic keratoses are a sensitive indicator of cumulative exposure to UVB radiation and increased risk of nonmelanoma skin cancers, particularly SCC.

The most common locations are chronically sun-exposed surfaces: face, ears, dorsal hands, and forearms. The dorsal hand lesions have a greater tendency toward a hyperkeratotic form and may appear clinically as cutaneous horns.

Types of actinic keratoses that can be recognized histologically include atrophic, acantholytic, bowenoid, and pigmented. As many as 25% of actinic keratoses will remit spontaneously, and predicting whether a given lesion will involute or become malignant is difficult. Indications for treatment include onset of symptoms, recent substantial growth, or undesirable appearance.

There are a number of treatment methods for actinic keratoses. For small lesions, cryotherapy with liquid nitrogen is very effective, with a 98.8% cure reported. Shave excision or electrodesiccation and curettage can also be performed on individual lesions.

For extensive, broad, or numerous lesions, topical 5 fluorouracil may be used. Fluorouracil, as a cream or solution, is applied twice daily, and treatment is stopped when a peak response is achieved, characterized by marked inflammation, oozing, crusting, or ulceration (approximately 4 to 6 weeks). Healing usually takes 3 to 6 weeks once treatment is stopped.

Cutaneous Horns

Cutaneous horn is the clinical term for a circumscribed conical, markedly hyperkeratotic lesion arising from a base that is usually erythematous and thickened. Cutaneous horns are seen most frequently on the face and scalp, but lesions also may occur on the hands.

Benign, premalignant, malignant, infectious, and autoimmune processes have all been documented as causes of cutaneous horns. Actinic keratoses accounted for the majority of lesions producing cutaneous horns followed by verruca vulgaris, SCC, and seborrheic keratoses. A deep shave or excisional biopsy with histologic examinations is necessary to determine the etiology and the appropriate therapy.

Verrucae

The most common verruca presenting on the hands is the verruca vulgaris. It is an elevated rounded papule with a rough "verrucous" surface and often contains black pinpoint dots that represent thrombosed capillaries. Lesions may be single or grouped. Periungual verrucae coalesce around the nail folds and can become fissured, inflamed, and tender. Mosaic or murmecia warts result from the coalescence of palmar warts into large plaques. Human papillomavirus types 1, 2, 4, and 7 are most frequently responsible for verrucae vulgaris.

Verrucae plana or flat warts are 1 to 3 mm, smooth, slightly raised, flat-surfaced papules. They are usually multiple and commonly present on the dorsal hands. Their color is flesh color to light brown, but more hyperpigmented lesions can occur and may be confused with other benign pigmented lesions. Human papillomavirus types 3 and 10 have most often been associated with flat warts.

Verruca vulgaris in children often spontaneously remits and may not require any therapy. Cryotherapy with liquid nitrogen by spray or cotton-tipped application is widely used but painful. Topical caustics and acids, such as salicylic acid, lactic acid, or trichloroacetic acid, peel skin and can be used alone or as an adjunct to cryotherapy. Retinoic acid has been used topically to treat flat warts and may function as a keratolytic or an irritant inducing remission. Curettage and electrodesiccation is also a popular method for verruca removal. It is a quick method requiring only one treatment; however, it may scar. Potentially scarring methods must be used cautiously, especially for periungual verrucae, which may destroy the matrix and the ability for normal nail formation. CO_2 laser has been used successfully in recalcitrant verrucae. Wart virus DNA is present in the "plume" from the surgical field, and precautions to prevent inhalation are necessary.

Arsenic Keratoses

Arsenic, once an ingredient in many medicinal solutions and still a component of insecticides, causes distinctive keratoses on the palms and soles. Arsenic keratoses are keratotic, 2- to 4-mm verrucous papules without surrounding inflammation.

Arsenic ingestion also produces carcinomas of the skin. Bowen's disease is the most common cutaneous carcinoma produced by arsenic, but SCC and superficial BCC also can occur. Treatment of arsenic keratoses is by cryotherapy, electrodesiccation and curettage, or topical application of 5-fluorouracil.

Keratoacanthomas

Keratoacanthoma (KA) is difficult to differentiate from SCC, which it resembles clinically and histologically. The solitary KA begins as a red, dome-shaped papule that expands rapidly and develops a central crater filled with a keratinous plug. KAs occur primarily on sun-damaged skin, with the central face, dorsal hands, and arms being most commonly involved. Lesions may occur in subungual regions. KAs usually reach their maximum size within only 6 to 8 weeks. Unlike SCCs, KAs often regress within months without therapy. Many investigators believe that these epithelial tumors are actually variants of SCC.

An increased incidence of KA is observed in immunosupressed patients. A viral etiology has also been suggested but not confirmed.

It can be difficult to distinguish KA from SCC based on histologic findings alone. Accurately differentiating between well-differentiated SCC and KA on clinical and histologic grounds may not be possible. The architecture of the lesion is important for diagnosis, and an excisional biopsy of the entire lesion is recommended. Many recommend treating suspect KAs or even all KAs as carcinomas.

KAs can be treated in a variety of ways. They may spontaneously involute, but the process may take up to a year, and the cosmetic result often is unacceptable. If the patient is immunosuppressed or SCC cannot be ruled out, surgical excision (with histologic examination) is recommended. Other reported successful treatments include electrodesiccation and curettage, intralesional 5-fluorouracil, intralesional bleomycin, and intralesional triamcinolone. Multiple lesions have been treated with methotrexate and etretinate. In giant KAs metacarpal amputation occasionally is required.

Bowen's Disease

Bowen's disease is an intraepidermal SCC or an SCC in situ that may ultimately become invasive. The risk of spread is relatively low (3% to 5%), and Bowen's disease may persist for years before becoming invasive.

Bowen's disease is usually a solitary lesion. Infrequently, the fingers, including the nail fold or nail bed, are involved.

The disease usually appears as a slowly enlarging erythematous scaling patch or plaque that often is sharply demarcated. Bowen's disease may resemble superficial BCC; however, it usually lacks a pearly border, telangiectasias, and a tendency to develop central atrophy.

Surgical excision is often required owing to extension down the outer root sheaths of hair follicles. Depending on the depth of involvement, cryotherapy, electrodesiccation and curettage, laser ablation, shave excision, and 5 fluorouracil may be alternative methods of treatment. Mohs' surgery may be indicated in lesions that are large or ill-defined, or in sites where preservation of tissue is important. For lesions of the distal fingers, Mohs' surgery or amputation may be indicated.

Nonmelanoma Carcinomas

BCC and SCC of the skin make up more than one third of all cancers in the United States, with about 600,000 new cases detected each year. Exposure to sunlight, particularly UVB radiation, is the principal cause of both BCC and SCC. Consequently, most lesions occur on sun-exposed skin. Although BCCs far outnumber SCCs on the facial skin, SCCs occur 3 times more often than BCCs on the hand. Appearance may vary and may mimic other lesions, such as ulcers or paronychia.

Immunosuppression greatly increases the risk of non-melanoma skin cancers, especially SCCs. SCCs may also show greater aggressiveness in such patients. The risk increases with the duration of immunosuppression and may result in significant long-term management problems.

Another important factor for developing a nonmelanoma skin cancer is a history of a previous nonmelanoma skin cancer. The estimated risk of developing 1 or more new skin cancers in patients with a prior history of BCC or SCC is 35% at 3 years and 50% at 5 years. Subsequent skin cancers tend to be of the same cell type as the previous one.

Squamous Cell Carcinomas

The majority of UV-induced SCCs develop on the arms, hands, head, and neck and are associated with other signs of solar damage such as actinic keratoses. SCCs most commonly present as a firm erythematous nodule with elevated borders and indistinct margins. Frequently the lesion ulcerates and/or becomes crusted. Occasionally, raised, fungoid, verrucous lesions without ulceration occur. Subungual SCCs are rare; the majority of these have been on the thumb or index finger. Diagnosis often is delayed because of the tumor's resemblance to a variety of benign conditions. SCCs usually grow locally but may invade the subcutis, muscle, or

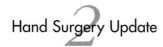

periosteum, and may grow along nerves, blood vessels, and lymphatic channels. Such malignancies may present as compression neuropathy, including carpal tunnel syndrome. SCC associated with ionizing radiation and scars usually occurs at the edges of affected sites. Those occurring in chronic ulcers may occur as a nonhealing plaque or nodule within the site, and biopsy is necessary to distinguish the SCC from the underlying condition.

Metastatic SCC is more common than metastatic BCC. Tumors developing in sites of chronic inflammation, scar tissue, radiation dermatitis, or in immunocompromised hosts have higher rates of metastasis. Regional lymph nodes are the most common site of metastasis, but liver, lung, bone, and brain metastases also occur. Despite aggressive treatment with surgery and adjuvant radiation therapy for lymph node metastasis, 5-year survival rates are between 14% and 39%.

Basal Cell Carcinomas

Approximately 80% of BCCs are found on the head and neck; they are much less common than SCC on the dorsal hand. Except in the basal cell nevus syndrome, lesions rarely occur on the palms. Five clinical types of BCC have been described: nodular ulcerative, superficial, morpheaform, cystic, and pigmented.

Nodular ulcerative BCC commonly is seen as a translucent flesh-colored or pearly papule with prominent telangiectasias and a rolled border. As the lesion enlarges, central ulceration and crusting can occur. Bleeding on slight injury is a common sign.

Superficial BCC usually occurs as a red, scaly macule or patch on the trunk and extremities—flat growths that exhibit little tendency to invade or ulcerate and enlarge slowly.

Morpheaform BCCs usually appear as a flat, indurated, white-to-yellow, ill-defined macule of plaque. As the lesion enlarges, it may become depressed, firm, and sclerotic, resembling a scar. The borders are not well defined, making therapy more difficult.

Cystic BCC frequently appears as a blue-gray cystic papule or nodule. These form as a result of disintegration of cells in the center of the tumor mass. Clinically, cystic BCCs can resemble eccrine or apocrine hydrocystomas.

Pigmented BCC differs from the noduloulcerative type only by the brown or black pigmentation contained in the lesion. Differentiation from other pigmented lesions, such as lentigines, seborrheic keratoses, and malignant melanoma, can be difficult.

The basal cell nevus carcinoma syndrome is an autosomal dominant disorder characterized by numerous BCCs, odontogenic cysts of the jaw, pitted depressions on the palms and soles, and anomalies of the ribs, spine, skull, and central nervous system. The palmar and plantar pits are 1 to 3 mm in diameter and histologically represent defective epithelium with increased propensity for forming BCC.

Metastatic BCC is very rare; the reported incidence ranges from 0.01% to 0.1%. Several factors increase the risk of recurrence for BCC. Tumors of the midface, ears, scalp, and forehead are associated with the highest risk of recurrence; upper extremity basal cell recurrence is low, less than 1%. BCCs larger that 6 mm in diameter recur more frequently than smaller ones. Histologic patterns of infiltration, sclerosis, or multifocality have higher rates of recurrence.

Treatment of Nonmelanoma Skin Carcinomas

Several treatment options, surgical and nonsurgical, are used for nonmelanoma cancers of the skin. No single treatment method is ideal for all lesions. Important factors in choosing a treatment include the histopathologic type, location, size of the tumor, whether the tumor is primary or recurrent, age of the patient, healing ability of the patient, the patient's medical condition, and the surgeon's personal preference. The most common methods include cryotherapy, electrodesiccation and curettage, topical or intralesional chemotherapy, excisional surgery, Mohs' surgery, and radiation therapy.

Excisional surgery is effective for all types of nonmelanoma skin cancers. The advantages of excision include the ability to check peripheral and deep margins histologically and optimization of wound placement and closure. If the margins are positive, reexcision is recommended. Repair of the defect can be done with primary closure, local flaps or skin grafts, or healing by secondary intention.

Mohs' surgery is generally the preferred treatment for tumors in high-risk areas, tumors with more aggressive histologic variants, larger lesions, lesions occurring in immunocompromised patients, and recurrent tumors. Repair of the defect is similar to repair in excisional surgery. Cure rates are high.

Cryosurgery uses liquid nitrogen delivered by a hand-held spray apparatus or a cryoprobe. It has been effectively used for many lesions, including BCC (especially superficial), Bowen's disease, and some SCCs. The obvious significant disadvantage of cryosurgery is the lack of histologic documentation of tumor removal.

Curettage and electrodesiccation also do not provide histologic confirmation of tumor (margin) removal, but are commonly and successfully used for many primary skin tumors. The bulk of the lesion is removed by curetting in multiple directions followed by careful electrodesiccation. The cycle is usually repeated 2 to 3 times, with depth and periphery of the tumor determined by the "gritty" sensation the normal dermis imparts to the curette. This treatment modality is appropriate for small, primary, superficial, or nodular ulcerative BCCs and SCCs with clearly defined borders.

Radiation therapy is useful for maximizing tissue preservation and for tumors not accessible to surgical excision. The technique is advantageous for elderly, debilitated, or other patients at higher risk of surgical complications. It is also appropriate as adjuvant therapy for large or ill-defined tumors or in tumors incompletely removed by surgical excision.

Laser therapy has been used as a treatment for some skin cancers. The carbon dioxide laser can be used in highly focused mode to excise lesions in a relatively bloodless fashion. It has been used primarily for superficial BCCs, but no comparative studies demonstrating an advantage of laser over traditional methods have been published.

Topical 5-fluorouracil may be successful in the treatment of superficial BCC and Bowen's disease but should not be used for nodular or deeper skin cancers. Its method of use was described in the "Actinic Keratoses" section. The rates of recurrence may be higher than for surgical and destructive procedures.

Intralesional bleomycin and intralesional interferon alpha are experimental treatment approaches for BCC and SCC. Photodynamic therapy is an investigational treatment in which a systemic photo sensitizer and nonionizing radiation are used to destroy tumor tissue preferentially. The uses for photodynamic therapy are under investigation and may be limited by generalized cutaneous photosensitivity lasting up to 4 weeks.

Prevention
Prevention is important in the treatment of nonmelanoma skin cancers. The use of sunscreens that block the majority of UVB radiation for the first 18 years of life could reduce the lifetime risk of nonmelanoma skin cancer by 78%.

Lymph Node Dissection
In SCCs and BCCs indications for lymph node dissection are controversial. The main indications for elective lymph node dissection are in patient staging. In instances of palpable nodes with a large primary lesion, lymph node biopsy at the epitrochlear or axillary region may be helpful in indicating which levels of amputation to perform. Elective epitrochlear axillary node dissection with locally confined tumor, that is, margins free of tumor after resection and reconstruction, need not be performed in SCCs and BCCs. The issue has not been well addressed in the upper extremity, but it is believed that local management will be sufficient for most SCCs and BCCs of the hand. In instances of massive tumors requiring digital, hand, or forearm amputation, epitrochlear and axillary node biopsy

can be considered to guide adjunctive treatment such as radiation and/or chemotherapy.

Melanomas of the Hand

Melanoma is a neoplastic disorder produced by malignant transformation of normal melanocytes. Melanocytes, the cells responsible for production of the pigment melanin, arise from neural crest tissue.

Historically, melanoma represented approximately 4% to 5% of all skin malignancies and 3% of carcinomas in general. In the United States this malignancy currently has an approximately 50% mortality. The actual incidence of melanoma is increasing more rapidly than that of any other malignancy. For the past decade, this rise has exceeded 90%. Since 1900, the lifetime risk has increased from 1 in 1,500 to a projected 1 in 90 by the year 2000. Death rates are also increasing for patients in the younger age groups.

Factors such as age, hormonal status, genetic predisposition, and environmental factors are said to be associated with melanoma. The specific role of UV light as an etiologic factor in melanoma is unresolved, but may be an ever-increasing risk factor with increased sun exposure to UVA as well as UVB lights, both of which are thought to be carcinogenic.

Melanoma rarely occurs before puberty, but cases of childhood and adolescent melanomas have been reported. Melanoma is also unusual in the noncaucasian population, with a caucasion to noncaucasion ratio of almost 20 to 1.

Histologic Types
There are 4 histologic types, each of which has distinctive features and clinical presentations. The 4 types are (1) lentigo maligna melanoma; (2) superficial spreading melanoma; (3) acral lentiginous melanoma; and (4) nodular melanoma. The first 3 have a junctional component, whereas nodular melanoma is entirely subjunctional.

Various clinical features distinguish each type of melanoma. Lentigo maligna is commonly seen in individuals in the sixth to eighth decade of life. Superficial spreading melanoma may occur on both sun-exposed and nonsun-exposed areas of the body. Nodular melanomas are characterized by vertical growth.

Prognostic Factors
The extent of the malignancy at the time of diagnosis is the most important prognostic indicator for survival. Patients classified as having stage I or primary disease have a better prognosis than those with regional spread of the disease involving transient lesions or involvement of first-order

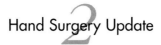
lymph nodes (stage II). Patients with distal disease involving metastasis to visceral organs or the skeleton have a poor prognosis (stage III).

In 1969, different histologic types of melanoma were documented. The importance of the level of invasion as described can be used for planning both surgical treatment and adjuvant systemic therapy (Table 1).

The importance of tumor thickness in terms of predicting the biologic behavior of melanoma was emphasized in 1970. Subsequently, multiple studies have indicated that tumor thickness is perhaps the most significant prognostic indicator.

One author suggested that thin melanomas (< 0.76 mm) were associated with localized disease and had a better that 90% cure rate. Patients with intermediate-thickness melanomas (0.76 to 4 mm) had increasing risk to subsequent regional or distant disease. Those with thick melanomas (> 4 mm) had at least an 80% risk of already having occult disease at the time of initial diagnosis. Tumor thickness and ulceration are the 2 pathologic factors that have the greatest statistical significance for prognosis.

Scattered reports in the literature discuss the biologic behavior of some types of melanoma as it relates to the hand. Other reports appear in publications written by oncologists, dermatologists, and general surgeons. However, there is no clear review of the behavior and treatment of malignant melanoma in the hand.

Cutaneous melanoma of the hand is a relatively rare clinical entity. As in all cases of melanoma, early detection of the lesion without significant invasion offers the best chance of survival. Factors such as clinically positive nodes at the time of diagnosis or distant metastasis predict poor prognosis.

Therefore, recommendations for elective lymph node dissection are as follows: (1) Lesions less than 1.5 mm have a low incidence of positive nodes; therefore, an elective lymph node dissection generally is not recommended. (2) Lesions that are 1.0 to 4.0 mm may benefit from dissection of the first-order lymph nodes in the upper extremity; epitrochlear nodes are rarely involved, and an axillary dissection might be considered in these patients. (3) In lesions greater than 4.0 mm thick there is a 70% probability of distant metastasis; therefore, elective lymph node dissection is of little value. The level of tumor invasion and tumor thickness remain the most significant prognostic indicators once the lesion is excised.

Subsequently, excisional biopsy to the level of the subcutaneous fat is recommended for all suspicious lesions not involving the subungual region. The nail area should be biopsied by removing the nail plate and performing an incisional biopsy of the lesion. Based on final pathology, amputation can then be done. This enables the pathologist to determine tumor thickness, levels of invasion, tumor ulceration, mitotic index, and microscopic satellitosis. Frozen sec-

Table 1

Criteria for levels of tumor invasion as it relates to skin histology

Level	Description
1	All tumor cells above basement membrane
2	Invasion into loose connective tissue of papillary dermis
3	Tumor cells at junction of papillary and reticular dermis
4	Invasion into reticular dermis
5	Invasion into subcutaneous fat

(Reproduced with permission from Peimer C (ed): *Surgery of the Hand and Upper Extremity*. New York, NY, McGraw-Hill Health Professions Division, 1996.)

tion is unreliable in melanoma and should not be used. Shave biopsy, curettage, or electrocoagulation are not recommended for a suspicious lesion.

Cutaneous primary lesions that are levels I and II should be excised with a 1- or 2-cm margin peripheral to the lesion and skin-grafted if primary tension-free closure is not possible. Subungual melanomas that involve the fingers should be amputated at the distal interphalangeal joint. Subungual lesions of the thumb should be amputated at the interphalangeal joint to preserve opposition and adequate function. Ray resection is rarely required unless there is transitory metastasis. Node excision can be considered for lesions 1.5 to 4.0 mm in thickness. If there is a local recurrence within 5 cm of the primary site, the lesion should be excised with a 3- to 5-cm new margin. In this instance, other methods of reconstruction of the defect may be required, such as free-tissue transfer for exposed depending structures such as tendon, nerve, or bone.

Metastasis

Metastasis occurs to long bones, small bowel, and central nervous system. Mean survival with bony metastasis is only a few months. For stage III disease, single or combination chemotherapy has been recommended. Radiation has been found to be helpful only as a palliative measure. Adjunctive treatment such as extremity perfusion and hyperthermia have been used with some success, but conclusions cannot be made in relation to melanoma of the hand.

The most important factor for the hand surgeon is to recognize melanoma in its various forms and to biopsy any hand lesion with discoloration or nodular appearance or any lesion involving the subungual area. Suspected subungual hematoma should be observed, and biopsy should be performed only if the lesion is persistent.

Lesions with deeper levels of invasion or of increased thickness and in noncaucasians generally have a poor prognosis. Elective node dissection should be reserved only for intermediate-thickness lesions. Radical ablative surgery usually is not indicated. In most cases, function can be preserved and adequate resection achieved if the basic guidelines are followed.

Kaposi's Sarcoma

Prior to the acquired immune deficiency syndrome (AIDS) epidemic, Kaposi's sarcoma had been an uncommon disease in North America. Kaposi's sarcoma historically was seen in men older than age 75 of Jewish and Mediterranean origin, in black Africans, and in patients compromised by immunodepressant medication.

Histologically, the Kaposi's sarcoma tumor in AIDS patients is indistinguishable from the classic forms. Kaposi's sarcoma is seen in 43% of homosexual males with AIDS but only in 11% of the other at-risk groups. The majority of Kaposi's sarcomas occur in the head and neck region; however, it has been seen in the hand in a patient with AIDS.

Tumors With Eccrine Differentiations

The differentiated distribution of eccrine glands and apocrine glands in the human body suggests that any sweat gland tumor found in the hand is of eccrine origin. Sweat gland tumors are uncommon, and the literature on sweat gland neoplasms of the hand consists largely of case reports or small series.

Porokeratotic eccrine ostial and dermal duct nevus is characterized by multiple punctuate pits and comedolike plugs usually appearing at birth and mostly on the palms and soles. The histologic picture consists of comedolike dilatations and comedolike lamellae involving the eccrine ostia and ducts.

Although syringoma is a relatively common adrenal tumor, syringoma of the hands rarely has been reported. Multiple syringomas that appeared as symmetric grouped erythematous papules limited to the dorsum of the proximal and middle phalanges of both hands have been reported.

Eccrine poromas occur most commonly on the feet but are found frequently on the hand and fingers. The usual clinical presentation is a firm, raised, or slightly pedunculated asymptomatic papule or nodule less than 2 cm in diameter. Other appearances include a cystic subcutaneous mass in the thenar region and a pedunculated papule with a surrounding dermatitis on the palm. Eccrine poromatosis is an unusual clinical variant consisting of multiple papules on the palm and soles.

Malignant Sweat Gland Tumors

Carcinomas of eccrine glands fall into 2 groups: those related to benign eccrine tumors and those considered primary eccrine carcinomas. Included in the first group are malignant eccrine poroma, malignant eccrine spiradenoma, malignant clear cell hidradenoma, and malignant chrondroid syringoma. Case reports in the literature describe instances of sweat gland carcinoma in the hand and provide little guidance as to their management. Removal with adequate margins and subsequent close follow-up are necessary; however, the roles of lymph node dissection, chemotherapy, and radiation are undefined.

Annotated Bibliography

Chakrabarti I, Watson JD, Dorrance H: Skin tumours of the hand: A 10-year review. *J Hand Surg* 1993;18B:484–486.

This 10-year retrospective study was performed to determine the incidence, distribution, histologic type, and behavior of skin tumors of the hand that were referred to a plastic surgery unit. The incidence of squamous cell carcinoma that required surgical excision was 5 cases per million per year.

Fink JA, Akelman E: Nonmelanotic malignant skin tumors of the hand. *Hand Clin* 1995;11:255–264.

This article provides an overview of basal and squamous carcinomas as well as Bowen's disease. Review of the literature is included, along with the entities of Merkel cell carcinoma, dermatofibrosarcoma protuberans, sweat gland tumors, and Kaposi carcinoma.

Glover MT, Niranjan N, Kwan JT, Leigh IM: Non-melanoma skin cancer in renal transplant recipients: The extent of the problem and a strategy for management. *Br J Plast Surg* 1994;47:86–89.

The authors describe their experience with a group of 291 patients, and describe the epidemiology of dysplastic changes in all sun-exposed areas. The subgroup of patients developed squamous cell carcinomas and required frequent surgery. Because of the virulent nature of some of these squamous cells, patient death is possible. Surveillance is very important in the management of these patients, particulary longstanding transplant patients on immunosuppressants.

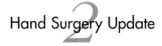

Haws MJ, Neumeister MW, Kenneaster DG, Russell RC: Management of nonmelanoma skin tumors of the hand. *Clin Plast Surg* 1997;24:779–795.

The authors of this review article go over the standard types of nonmelanoma skin tumors including squamous cell and basal cell. The article is well illustrated with a good bibliography.

Milanov NO, Shilov BL, Tjulenev AV: Surgical treatment of radiation injuries of the hand. *Plast Reconstr Surg* 1993;92:294–300.

In this study from Russia, the authors describe treatment of 12 patients with severe radiation damage to the hands. Coverage with flaps was the usual procedure. Aggressive debridement and immediate coverage with well-vascularized flaps can result in adequate wound healing and extremity salvage.

Sau P, McMarlin SL, Sperling LC, Katz R: Bowen's disease of the nail bed and periungual area: A clinico-pathologic analysis of seven cases. *Arch Dermatol* 1994;130:204–209.

The authors describe 7 cases of Bowen's disease and the role of human papilloma virus in the bowenoid changes. Bowen's disease in the nail bed can present flammatory as well as neoplastic condition. Mohs' micrographic surgery has been recommended to preserve tissue and function.

Slingluff CL Jr, Stidham KR, Ricci WM, Stanley WE, Seigler HF: Surgical management of regional lymph nodes in patients with melanoma: Experience with 4682 patients. *Ann Surg* 1994;219:120–130.

This review article describes the Duke melanoma database of 4,682 patients. The median follow-up was 4.7 years. The data suggested a significant incidence of metastases to contralateral in lymph nodal basins. A lymphoscintigraphy could be justified for the preoperative evaluation of patients with elective lymph node dissections. However, many patients who underwent a lymph node dissection demonstrated no apparent impact on survival.

Thompson SC, Jolley D. Marks R: Reduction of solar keratoses by regular sunscreen use. *N Engl J Med* 1993;329:1147–1151.

The authors describe the incidence of mortality from skin cancer, which is increasing in many countries. This study examined the use of sunscreen in reducing solar keratoses that are precursors to cutaneous carcinomas. Regular use of sunscreen prevented the development of these keratoses and, by implication, reduced the risk of skin cancer in the long term.

Tseng JF, Tanabe KK, Gadd MA, et al: Surgical management of primary cutaneous melanomas of the hands and feet. *Ann Surg* 1997;225:544–553.

In this study of 116 patients with melanoma of the hands (n = 26) and feet (n = 90), those patients with a melanoma of less than 1.5 mm had a lower incidence of nodal metastases and can be treated with a 1-cm margin. Thicker melanomas are associated with a higher rate of systemic spread. A 2-cm margin of resection and interoperative lymphatic mapping followed by lymphadenectomy, depending on the presence or absence of a sentinel node, is recommended.

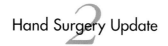

Chapter 36
Management Principles of Aggressive Tumors of the Hand and Forearm

Brian E. McGrath, MD

Introduction

Diagnosis of malignant and benign soft-tissue lesions in the hand and forearm is difficult due to their insidious growth and rare occurrence (4% malignant and 15% benign). Although the term "aggressive" refers to the higher spectrum of biologic activity that this group of neoplasms demonstrate, their rate of growth and host response pales in comparison to many infections or inflammatory conditions. Frequently, aggressive benign or malignant soft-tissue neoplasms present with little more than a slow-growing nonpainful mass; similar lesions in bone usually present with pain.

Although masses in the hand are more easily detected secondary to their relatively superficial location and are smaller in size at presentation, their metastatic potential and the consequent loss of prehensile hand function should not be underestimated. Over the last 5 years, advances in medicine have significantly enhanced our ability to care for patients with aggressive lesions of the hand and forearm. Diagnostic imaging has improved, both in quality of images and their interpretation; immunohistochemical and cytogenetic analysis have improved the characterization and subclassification of bone and soft-tissue tumors; adjuvant therapies, such as radiation therapy and chemotherapy, have improved local control of the disease process; and tissue processing has advanced to allow reliable immunohistochemical and cytogenetic analyses of core biopsies and fine needle aspirates.

Staging

The principles of staging aggressive soft-tissue and bone neoplasms were adequately outlined in the first edition of this book; only a few comments need be added. First, the entire staging of the lesion, including history and physical examination and all imaging studies, must precede the biopsy. Second, the biopsy should be performed through the most direct, limited exposure, using the surgeon's preferred technique and contaminating the fewest "expendable" structures with the biopsy tract. Excisional biopsy is not recommended if vital structures are at risk of contamination (Fig. 1). Finally, the staging system adopted by the Musculoskeletal Tumor Society from Enneking and associates does not incorporate tumor size as a variable affecting outcome. Several recent studies using the Hajdu and American Joint Committee on Cancer (AJCC) staging systems have identified tumor size as an important factor in patient survival. Although the application of these staging systems further subdivides and fragments the already small numbers of patients reported in most series of hand tumors, thereby making statistical comparison of stage difficult, tumor size should be considered in any outcome discussion.

Imaging

Imaging techniques such as computed tomography (CT) and magnetic resonance imaging (MRI) have improved dramatically in the last decade. High resolution CT and software "image reconstruction" packages aid preoperative planning for bone lesions. Improved MRI sequences, enhanced with gadolinium, and more experienced musculoskeletal radiologists have improved the identification of anatomic structures, narrowed the preoperative differential diagnosis, and enhanced the definition of tumor margins for both soft-tissue and bone lesions. These improvements allow the oncologic surgeon to cut much closer than the conventional 4- to 5-cm bone margin and the 1- to 2-cm soft-tissue margin without risking an increase in local recurrence. Closer, negative margins decrease the functional loss in an extremity, but require intensive preoperative planning by a multidisciplinary team including a musculoskeletal radiologist, radiation oncologist, hand surgeon, and oncologic surgeons.

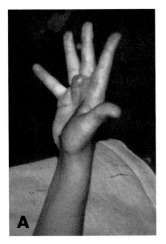
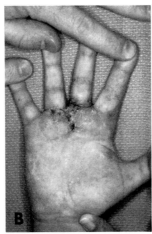
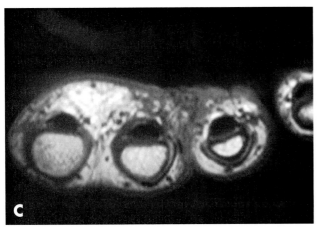
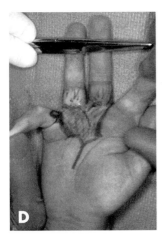
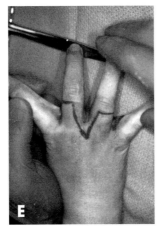

Figure 1

A, Right hand of a 9-year-old boy with a third web space epithelioid sarcoma. **B,** Hand after excisional biopsy through a Y-incision. **C,** MRI revealing the third web space tumor bed and residual tumor. **D** and **E,** Preoperative planning of double ray resection required to obtain negative margins.

Radiation Therapy and Chemotherapy

Although the mainstay of treatment for aggressive soft-tissue and bone tumors of the hand and forearm is surgery, the judicious use of radiation therapy and chemotherapy can improve local control and survival. Radiation therapy is the most widely used form of adjuvant therapy and has been shown to improve local control of malignant lesions when surgical margins are less than 1 cm. Careful planning by an experienced radiation oncologist relies heavily on 3-dimensional analysis of dosimetry to deliver appropriate ionizing energy to the tumor or tumor bed and spare as much normal tissue as possible. Many new simulation techniques have been reported recently. Palliative external beam radiation is used with patients with painful metastatic lesions to the hand and forearm. Preoperative (ie, neoadjuvant) radiation therapy is commonly employed when the lesion is close to vital, preservable structures. Although brachytherapy has also been shown to have a useful role in the management of soft-tissue sarcomas of the hand, it is often difficult to employ, requires extensive planning, and usually requires some additional soft-tissue coverage.

The role of chemotherapy in the treatment of osteogenic sarcoma, Ewing's sarcoma, and rhabdomyosarcoma has been well documented in the literature; however, current chemotherapy methods have not been proven to improve survival of patients with nonrhabdomyosarcoma soft-tissue sarcomas of the hand.

Biopsy

Biopsy of a potentially malignant lesion should be planned as carefully as the definitive resection surgery. It should be possible to incorporate the biopsy tract into the planned resection incision to allow for its complete resection with the tumor. Open incisional biopsy with intraoperative frozen section, reviewed by an experienced musculoskeletal pathologist, remains the gold standard. Improved cytopathologic tissue processing techniques have advanced the role of fine needle aspiration in the diagnosis and treatment of sarcomas. Cytopathology requires greater attention to detail by both the surgeon and pathologist to ensure that an accurate diagnosis is made. Reliable immunohistochemical and cytogenetic evaluations have been reported from academic centers devoted to fine needle aspiration. A few centers have reported reliable immunohistochemical and cytogenetic evaluations of biopsy samples obtained by fine needle aspirates.

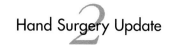
Cytogenetics and Immunohistochemistry

The greatest advances in the care of patients with sarcoma are occurring in the fields of cytogenetics and immunohistochemistry. Abnormal genes and fusion proteins have been identified in many sarcomas. The presence or absence of these abnormal products may lead to the reclassification or subclassification of the traditional histology-based staging systems. The chromosomal translocations seen in Ewing's sarcoma and rhabdomyosarcoma have been well described in all anatomic locations of the "small round blue cell tumors." These original cytogenetic abnormalities have allowed us to better differentiate among small round blue cell tumors. Unfortunately, this type of analysis takes time to prepare and process. Currently, these data are usually available only after treatment has commenced and are used to confirm the diagnosis and help design future treatment protocols. Other cytogenetic abnormalities are seen in synovial cell sarcomas, myxoid liposarcomas, myxoid chondrosarcomas, and clear sarcomas. Many other lesions have cytogenetic abnormalities yet undiscovered that may lead to improved classification and diagnosis, staging, and treatment.

Many advances in immunohistochemistry have been made over the last 5 years. This type of analysis helps classify less differentiated tissue. The difficult differential diagnosis of an epithelioid sarcoma has been improved by using immunohistochemical analysis of epithelioid membrane antigen, vimentin positivity with internal control, and high and low molecular weight cytokeratins. Cluster designation (CD) 99 identifies a surface glycoprotein encoded by the MIC2 gene that is overexpressed in Ewing's sarcoma. Antibodies to primitive muscle markers, such as MYO-D1, have helped to classify previously unclassifiable tumors as embryonal rhabdomyosarcoma.

Aggressive Tumor Types

Fibromatosis
A group of fibroblastic tumors that are locally invasive but do not metastasize, fibromatosis has been classified into superficial and deep groups. The superficial group arises from the fascia and rarely invades deep structures of the hand (eg, Dupuytren's disease). The deep group is generally referred to as aggressive fibromatosis.

Extra-abdominal desmoid/aggressive fibromatosis is only rarely encountered in the hand and forearm. The presenting symptoms of this often slow-growing mass may be pain/dysesthesia or restriction of motion. Plain radiographs may suggest a cortical erosion, but are otherwise unhelpful. MRI demonstrates the extent of the mass and its involvement with the neurovascular structures, but is seldom diagnostic. Pentavalent technetium-99m dimercaptosuccinic acid avidity and a lack of gallium-67 citrate uptake, combined with 1 relative isointense T1-weighted and hyperintense T2-weighted images compared to skeletal muscle, have been shown to be a diagnostic criterion for extra-abdominal desmoid.

Treatment of aggressive fibromatosis is nonetheless vexing. This is a benign disease, but one with a great propensity for local recurrence and extension. Complete surgical excision is the goal of therapy, but some lesions are functionally unresectable. Dosage of 50 to 60 Gy of external beam radiation therapy has been successfully used to treat nonresectable primary disease and microscopic residual following attempted surgical resection. A 25% local recurrence rate is expected when approximately 56 Gy of external beam radiation is applied to unresectable disease, while lower recurrence rates are expected with 50 Gy of external beam radiation following gross surgical resection. Complications from external beam radiation with doses less than 56 Gy are 5% over 15 years. Low-dose vinblastine and methotrexate have also been effective in treating nonresectable fibromatosis.

Giant Cell Tumor of Bone
Giant cell tumor of the distal radius represents the third most common site of giant cell tumor of bone, with an incidence of roughly 10%, while the incidence of giant cell tumor of the small bones of the hand ranges from 2% to 5%. Histologic evaluation has not been shown to be predictive of the biologic behavior of the lesion except for the rare diagnosis of a malignant variant of giant cell tumor. The treatment philosophy for the distal radius and the small bones of the hand is only controversial in that the goal of treatment is complete excision of the lesion to minimize local recurrence while preserving maximum function and durability of the residual hand.

The high rate of local recurrence of distal radius and hand giant cell tumor (25% to 80%) has been associated with less than aggressive removal of the lesion in an effort to maintain function. This has led many surgeons to treat these lesions with a more aggressive, en bloc resection followed by reconstruction with intercalary grafts, arthrodesis, osteoarticular allograft, or prosthetic replacement. The rate of local recurrence following wide resection is clearly lower, but the consequent loss of motion or stability of the wrist or digit following such reconstruction may be a high price to pay. The current strategy for treatment of giant cell tumor of the distal radius and small bones of the hand is based on the degree or percentage of bone loss secondary to the lesion. Tumors with extensive cortical bone loss or extraosseous extension should be resected and reconstructed as needed, while lesions with minimal cortical destruction and negligible extraosseous extension may be treated with an extended curettage (including power burr and electric cautery through a large cortical window, with or without adjuvant phenol cryotherapy or exothermic heat necrosis with bone cement). Following curettage of the lesion, the defect can be reconstructed with suitable material (eg, cement, allograft, autograft, demineralized bone, or bone substitutes). Follow-up should be frequent (every 3 to 4 months) for several years, and include radiographic studies appropriate to detect local recurrence prior to symptoms, significant bone loss, or extraosseous extension. Rare cases of pulmonary metastasis of benign giant cell tumors have been reported and appear to be more common from upper extremity lesions and following local recurrences.

Rhabdomyosarcoma

Although rhabdomyosarcomas constitute only 5% to 15% of sarcomas occurring in the hand and forearm, they represent the most common soft-tissue sarcoma from childhood to young adulthood. The tumor arises from mesenchymal origin and differentiates towards striated skeletal muscle. It is subclassified into 1 of 3 types—embryonal, alveolar, and pleiomorphic. The most common presenting symptom is pain, but numbness or paresthesia secondary to local nerve compression may be present.

Alveolar rhabdomyosarcoma is the most common subtype to occur in the hand, but represents the second most common type of rhabdomyosarcoma overall. The patient is generally 10 to 25 years of age. The mass often develops between the metacarpals on the dorsal or palmar surface. Embryonal rhabdomyosarcoma is the most common variant (70%), but is the second most common type to appear in the hand. It most often arises as a small mass along a flexor tendon.

Rhabdomyosarcoma is one of the "small round blue cell" tumors. The more differentiated cells resemble rhabdomyoblasts, and are more elongated with recognizable transverse striations in the cytoplasm. The predominant feature of alveolar rhabdomyosarcoma is the formation of "islands" with central paucity of cells resembling alveoli. Embryonal rhabdomyosarcoma demonstrates considerable variability of skeletal muscle differentiation. Small round blue cells prevail, with occasional rhabdomyoblastic differentiation. The clinical staging of rhabdomyosarcoma is outlined in Table 1.

Treatment for rhabdomyosarcoma requires a multidisciplinary team, including the pediatric oncologist, a surgical oncologist, and the radiation oncologist. Several protocols have

Table 1

Clinical staging of rhabdomyosarcoma

Group 1	Localized disease, completely resected
Group 2	Grossly resected tumor with microscopic residual disease but with regional lymph node metastasis
	Grossly resected tumor (regional lymph node involvement and/or extension of tumor into an adjacent organ) without microscopic residual disease
	Grossly resected tumor with microscopic residual disease but with regional lymph node metastasis
Group 3	Incomplete resection or biopsy of primary tumor with gross residual disease
Group 4	Distant metastatic disease present at time of diagnosis

(Reproduced with permission from Enzinger FM, Weiss WE: *Soft Tissue Tumors.* St. Louis, MO, CV Mosby, 1988, p 481.)

been assessed and additional agents are added to protocols regularly. Vincristine, actinomycin D, cyclophosphamide, adriamycin, and cis-platinum are the chemotherapy agents currently used on Intergroup Rhabdomyosarcoma Study (IRS) trial. Local control of the disease is obtained by surgical resection, radiation, or a combination. Five-year survival ranges from 75% for patients in groups 1 and 2 to 20% for group 4 patients.

Soft-Tissue Sarcomas of the Hand

Although soft-tissue sarcoma of the hand is usually a small nonpainful mass at presentation, the lethal potential should not be underestimated. Soft-tissue sarcomas in the hand represent 3% to 5% of all soft-tissue sarcomas. The four most common histologic subtypes in the hand are synovial cell sarcoma, malignant fibrous hysticytoma (MFH), epithelioid sarcoma, and rhabdomyosarcoma. The histologic subtypes and the location of these lesions have both been implicated in their relatively high incidence rate of regional lymph node metastasis (10% to 20%). Evaluation of the regional nodal basins with a thorough physical examination and appropriate imaging studies as well as biopsy of any suspicious nodes is advised. Local recurrence has been associated with less than wide surgical margins. The treatment of soft-tissue sarcomas of the hand should be based on the grade, stage, and size of the lesion. Both high- and low-grade

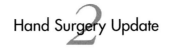

lesions require a wide surgical margin, and judicious use of adjuvant radiation therapy for margins less than 1 cm. Limb salvage and limb ablative surgeries following local recurrence in patients without metastasis have been shown to be effective and support the argument for nonablative primary surgery in carefully selected patients. The 5-year survival for patients with soft-tissue sarcoma of the hand and forearm ranges from 50% to 80% in recently reported studies.

Epithelioid Sarcoma

Epithelioid sarcoma is a malignant lesion that is often confused with granulomatous processes and with squamous cell carcinoma. Its most common location is in the hand, and it is the second or third most common soft-tissue sarcoma after synovial cell sarcoma and/or MFH in the most recently reported studies of hand and forearm sarcomas. Epithelioid sarcoma presents as a small, painless nodule. Histologically, it is represented by proliferation of large cells of polygonal shape, with ample cytoplasm and large vesicular nuclei. Cells form nodules that often contain central areas of necrosis resembling granulomatous disease. Immunohistochemical analysis with epithelial membrane antigen, high- and low-weight cytokeratins, and vimentin with internal control assist the pathologist.

Epithelioid sarcomas have a relatively high rate of metastasis to regional lymph nodes and lung. Treatment requires wide surgical resection with tailored adjuvant or neoadjuvant radiation therapy. Thorough examination of the regional lymph nodes, detailed imaging studies, and perhaps sentinel lymph node biopsy (a common practice in breast and melanoma surgeries) should be conducted.

Osteosarcoma

Unlike soft-tissue sarcomas of the hand, osteosarcoma occurring in the small bones of the hand has been reported to carry a more favorable prognosis than its more common long-bone counterpart. Osteosarcoma of the hand represents only 0.2% of all osteosarcomas, with a median age of 42 years. Marginal resection results in a high rate of local recurrence. Treatment goals are wide surgical resection and adjuvant chemotherapy for high-grade disease.

Chondrosarcoma

Chondrosarcoma remains a rare primary tumor in the hand. However, in the presence of multiple hereditary exostosis, enchondromatosis (Ollier's disease), or Maffucci's syndrome, the degeneration of a previously benign cartilage tumor to malignancy is less rare. Strict attention to rapid changes in size and pain associated with a longstanding benign cartilage tumor is important. Radiologic findings of cortical destruction, a soft-tissue mass, and a permeative lytic pattern have been associated with malignancy. Complete surgical excision remains the treatment of choice for chondrosarcomas. Metastasis has been associated with the uncommon high-grade lesions.

Metastatic Carcinoma

Carcinoma metastases to the bones in the hands is reported to represent only 0.01% of all bony metastasis. Lung cancer remains the most common form of acrometastasis, followed by the kidney. Needle biopsy should be performed following a complete work-up of the patient with an unknown primary. Palliative radiation therapy or excision should be tailored to the patient's needs.

Summary

The diagnosis, staging, treatment, and primary reconstruction for bone and soft-tissue tumors of the upper limb require a team of experienced specialists. Patient survival and functional outcome are optimized by referral of patients with these unusual lesions to appropriate centers for evaluation, diagnosis, and care.

Annotated Bibliography

Introduction

Dell PC, Stern PJ: Benign and malignant neoplasms of the upper extremity, in Peimer CA (ed): *Surgery of the Hand and Upper Extremity.* New York, NY, McGraw-Hill, 1996, pp 2231–2264.

In this thorough description of benign and malignant neoplasms that occur in the upper extremity, the authors painstakingly review each and every aspect of disease from diagnosis through treatment and outcome.

Fleegler EJ: An approach to soft tissue sarcomas of the hand and upper limb. *J Hand Surg* 1994;19B:411–419.

The author reviews general guidelines for evaluation of masses in the hand and upper extremity with special emphasis on the regional nodal basin. The most common soft-tissue sarcomas of the hand and upper extremity are described—MFH, synovial cell sarcoma, rhabdomyosarcoma, and epithelioid sarcoma.

Imaging

Kransdorf MJ, Murphey MD: MR imaging of musculoskeletal tumors of the hand and wrist. *Magn Reson Imaging Clin N Am* 1995;3:327–344.

This is a review of 3,016 cases of hand and wrist tumors seen at the AFIP over 10 years. The authors concluded that a specific diagnosis could be made or strongly suspected based on the imaging characteristics of many benign lesions, but MRI of most malignant lesions was nonspecific.

Radiation Therapy and Chemotherapy

Bray PW, Bell RS, Bowen CV, Davis A, O'Sullivan B: Limb salvage surgery and adjuvant radiotherapy for soft tissue sarcomas of the forearm and hand. *J Hand Surg* 1997;22A:495–503.

In this prospective report of 25 patients with soft-tissue sarcoma of the hand and forearm, treatment goals were to achieve adequate oncologic margins and to maximize the function of the extremity. The goal of the surgery was to achieve a wide margin. Radiation was advised for gross surgical margins that were less than 1 cm. The total dose for high-grade was 66 Gy divided into two Gy fractions, and 50 to 60 Gy for low-grade tumor. Preoperative radiation was used for patients with tumors that involved the vital neurovascular structures. Follow-up average was short, but only 3 patients developed local recurrence.

Li C, Crawford S, Mundt AJ, Vijayakumar S: Computer-aided treatment design of a distal upper extremity soft tissue tumor with electron beam radiotherapy. *Med Dosim* 1993;18:143–148.

This article provides a detailed description of an innovative approach to deliver a uniform dose of electron beam radiation to a 6-cm first web space soft-tissue sarcoma.

Cytogenetics and Immunohistochemistry

Kilpatrick SE, Garvin AJ: Recent advances in the diagnosis of pediatric soft-tissue tumors. *Med Pediatr Oncol* 1999;32:373–376.

The authors describe their experience using immunohistochemistry, cytogenetics, and molecular events to diagnose soft-tissue sarcoma in children.

Fibromatosis

Ballo MT, Zagars GK, Pollack A: Radiation therapy in the management of desmoid tumors. *Int J Radiat Oncol Biol Phys* 1998;42:1007–1014.

Describing their experience with 75 patients with aggressive fibromatosis, the authors review the indications for radiation therapy with unresectable and resectable disease. They provide an in-depth review of their experience with radiation therapy with regard to dose and complications.

Kobayashi H, Kotoura Y, Hosono M, et al: MRI and scintigraphic features of extraabdominal desmoid tumors. *Clin Imaging* 1997;21:35–39.

The authors describe their experience using technetium bone scans combined with gallium scans and conventional MRI sequences to diagnose extra-abdominal desmoid tumors.

Giant Cell Tumor

Athanasian EA, Wold LE, Amadio PC: Giant cell tumors of the bones of the hand. *J Hand Surg* 1997;22A:91–98.

The authors describe a lengthy experience with patients who had giant cell tumors of bone in the hand. Local recurrence was seen after 11 of 14 intralesional procedures involving curettage or curettage and bone grafting. Local recurrence dropped to 36% with excision of the lesion either by wide excision, amputation, or ray resection. They also observed 2 pulmonary metastases following or concurrent with local recurrences.

Chatterjee ND, Kundu S, Mondal PK, Chatterjee S, Sarkar N, Singh B: Giant cell tumour of short bones of hand. *J Indian Med Assoc* 1995;93:149–150.

The authors describe the treatment of giant cell tumors of the short bones of the hand. This in-depth presentation of 3 cases details the incidents and recommended treatment.

Vander Griend RA, Funderburk CH: The treatment of giant-cell tumors of the distal part of the radius. *J Bone Joint Surg* 1993;75A:899–908.

Twenty-three patients with giant cell tumor of the distal radius were evaluated to develop a treatment selection criteria. Interosseous lesions with minimal cortical perforation were treated effectively with curettage and cement packing. Patients with extensive extraosseous desease were best treated with wide resection.

Rhabdomyosarcoma

Giannakopoulos PN, Sotereanos DG, Tomaino MM, Goodman MA, Herndon JH: Benign and malignant muscle tumors in the hand and forearm. *Hand Clin* 1995;11:191–201.

The authors reviewed the evaluation, classification, treatment, and outcome of benign and malignant muscle tumors found in the hand and forearm. A detailed review of leiomyosarcoma and rhabdomyosarcoma is presented.

Soft-Tissue Sarcoma

Brien EW, Terek RM, Geer RJ, Caldwell G, Brennan MF, Healey JH: Treatment of soft-tissue sarcomas of the hand. *J Bone Joint Surg* 1995;77A:564–571.

A retrospective series of 23 patients with predominantly high-grade soft-tissue sarcoma of the hand were compared to a similar group of soft-tissue sarcomas of the extremity. The authors concluded that the rate of survival of the patients with soft-tissue sarcoma of the hand less than 5 cm was significantly worse than that of 152 patients who had a similar tumor at another extremity site. This difference in survival was not present when the authors controlled to the high rate of positive surgical margins in patients with soft-tissue sarcomas of the hand.

Johnstone PA, Wexler LH, Venzon DJ, et al: Sarcomas of the hand and foot: Analysis of local control and functional result with combined modality therapy in extremity preservation. *Int J Radiat Oncol Biol Phys* 1994;29:735–745.

This article is a retrospective review of 28 patients with soft-tissue sarcoma of the hand and foot—15 cases of Ewing's sarcoma, 7 cases of rhabdomyosarcoma, and 6 cases of nonrhabdomyosarcoma. All surgical treatment was limb-sparing except for 2 patients who underwent ray resection for hand sarcomas. The Ewing's sarcoma patient group was given 50 Gy, rhabdomyosarcoma group 54 Gy, and the nonrhabdomyosarcoma group 63 Gy. Local control at 5 and 10 years was 84% for Ewing's sarcoma, 100% for rhabdomyosarcoma, and 100% for nonrhabdomyosarcoma. The authors concluded that a prudent management course would be to defer amputation for the management of local recurrence.

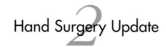

Osteosarcoma

Okada K, Wold LE, Beabout JW, Shives TC: Osteosarcoma of the hand: A clinicopathologic study of 12 cases. *Cancer* 1993;72:719–725.

In this case report on osteosarcoma of the hand, the median age was 45 years. The 12 patients had 7 tumors in the phalanges and 6 in the metacarpals. Radiographic findings were similar to that seen in other skeletal locations of osteosarcoma. Only 1 patient died of metastatic disease. Early detection of the tumor may be responsible for the good prognosis with osteosarcoma of the hand.

Sugano I, Tajima Y, Ishida Y, et al: Phalangeal intraosseous well-differentiated osteosarcoma of the hand. *Virchows Arch* 1997; 430:185–189.

This is a very detailed case report of a well differentiated intraosseous osteosarcoma of the phalanx, including radiographic, histologic, and immunohistochemical analysis.

Chondrosarcoma

Meneses MF, Unni KK, Swee RG: Bizarre parosteal osteochondromatous proliferation of bone (Nora's lesion). *Am J Surg Pathol* 1993;17:691–697.

The authors describe in detail 65 cases of bizarre parosteal osteosarcomatosis proliferations of bone; 36 of the lesions occurred in the hand. They stress the radiographic differences between exostosis and bizarre parosteal osteosarcomatosis proliferations—the lack of medullary confluence with the lesions as seen in osteochondroma. The lesions are composed of cartilage, bone, and spindle cells. All components lack malignant features. Local recurrence was common, but no metastases were seen.

Ogose A, Unni KK, Swee RG, May GK, Rowland CM, Sim FH: Chondrosarcoma of the small bones of the hands and feet. *Cancer* 1997;80:50–59.

The authors describe their experience with 88 chondrosarcoma involving the hands. They found that the radiographic findings of cortical destruction, soft-tissue mass, or permeative pattern was consistent with a diagnosis of malignancy.

Saunders C, Szabo RM, Mora S: Chondrosarcoma of the hand arising in a young patient with multiple hereditary exostoses. *J Hand Surg* 1997;22B:237–242.

The authors documented the case of a 21-year-old man with multiple hereditary exostosis who developed malignant degeneration of a previously benign thumb lesion. A thorough review of the literature is also presented.

Metastatic Disease

Abrahams TG: Occult malignancy presenting as metastatic disease to the hand and wrist. *Skeletal Radiol* 1995;24:135–137.

The authors report 3 cases of occult malignancy presenting as metastasis to the hand and wrist. They stress the importance of considering metastasis as a diagnosis when faced with any aggressive lytic or blastic lesion of the hand or wrist in a patient over 40.

Castello JR, Garro L, Romero F, Campo M, Najera A: Metastatic tumors of the hand: Report of six additional cases. *J Hand Surg* 1996;21B:547–550.

This report of 6 cases of metastatic disease to the hand includes 2 from lung, 1 from kidney, 1 of the hard palate, 1 from the larynx, and 1 of the pharynx. Treatment was palliative in all cases. Two of the patients had metastasis with the first sign of malignant disease. Median survival was only 7 months.

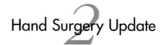

Chapter 37
Benign, Aggressive, and Malignant Neoplasms

Paul Dell, MD

Introduction

It would be impossible to review the subject of benign and malignant tumors of the musculoskeletal system in its entirety in one chapter. Because common clinical presentation, histology, and treatment are discussed in standard textbooks, this chapter will focus on areas in which significant advancements in tumor surgery have been made. Advances in imaging, which is essential for proper staging of tumors, are reviewed in the chapter on that topic.

Wrist Ganglion

The dorsal wrist ganglion typically arises from the scapholunate ligament and is found between the dorsal capsule and the scapholunate joint. Classical care of a ganglion recalcitrant to conservative care includes open excision, specifically excising the stalk, which attaches the cystic portion to the capsule. It has been suggested that it may be necessary to excise only the stalk, leaving the main cyst in situ. Complications associated with surgical excision include loss of palmar flexion secondary to dorsal scarring and scapholunate instability secondary to excessive scapholunate ligament excision.

Arthroscopic excision of the stalk has been described. Using standard arthroscopic instrumentation and principles, a wrist scope is placed in an ulnar portal directed radial to the dorsal aspect of the scapholunate ligament. In a series of 18 patients, the ganglion stalk was seen approximately 60% of the time. When a needle is placed through the ganglion and into the stalk, the origin may be seen more clearly. A radial portal is established, typically the standard 3/4 portal. Approximately 1 cm of the dorsal capsule is resected with a power shaver. No recurrences were reported at 16 months' follow-up.

Arthroscopic resection of a ganglion stalk accomplishes the objectives of surgical excision with much less invasive technique. Care should be taken to avoid injury to the extensor tendons and the scapholunate ligament. The long-term results are unknown at this time and further evaluation of this technique is needed. Only overt ganglia should be addressed arthroscopically.

Osteoid Osteoma

Osteoid osteoma is a benign bone-forming lesion with a predilection for the cortex of the shafts of long bones. Classically, patients complain of pain that is characteristically described as dull and aching, typically worse at night. Pain relief with nonsteroidal anti-inflammatory agents is often prompt. By definition, osteoid osteomas are less than 2 cm in diameter and composed of abnormal osteoid and osteoblasts surrounded by a rim of reactive bone. The nidus sometimes is difficult to isolate but improvements in preoperative evaluation, which include computed tomography (CT), particularly when supplemented with intravenous contrast, have proven helpful in isolation. Imaging defines the location of the nidus precisely to reduce the possibility of incomplete resection. Treatment classically has been en bloc excision. However, the amount of bone that must be removed in an excisional procedure is often substantial, and surgical localization may be unsuccessful if an intense periosteal reaction is present.

A variety of techniques other than en bloc excision have been reported recently. CT-guided percutaneous excision using 14-gauge bone biopsy needles resulted in resolution of symptoms in 14 of 16 patients, with no complications. Percutaneous methods of producing thermal necrosis within the lesion have included the use of laser photocoagulation and radiofrequency ablation. In the former, a CT-guided fiber was introduced into the nidus through an 18-gauge needle. Coagulative necrosis was seen in a well-defined area at the tip of the fiber, measuring 5 to 9 mm. Radiofrequency ablation uses an electrode introduced into the lesion through a biopsy tract, similarly producing a 1-cm sphere of thermonecrosis. No attempt was made to remove the lesion with either technique. With both of these techniques, symptoms were completely resolved in 90% of the patients. There was no curtailment in activities, and no recurrences were noted in those successfully treated patients.

Soft-Tissue Sarcoma

Soft-tissue sarcomas represent fewer than 1% of all newly diagnosed malignant tumors. Sixty percent occur in extremities, two thirds occur in the lower extremity, usually the thigh, and one third occur in the upper extremity, most commonly in the arm. Histologically, soft-tissue sarcomas are a heterogenous group of tumors representing approximately 30 different types.

The treatment and prognosis of soft-tissue sarcomas depend more on tumor site, tumor size, and histologic malignancy grade than on exact histologic type. Deeply seated tumors of both intermediate and high grade histologic types have a poor prognosis because of the general increase in size before detection and the proximity to neurovascular bundles. Deeply seated intermediate-grade tumors measuring greater than 10 cm have a higher incidence of metastases and a lower 5-year survival than a group of tumors that are more superficially located, smaller in size, but of comparable histologic type. However, in high-grade tumors, deeply seated lesions measuring greater than 5 cm have a much poorer prognosis than more superficial, smaller lesions. Thus, the tumor size that is significant for prognosis of patients with soft-tissue sarcoma is different among intermediate- (10 cm) and high-grade (5 cm) tumors. In addition to tumor size and location, tumor necrosis and vascular invasion have emerged as strong prognostic factors. Large high-grade sarcomas are more likely to be necrotic as a result of inherent factors related to tumor growth.

Specific chromosomal changes have been detected in some types of soft-tissue sarcomas, specifically synovial sarcoma, liposarcoma, and alveolar rhabdomyosarcoma. These chromosomal changes may be helpful in classification, but the prognostic significance is unclear at this point.

Treatment

Surgery alone, surgery combined with radiotherapy, surgery combined with brachytherapy, or radiotherapy alone have been advocated in the treatment of soft-tissue sarcomas. The surgical objective is to achieve adequate surgical margins for good local tumor control. Local recurrence of 60% can be expected with marginal excision. Wide excision, which includes several centimeters of normal tissue, decreases the risk of local recurrence to approximately 20%. Fewer than 10% of patients with soft-tissue sarcomas in the extremities undergo amputations. Generally, amputations are indicated for tumors that infiltrate the skeleton or neurovascular bundle.

Postoperative radiotherapy, in combination with surgery, is the most common method for treatment of soft-tissue sarcomas. For this treatment to have a reasonable prognosis, all macroscopic disease must be adequately excised. Occasionally, it is impossible to achieve adequate surgical margins for large, deep intramuscular sarcomas. In these cases, preoperative radiotherapy may be helpful for preservation of the limb. Theoretically, preoperative radiotherapy inactivates tumor cells to reduce metastatic potential and decreases tumor volume. A smaller volume of irradiation is necessary preoperatively compared to that needed for the larger postoperative wound bed. Irradiation causes formation of a dense pseudocapsule that facilitates surgical excision.

Preoperative irradiation has been reported to cause extensive tumor necrosis in 75% of 27 patients. Using a similar irradiation protocol and assessment of necrosis, extensive necrosis was found in only 35% of cases. Although it is somewhat difficult to compare the results of these 2 studies because of patient selection, the more recent report includes patients that would be most appropriate for preoperative irradiation. Overtly, these were patients with large sarcomas that were adjacent to neurovascular structures or were in anatomic areas that rendered limb-salvage surgery difficult. However, these patients are the very specific subgroup that are candidates for preoperative radiotherapy.

Postoperative radiotherapy and surgery represent the most common combination of treatments for extremity soft-tissue sarcomas. When compared to postoperative radiotherapy, preoperative irradiation was not associated with any benefit in terms of relapse-free survival, overall survival, or actuarial local control. However, there was a significantly higher incidence of major wound complications among patients treated with preoperative irradiation. The advantages of postoperative radiotherapy include no delayed wound healing and a tumor specimen that would not be affected by any response to irradiation. Generally recommended radiotherapy doses range between 60 and 70 Gy for 6 to 7 weeks. Local recurrence rates of between 10% and 20% have been reported. A distinct disadvantage of postoperative therapy is the occurrence of wound complications that may delay radiotherapy timing, thereby allowing residual microscopic disease to proliferate, perhaps altering the patient's prognosis. Preoperative irradiation should be reserved for those situations in which the tumor is initially thought to be resectable. Chemotherapy has not been successful in treating localized soft-tissue sarcomas. Following irradiation, the patient should be restaged and final decision made as to appropriateness of limb-salvage surgery.

Brachytherapy gives excellent local control with the advantage of a short overall treatment time. A combination of adequate surgery and brachytherapy is highly effective in improving local control for high-grade tumors, independent of size and location in the extremity. However, no effect has been shown in preventing distant metastases or in prolonging survival in high-grade tumors. Brachytherapy offers several theoretical advantages in the management of soft-tissue sarcomas. The application of radiation sources directly into the tumor bed permits the administration of a high dose to the target area, while sparing adjacent normal uninvolved structures. Immediate postoperative application has the theoretical advantage of treating tumor cells before dense scarring, which occurs with the completion of wound healing, the usual time when postoperative irradiation is started. Brachytherapy is limited by the size of the implant, 20 to 25×10 cm. Wound closure requires planning to avoid undue tension over the catheters. To diminish wound complications, the radioactive material is not loaded into the catheter until 5 to 6 days after surgery; this permits the initiation of wound healing. A dose of 45 Gy in 4 or 5 days at 0.5 cm from the plane of the source usually is prescribed.

Selected small soft-tissue sarcomas can be managed by wide excision alone. Sarcomas smaller than 5 cm that were located superficially in the extremity and treated with wide local excision had the same recurrence rate and survival rate in patients treated with and without postoperative radiotherapy.

Although adequate resection margins can be achieved in certain locations, lesions around the elbow are invariably difficult to excise. Radiotherapy remains the essential component of the limb-sparing approach to such tumors. Soft-tissue sarcomas of the hand were once believed to be treated best by amputation alone because radiotherapy was believed to cause unacceptable morbidity. With attention to radiation technique, however, function can be preserved, even with doses of 60 Gy or higher. Nearly 90% of the patients with sarcoma of the forearm and hand who were treated by limb salvage and adjuvant radiotherapy and survived were able to return to occupational activities of daily living with no or minimal functional limitation. With careful design of treatment fields, a significant functional limitation resulting from adjuvant radiotherapy was found to be uncommon.

Indications for radiotherapy alone for soft-tissue sarcoma are limited to patients with locally advanced inoperable, or recurrent, metastatic disease. The aim of treatment is palliation.

Treatment After Unplanned Resection

It is not unusual for patients who have had an incisional biopsy or unplanned resection of a lesion to present with a subsequent diagnosis of soft-tissue sarcoma. Unplanned excisions without adequate preoperative staging frequently lead to inadequate surgical excisions. The margins of the resection are difficult to assess accurately, and it is impossible to estimate the extent of residual tumor. If residual tumor load is known to be small, it would be safe to manage the patient with irradiation alone. However, if there is substantial burden of residual sarcoma in the wound, additional wide resection of the previous operation site should be advised. In a recent study, at least one third of the patients who had no detectable tumor on physical examination or cross-sectional imaging after an unplanned excision had residual sarcoma on histologic examination of the specimen obtained at repeat resection. With such a high predilection for persistence of disease, it is recommended that a repeat wide excision be performed after staging studies. These studies indicate that emphasis should be placed on careful preoperative staging before the index procedure. To avoid unplanned excisions, all patients who have a subfascial mass should have cross-sectional imaging of the local site as well as incisional or needle biopsy before resection is attempted. In one study, microscopic residual tumor was found in 49% of tumor beds after marginal excision following primary excision without staging. No recurrences were noted in patients who underwent wide local excision of the tumor or of the previous operation site.

Malignant Bone Lesions

Osteosarcoma

In the prechemotherapy era, osteosarcomas treated by ablative surgery alone had a dismal prognosis. Five-year survival figures published before 1972 were consistently reported at 20%. The literature is replete with chemotherapy trials that have proven beyond doubt the superiority of adjuvant/neoadjuvant multiagent combination chemotherapy over surgery alone. Chemotherapeutic agents found effective in osteogenic sarcoma include adriamycin, cisplatin, high dose methotrexate (HDMTX), bleomycin, cyclophosphamide, and ifosfamide. New chemotherapeutic agents are added regularly, and dosages and timing are manipulated frequently.

The use of preoperative chemotherapy was initially reported in 1979. When compared to adjuvant chemotherapy alone, the use of neoadjuvant chemotherapeutic agents had a 2-year disease-free survival rate of 70%. Subsequently, neoadjuvant therapy has been used with increasing frequency in recent years. This approach may facilitate limb-salvage procedures and allow the oncologist to customize postoperative chemotherapy based on tumor response. Tumors perilously close to neurovascular bundles may become resectable following chemotherapy, thus avoiding limb ablation.

Adjuvant chemotherapy is used postoperatively to eliminate micrometastases that might be present. Most current chemotherapy regimens incorporate adriamycin, cisplatin, and HDMTX. The combination of bleomycin, cyclophosphamide, and actinomycin D is also widely used. The primary toxic effects of methotrexate are myelosuppression or gastrointestinal mucosal inflammation. These typically occur 5 to 10 days after the dose, but can be prevented by the administration of lucovorin and, more recently, the use of granulocyte colony stimulating factor. Nephrotoxicity as a result of HDMTX can delay drug clearance and markedly enhance the toxic effects of methotrexate.

In an attempt to determine the prognostic factors that influence disease-free survival in patients with nonmetastatic osteosarcoma of the extremities, literature published since the early l970s was reviewed. This time was chosen to represent the start of the chemotherapeutic era. Diagnostic variables evaluated included age, sex, anatomic tumor location, tumor size, and tumor necrosis as a response to neoadjuvant chemotherapy. Although tumor size and necrosis following neoadjuvant chemotherapy were significant prognostic variables in relation to survival in univariate analysis, only tumor necrosis maintained its significance in multivariate analysis.

In a recent review of 268 patients with nonmetastatic osteosarcoma of the extremity, neoadjuvant chemotherapy consisted of 4 courses of HDMTX and 1 course of bleomycin, cyclophosphamide, and dactinomycin (DCD). Adjuvant chemotherapy was dictated by histologic response to preoperative chemotherapy. Good responders (those with less than 5% residual viable tumor) were treated postoperatively with HDMTX, DCD and doxorubicin (DOX). The poor histologic responders were treated with DCD, DOX, and cisplatin. Tumors from 206 patients were evaluated for histologic response. Of these 206 patients, 118 (57%) underwent amputation; 88 (43%) had limb salvage surgery. Amputations were performed more often for large tumors and for patients whose neoadjuvant therapy was terminated because of local progression in size of the lesion. Good histologic responders had an 8-year postoperative event-free survival rate of 87%; those with a poor histologic response had an 8-year postoperative event-free survival rate of 46% and a survival rate of 52%. Unfortunately, only 58 (28%) of the 206 patients whose histologic response could be assessed displayed a good histologic response to neoadjuvant chemotherapy, while 148 (72%) had a poor histologic response. Additionally, 11 patients developed early distant metastases while in the neoadjuvant phase of their care.

Gadolinium-enhanced magnetic resonance (MR) may be helpful to evaluate the degree of vascularity or necrosis following chemotherapy. After routine MR imaging, subtraction MR was performed in the same plane with gadolinium enhancement. Subtraction images were created by subtracting precontrast images from enhanced T1-weighted images. In a similar fashion, the effect of neoadjuvant therapy on tumors has been measured by scanning with fluorine-18-fluorodeoxyglucose positron emission tomography. In both techniques, the initial results need to be further substantiated.

When detectable pulmonary metastases occur after the index treatment of extremity osteosarcomas, they frequently are located in the periphery of the lung and are amenable to surgical excision. For the patient to be a candidate for pulmonary resection, the primary tumor site has to be completely controlled and no other metastatic lesions noted. Neoadjuvant and adjuvant chemotherapy at the time of pulmonary wedge resection has extended the 5-year survival by 23%. The risk of metastases is directly related to complete resection of the primary tumor. Tumor-free margins must be obtained at the index procedure. Interestingly, neoadjuvant chemotherapy and metastatic nodule necrosis is not a prognostic factor as it is in the primary tumor resection. Patients with metastases to bone uniformly do poorly.

Approximately 20% of patients with osteosarcoma have radiologically detectable pulmonary metastases at their initial evaluation. In a report of 19 patients presenting with pulmonary metastases, lung metastases disappeared in 3 patients after primary chemotherapy. In the remaining 16 patients, a simultaneous resection of the primary and metastatic tumors was performed after chemotherapy. Of the patients that achieved radiologic remission at a 30-month follow-up, 55% remained continuously free of disease. A strong correlation was found in these patients between degree of necrosis of the primary tumor and metastatic tumor. All patients received a neoadjuvant course of HDMTX, cisplatin, DOX, and ifosfamide. Postoperative chemotherapy began approximately 2 weeks after surgery, utilizing the same agents.

Ewing's Sarcoma

Before the use of adjuvant chemotherapy for the treatment of Ewing's sarcoma, the 5-year survival for these patients was approximately 10%. Surgery was reserved principally for local control if the lesion was in a resectable area, such as the fibula. A combination of vincristine, adriamycin, and cyclophosphamide has formed the basis for standard chemotherapy treatment for Ewing's sarcoma. Because aggressive chemotherapy has dramatically improved the prognosis of patients with Ewing's sarcoma, the issue of local control has become more important. In patients who have primary lesions in areas that are not resectable, twice daily radiotherapy has been initiated to improve local control and to maintain function after treatment. The dose of twice daily radiotherapy varied

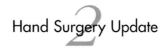
depending on the response of the soft-tissue component of the tumor to chemotherapy and ranged from 50 to 60 Gy at 1.8 to 2 Gy per fraction. After the initial radiotherapy treatment, chemotherapy was started in all cases.

There appears to be a strong relationship, perhaps even a common cell of origin, between Ewing's sarcoma and primitive neuroectodermal tumor of bone. Chromosomal translocation has been identified in both as well as high levels of cholene acetyl transferase activity. Although Ewing's sarcoma has no unique antigenic properties, negating any benefit of immunohistochemistry, identification of specific chromosomal aberrations has recently been recorded. Transcripts have been found in all cell lines and tissue samples of Ewing's sarcoma but not in any other tumors, thereby aiding in diagnosis. Early diagnosis is important to tailor the appropriate chemotherapeutic course.

Wound Healing Complications After Musculoskeletal Sarcoma

There is a high rate of wound healing complications associated with musculoskeletal sarcoma resections. Wound complications range from 5% to 35% and are anticipated in individuals undergoing resection. The procedures are lengthy and involve extensive exposures. Frequently, these patients have received preoperative chemotherapy and/or radiation therapy and may be systemically ill. The patient's nutritional status should be evaluated by serum albumin levels. A good nutritional status for wound healing would be defined as serum albumin levels greater than 3.5 g/dl. Specific factors that have been associated with wound healing complications include allogeneic blood transfusions, preoperative chemotherapy and radiotherapy, and large undermining of skin flaps. Allogeneic blood transfusions may depress immune competence and, therefore, alter wound healing. In most sarcoma resections, there is significant undermining of skin and, therefore, devascularization of skin flaps, which results in greater tension on the directly closed wound. Concomitantly, there is a large surgical dead space that is a site for hematoma or seroma in the postoperative period.

Preoperative radiotherapy obviously affects vascularity of the skin flaps and decreases their mobility. It is mandatory in prevention of wound complications to thoroughly plan the surgical procedure, which may and often does include transfer of vascularized tissue into the defect left by tumor resection. Tissue transfer decreases skin tension and obliterates dead space. Particularly useful in preoperative irradiation, vascularized tissue transferred from outside the field of irradiation provides a healthier basis for wound healing.

Extremity Reconstruction

Advances in adjuvant therapy and surgical techniques have made limb-sparing surgery an option in up to 80% of patients with malignant tumors. Successful limb-sparing surgery employs the established principles of oncology surgery. Tumor resection must be achieved with a wide surgical margin. Skeletal reconstruction of massive defects has included autogenous grafts, arthrodeses, allografts, composite allografts, and endoprosthetic replacements. Following skeletal reconstruction, local muscle flaps or free-tissue transfers are necessary to cover and close the resection site. Local rotational flaps or free flaps have dramatically decreased the rates of local wound complication and infection. Malignant lesions of the hand are unusual and are typically handled by subtotal amputation. The anatomic peculiarities of the elbow make it difficult to accomplish the surgical objectives of tumor resection without compromise of joint, nerve, or vascular structures. Consequently, in the upper extremity the limb-sparing surgery is reserved for malignant lesions of the humerus. In a report of prosthetic replacement in 29 proximal humeri, only 3 (approximately 10%) underwent revision. Additionally, there was 1 local recurrence of tumor, and 1 patient underwent amputation because of infection. Prosthetic replacement of the humerus resulted in higher functional scores when compared to the lower extremity.

Immediate free-tissue transfer provides an excellent, well-vascularized soft-tissue envelope over bone reconstruction, particularly in previously irradiated fields. With reported patency of 97%, the survival rate of free flaps is similar to that in traumatic reconstructions. Free flaps obviously also are indicated where large soft-tissue sarcomas have been excised. Flaps tolerate irradiation well and provide a suitable bed under which tendon transfers may be performed. Free flaps decrease wound complications and allow earlier healing, thereby permitting the oncologist to proceed with adjuvant therapy and enhancing the efficacy of limb-salvage surgery.

Annotated Bibliography

Ganglion

Osterman AL, Raphael J: Arthroscopic resection of dorsal ganglion of the wrist. *Hand Clin* 1995;11:7–12.

Eighteen dorsal wrist ganglia were arthroscopically excised without recurrence. The technique is described.

Osteoid Osteoma

Gangi A, Dietemann JL, Gasser B, et al: Interstitial laser photocoagulation of osteoid osteomas with use of CT guidance. *Radiology* 1997;203:843–848.

The authors describe thermal destruction of nidus using a high-power semiconductor diode laser with an optical fiber.

Roger B, Bellin MF, Wioland M, Grenier P: Osteoid osteoma: CT-guided percutaneous excision confirmed with immediate follow-up scintigraphy in 16 outpatients. *Radiology* 1996;201:239–242.

The osteoid osteoma nidus was removed in 14 of 16 patients without complication using 14-gauge biopsy cutting needles.

Rosenthal DI, Springfield DS, Gebhardt MC, Rosenberg AE, Mankin HJ: Osteoid osteoma: Percutaneous radio-frequency ablation. *Radiology* 1995;197:451–454.

A small radiofrequency electrode was introduced into the lesion through the biopsy track. No attempt was made to remove the lesion.

Soft-Tissue Sarcoma

Bray PW, Bell RS, Bowen CV, Davis A, O'Sullivan B: Limb salvage surgery and adjuvant radiotherapy for soft tissue sarcomas of the forearm and hand. *J Hand Surg* 1997;22A:495–503.

Local recurrence was related to original marginal excision. Minimal functional limitations were noted in activities of daily living.

Cheng EY, Dusenbery KE, Winters MR, Thompson RC: Soft tissue sarcomas: Preoperative versus postoperative radiotherapy. *J Surg Oncol* 1996;61:90–99.

Twenty-eight patients underwent preoperative irradiation and 33 patients underwent postoperative therapy. A higher incidence of wound complications without any benefit was found in those patients receiving preoperative radiation.

Geer RJ, Woodruff J, Casper ES, Brennan MF: Management of small soft-tissue sarcoma of the extremity in adults. *Arch Surg* 1992;127:1285–1289.

Small, superficial soft-tissue sarcomas may be amenable to wide excision without radiotherapy.

Gibbs CP, Peabody TD, Mundt AJ, Montag AG, Simon MA: Oncological outcomes of operative treatment of subcutaneous soft-tissue sarcomas of the extremities. *J Bone Joint Surg* 1997;79A:888–897.

Sixty-two patients had primary surgery without staging; 59 patients had either palpable or microscopic recurrence. All patients underwent a wide excision following staging; there was no recurrence.

Harrison LB, Janjan N: Brachytherapy in sarcomas. *Hematol Oncol Clin North Am* 1995;9:747–763.

This historical review of brachytherapy also provides comparison to effectiveness of external beam therapy.

Hew L, Kandel R, Davis A, O'Sullivan B, Catton C, Bell R: Histological necrosis in soft tissue sarcoma following preoperative irradiation. *J Surg Oncol* 1994;57:111–114.

Forty-eight patients with soft-tissue sarcoma that had adverse features for limb-salvage surgery were treated by preoperative irradiation followed by surgery. Only 17 patients (35%) demonstrated greater than 80% tumor necrosis, and that extensive necrosis was more likely to be found in liposarcomas.

Hilaris BS, Bodner WR, Mastoras CA: Role of brachytherapy in adult soft tissue sarcomas. *Semin Surg Oncol* 1997;813:196–203.

Brachytherapy and surgery were found to be highly effective in improving local control. However, no effect was shown in preventing distant metastases, suggesting that perhaps adjuvant irradiation may be additionally beneficial.

Nakanishi H, Tomita Y, Ohsawa M, et al: Tumor size as a prognostic indicator of histologic grade of soft tissue sarcoma. *J Surg Oncol* 1997;65:183–187.

One hundred sixty-two patients with soft tissue sarcomas were divided into intermediate or high grade histologic type. Tumor size was found to be a strong prognostic indicator but differed dependent on histologic grading.

Ngan SY: Radiotherapy in soft tissue sarcoma of the extremities. *Acta Orthop Scand* 1997;273(suppl):112–116.

This is a review of the different modalities of care in the treatment of soft-tissue sarcomas.

Noria S, Davis A, Kandel R, et al: Residual disease following unplanned excision of soft-tissue sarcoma of an extremity. *J Bone Joint Surg* 1996;78A:650–655.

Sixty-five patients were referred for additional management after an unplanned soft-tissue sarcoma excision. There was no way to predict which patients would have residual tumor and advised repeat excision.

Willett CG, Schiller AL, Suit HD, Mankin HJ, Rosenberg A: The histologic response of soft tissue sarcoma to radiation therapy. *Cancer* 1987;60:1500–1504.

Following resection of soft-tissue sarcomas, the extent of histologic nerosis in the specimen was recorded and graded.

Osteosarcoma

Bacci G, Mercuri M, Briccoli A, et al: Osteogenic sarcoma of the extremity with detectable lung metastases at presentation: Results of treatment of 23 patients with chemotherapy followed by simultaneous resection of primary and metastatic lesions. *Cancer* 1997;79:245–254.

The combination of aggressive chemotherapy with resection of the primary and metastatic lesions permitted a free of disease interval of 30 months in 55% of patients. Patients who never achieved a tumor-free status died within a few months.

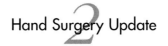
Davis AM, Bell RS, Goodwin PJ: Prognostic factors in osteosarcoma: A critical review. *J Clin Oncol* 1994;12:423–431.

The extent of tumor necrosis after neoadjuvant chemotherapy was found to be the most sensitive prognostic factor in evaluating children with osteosarcoma.

Jones DN, McCowage GB, Sostman HD, et al: Monitoring of neoadjuvant therapy response of soft-tissue and musculoskeletal sarcoma using fluorine-18-FDG PET. *J Nucl Med* 1996;37:1438–1444.

Changes in accumulation of fluorodeoxyglucose in tumors after neoadjuvant chemotherapy may be helpful in demonstrating response to therapy.

Provisor AJ, Ettinger LJ, Nachman JB, et al: Treatment of non-metastatic osteosarcoma of the extremity with preoperative and postoperative chemotherapy: A report from the Children's Cancer Group. *J Clin Oncol* 1997;15:76–84.

Postoperative chemotherapy was tailored to the histologic response achieved after neoadjuvant chemotherapy. Survival and disease-free interval were found to be directly related to histologic response.

Wada T, Isu K, Takeda N, Usui M, Ishii S, Yamawaki S: A preliminary report of neoadjuvant chemotherapy NSH-7 study in osteosarcoma: preoperative salvage chemotherapy based on clinical tumor response and the use of granulocyte colony-stimulating factor. *Oncology* 1996;53:221–227.

Human granulocyte colony-stimulating factor was used to prevent leukocytopenia and to increase the dose intensity of the chemotherapy.

Ward WG, Mikaelian K, Dorey F, et al: Pulmonary metastases of stage IIB extremity osteosarcoma and subsequent pulmonary metastases. *J Clin Oncol* 1994;12:1849–1858.

Aggressive pulmonary resection of metastatic osteosarcoma, when combined with preoperative and postoperative chemotherapy, can significantly prolong survival. Bone metastasis has a dismal prognosis.

Ewing's Sarcoma

Bolek TW, Marcus RB Jr, Mendenhall NP, Scarborough MT, Graham-Pole J: Local control and functional results after twice-daily radiotherapy for Ewing's sarcoma of the extremities. *Int J Radiat Oncol Biol Phys* 1996;35:687–692.

Functional results were improved after twice-daily radiation in a group of 37 patients.

Eggli KD, Quiogue T, Moser RP Jr: Ewing's sarcoma. *Radiol Clin North Am* 1993;31:325–337.

Authors present a review of pertinent clinical histologic presentations and therapeutic modalities for Ewing's sarcoma.

Scotlandi K, Serra M, Manara, MC, et al: Immunostaining of the p 30/32 mic2 antigen and molecular detection of EWS rearrangements for the diagnosis of Ewing's sarcoma and peripheral neuroectodermal tumor. *Hum Pathol* 1996;27:408–416.

Detection of EWS fusion transcripts enabled early diagnosis of Ewing's and proper management.

Postoperative Wound Complications

Chmell MJ, Schwartz HS: Analysis of variables affecting wound healing after musculoskeletal sarcoma resections. *J Surg Oncol* 1996;61:185–189.

Preoperative chemotherapy, depressed preoperative hematocrit, and allogenic blood transfusions were found to affect wound healing outcomes.

Peat BG, Bell RS, Davis A, et al: Wound-healing complications after soft-tissue sarcoma surgery. *Plast Reconstr Surg* 1994;93:980–987.

Preoperative irradiation, smoking, vascular disease, and extent of soft-tissue dissection influenced wound healing. Vascularized tissue transfer was often planned when patients had received preoperative irradiation.

Limb Salvage

Cordeiro PG, Neves RI, Hidalgo DA: The role of free tissue transfer following oncologic resection in the lower extremity. *Ann Plast Surg* 1994;33:9–16.

Fifty-nine free flaps had an overall success rate of 96.6%. The most common flap was musculocutaneous.

Heiner J, Rao V, Mott W: Immediate free tissue transfer for distal musculoskeletal neoplasms. *Ann Plast Surg* 1993;30:140–146.

Ten patients were treated for soft-tissue sarcoma distal to the elbow or knee.

Malawer MM, Chou LB: Prosthetic survival and clinical results with use of large-segment replacements in the treatment of high-grade bone sarcomas. *J Bone Joint Surg* 1995;77A:1154–1165.

Eighty-two patients underwent limb-sparing surgery with prosthetic reconstruction. When compared to lower extremity reconstruction, the proximal humerus had the highest functional score and was associated with the least complications.

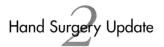

Hand Surgery Update 2

Section IX
Pediatric Hand

Chapter 38
Trauma and Infection in the Hand and Wrist in Children

Chapter 39
Congenital Anomalies

Chapter 40
Spasticity and Cerebral Palsy

American Society for Surgery of the Hand

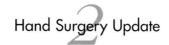

Chapter 38
Trauma and Infection in the Hand and Wrist in Children

387

Ronald C. Burgess, MD

Introduction

The child's hand has open physes and its soft tissues and skeletal structures have different tolerance to stress when compared to the adult hand. In addition, it frequently is difficult to establish an accurate diagnosis in the immature patient.

Mechanism of Injury

Child abuse must regrettably be remembered as a source of hand injury in our society. Direct impact as the child attempts to protect his or her face is responsible for most adult-inflicted hand trauma in children.

Athletic activities, such as gymnastics or platform diving, contribute to injury to the wrist and hand. Repetitive compression trauma to the immature wrist can cause physeal widening, cystic changes within the distal radius and carpal bones, and metaphyseal beaking of the distal radius. If continued, these same stresses may lead to premature growth arrest of the distal radius with ulnar overgrowth and impaction as the source of wrist pain. Loose bodies within the radiocarpal joint, ligamentous injuries, and synovitis are also found with repetitive impact loading.

Principles of Management

A honed index of suspicion is needed in caring for the injured hand in the child. Careful physical examination, anticipation of injury based on mechanism and location of symptoms, comparison radiographs, and repeat examination after a few days of splinting should allow accurate diagnosis. Penetrating injury in the child is often best evaluated under anesthesia with preparations to repair all possible injured structures.

Flexor Tendon Injury

Injury to the flexor tendons can be inferred from the resting posture of the digit (Fig. 1). Partial injury may also

cause an altered stance of the finger but is more likely to be discovered late. Early exploration of suspicious wounds may be needed to ascertain the status of underlying structures.

Zone II flexor tendon injuries in children remain problematic. Because the worst early complication following flexor tendon repair is rupture, repair of digital flexor tendons in children is best protected by immobilization for 3 to 4 weeks. In a large group of children with zone II flexor tendon injuries, there was no benefit of an early mobilization program compared to immobilization for 3 to 4 weeks in a young child. However, immobilization beyond 4 weeks resulted in greater stiffness. Controlled mobilization in selected older children may have merit. Motion may improve slightly with growth and continued use of the digit.

Results of late digital flexor tenolysis in a child younger than 10 years of age were disappointing. There have been no recent studies comparing the results of flexor tendon reconstruction with direct repair. Because the improved results in adults following flexor tendon repair are related to early, controlled mobilization, children may be better candidates for tendon grafting.

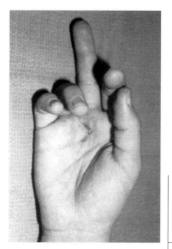

Figure 1

The loss of the normal cascade of the fingers is evidence of flexor tendon laceration in this small laceration of the palm.

Skeletal Injury

The most common location for physeal injury is in the child's hand. Salter-Harris type II pattern is the most common, followed by Salter-Harris type III. Salter Harris type II was the predominant injury at the metacarpophalangeal joint; Salter-Harris type III was more common at the proximal interphalangeal joint. Multiple physeal injuries in the same hand do occur. Indications for surgical intervention include displacement of articular surfaces, especially in condylar and subcondylar fractures, entrapment of fragments, and inability to obtain or maintain a reduction (Fig. 2). Complications of these injuries, although uncommon, include angulation, deformity, entrapment of adjacent tendons, and premature closure of growth plates (Fig. 3). There is limited ability to remodel angulation; rotational deformity does not remodel. Osteochondral grafting for articular defects using parts of the carpometacarpal articulation of the index or long finger appear to have some usefulness in replacing lost bone and cartilage stock.

Two cases of physeal fracture dislocations of the distal phalanx have been reported. The distal phalangeal epiphysis was displaced by the pull of the extensor tendon to the dorsal aspect of the distal interphalangeal (DIP) joint. In each the diagnosis was made late, and the presenting complaint was a dorsal mass at the DIP joint.

Carpal injuries do occur in children and must be suspected in cases in which symptoms fail to resolve (Fig. 4). Imaging studies comparing injured and uninjured sides are most helpful in assessing injuries to areas with unossified skeletal structures.

Injury to the distal end of the forearm in the child may involve a Galeazzi type lesion. The injury to the ulnar side of the wrist may be ligamentous (a Galeazzi lesion) or transphyseal (a Galeazzi equivalent lesion). Recognition of the physeal injury may be difficult, and open treatment may be necessary. Growth arrest following transphyseal fracture is rare but will result in progressive deformity if not recognized. Long-term follow-up of physeal injuries should help identify those children before significant deformity develops.

Thermal Injury

The most common cause of burn injury to the child's hand is the household iron. Most of the burn injuries were accidental although abuse occurred in 7% in 1 series. Treatment and reconstruction of the burned hand and thumb observe the same principles in children as in adults: active motion during healing of superficial burns, early excision of deeper

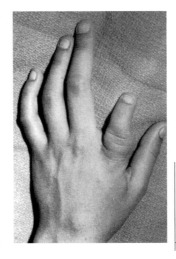

Figure 3
An infected open fracture of the proximal phalanx of the index finger as a toddler led to growth arrest and significant deformity at maturity.

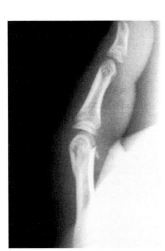

Figure 2
The distal spike of the proximal fragment is displaced into the subcondylar fossa and will prevent flexion unless the fracture is reduced.

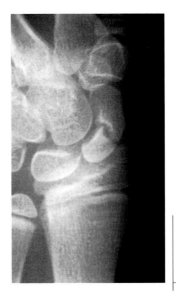

Figure 4
This 4-month-old fracture of the scaphoid in a 9-year-old healed with 3 additional months of casting.

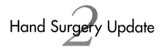

burns, coverage with skin graft (full thickness if possible), and temporary wire fixation of joints to prevent contractures. Factors related to poor outcome include burns to the thumb-index web space, poor compliance with care, deeper burns, and dorsal burns (Fig. 5).

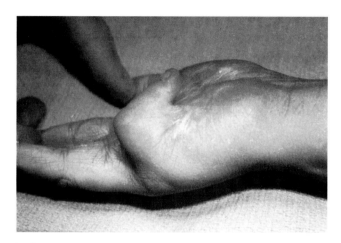

Figure 5

A palmar burn at age 2 was treated with dressing changes; there was progressive flexion deformity of the little finger by age 11.

Infections

Osteomyelitis of the distal forearm resulted in acquired radial clubhand deformity. Surgical reconstruction included bone grafting, centralization, and Ilizarov lengthening in order to improve appearance and maintain mobility. Residual forearm shortening is significant when the growth arrest occurred early.

Pediatric herpetic infections of the hand are most commonly found in younger patients with oral lesions. Finger or thumb sucking is the associated behavior in these children. Initial symptoms are tingling and pain at the site of infection. The characteristic vesicular eruption appears with clear fluid on an erythematous but unswollen base. Over 1 to 2 weeks, the fluid may become turbid and will develop a crust with desquamation and healing of the skin. Treatment is nonsurgical and symptomatic, with precautions to prevent cross infection within the household. Antibiotics are needed for bacterial superinfection only.

Microvascular Reconstruction

Principles of reconstruction are similar in children and adults. In severe posttraumatic injuries, reconstruction of the thumb with toe-to-hand transfer provides the best

pinch and grasp. Secondary tenolysis is anticipated in the preoperative counseling.

Annotated Bibliography

Mechanism of Injury

Johnson CF, Kaufman KL, Callendar C: The hand as a target organ in child abuse. *Clin Pediatr* 1990;29:66–72.

Sixty-five percent of pediatric hand abuse lesions are the result of contusion, often in an older child trying to protect his or her face.

le Viet DT, Lantieri LA, Loy SM: Wrist and hand injuries in platform diving. *J Hand Surg* 1993;18A:876–880.

Wrist injuries are commonly seen in competitive divers, and the mechanism of injury is discussed.

Principles of Management

Iconomou TG, Zuker RM, Michelow BJ: Management of major penetrating glass injuries to the upper extremities in children and adolescents. *Microsurgery* 1993;14:91–96.

This is an overview of the treatment of penetrating trauma in children.

Flexor Tendon Injury

Birnie RH, Idler RS: Flexor tenolysis in children. *J Hand Surg* 1995;20A:254–257.

Patients in the first decade of life had minimal improvement in active motion following flexor tenolysis.

Grobbelaar AO, Hudson DA: Flexor tendon injuries in children. *J Hand Surg* 1994;19B:696–698.

The results of flexor tendon repair in children using mobilization techniques were very satisfactory. None of the patients had subsequent tenolysis.

O'Connell SJ, Moore MM, Strickland JW, Frazier GT, Dell PC: Results of zone I and zone II flexor tendon repairs in children. *J Hand Surg* 1994;19A:48–52.

There was no benefit of early mobilization protocols in children compared to immobilization for 3 to 4 weeks. Immobilization beyond 4 weeks resulted in an appreciable deterioration of function.

Skeletal Injury

Caputo AE, Watson HK, Nissen C: Scaphoid nonunion in a child: A case report. *J Hand Surg* 1995;20A:243–245.

A scaphoid nonunion in a 9-year-old boy was successfully treated surgically.

Cook PA, Kobus RJ, Wiand W, Yu JS: Scapholunate ligament disruption in a skeletally immature patient: A case report. *J Hand Surg* 1997;22A:83–85.

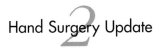
The authors describe a scapholunate ligament rupture in a 14-year-old boy following a fall.

Fischer MD, McElfresh EC: Physeal and periphyseal injuries of the hand: Patterns of injury and results of treatment. *Hand Clin* 1994;10:287–301.

This is a review of 1,048 hand fractures in 1,021 patients.

Ishida O, Ikuta Y, Kuroki H: Ipsilateral osteochondral grafting for finger joint repair. *J Hand Surg,* 1994;19A:372–377.

An osteochondral graft obtained from the base of the second or third metacarpal was used to reconstruct osteochondral defects of the interphalangeal joints.

Letts M, Rowhani N: Galeazzi-equivalent injuries of the wrist in children. *J Pediatr Orthop* 1993;13:561–566.

Separation of the distal ulnar growth plate with displacement of the ulnar metaphysis was more common that the classic Galeazzi fracture at this children's hospital. A classification of the Galeazzi injury complex in children is provided to facilitate diagnosis and management. The authors recommend reduction with the forearm in full supination in an above-elbow cast.

Light TR, Bednar MS: Management of intra-articular fractures of the metacarpophalangeal joint. *Hand Clin* 1994;10:303–314.

Displaced intra-articular fractures often require open reduction and internal fixation.

Ray TD, Tessler RH, Dell PC: Traumatic ulnar physeal arrest after distal forearm fractures in children. *J Pediatr Orthop* 1996; 16:195–200.

This rare growth arrest following growth-plate fractures can result in progressive deformity.

Waters PM, Benson LS: Dislocation of the distal phalanx epiphysis in toddlers. *J Hand Surg* 1993;18A:581–585.

Two cases of physeal fracture-dislocation of the distal phalanx were originally undiagnosed and presented as a dorsal mass in a foreshortened digit with decreased DIP joint motion.

Thermal Injury

Batchelor JS, Vanjari S, Budny P, Roberts AH: Domestic iron burns in children: A cause for concern? *Burns* 1994;20:74–75.

A review of 26 children with contact thermal burns to the hand showed 46% to have been caused by irons.

Brown RL, Greenhalgh DG, Warden GD: Iron burns to the hand in the young pediatric patient: A problem in prevention. *J Burn Care Rehabil* 1997;18:279–282.

Iron burns to the hand occurred most commonly in male children younger than 2 years. Fifteen percent of the 82 patients in this series required grafting.

Kurtzman LC, Stern PJ, Yakuboff KP: Reconstruction of the burned thumb. *Hand Clin* 1992;8:107–119.

This is a review of skin grafting, local flap, and distant flap treatments for burns of the thumb.

Vasseur C, Martinot V, Pellerin P, Herbaux B, Debeugny P: Palmar burns of the hand in children: 81 cases. *Ann Chir Main Memb Super* 1994;13:233–239.

This is a review of 81 children treated with conservative care and occasional use of both contracture releases and skin grafts.

Infections

Ono CM, Albertson KS, Reinker KA, Lipp EB: Acquired radial clubhand deformity due to osteomyelitis. *J Pediatr Orthop* 1995;15:161–168.

The authors review 9 patients with this rare complication.

Walker LG, Simmons BP, Lovallo JL: Pediatric herpetic hand infections. *J Hand Surg* 1990;15A:176–180.

Fourteen cases were seen in children younger than 6 years old.

Microvascular Reconstruction

Cooney WP III, Wood MB: Microvascular reconstruction of congenital anomalies and post-traumatic lesions in children. *Hand Clin* 1992;8:131–146.

This is a review of microvascular techniques used in children.

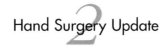

Chapter 39
Congenital Anomalies

391

Paul R. Manske, MD

Embryology

Relatively little is known about the pathophysiologic events that occur during the embryologic development of the upper extremity limb bud and lead to the anomalous conditions in the newborn. Several important investigative studies in laboratory animals have been performed. A mutagenic agent (myleran) was administered to pregnant rats at various time periods, and the resultant fetuses were examined grossly and histologically. Ulnar deficiency was induced in Gun:Wistar rats when myleran was administered on the ninth and tenth days of pregnancy, and radial deficiency was induced by administering this drug to WKAH/HKm rats on days 10 and 11. Central deficiency, along with central polydactyly and osseous syndactyly, was induced by myleran administration to Gun:Wistar rats on days 10 to 11.5 of pregnancy. Thus, the timing of the administration of the mutagenic agent appears to be critical to the development of specific types of longitudinal deficiency. However, the presentation of ulnar deficiency only in Gun:Wistar rats, and radial deficiency only in WKAH/HKm rats also suggests the predisposition of genetic factors.

The mortality rate was higher when the myleran was administered on the ninth and tenth days (ie, the period producing ulnar deficiency) than when administered on days 10 and 11 (ie, the period producing radial deficiency). This information potentially explains why ulnar deficiency is not observed as frequently as radial deficiency in newborns.

The size of the limb bud in longitudinally deficient fetuses was smaller and developed asymmetrically compared to unaffected controls. Furthermore, the density of mesenchymal cells in the deficient limb buds was lower than in control animals. The investigators postulated that the mutagenic agents affect principally the mesenchymal cells. These studies are important for the future understanding of longitudinal limb deficiency.

Finally, the association of central deficiency (cleft hand), along with central polydactyly and osseous syndactyly of the central digits was observed in litter mates from pregnant rats. This observation indicates that the seemingly disparate conditions of deficiency (failure of formation), polydactyly (formation of extra parts), and syndactyly (failure of differentiation)

can all result from a single mutagenic insult and are interrelated. The specific clinical manifestation is probably a result of magnitude of the insult, rather than a result of the occurrence of multiple or separate insults. This experimental observation corresponds to the established interrelationship between cleft hand, central polydactyly, and osseous syndactyly that is often seen in the clinical presentation of central deficiency. A similar clinical observation was made on a newborn infant with bilateral radial abnormalities—radial club hand on one side and radial polydactyly on the other. Heretofore, reports of radial polydactyly in association with radial deficiency have been rare in contrast to the frequent observation of this phenomenon in central deficiency.

During embryonic development, the overlying ectoderm of the limb bud undergoes thickening, forming a longitudinal apical ectodermal ridge (AER) by the fifth week in the human embryo. The interaction between the AER and the underlying mesoderm plays an important role in the proximal-distal differential development of the limb. Mutagenic insults to the superior, central, or inferior regions are believed to produce radial, central, or ulnar deficiencies, respectively. A subpopulation of mesenchymal cells on the inferior border of the limb bud constitute the zone of polarizing activity (ZPA), and are responsible for giving the hand its radial-ulnar orientation. In normal development, the ZPA produces varying concentration gradients of morphogens that affect the development of both the ulnar and radial aspects of the limb. It is likely that mutagenic insults in the region of the ZPA are also responsible for resultant congenital anomalies. In past experiments, transplantation of the ZPA cells from the inferior margin to the superior margin on the embryonic chick limb bud resulted in ulnar duplication of the normal limb. It is postulated that the mirror hand is in fact caused by duplication and abnormal positioning of the ZPA during embryogenesis. This also explains the frequent observation of abnormal thumb development in patients with ulnar deficiency; it has been postulated that a mutagenic insult in the region of the ZPA on the inferior margin of the limb bud can produce both a deficiency of the ulnar structures and a coexisting abnormality of the thumb and radial structures of the hand.

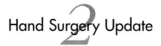

Table 1
Congenital hand classification

Category	Description
I	Failure of formation of parts (arrest of development)
II	Failure of differentiation (separation) of parts
III	Duplication
IV	Overgrowth (gigantism)
V	Undergrowth (hypoplasia)
VI	Congenital constriction band syndrome
VII	Generalized skeletal abnormalities

Classification

Until the abnormal pathophysiologic events of the developing limb bud are more clearly defined, the classification of upper extremity anomalies will continue to be based on the gross morphologic presentation. Although there are critics of the 7 classification categories established many years ago by Swanson (Table 1), no reasonable alternative has been proposed. Consequently, the general groupings of that classification system remain in place. Recent articles on the classification of congenital hand deformities have focussed on further defining conditions in this established grouping.

Radial Longitudinal Deficiency
The hypoplastic thumb, representing a spectrum of first ray deficiencies, was initially recognized by Mueller and subsequently classified into 5 types. In a review of 98 patients with 160 hypoplastic thumbs, 139 thumbs could be classified (Table 2). Fifty-nine percent of the hypoplastic thumbs had associated dysplasia of the radius; 86% had other congenital abnormalities, including 44% who had a recognized syndrome or association such as Holt-Oram or VATER (vertebral segmental and fusion abnormalities, anal atresia, tracheoesophageal fistula, esophageal atresia, renal abnormalities, and radial ray deficiencies).

The type III hypoplastic thumb subsequently was further divided into A and B subtypes. In contrast to the well-defined features of type II thumbs (thumb-index web narrowing,

thenar muscle hypoplasia, and instability of the ulnar collateral ligament at the metacarpophalangeal joint) and the well-defined features of the type IV pouce flotant, the deficiencies of type III thumbs had not been as well defined. Previously published articles noted more severe type II deficiencies, as well as abnormalities of the extrinsic thumb muscles and osseous deficiencies of the proximal base of the first metacarpal.

It was proposed that type IIIA thumbs include extrinsic tendon abnormalities and a stable first metacarpal base, while type IIIB thumbs include extrinsic tendon abnormalities and a deficient-unstable first metacarpal base. The rationale behind the proposed subclassification was not simply to further define the spectrum of abnormalities, but to recognize that type IIIA thumbs can be surgically reconstructed (as can types I and II), while type IIIB thumbs are treated by ablation and index finger pollicization, similarly to type IV and V thumbs.

In addition, identification of 3 principal extrinsic tendon abnormalities was based on a series of 13 patients and the combined reports of another 41 patients. These anomalies include absent extensor pollicis longus, absent or aberrant displacement of the flexor pollicis longus, and tendinous interconnections between the extrinsic flexor and extensor systems.

Other authors further defined more proximal type IIIA abnormalities in the hands and distal forearms of 11 patients, identifying duplication of radial musculotendinous units, anomalous muscles between the thumb and index rays, and

Table 2
Incidence of hypoplastic thumb (n = 139)

Type*	Number of thumbs	%
I	6	4.3
II	20	14.4
IIIA	27	19.4
IIIB	5	3.6
IV	31	22.3
V	50	36.0

*Modified Blauth classification

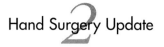
abnormal insertions or dense adhesions along the course of the extrinsic radial tendons. These authors recommended that in order to perform adequate surgical reconstruction, an extensive approach from the thumb to the radial aspect of the distal forearm of type IIIA patients was necessary to divide all of the abnormal connections, reorient the tendons, and lyse adhesions.

Ulnar Longitudinal Deficiency

Deficiencies of the ulnar aspect of the upper extremity (often descriptively referred to as ulnar club hand) have heretofore been classified according to the radiologic appearance of the ulna; these forearm/elbow radiologic features include ulnar hypoplasia, partial ulnar aplasia, complete absence of the ulna, radial head dislocation, and radiohumeral synostosis. However, these classification schemes do not address hand abnormalities, which have been reported in up to 80% of ulnar deficient extremities. Furthermore, 55% to 75% of the surgical procedures on the ulnar deficient extremity are performed on the hand rather than forearm. Although hand abnormalities have been classified according to the number of missing ulnar rays, this classification does not consider the frequent occurrence of thumb abnormalities; previous articles indicated a 64% to 100% incidence of thumb and radial side hand abnormalities. The involvement of the radial side of the hand and ulnar deficiency are thought to be related to an embryologic insult to the cells in the ZPA as described in the previous section.

In a review of 55 ulnar deficient extremities, the occurrence of thumb and thumb web abnormalities was noted in 73%. Moreover, the majority (53%) of recommended surgical procedures involved the thumb. Consequently, the authors proposed a classification scheme for the hand in ulnar deficient extremities; it is based on the characteristics of the thumb web space (Table 3). They proposed that the hand classification be added (as an alphabetic letter) to the forearm/elbow classification (as a Roman numeral), and they provided surgical recommendations based on the hand classification. Types C and D required the most (81%) recommended surgical procedures. No correlation was noted between the hand abnormalities and/or the number of surgical procedures and the previously recognized elbow/forearm abnormalities.

Central Longitudinal Deficiency

Previous classification of central deficiency (cleft hands) has been based on the characteristics of the cleft. Barsky's classification distinguished between the typical cleft (central deficiency with presentation of normal marginal digits) and the atypical cleft (central rays reduced to nubbins and short rudimentary marginal rays); however, the atypical cleft hand

Table 3
Classification of ulnar deficiency

Type	Deficiency	Number of hands
A	Normal first web and thumb	15
B	Mild first web space narrowing	10
C	Moderate to severe first web and thumb deficiency, including loss of opposition, malrotation of the thumb into the plane of the other digits, thumb-index syndactyly, absent extrinsic tendons	20
D	Absent thumb	10
	Total	55

(Reproduced with permission from Cole RJ, Manske PR: Classification of ulnar deficiency according to the thumb and first web. J Hand Surg 1997;22A:479–488.)

is no longer considered a central deficiency, but rather a transverse deficiency and a form of symbrachydactyly. Several authors have classified the cleft hand according to the number of deficient central bony elements. Finally, the association between central deficiency and central polydactyly-osseous syndactyly has been recognized and incorporated as subtypes into the cleft hand classification.

A new central deficiency classification was proposed in a recent article, but it was still based on the features of the cleft. The simple cleft hand had complete absence of the middle ray; the complex cleft hand was characterized by syndactyly (including the first and second rays) and transverse bony polydactyly; and extensive cleft hands featured aplasia of the radial structures of the hand.

Previous authors recognized that adequate surgical reconstruction of the thumb web space was the most important objective in reconstruction of the hand with a central cleft deficiency. Furthermore, several techniques have been described that reconstruct the thumb web using skin transposed from the cleft. However, the thumb and thumb web features of the cleft hand have not been incorporated into the classification of this anomaly. A proposed classification of the hand with a central deficiency is based on the progressive narrowing of the thumb web space (Fig. 1). Type I has a normal web; type II features a narrowed web; in type III, the web is obliterated and the thumb and index rays are

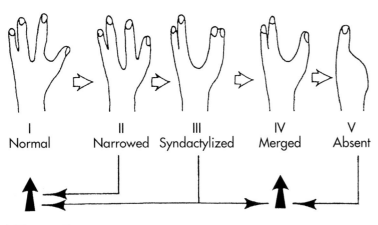

Figure 1

Schematic drawing of progressive narrowing of the thumb-web space in central deficiency. (Reproduced with permission from Manske PR, Halikis MN: Surgical classification of central deficiency according to the thumb web. J Hand Surg 1995;20A:687–697.)

syndactylized; in type IV, the index ray is suppressed and the thumb web is merged with a cleft; and in type V, the thumb elements are also suppressed and the thumb web is absent. In a review of 46 hands with central deficiency, the progressive narrowing of the thumb web correlated with the progressive severity of the central defects.

Surgical recommendations were guided by this classification scheme. The normal type I hand required no thumb web reconstruction, only cleft closure with local tissue reduction of the intermetacarpal space and excision of the polydactylous bony elements when present. Type II hands required reconstruction of the thumb web using local pedicle flaps or pedicle flaps from the cleft in more severe cases, in addition to the cleft closure as noted above. Type III required syndactyly release and reconstruction of the thumb web using skin grafts and pedicle flaps from the cleft and usually required a more extensive cleft closure often requiring transposition of the index metacarpal. Alternatively, the index finger bony elements could be excised, thereby obtaining a merged rather than a normal web space. Type IV hands usually required no surgical reconstruction of a thumb web, although removal of tissue from the web space along with stabilization of the metacarpophalangeal (MCP) joint was often required. In type V hands, metacarpal lengthening or toe to hand transfer should be considered.

Symbrachydactyly

The morphologic features of symbrachydactyly include elements of both transverse deficiency (hypoplasia or aplasia of phalanges) and syndactyly (webbed digits). The relationship

of symbrachydactyly to transverse terminal deficiency and syndactyly was examined to determine whether symbrachydactyly should be classified as a form of transverse deficiency (failure of formation) or syndactyly (failure of differentiation). The authors compared various clinical features of 53 patients with symbrachydactyly (intercalated phalangeal hypoplasia or aplasia and web digits) to 113 patients with terminal digital hypoplasia or aplasia and 129 cases of syndactyly. They noted similar clinical features between symbrachydactyly and terminal deficiency with respect to sex ratio, bilaterality, inheritance patterns, and associated anomalies of the feet and other organs; however, all clinical features between symbrachydactyly and syndactyly were different except for a similar sex ratio. They concluded that symbrachydactyly is a mild form of transverse arrest, rather than a form of syndactyly. Tri-, di-, and monophalangeal symbrachydactyly and adactyly with nubbin digits are a spectrum of sequential anomalous conditions. These observations support previous observations regarding the classification of this condition.

Apert Acrosyndactyly

The characteristics of the hand in Apert acrosyndactyly include (1) a short radially deviated thumb, (2) complex syndactyly of the second, third, fourth, and sometimes the fifth digit, and (3) symbrachyphalangism. Previously reported treatment includes early separation of the border digits, particularly the thumb; creation of an adequate thumb web space for independent thumb function; separation of the central digits, creating either 4-fingered (5-digit) or 3-fingered (4-digit) hands. However, no guidelines exist as to which type of hand to reconstruct and which ray to resect to accomplish this.

Previous classifications have been descriptive, according to the complexity and severity of the presentation. A classification system was proposed to facilitate the decision-making in the surgical reconstruction of the hand, based on the authors' experience with 28 Apert acrosyndactyly hands in 14 patients (Fig. 2). In the type I deformity, there is little or no angular deformity at the digital MCP joints, with nearly parallel alignment of the metacarpals and proximal phalanges. The distal bony syndactyly is isolated to the distal phalanx with a separate distal phalanx of digit 5. All type II deformities have MCP joint angular deformity of varying degrees. In type IIA there is mild angular deformity at the MCP joints, which is distinguishable from type I by more extensive complex bony syndactyly. In type IIB digit 2 is markedly pronated and lies in the plane of the thumb; the MCP joint of digit 2 is apex

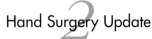

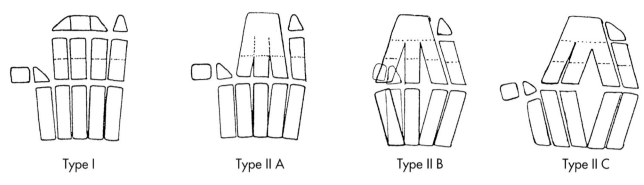

Type I   Type II A   Type II B   Type II C

Figure 2

Schematic drawing of proposed classification for Apert acrosyndactyly. (Reproduced with permission from Van Heest AE, House JH, Reckling WC: Two-stage reconstruction of Apert acrosyndactyly. *J Hand Surg* 1997;22A:315–322.)

radially angulated, and the MCP joints of digits 4 and 5 are apex ulnarly angulated. In type IIIC digit 4 is markedly supinated and lies in the plane of digit 5; there is apex radial angulation of MCP joints 2 and 3 and apex ulnar angulation of MCP joints 4 and 5.

The authors' surgical recommendations include 2-stage reconstructive procedures for all types; the surgical procedures are directed toward digital separation, ray resection, and correction of the delta deformity of the thumb. In type I, a thumb and 4-fingered hand is created. In type IIA, the third ray is resected, creating a 3-fingered hand. In type IIB, the second ray is resected, creating a 3-fingered hand; in type IIIC, the fourth ray is resected, creating a 3-fingered hand.

Fetal Ultrasonography in the Diagnosis of Congenital Hand Anomalies

The use of ultrasonography to detect intrauterine congenital anomalies of the hand and upper extremity is emerging as an important diagnostic technique. Scattered reports of intrauterine detection of congenital hand defects detected by ultrasonography have appeared in the recent medical literature. These include the cleft hand, amniotic band syndrome, the windblown hand seen in Freeman-Sheldon syndrome, the trident hands seen in achondroplasia, radial club hand and phocomelia, clinodactyly, syndactyly, polydactyly, hypoplastic digits, and Simian creases.

The evaluation of fetal hands is not included in the obstetric ultrasonographic screening guidelines of either the American Institute of Ultrasound in Medicine or the American College of Obstetricians and Gynecology as of 1991 and

1993. At Ohio State University, the evaluation of fetal hands was included on 215 obstetric patients referred for ultrasonographic examination; 101 were referred for routine assessment of fetal growth and 114 were "at risk" patients for potential increased anomalies. The ultrasonographic evaluation of both hands was accomplished in 188 (87%) of the fetuses within the maximally allotted 5-min time period. The mean additional screening time for both hands was 2.2 minutes. Previously undiagnosed hand abnormalities were noted on ultrasound examination and subsequently confirmed at delivery in 6 patients; 2 additional children had abnormalities at delivery that were not detected by ultrasonography; there were no false positive examinations. The routine inclusion of fetal hand abnormalities at the time of obstetric ultrasonography is advised; most hand surgeons would likely support this position.

Microvascular Free-Tissue Transfer and Congenital Hand Anomalies

For many years, microvascular free-tissue transfer has been an accepted technique for reconstruction of acquired traumatic defects, mostly in adult hands. However, there has been a reticence to apply this technique to the reconstruction of congenital deficiencies in children. This likely relates to several factors, including the absence of normal proximal anatomic structures (tendons, nerves, bones and joints, arteries and veins) to which the transferred part can be joined, particularly in radial, central, or ulnar longitudinal deficiencies; the absence of "cortical representation" of the deficient part in the brain; and the concern about the very small diameter of the vessels in the infant. Recently, several surgeons have advocated microvascular tissue transfer for congenital anomalies, reporting good results.

Whole Digit Transfers

The most frequent report is free-tissue transfer of toes from the foot to the hand. Initially the technique was applied to patients with ring constriction syndrome, based on the concept that in utero amputation did not affect the growth and development of the structures proximal to the amputation site. However, this observation of normal proximal anatomy has also been noted in patients with transverse arrest and symbrachydactyly. Although the proximal structures may be hypoplastic, they are sufficiently present to produce useful function following transfer.

One group reported approximately 70 microvascular toe transfers in 40 children, principally with symbrachydactyly, transverse arrest, complex syndactyly, and ring constriction syndrome. The second toe transfers were used to supplement rudimentary digits already present in the hand. The operations were performed at 6 months to 14 years of age. The authors' preferred age at operation is between 2 and 5 years, which gives the family sufficient time to come to terms with the condition and the decision for undertaking the surgical procedure, but completes the surgery before the child goes to school. There was no evidence of increased function or performance when the surgery was carried out at a younger age. The objective of the surgical procedure was to facilitate pinch of small and/or large objects and to augment grasping power by the lengthened or additional digits; the enhancement of hand aesthetics was a less important objective. The thumb was the most frequent recipient ray. The second toe was the most frequent donor. It was transferred on a single artery, the first dorsal interosseous in two thirds of the patients and the plantar system in one third. In 25 children, 2 second toes were transferred, 1 from each foot; the authors now perform this 2-toe transfer at a single operation.

All transferred digits survived. In 4 transfers, there was premature closure of the physis. The length of the transferred toes averaged 91% of the contralateral toe at follow-up. All but 3 patients developed active movement of the transferred toe, averaging 60° active motion at each joint. The transfer enhanced grip of small and large objects against resistance in 50% to 75% of the patients. Two-point discrimination was noted to be an average 5 mm, but Semmes-Weinstein monofilament testing showed 28% of the digits had only protective sensibility. Eighty-five percent of the parents and children thought the transfer improved the appearance of the hand.

Another author reported 16 second toe to hand vascularized tissue transfers in 16 patients, again primarily for

monodactylous symbrachydactyly. The objective of the procedure was to improve function by providing pinch and grasp, not to improve the aesthetic appearance. The age of the patients ranged from 10 months to 16 years. The transfers were based on a single artery in only 21% of cases, and 2 to 4 arteries in the remaining patients. One procedure failed; 86% of the growth plate remained open at follow-up (average 4.2 years). Two-point discrimination averaged 5 mm, but active range of motion of the digit as a whole was only 48°.

Vascularized transfer of the second toe to the anterior aspect of the forearm ("stub" operation) was described for patients with only the carpus present. This modification of an earlier described procedure provides pinch function to the peromelic hand. The second metatarsal is placed subperiosteally on the anterior radius. The extensor and flexor tendons of the transferred toe are sutured to the numerous digital flexor tendons of the forearm, but not to the wrist flexor tendons. The transfer is vascularized by anastomosis of the plantar and dorsal metatarsal arteries to the radial artery. In 6 patients operated on at 11 to 21 months of age, the transferred toes were viable, and the physis remained open at 1- to 9-year follow-up. The mobility of the toe averaged 40°, and carpus motion averaged 52°.

Yet another author used microvascular transfer to restore function of 18 adactylous hands in children 2 to 12 years old, preferring an age of 2 to 4 years at the time of surgery. This author performed only a single toe transfer, but included all 3 joints in most patients. The transfer was based on various toe arteries, but the plantar II/III intermetatarsal artery is preferred. Five patients required early reoperation for vascular compromise, and a secondary tenolysis was performed in 4 patients. Linear growth of the phalanges was normal, but impaired metatarsal head growth was noted in at least 2 patients. All but 1 of the 3 tissue transfers remained viable, and 14 patients had improved grasp-pinch function.

In a report of 30 vascularized toe transfers for the more severe forms of symbrachydactyly, 25 were successful and 5 showed complete or partial necrosis. In the monodactylous form of symbrachydactyly, the transfer was frequently performed on the ulnar side, with the surgeon using conventional distraction lengthening techniques on the radial ray; all patients had improved functional results. In the peromelic form, it was important that the basal carpometacarpal joint of the thumb was present in order to consider toe transfer.

In the largest series, 103 microvascular toe to hand transfers in 66 pediatric patients at the Institute for Orthopaedic Diseases in St. Petersburg were reported; 49 patients had congenital conditions including brachydactyly, ectrodactyly,

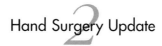

and adactyly. The donor digit was the second toe in most cases, but the fifth toe and a composite of the second and third toes also were used. Toe transfers were performed from both feet in 20 patients. When multiple toes were transferred, the authors preferred to anastomose the donor arteries to the radial and ulnar arterial system by dividing and performing the anastomosis to both ends of the palmar arch. The reported results are sketchy, but aesthetics and function were noted to be improved.

These are technically demanding procedures and should be performed only by surgeons with extensive experience with microsurgical techniques, who are knowledgeable about pediatric hand surgery. Although these techniques hold much promise, they have not supplanted more conventional techniques of distraction lengthening and nonvascularized toe phalangeal transfers, particularly in patients with rudimentary metacarpals and/or phalanges. Several authors propose use of these conventional techniques (either to the transferred digit or to adjacent digits) to augment the function of the free-tissue transfer.

Another group reported results of 73 nonvascularized proximal and middle toe phalangeal grafts to the hand of children with congenital defects. The results were dependent on the age of the child at transfer. The physes remained open in 94% of those operated on before reaching 1 year of age, in 71% of those operated on at 1 to 2 years, and 48% of those older than 2 years. Open physes were noted significantly more often in patients that had ligament reattachment at the time of surgery. Growth rates showed similar age dependency; they were 1 mm/year for patients operated on when younger than 2 years, and 0.5 mm/year for patients operated on when older than 2 years. However, the growth rate of the transferred digit was only 71% that of the contralateral toe in 17 patients for whom radiographs of the opposite foot had been obtained; this is in contrast to a previously reported figure of 91%.

Metacarpal bone lengthening was reported in patients with brachydactyly and ring constriction syndrome. Seven metacarpals were lengthened by single-stage intercalary lengthening using iliac crest bone graft and internal fixation; 6 metacarpals were lengthened by distraction techniques (0.5 to 1.0 mm/day for 13 to 34 days) using an external fixator, followed by iliac crest bone grafting and internal fixation. The patients averaged 7.7 years of age (3 to 17 years) at the time of surgery. The single-stage procedure provided 2 to 20 mm of length, averaging 4.7 mm or 18% of the initial length of the bone. The distraction lengthening technique provided 12 to 30 mm of length, averaging 17 mm or 58% of the initial length of the bone. Complications from the single-stage procedure included subsequent shortening of the bone by more than 2 mm in 3 patients and a flexion deformity at the osteotomy

site in 1. The only distraction lengthening complication was transient disturbance of sensibility in 1 patient.

Thumb-Index Web Space

The use of a free-tissue groin flap transfer was advocated to resurface the thumb-index web space in cases of severe deficiency, such as thumb-index syndactyly, complex acrosyndactyly, Apert acrosyndactyly hand, and the ulna-deficient hand. Although the superficial circumflexed iliac artery vascular pedicle of the groin flap is short, it has the same diameter as the recipient radial artery and the anastomosis is easily performed in the anatomic snuff box. The advantages of the groin flap are that the tissue is thin and pliable and the donor site is expendable. Consequently, the authors prefer this to conventional resurfacing flaps, such as the dorsal transposition flap, the radial forearm flap, and the posterior interosseous flap for the thumb-index web space.

Use of the microvascular flap to resurface the thumb web is an emerging technique that has not replaced the more conventional techniques. Two investigators reviewed their 20-year experience with dorsal transposition flaps in 46 hands of 38 patients with congenital thumb web narrowing. The longitudinal flap, which is transposed from the radial aspect of the dorsum of the hand and index finger into the thumb-index space was used in 13 radial club hands, 6 hands with symbrachydactyly, 5 with acrosyndactyly, 5 with triphalangeal thumbs, 4 with Poland syndrome, 4 with arthrogryposis, and 9 hands with various other conditions. There was no postoperative flap necrosis in any case. The preoperative first web space angle increased from an average 8° to 67°. Inadequate or incomplete correction, hypertrophic scarring, or infection was noted in 37% of cases, most frequently in those patients with thumb-index syndactyly associated with symbrachydactyly. Generally speaking, aesthetic results were acceptable, and patient satisfaction was high.

The severe narrowing of the thumb-index web space in 4 hands with Apert acrosyndactyly was treated using tissue expanders before the reconstructive procedure. In all extremities, the need for skin grafts to reconstruct the web space at subsequent surgical release of the thumb was minimized. In contrast to previous reports of this technique in the pediatric population, there were no complications, infections, skin necrosis, or loss of expander. The report emphasized placement of the expanders in the first 6 months of life, use of small volume (5 ml) expanders, and leaving the port externalized and exposed to prevent repeated injections through the skin.

Distally based fasciocutaneous island flaps from the forearm were advocated as a means to reconstruct the thumb-index space in 18 extremities (Freeman-Sheldon syndrome, hypoplastic thumb, arthrogryposis, 5-fingered hand). The radial forearm flap was preferred and used in 16 cases; the posterior interosseous flap was used in 2 patients who had weak or absent radial pulses on palpation and/or had previous surgical release of the first web space. Superficial skin loss occurred in 1 extremity; the remaining results were excellent, and the distal island pedicle flap provided good skin coverage and adequate release. An advantage was the minimal scars on the dorsum of the hand.

Treatment of Other Congenital Conditions

Radial Clubhand

Two rather clever surgical techniques have been proposed for the treatment of the radial clubhand. The first was distraction lengthening (up to 1 mm/day) of the radially deviated hand using a dual-post external fixator before radialization or centralization of the carpus on the distal ulna to stretch the tight soft-tissue radial structures. The device was distracted for 2 to 4 weeks and left in place for an additional 2 to 3 weeks; it was removed 1 day before the definitive procedure. Its placement allowed adequate realignment without carpal bone resection of the carpus in 5 of 6 clubhands and 38° improvement in the radial angulation. This result compared to attainment of adequate alignment without carpal bone resection in only 1 of 6 patients treated without the distraction technique, and only 19° improvement in radial angulation. There was little difference (17 mm versus 16 mm) between the 2 groups in the radial translation of the carpus.

The second technique was the proposed use of a bilobed skin flap on the dorsum of the hand for surgical exposure at centralization, transposing the redundant ulnar skin to the area of skin deficiency on the radial side of the wrist. A skin flap with ulnar and distal lobes on a common proximal pedicle was transposed distally and radially (respectively), closing the resultant ulnar-sided defect as a transverse incision. This flap provided excellent surgical exposure for the 6 reported centralization procedures, was effective in transposing the skin, and resulted in no flap necrosis.

Reconstruction of the Duplicated Thumb

Several articles review the aesthetic and functional results following surgical treatment of the duplicated thumb and suggest that proper surgical reconstruction may be more difficult than previously noted. One group reviewed 76 duplicated thumbs operated on at the Honolulu Shriners Hospital from 1925 to 1991. The thumbs were distributed among the 7 Wassel categories, which is comparable to previous reports.

Three basic surgical procedures were performed, including simple ablation, ablation with reconstruction of the preserved thumb, and central wedge resection (Bilhaut-Cloquet procedure); the specific surgical technical details were not presented. An acceptable or unacceptable outcome was determined postoperatively, based on the presence of joint laxity, angular deformity, functional deficit, and unsightly appearance. Half of the simple excisions, as well as half of the excisions with reconstructed thumbs, had an unacceptable outcome, primarily because of joint angulation and instability. All of the central wedge resection thumbs were considered unacceptable.

In a more detailed study, another group evaluated the surgical outcome of 106 duplicated thumbs that bifurcated at the MCP joint (Wassel type IV), dividing them into 4 types. Type A (16%) had a wide cartilaginous connection between the phalanges; type B (68%) had 2 separate proximal phalanges; type C (6%) had a cartilaginous connection to the metacarpal; and in type D (10%), the smaller (excised) thumb was attached only by a fibrous connection to the joint capsule. These authors also evaluated the outcome with respect to relative size of the excised digit (as measured by the sagittal cross-sectional area on radiographs) and to the presence of 3 phalanges in the preserved digit. In general, the surgical procedure included excision of the radial digit, reposition of the abductor pollicis brevis to the dorsum of the MCP joint, reconstruction of the radial collateral ligament, a corrective closing wedge osteotomy of the metacarpal when required, and an appropriate skin flap closure.

The reconstructed thumbs were evaluated as good, fair, or poor according to previously published criteria of Tada; these criteria included range of MCP and interphalangeal motion, stability, alignment, and aesthetics. Good results were obtained in only 50% of the type A and C thumbs (having cartilaginous connections to either the adjacent phalanx or metacarpal). However, good results were obtained in 80% of the type B and D thumbs (having separate proximal phalanges or fibrous connections to the joint capsule). The presence of 3 phalanges in the preserved digit produced a fair result in almost all cases. Finally, when the size of the excised digit was more than 75% of the preserved digit, the results were fair or poor in more than 90% of the cases.

Camptodactyly

Camptodactyly is a congenital flexion deformity of the proximal interphalangeal (PIP) joint, usually affecting the small finger. Although abnormal anatomic features of the flexor digitorum sublimis and lumbrical muscles have been found to occur in some cases, there is no unanimity of opinion as to whether surgical treatment is better than splinting, or

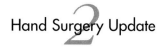

whether surgical treatment should consist only of releasing the tethered structures on the flexor side of the joint or should also include balancing the flexor and extensor forces by tendon transfer.

In an attempt to address the treatment of camptodactyly by classifying the deformity into 3 types, one group reviewed their experience with 59 PIP joints with camptodactyly. Type I deformities (24 joints) were isolated anomalies of the small finger PIP joint identified and treated in infancy. Type II deformities (5 joints) were also isolated small finger PIP joints, but patients did not present for treatment until the adolescent years. Type III deformities (30 joints) were more severe contractures seen at birth, which always involved multiple digits on the same hand, were often bilateral, and were associated with other congenital anomalies.

All patients were treated initially with daily splinting of the contracture (15 to 18 hours for infants, 10 to 12 hours for older children), as well as frequent passive stretching exercises until full passive extension was obtained. All patients with type I deformities responded well to the splinting protocol, with an average of improvement of the flexion contracture from 23° to 4° at an average 3-year follow-up. The 5 joints with type II deformities did not respond as well to splinting. Only 1 joint obtained complete correction with meticulous attention to the splinting protocol. Two joints had worsening of the flexion contracture, but compliance to the splinting was marginal. Two joints required surgical correction (the specific technique not indicated) with poor postoperative correction; again, the patients were not compliant with either the pre- or postoperative splinting programs. Type III deformities were generally responsive to splinting; nearly full extension was obtained in 24 of the 30 digits. Six digits with more severe contractures (over 50°) had surgical correction with improvement to 0° to 9° extension lag.

Although the authors concluded that camptodactyly should be considered primarily a nonsurgical condition, this conclusion is applicable principally to smaller contractures in infants and young children. The issue as to what to do with severe contracture seen in older children, especially those that are refractory to splinting treatment or in noncompliant patients, is still not clearly defined.

In another report, 59 patients with 83 camptodactylous PIP joints were treated by (1) manipulation alone, (2) static and dynamic extension splints, or (3) surgical tenoarthrolysis (without tendon transfer) of the tethering structure on the volar aspect of the joint and a dorsal rotation skin flap followed by extension splinting. Eleven of 20 manipulated joints improved; 14 of 24 splinted joints improved; and 30 of 39 surgically treated joints improved. These results provide general guidelines for treatment, but emphasize the need for individualization. Mild forms can be treated with splinting; in younger children with more severe deformity, surgical release of the contracture without tendon transfer corrects the deformity; and adolescents do not respond well to surgical release.

Constriction Band Syndrome

The clinical manifestations of 88 patients with constriction band syndrome of the hand were reviewed by another team. Digital band indentation occurred in 109 digits in 81 patients. The thumb was least involved, likely reflecting its shorter length and adducted position in the palm. Syndactyly was present in 46 patients; the middle, ring, and index fingers were most often involved, followed by the small finger; the thumb was involved in only 1 patient. Thirty-three of the 46 patients also had distal amputation of the digits, thereby suggesting that the band had pulled the adjacent digits together causing necrosis of the distal tissue and syndactyly of the proximal component. Forty-seven patients had a total of 231 digital amputations, again affecting principally the long, ring, and index fingers followed by the small finger; the thumb was the least involved.

In this same group of patients, there were only 138 lower-limb amputations. In contrast to the reduced involvement of the thumb, the more prominent hallux was the toe most commonly affected.

Fourth and Fifth Metacarpal Synostosis

In a report on treatment of 9 cases of congenital synostosis of the fourth and fifth metacarpals, the underlying diagnoses included ulnar deficiency, cleft hand (central deficiency), and symbrachydactyly. In all cases, the small finger was hypoplastic and the middle phalanx in particular was short. Surgical reconstruction was performed on 4 cases; it consisted of splitting of the common synostosed metacarpal and placement of an autogenous iliac crest bone block to maintain the intermetacarpal space. The appearance of the hand was improved in all 4 cases.

A group of 99 fourth and fifth metacarpal synostoses were reviewed as part of a larger series of 152 hands with various combinations of metacarpal synostosis. The fifth metacarpal was short in all cases, the small finger was hypoplastic and could not be abducted as a result of the skeletal deformity and the absent third palmar interosseous muscle. Amputation was performed when the fifth digit was severely hypoplastic, abducted, and nonfunctional. The investigators preferred, however, to surgically realign a functioning small finger. A longitudinal osteotomy of the common metacarpal and a transverse osteotomy of the ulnar component were performed to give proper longitudinal alignment to the fifth digital ray and to transpose it distally. The corrected position of the osteotomized bone was maintained with a bone graft block from the iliac crest, taking care not to injure the physeal growth plate. The radial collateral ligament of the small finger was reconstructed when there was complete distal synostosis of the fourth and fifth metacarpals with a common MCP joint; a segment of extensor tendon was attached to the metacarpal head and the base of the proximal phalanx using transosseous sutures. The extensor tendons were aligned by transposing a tendinous slip from the ring finger to the extensor aponeurosis of the small finger or by transposing the inserting slip of the common extensor tendon of the small finger proximally to the ring finger extensor tendon. Although the alignment of the small finger was improved, the hypoplastic digit usually continued to be stiff at the MCP joint and did not have a normal appearance.

Psychology of Congenital Anomalies

Several interesting studies have appeared in the recent literature regarding the psychological aspects of congenital anomalies. These will be very important to the hand surgeon who realizes that these congenital abnormalities impact the lives of patients far beyond the limitations of the functional anatomic deficits.

Parental Adjustment to Hand Anomalies

The birth of a child with visible disfigurement requires parental adjustment to the condition. The parents' response is important not only for their well being, but is also considered important to the child's psychosocial development. Parents of 34 children born with various forms of digital deficiencies that caused some degree of cosmetic and functional impairment were interviewed when the children were 6 months to 13 years of age. None of the anomalies were apparent on prenatal examination. No parent had received psychological counseling since the birth of the child.

The initial period of grieving and stress (denial, guilt, anger, shock, tearfulness) on the birth of the child resolved within several days in approximately half of the parents; however, it lasted weeks and months in one fourth and took years or never came to resolution in 26% of the parents.

Fifty-three percent of the parents adjusted adequately to their child's deformity; they experienced little or no anxiety when they took their babies out for social activities, and 62% freely took and displayed photographs of the child. However, 47% acknowledged anxiety when taking the baby out, sometimes covering and hiding the part, and 38% took photographs but kept the deformed part (or the photographs themselves) hidden. Forty-four percent of the parents

thought the disfigurement produced strains and arguments in their marital relationship, and 18% would not consider having more children as a result of the experience.

There was no significant correlation between the parents' ability to adjust with respect to the age of the child, the sex of the child, the social status of the parents, or the severity of the deformity. The factor that was significant in parental adjustment was the perceived support from their extended family. Well-adjusted parents experienced strong family support in 95% of the cases, while parents who adjusted poorly experienced strong family support in only 13% of cases.

Surgical Decision Making by Parents and Children

The same group of families was used to analyze the decision-making process in deciding whether the child should have a major reconstructive surgical procedure. The surgical procedure in this study always entailed toe to hand free-tissue transfer, but it is arguable that the results can be applied to other major surgical procedures on the congenital hand as well. The parents of 27 of the 34 children elected to have the surgical procedure. Parents were interviewed and completed a questionnaire. As anticipated, parents regarded themselves, along with the surgeon and a facilitating counselor, as the primary decision makers; when the child was older than 6 years of age, the decision-making pattern also included the child. The factors that influenced the parents to have surgery were related principally to the communication process with the medical personnel, including the surgeons' general approach to the problem and the information and counseling they received from health care providers. Of less importance were their own perception of the child's appearance and function or their own anxieties about the surgical procedure. This information heightens the responsibility of health care providers in presenting information in a complete, yet neutral and objective manner.

Psychological Impact of Major Surgery on Children and Parents

Finally, the psychological impact of a major surgical reconstructive procedure on 14 of the above noted children at 2 years after surgery was investigated. The research tools involved a semistructured interview and measurement questionnaires for anxiety, depression, and social dysfunction.

In general, the surgery had no profound impact on the overall emotional state of the parents. For well-adjusted parents, the preoperative scores were low (reduced anxiety, depression, social dysfunction) and remained so postoperatively. On the other hand, poorly adjusted parents had substantially higher scores preoperatively; postoperatively there was reduction in

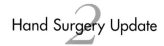
the depression scores but anxiety and social dysfunction scores remained high. However, poorly adjusted parents had increased positive thinking about the child postoperatively, focusing more on the child and less on themselves.

For the children, the surgical procedure produced generalized reduction in distress and concern about their hands. However, the results were related in great part to the level the parents had adjusted to the congenital condition. Children of well-adjusted parents had fewer behavioral and social competence problems preoperatively, which continued postoperatively. Children of poorly adjusted parents had worse behavioral and social competence scores preoperatively and had greater levels of distress and concern about their condition; there was postoperative improvement in the scores, but they remained higher than those of their counterparts. This information underlines the important role that parents have in enabling children with congenital anomalies to deal with their condition both before and after surgery.

There was a high degree of (negative) correlation between function and the child's level of distress and self-consciousness. Stated positively, surgical procedures that improve hand function are likely to improve the child's self image. Conversely, there was no correlation between the child's appearance and level of self-consciousness; this suggests that surgical procedures to improve aesthetics may have limited psychological impact on the child.

Finally, the assessment of the child's appearance and function by a panel of concerned but noninvolved "experts" (including pediatricians, teachers) showed no correlation to the assessment of appearance and function by the parent and the child.

Annotated Bibliography

Embryology

Cole RJ, Manske PR: Classification of ulnar deficiency according to the thumb and first web. *J Hand Surg* 1997; 22A:479–488.

The authors of this review of 55 cases of ulnar deficiency propose a classification system based on characteristics of the thumb and thumb web space. The frequent occurrence of thumb abnormalities in the ulnar deficient hand is thought to be caused by a mutagenic insult to the ZPA.

Hersh JH, Dela Cruz TV, Pietrantoni M, et al: Mirror image duplication of the hands and feet: Report of a sporadic case with multiple congenital anomalies. *Am J Med Genet* 1995; 59:341–345.

This case report discusses pathophysiology of mutagenic insult to the zone of polarizing activity.

Ogino T: Congenital anomalies of the hand: The Asian perspective. *Clin Orthop* 1996;323:12–21.

This is another review of experimental studies in pregnant rats that define the response to administering mutagenic agents at various time periods.

Ogino T, Kato H: Clinical and experimental studies on teratogenic mechanisms of congenital absence of digits in longitudinal deficiencies. *Cong Anom* 1993;33:187–196.

This is a review of experimental studies in pregnant rats that define the response to administering mutagenic agents at various time periods.

Rotman MB, Manske PR: Radial clubhand and contralateral duplicated thumb. *J Hand Surg* 1994;19A:361–363.

This case report identifies a patient with failure of formation on one upper extremity and formation of extra parts on the opposite upper extremity.

Classification

Radial Longitudinal Deficiency

Graham TJ, Louis DS: A comprehensive approach to surgical management of the type IIIA hypoplastic thumb. *J Hand Surg* 1998;23A:3–13.

This is a more extensive definition of hand and forearm musculotendinous abnormalities in 11 type IIIA hypoplastic thumbs.

James MA, McCarroll HR Jr, Manske PR: Characteristics of patients with hypoplastic thumbs. *J Hand Surg* 1996;21A: 104–113.

The authors review characteristics and associated anomalies of 160 hypoplastic thumbs.

Manske PR, McCarroll HR Jr, James M: Type III: A hypoplastic thumb. *J Hand Surg* 1995;20A:246–253.

This is a subclassification of type III hypoplastic thumbs into subtype A, those having extrinsic tendon abnormalities and a stable metacarpal base, and subtype B, which have extrinsic tendon abnormalities and an unstable metacarpal base. Type IIIA is reconstructible, while type IIIB should be treated by ablation and pollicization.

Central Longitudinal Deficiency

Glicenstein J, Guero S, Haddad R: Median clefts of the hand: Classification and therapeutic indications apropos of 29 cases. *Ann Chir Main Memb Super* 1995;14:253.

Manske PR, Halikis MN: Surgical classification of central deficiency according to the thumb web. *J Hand Surg* 1995; 20A:687–697.

These 2 articles provide classification of cleft hand based on the characteristics of the thumb-index web space.

Symbrachydactyly

Miura T, Nakamura R, Horii E: The position of symbrachydactyly in the classification of congenital hand anomalies. *J Hand Surg* 1994;19B:350–354.

This is a review of clinical features of 53 symbrachydactyly patients compared to 113 patients with terminal digital hypoplasia or aplasia (transverse arrest) and 129 patients with syndactyly. The clinical features of the symbrachydactyly patients were similar to those of the transverse arrest patients.

Apert Acrosyndactyly

Van Heest AE, House JH, Reckling WC: Two-stage reconstruction of apert acrosyndactyly. *J Hand Surg* 1997;22A:315–322.

This classification of Apert acrosyndactyly is based on the experience of 14 bilaterally affected patients. The classification presents guidelines for surgical treatment.

Fetal Ultrasonography in the Diagnosis of Congenital Hand Anomalies

Reiss RE, Foy PM, Mendiratta V, Kelly M, Gabbe SG: Ease and accuracy of evaluation of fetal hands during obstetrical ultrasonography: A prospective study. *J Ultrasound Med* 1995; 14:813–820.

Ultrasonographic evaluation of fetal hands of 215 obstetrical patients was accomplished within the allotted 5 minutes in 188 fetuses. Six previously undiagnosed hand abnormalities were noted. There were 2 false negative examinations and no false positives.

Microvascular Free-Tissue Transfer and Congenital Hand Anomalies

Whole Digit Transfers

Buck-Gramcko U, Buck-Gramcko D: Free toe transplantation in congenital hand defects. *Handchir Mikrochir Plast Chir* 1995; 27:181–188.

This is a report of 30 vascularized toe transfers for more severe forms of symbrachydactyly.

Foucher G: Second-toe-to-finger transfer in hand mutilations. *Clin Orthop* 1995;314:8–12.

The author reports experience with 16 vascularized second toe transfers to the hand for monodactylous symbrachydactyly.

Foucher G: The "stub" operation: Modification of the Furnas and Vilkki technique in traumatic and congenital carpal hand reconstruction. *Ann Acad Med Singapore* 1995;24:73–76.

Treatment of peromelic hand by free-tissue toe transfer to the anterior forearm to provide a pinch mechanism is described.

Kay S, Coady M: The role of microsurgery and free tissue transfer in the reconstruction of the pediatric upper extremity. *Ann Acad Med Singapore* 1995;24:113–123.

The authors review 70 microvascular toe transfers to the hand in children for digital deficiencies. Additional free-tissue transfers include reconstructing the thumb-web interspace, joint transfers, and bone transfers to treat pseudarthrosis.

Kay SP, Wiberg M: Toe to hand transfer in children: Part 1. Technical aspects. *J Hand Surg* 1996;21B:723–734.

The authors describe technical aspects of microvascular toe transfer to the hand in 40 pediatric patients with congenital anomalies.

Kay SP, Wiberg M, Bellew M, Webb F: Toe to hand transfer in children: Part 2. Functional and psychological aspects. *J Hand Surg* 1996;21B:735–745.

The authors discuss functional and psychological results of microvascular toe transfer in 40 patients with congenital anomalies.

Ogino T, Kato H, Ishii S, Usui M: Digital lengthening in congenital hand deformities. *J Hand Surg* 1994;19B:120–129.

The authors present results of single-stage lengthening and distraction lengthening techniques for shortened metacarpals and brachydactyly and ring constriction syndrome.

Radocha RF, Netscher D, Kleinert HE: Toe phalangeal grafts in congenital hand anomalies. *J Hand Surg* 1993;18A:833–841.

Results of 73 nonvascularized toe phalangeal transfers to the hand are reported. Ninety-four percent of the physes remained open when the surgery was performed at 12 months or less, with reduced physeal viability than when surgery was performed at a later time.

Shvedovchenko IV: Toe-to-hand transfers in children. *Ann Plast Surg* 1993;31:251–254.

The author reports 103 microvascular toe-to-hand transfers in children.

Vilkki SK: Advances in microsurgical reconstruction of the congenitally adactylous hand. *Clin Orthop* 1995;314:45–58.

This is a report of 18 microvascular toe transfers for the congenitally adactylous hand.

Thumb-Index Web Space

Coombs CJ, Mutimer KL: Tissue expansion for the treatment of complete syndactyly of the first web. *J Hand Surg* 1994;19A: 968–972.

The use of tissue expander as pretreatment to reconstruct the thumb-index web space is discussed.

Friedman R, Wood VE: The dorsal transposition flap for congenital contractures of the first web space: A 20-year experience. *J Hand Surg* 1997:22A:664–670.

This is a report of the conventional dorsal transposition flap to increase the span of the thumb web space in 46 patients with congenital deficiency. Results in general were good, except for patients with symbrachydactyly.

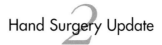
Upton J, Havlik RJ, Coombs CJ: Use of forearm flaps for the severely contracted first web space in children with congenital malformations. *J Hand Surg* 1996;21A:470–477.

The authors report excellent results of radial forearm pedicle flap and posterior interosseous pedicle flap to treat the severely narrowed thumb-web space in various congenital conditions.

Treatment of Other Congenital Conditions

Radial Clubhand

Evans DM, Gateley DR, Lewis JS: The use of a bilobed flap in the correction of radial club hand. *J Hand Surg* 1995;20B:333–337.

The authors describe a bilobed rotational flap, which transposes excess skin and soft tissue from the radial to the ulnar side of the wrist.

Nanchahal J, Tonkin MA: Pre-operative distraction lengthening for radial longitudinal deficiency. *J Hand Surg* 1996;21B:103–107.

Use of a Kessler longitudinal distraction device facilitated the realignment of the radial clubhand on the ulna without resection of the carpal bones.

Reconstruction of the Duplicated Thumb

Horii E, Nakamura R, Sakuma M, Miura T: Duplicated thumb bifurcation at the metacarpophalangeal joint level: Factors affecting surgical outcome. *J Hand Surg* 1997;22A:671–679.

Evaluation of 106 duplicated thumbs that bifurcated at the MCP joint indicated that good results were associated with 2 separate phalanges and the presence of a rudimentary duplicated thumb attached by fibrous tissue to the MCP joint capsule; poor results were associated with a cartilage connection of the duplicated phalanges to each other or to the metacarpal and with an excised thumb that was more than 75% as large as the preserved one.

Townsend DJ, Lipp EB Jr, Chun K, Reinker K, Tuch B: Thumb duplication, 66 years' experience: A review of surgical complications. *J Hand Surg* 1994;19A:973–976.

A review of 66 duplicated thumbs treated surgically between 1925 and 1991 indicated an unacceptable outcome, as determine by joint laxity, angular deformity, functional deficits, and appearance in more than half of the patients.

Camptodactyly

Benson LS, Waters PM, Kamil NI, Simmons BP, Upton J III: Camptodactyly: Classification and results of nonoperative treatment. *J Pediatr Orthop* 1994;14:814–819.

Review of nonoperative splinting as treatment for camptodactyly indicates that it is most effective for smaller contractures in young children.

Glicenstein J, Haddad R, Guero S: Surgical treatment of camptodactyly. *Ann Chir Main Memb Super* 1995;14:264–271.

Review of 70 camptodactylous PIP joints indicates that splinting alone is effective for mild contractures, surgical release of the flexion deformity without tendon transfer followed by splinting is effective in more severe cases, and adolescents to not respond well to operations.

Constriction Band Syndrome

Light TR, Ogden JA: Congenital constriction band syndrome: Pathophysiology and treatment. *Yale J Biol Med* 1993;66:143–155.

Review of clinical manifestations of 88 patients with constriction band syndrome indicates increased band formation, amputation, and syndactyly are found in the index, long, and ring fingers, with less involvement of the small, and minimal involvement of the thumb. The thumb was thought to be protected by its shorter length and adducted position in the palm.

Fourth and Fifth Metacarpal Synostosis

Buck-Gramcko D, Wood VE: The treatment of metacarpal synostosis. *J Hand Surg* 1993:18A:565–581.

This is a report of 99 patients with fourth and fifth metacarpal synostosis. Functionless fifth digits were treated by amputation. Functioning digits were realigned by longitudinal splitting of the common metacarpal and distal transposition of the fifth metacarpal, along with radial collateral ligament reconstruction and tendon transfers.

Ogino T, Kato H: Clinical features and treatment of congenital fusion of the small and ring finger metacarpals. *J Hand Surg* 1993;18A:995–1003.

This a report of 4 patients with synostosis of the fourth and fifth metacarpals treated by longitudinal division of the common metacarpal and placement of a bone block to maintain the alignment. Appearance of the hand was improved.

Psychology of Congenital Anomalies

Bradbury ET, Hewison J: Early parental adjustment to visible congenital disfigurement. *Child Care Health Dev* 1994;20:251–266.

Psychological evaluation by questionnaire and interview of the parents of 34 children born with congenital anomalies is presented. There was no significant correlation between the parents' ability to adjust to the condition and the age of the child, sex of the child, social status of the family, or severity of the deformity. The only significant factor in parental adjustment was the perceived support from the extended family.

Bradbury ET, Kay SP, Hewison J: The psychological impact of microvascular free toe transfer for children and their parents. *J Hand Surg* 1994;19B:689–695.

This is an evaluation of the psychological impact of a major reconstructive procedure for congenital hand deformities. Well-adjusted parents and their children will respond well, while poorly adjusted parents and the affected children will not respond as well postoperatively.

Bradbury ET, Kay SP, Tighe C, Hewison J: Decision-making by parents and children in paediatric hand surgery. *Br J Plast Surg* 1994;47:324–330.

Evaluation of families whose children were undergoing major reconstructive surgery for congenital deficiencies indicates that parents are principally influenced in the decision-making process by the communication with the surgeon and other health care workers, and are less influenced by the child's appearance or their own anxieties about the surgical procedure.

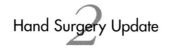
Chapter 40
Spasticity and Cerebral Palsy

Marybeth Ezaki, MD

Cerebral palsy (CP) is the common name given to a non-progressive, static encephalopathy that is present from birth and affects children with a wide range of neurologic deficits. Spasticity is the most common motor disorder in CP. Patterns of limb involvement include hemiplegia, diplegia (bilateral lower limb involvement), and quadriplegia. Developmental delay and intellectual impairment range from minimal to severe.

Etiology and Diagnosis

The overall prevalence of CP is 1.5 to 2.0 per 1,000 live births. A common misconception is that all forms of CP are related to or caused by perinatal anoxia or difficulty with delivery. The number of children affected by CP has not fallen with improvements in obstetrical care. Difficult delivery and birth injury are infrequent causes of CP; in fact, coexistence of brachial plexopathy—often associated with a difficult delivery—with CP is rare. Different clinical forms of CP are likely to be associated with different potential etiologies. Spastic diplegia, in which both lower limbs are involved with or without upper limb involvement, is the common form of motor involvement in children born preterm. The brain of the very immature infant is thought to be more susceptible to hypoxia. Residual paraventricular leukomalacia is found on brain imaging in these children. The extrapyramidal tracts of the lower limbs lie in a paraventricular position and are affected bilaterally by intraventricular hemorrhage, which occurs frequently in the small premature neonate.

An estimated 60% of all CP cases have a prepartum etiology. Spastic hemiplegia is the common motor dysfunction in these children. A significant number of cases have no perinatal risk factors and no history of prematurity. Imaging studies on these children are likely to show evidence of cerebral malformations or earlier antenatal lesions.

Based on statistical evidence and the strong associated risk of twin pregnancy, a recent hypothesis implicates the "vanishing twin syndrome" as a cause of spastic CP. In the surviving twin of a pregnancy in which one twin is stillborn, the risk of CP is 50 to 100 times higher than in a singleton pregnancy. In these cases *fetus papyraceous* (a macerated fetus) can be identified. In ultrasound studies of multiple gestation pregnancies diagnosed in the first trimester, the incidence of a vanishing twin ranged from 10.5% to 100%. Extrapolation from studies on the prevalence of twinning, rates of loss of multiple gestation pregnancies, prevalence of CP, types of CP, and associated risks of twinning and CP suggests that the vanishing twin in the first or second trimester may explain the etiology of some cases of spastic CP.

Association of growth retardation and other dysmorphic features with some cases of CP suggests that other genetic or syndromic factors may be involved.

Sensory Deficiencies

Sensation is altered or deficient in the majority of children with CP. Although evaluation of the sensory deficit is difficult, one group found that 88% percent of hemiplegic children had significant impairments in at least one sensory modality that included somatosensory-evoked potentials. Hemiplegic children who received intensive occupational therapy that concentrated on motor skills alone did not show improvement in their performance.

Effect of Spasticity on Growth

A progressive, nonproportional and unpredictable limb-length discrepancy is a common finding in spastic hemiplegia. The size of the limb as well as the overall rate of maturation are affected. The etiology for this is not related to the overall nutritional status of the child. Delays in skeletal maturation on the affected side compared to the nonspastic side averaged 7.3 months in one study. Another investigator found a correlation between severity of sensory impairment and degree of growth impairment in the affected limb.

Treatment

A recent review article on the orthopaedic management of limb problems in children with CP devoted only one paragraph to the upper limb. The author stated that fewer than 5% of these children would benefit from surgical reconstruction.

Most surgical treatment in CP is focused on the lower limb. In general, if the child has volitional use of the hand, surgical intervention can potentially lessen deformity and improve function.

The establishment of reasonable pretreatment goals is the basis for successful outcome. Goals of treatment in the spastic limb include improvement of function, decrease of deformity, improvement of appearance, and facilitation of custodial care. Volitional use of the hand before surgery is the best predictor of functional improvement after a change in its position. However, a change in the position of even a minimally functional hand can significantly alter its role as an assist hand and improve the overall well-being of the child by normalizing appearance and lessening the social stigma of spasticity in children who are not mentally or developmentally delayed.

Nonsurgical Treatment

Nonsurgical treatment of spasticity is directed toward prevention of contractures, splinting for positional improvement, and hand therapy to improve dexterity and pattern use. Inhibitory casting and aggressive splinting do not improve the results of standard therapy intervention. There is no evidence that any one type of therapy is more beneficial than others. In a recent review article, the authors found no definitive effect of therapy protocols that varied timing, frequency, and type of intervention.

Newer forms of nonsurgical treatment for spasticity include muscle relaxants, such as baclofen, and botulinum toxin to effect a decrease in spasticity.

Baclofen Baclofen is a muscle relaxant and antispasmodic released by the Food and Drug Administration (FDA) for treatment of spasticity caused by multiple sclerosis or spinal cord injury in adult patients. Baclofen is used "off label" most often in generalized spasticity or in cases of lower limb spasticity. In CP, production of excitatory neurotransmitters exceed that of inhibitory neurotransmitters. Inhibitory neurons are deficient or impeded in releasing γ-aminobutyric acid (GABA), the inhibitory neurotransmitter. There is excessive stimulation of alpha motor neurons, resulting in spasticity. This can be reduced by posterior rhizotomy, a surgical procedure that interrupts excitatory neurons, or by medications that increase the concentration of GABA or other inhibitors. Baclofen binds with the GABA receptors in the superficial layers of the spinal cord, substituting for the inhibitor and allowing intrinsic levels of GABA to rise. Baclofen crosses the blood-brain barrier poorly; oral delivery is less effective than intrathecal administration. Continuous intrathecal infusion achieves therapeutic levels with lower overall dosages. Four groups

of patients will potentially benefit from intrathecal baclofen: (1) patients in whom a selective rhizotomy is contraindicated because they depend on a certain degree of spasticity for ambulation; (2) older patients who do not have potential to learn better gait patterns, and have lower limb spasticity; (3) patients who have discomfort from their spasticity; and (4) patients who require relief from their spasticity to facilitate custodial care. Implantation of a pump and a reservoir of baclofen for continuous release appears to be an effective form of treatment for certain forms of lower-limb spasticity.

Botox® Botulimun toxin A (Botox®) appears to be useful in some forms of CP, although it is specifically released by the FDA only for treatment of strabismus and blepharospasm associated with dystonia in patients over 12 years of age. Botulinum toxin prevents the release of acetylcholine at the neuromuscular junction, thereby interfering with muscle contraction. Recovery from a nonlethal dose is by nerve terminal sprouting, which occurs over a course of approximately 3 months. During the period of partial paralysis of the selected muscles, a decrease in spasticity and ability to stretch out contractures can improve function. In a randomized, double-blind study, one group compared botulinum toxin with sterile saline and found improvement in elbow and thumb extension, elbow and wrist flexor tone, and grasp and release. They conclude that the ideal patient is one with marked flexor spasticity, no contracture, and some volitional control of the limb. Contraindications appear to be fixed contractures, lack of volitional control or lack of spasticity. Repeated injections may be required as muscle recovery occurs. Potential problems include the development of antibodies to Botox® and the cost of treatment.

Surgical Treatment

The surgical treatment of upper limb spasticity in CP is limited to what can be done at the musculoskeletal level for a primary central neurologic problem. Unacceptable position of the limb is an indication for surgical care but the goals must be clearly defined preoperatively. The goals of surgical treatment can be broadly grouped as position changes to improve either function or appearance and position changes to facilitate hygiene or custodial care. Most surgical procedures are designed to release contractures and restore balance by combinations of soft-tissue releases and tendon transfers where possible, or by arthrodesis where soft-tissue procedures are inadequate. Selective neurectomy also has a place in the treatment of spasticity. Rhizotomy is usually reserved for cases of uncontrolled spasticity in the lower limbs.

The typical posture of upper limb spasticity is one of elbow, wrist and finger flexion, and forearm pronation.

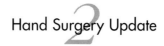
Wrist flexion contracture is common, and balance is difficult to achieve. One group described selective releases of wrist and finger flexors and transfers to augment wrist extension. Transfer of extensor carpi ulnaris rather than the flexor carpi ulnaris to the extensor carpi radialis brevis is often more beneficial because of the in-phase nature of this motor. Some wrist flexion is needed to allow finger extension in the majority of these children. For severe wrist flexion contractures, especially in the nonfunctional hand, wrist arthrodesis and releases of extrinsic and intrinsic finger contractures can offer a solution to hygiene and care problems.

Thumb-in-palm deformity is common. In a report on 59 patients with this deformity, the authors defined the deforming forces as to adductor, and intrinsic tightness and weakness of the extensors and abductors. They recommend addressing each in turn, and offer a classification for the deformity based on the structures involved. Another team recommends rerouting the extensor pollicis longus through the first dorsal compartment to augment thumb abduction.

Annotated Bibliography

Krageloh-Mann I, Petersen D, Hagberg G, Vollmer B, Hagberg B, Michaelis R: Bilateral spastic cerebral palsy: MRI pathology and origin. Analysis from a representative series of 56 cases. *Dev Med Child Neurol* 1995;37:379–397.

Magnetic resonance imaging findings in different clinical forms of CP can be correlated with antenatal and perinatal etiology for the neurologic dysfunction. In cases of spastic diplegia, or bilateral spastic forms of CP, evidence of paraventricular leukomalacia, which affects the extrapyramidal tracts to the lower limbs, characteristically correlates with perinatal insult to the cerebral cortex.

Pharoah PO, Cooke RW: A hypothesis for the aetiology of spastic cerebral palsy: The vanishing twin. *Dev Med Child Neurol* 1997;39:292–296.

In this fascinating paper, the authors hypothesize that the death of a monochorionic cotwin after the eighth week of gestation may explain spastic CP of unknown etiology. This "vanishing twin syndrome" is a recognized phenomenon. CP prevalence rates have not declined with improvements in obstetric care. The death of a cotwin during the second half of gestation is recognized as an important risk factor for spastic hemiplegia in the surviving twin. Statistical evidence of multiple gestation from first trimester ultrasound with subsequent delivery of a singleton pregnancy is presented to support the hypothesis.

Sensory Deficiencies

Cooper J, Majnemer A, Rosenblatt B, Birnbaum R: The determination of sensory deficits in children with hemiplegic cerebral palsy. *J Child Neurol* 1995;10:300–309.

Sensory impairments have long been known to influence the potential for use of an involved hand, but specific sensory testing is difficult in children with CP. The authors evaluated stereognosis, 2-point discrimination, proprioception, pressure sensitivity, directionality, and somatosensory-evoked potentials. Significant abnormalities in sensation were found in 88% of hemiplegic children.

Van Heest AE: Congenital disorders of the hand and upper extremity. *Pediatr Clin North Am* 1996;43:1113–1133.

Sensory deficits are present in the majority of children with spastic hemiparesis. Size discrepancy also correlates with sensory capabilities.

Yekutiel M, Jariwala M, Stretch P: Sensory deficit in the hands of children with cerebral palsy: A new look at assessment and prevalence. *Dev Med Child Neurol* 1994;36:619–624.

Sensory deficits appear to be responsible for a significant portion of the functional deficit in children with CP. Attempts to improve function with therapy focused only on improved motor function have been unsuccessful.

Effects of Spasticity on Growth

Roberts CD, Vogtle L, Stevenson RD: Effect of hemiplegia on skeletal maturation. *J Pediatr* 1994;125:824–828.

Using the Fels method in a study of 19 well-nourished children with spastic hemiplegia, the authors found delayed skeletal maturation as well as underdevelopment of the affected side compared with the uninvolved side. Twelve of the 19 children showed a delay of 6 months or more in skeletal age. The etiology for this nonnutritional growth delay may be related to decreased functional use, neurotrophic or circulatory factors, or sensory deficit.

Treatment

Albright AL: Intrathecal baclofen in cerebral palsy movement disorders. *J Child Neurol* 1996;11(suppl 1):S29–S35.

The author discusses the mechanism by which baclofen affects spasticity, and outlines the rationale, indications, and protocols for intrathecal baclofen.

Corry IS, Cosgrove AP, Walsh EG, McClean D, Graham HK: Botulinum toxin A in the hemiplegic upper limb: A double-blind trial. *Dev Med Child Neurol* 1997;39:185–193.

This randomized, prospective double-blind study compared the results of Botulinum toxin A and normal saline injected into the upper limbs of children with spasticity. Beneficial effects were seen in range of motion and function. The authors discuss the indications, risks, and techniques.

DeLuca PA: The musculoskeletal management of children with cerebral palsy. *Pediatr Clin North Am* 1996;43:1135–1150.

The author of a review article on the orthopaedic management of limb problems in children with cerebral palsy devoted only 1 paragraph to the upper limb, and stated that fewer than 5% of these children would benefit from surgical reconstruction.

Law M, Russell D, Pollock N, Rosenbaum P, Walter S, King G: A comparison of intensive neurodevelopmental therapy plus

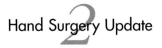

408   Spasticity and Cerebral Palsy

casting and a regular occupational therapy program for children with cerebral palsy. *Dev Med Child Neurol* 1997; 39:664–670.

In a review of published literature, the authors found no definitive effect of therapy protocols that varied timing, frequency, and type of intervention. They found no difference in hand function or quality of upper limb movement in a comparison of 2 treatment groups (intensive therapy plus casting and standard occupational therapy intervention).

Pomerance JF, Keenan MA: Correction of severe spastic flexion contractures in the nonfunctional hand. *J Hand Surg* 1996; 21A:828–833.

Wrist arthrodesis in combination with soft-tissue releases and transfers can help resolve hygiene problems and facilitate care in patients with severe wrist flexion contractures.

Rayan GM, Saccone PG: Treatment of spastic thumb-in-palm deformity: A modified extensor pollicis longus tendon rerouting. *J Hand Surg* 1996;21A:834–839.

The authors describe indications, technique, and results of rerouting the extensor pollicis longus through the first dorsal compartment to add abduction to the thumb.

Sakellarides HT, Kirvin FM: Management of the unbalanced wrist in cerebral palsy by tendon transfer. *Ann Plast Surg* 1995;35:90–94.

Indications and treatment in 60 cases of children with wrist flexion contractures are described.

Sakellarides HT, Mital MA, Matza RA, Dimakopoulos P: Classification and surgical treatment of the thumb-in-palm deformity in cerebral palsy and spastic paralysis. *J Hand Surg* 1995;20A:428–431.

Children with thumb-in-palm deformity have different combinations of deforming forces resulting in subtypes of spastic thumbs. The authors attempt to define the deformity forces and recommend specific procedures to rebalance the thumb. The classification used in this series of 59 patients is based on weak extensor pollicis longus, contracted thenar muscles, weak abductor pollicis longus, and multiple deformities.

Van Heest AE: Congenital disorders of the hand and upper extremity. *Pediatr Clin North Am* 1996;43:1113–1133.

In a review article on congenital upper limb problems that include CP, the author states that if the child has volitional use of the hand, surgical intervention can potentially lessen the deformity and improve function.

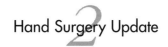

Section X
Other Conditions

American Society for Surgery of the Hand

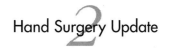

Chapter 41
Infections

Elizabeth Anne Ouellette, MD

Introduction

Hand infections are influenced by both local and systemic factors. Local factors include the location, nature, and severity of tissue disruption; the virulence of the pathogen; and the amount, type, and location of any foreign material in the wound. The potential for infection may also be influenced by prior injury to the limb, chronic edema and impaired circulation, or prior surgical excision of axillary lymph nodes. Systemic factors include the presence of systemic disease, such as diabetes, rheumatoid arthritis, systemic lupus erythematosus, or human immunodeficiency virus (HIV) infection; chronic use of medication that may predispose to infection (eg, cortisone); and the use of immunosuppressive medication.

Etiology and Incidence
Approximately 60% of hand infections are a result of trauma, 25% to 35% result from human bites, 10% to 15% result from drug abuse, and 5% to 10% result from animal bites. The most common types of hand infections are cellulitis and paronychia/eponychia, which each have an incidence of about 35%. Felons account for approximately 15% of hand infections and tenosynovitis for about 10% (Fig. 1). Abscesses of deep spaces of the hand and septic arthritis each have an incidence of about 2%. Osteomyelitis is seen in only about 1% of hand infections.

Causative Organisms

The organisms most likely to cause a given hand infection can often be predicted from the location of the infection, the course of its development, the initiating injury such as puncture wound or bite, and the status of the host. Organisms most frequently isolated in hand infections are listed in Table 1. About 65% of hand infections are caused by aerobic organisms. *Staphylococcus aureus*, isolated in about 35% of infections, is the most common organism. Other aerobic organisms such as α-hemolytic streptococci and group A β-hemolytic streptococci are also common. Gram-negative bacilli are uncommon but may be isolated in special circumstances, such as from contaminated wounds or from wounds in patients

who are drug abusers or have an altered immune status. Chronic or indolent infections may be caused by fungi or mycobacteria. Septic arthritis and osteomyelitis are often caused by *S aureus* and streptococci. Gonococcal infection may be a rare cause of tenosynovitis or a septic joint.

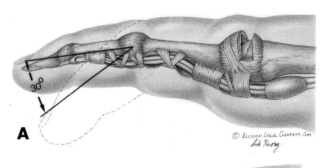

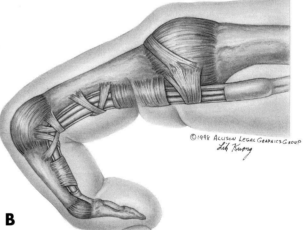

Figure 1

Flexor tenosynovitis, seen in about 10% of hand infections, is most common in the index, long, and ring fingers and is usually due to a penetrating injury. *Staphylococcus aureus* is the most common pathogen isolated, but frequently a mix of aerobic and anaerobic bacteria are identified. The poorly vascularized tendon sheath, which is rich in synovial fluid, provides an ideal environment for infection. **A,** The finger has a resting position of 30° of flexion secondary to swelling of the synovium of the flexor digitorum profundus and flexor digitorum sublimis tendons and effusion within the metacarpophalangeal, proximal interphalangeal, and distal interphalangeal joints. **B,** Full flexion in an uninfected finger with normal synovium and joints. (© Allison Legal Graphics Group, 1998.)

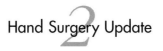
Table 1
Empiric antibiotic therapy used in common infections of the hand*

Situation/Type of Infection	Organism	Empiric Antibiotic Therapy
Simple laceration or open phalangeal fracture (no crush, contamination, soft-tissue loss, use of ORIF, or treatment delay)		None necessary with adequate surgical care
Deep infections in immunocompromised patients (patients with diabetes, HIV-positive patients, or patients with systemic lupus erythematosus or malignancies)	Multiple organisms: *Staphylococcus aureus*, gram-negative bacteria	Aminoglycoside and/or second- or third-generation cephalosporin
Human bites	α- and β-hemolytic streptococci, *Eikenella corrodens*, *S aureus, S epidermidis, Neisseria* species, anaerobes	Combination penicillin/gentamicin/cephalosporin of choice
Animal bites	*Pasteurella multocida, S aureus, S pyogenes, Streptococcus viridans,* α-hemolytic streptococcus, *Bacteroides* species	Same as human bite
Pin track infections with use of percutaneous pins/external fixators	Usually *S aureus* or *S epidermidis*	Cephalosporin of choice
Necrotizing fasciitis	Group A β-hemolytic streptococcus, staphylococcus, gram-negative aerobes, anaerobes	Penicillin 2 million U every 2 hr intravenously or clindamycin and gentamicin
Mycobacterial infections†	*Mycobacterium tuberculosis*	Isoniazid 10 to 15 mg/kg/day, up to 300 mg/day; rifampin 10 to 15 mg/kg/day up to 600 mg/day plus pyrazinamide and ethambutol
	Runyon group I *M marinum* *M kansasii*	As above, or ciprofloxacin, minocycline, doxycycline with ethambutol and rifabutine
	Runyon group III *M avium-intracellulare* *M terrae*	Multiple drug therapy, including ethambutol, cycloserine, imipenem, clofazamine, amikacin, ciprofloxacin, or ethionamide
	Runyon group IV *M fortuitum* *M chelonei* *M ulcerans*	Amikacin or kanamycin; doxycycline or minocycline
Gonococcal infections	*Neisseria gonorrhoeae*	Ceftriaxone or penicillin (clindamycin if allergic)
Fungal infections		
Cutaneous	*Trichophyton* species *Microsporum* species *Candida albicans*	Topical antifungicides
Subcutaneous	*Sporothrix schenckii*	Potassium iodide oral solution (saturated) 1 g/ml; begin with 5 to 10 drops orally 3 times a day, gradually advancing to 40 to 50 drops 3 times a day
Deep infections	*S schenckii*	Intravenous amphotericin B
	Blastomycosis, coccidioidomycosis, histoplasmosis, and maduromycosis	Intravenous amphotericin B††
Herpetic infections (herpetic whitlow)	*Herpes simplex*	Observation; or oral or intravenous acyclovir, usually in immuno-compromised patients
Open contaminated wounds	α-hemolytic streptococcus, staphylococcus, anaerobes, gram-negative bacilli	Cefazolin 1 g every 8 hr, penicillin G 2 million U every 4 hr (bite wounds, animal exposure), and gentamicin (severe crush, contamination)
Cestode infection	*Cysticercus cellulosa* (larval form of *Taenia solium*)	Antihelminthic agent††
Antibiotic resistance in immunocompromised and occasionally in healthy patients	Methicillin-resistant *S aureus*, group A β-hemolytic streptococcus	Vancomycin 500 mg intravenously every 6 hr

*Empiric antibiotic therapy given in this table is meant as a guideline only. Antibiotic therapy should be targeted as specifically as possible as soon as culture and sensitivity results have been obtained.
†Recommend treatment by infectious disease specialist
††Consult infectious disease specialist
ORIF, open reduction and internal fixation; HIV, human immunodeficiency virus.
(Adapted with permission from Bishop AT: Infections, in Manske PR (ed): *Hand Surgery Update*. Rosemont, IL, American Academy of Orthopaedic Surgeons, 1996, pp 395–404.)

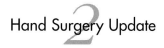

General Treatment Principles

The location of the infection; the extent of its spread; the existence of swelling, warmth, tenderness, lymphangiitis, and lymphadenitis; joint involvement; the initiating event; and the status of the host are determined by careful history and physical examination. Knowledge of the position of the hand at the time of injury may be helpful in predicting which anatomic spaces may be involved, especially in bite wounds. Examination should include an attempt to identify any abscess requiring drainage. Fluctuance on the dorsum of the hand may be difficult to assess, because the loose connection between the skin and underlying tissues allows swelling even in the absence of infection. Radiographs, a complete blood count, and the erythrocyte sedimentation rate usually are obtained.

Key elements of management are surgical drainage, splinting, elevation, rest, antibiotic use, and early rehabilitation. Infections seen very early in their course are sometimes treatable with antibiotics, splinting, and elevation alone. Most hand infections, including all those with any sign of suppuration, require surgical drainage. Established deep infections and those involving tendon, joint, or bone may require hospital admission for multiple surgical debridements and administration of intravenous antibiotics. Use of a general or regional anesthetic is recommended, especially for deep infections. A local anesthetic may not function in the septic environment, and its infiltration may contribute to the swelling and spread the infection.

The surgical incision will depend on the specific infection and location. In general, the incision should be parallel to neurovascular structures and as limited as possible. The deeper structures should be spread with blunt dissection to avoid injury to nerves, vessels, and tendons. Copious irrigation decreases contamination from opening the wound. Exposed joints or flexor tendons should be covered, but otherwise it is generally recommended that most hand wounds be left open initially and be allowed to heal by secondary intention. Placement of incisions such that tendons are not left in open wounds is best. An example is a midaxial incision in the digits, which allows adequate drainage from both the flexor and extensor sides as well as from any involved joint; yet it maintains coverage of any flexor or extensor tendons.

Whenever possible, culture of fluid or tissue is essential for appropriate targeting of antibiotic therapy. Gram's stain, culture, and antibiotic sensitivity determinations should be obtained. The laboratory should specifically be requested to culture for aerobic and anaerobic bacteria, for mycobacteria including *Mycobacterium tuberculosis*, and for fungi. In some cases testing for gonococci and for viruses may be requested.

Initial antibiotic therapy is empiric and depends on the Gram's stain and the organism most likely to cause the infec-

tion. The possibility of mixed flora should always be considered, especially in bite wounds and in immunocompromised patients. Empiric antibiotic treatment recommendations for some common hand infections are given in Table 1. Because of constant changes in available antibiotics and the variations in patient conditions and wound flora, this table is meant as a guide only. The assistance of an infectious disease specialist in the diagnosis and treatment of the infection may be advisable in difficult or unusual cases. Antibiotic therapy should be directed toward specifically cultured organisms as soon as laboratory results are obtained.

Postoperative splinting helps prevent secondary contractures of the joint. The hand should be elevated and splinted in the "safe" position, with the wrist in 30° to 50° extension, the metacarpophalangeals joint in 50° to 90° of flexion, and the interphalangeal joints in 0 to 10° of flexion. Palmar abduction of the thumb to the index metacarpal should be maximal. Active motion of the digits is begun as soon as possible. The dressing should be easily removable to allow frequent wound inspections. Further debridement may be necessary in cases of extensive infection. The wound may be closed secondarily once drainage has cleared and granulation tissue appears.

Infections in Patients With an Altered Immune Status

Infections in Patients With Diabetes
It is well known that patients with diabetes have both impaired immune reactions and an increased incidence of vascular related complications. The patient's predisposition to sepsis is well recognized and may cause significant morbidity. Although precise comparative numbers are not available, serious hand infections appear to be more common in patients with diabetes than in the general population—twice as prevalent, according to some estimates. The tissue response to infection and the ability to heal deep wounds may also be decreased. The worst complications from infections are seen in patients with chronic renal failure sufficient to require dialysis or renal transplantation.

Four situations or types of infections seen almost exclusively in patients with diabetes have been outlined: subepidermal infections, subcutaneous extrafascial dissecting infections, infections in wounds or after injections, and gangrene associated with infection. Subepidermal infections are essentially pus-filled blisters that may be small or very extensive. Although there may a deeper underlying infection, the condition can be treated easily by draining and debriding the blisters and administering appropriate antibiotics. The causative organism usually is *S aureus*. Subcutaneous extrafascial dissection infections may be extensive under the hand's surface without ever involving muscles or extensor tendon compartments and are clearly different from necrotizing fasciitis and myositis. These infections respond well to adequate surgical drainage. The skin must be incised throughout its full length when erythematous and especially when indurated to prevent an undrained portion of the infection from breaking into underlying tendon sheaths or joints. Even in patients with diabetes, infections in surgical wounds of the hand and wrist are extremely rare, especially in the absence of percutaneous pins or other hardware. Infection at injection sites in these patients have been reported, particularly after cortisone injections. Necrosis is most likely to be encountered in diabetic patients with chronic renal failure and peripheral neuropathy. Lacking the pain that drives the nondiabetic patient to seek medical attention, these patients may not realize the severity of the problem until their digits are frankly necrotic. Early and adequate surgery is essential in the patient with chronic renal failure because the severity and extent of the infection are almost always underestimated initially. Part of the severity may result from synergistic infection such as *S aureus* and *Pseudomonas*. Failure to amputate a single digit or ray early may lead to additional necrosis, especially if the blood supply to adjacent fingers is lost because of swelling and tissue destruction.

A review of 25 hand infections in adult patients with diabetes revealed that the highest incidence was in patients between the ages of 40 and 49 years. This age group constitutes an active group of individuals who are economically engaged in the work force or active in homemaking activities. Tissue sepsis was confined to the soft tissues in all patients and localized to the digits in 50% of patients. Predominately gram-negative organisms were cultured from the wounds, and multiple organisms were cultured in 55% of patients. *S aureus*, the most common causative organism in nondiabetic hand infection, was cultured in only 36% of patients. These findings confirm other reports that gram-negative infections and infections with multiple organisms are more common in diabetic patients than in nondiabetic patients. In contrast to foot infections that occur in older patients and tend to recur, the hand infections tended to be one-time events that resolved without recurrence when treated with early aggressive management consisting of adequate drainage and debridement along with parenteral combination antibiotic therapy.

In a review of local and national data on patients admitted to the hospital with codiagnoses of diabetes mellitus and hand infection, it was found that most of these hand infections were nonspecific, confined to the soft tissues, and responsive to broad spectrum parenteral antibiotic therapy. In the national group of 688 patients admitted to the Department of Veterans Affairs Medical Centers with diabetes and hand infections, only 20% had deep infections requiring surgery, and only 2.2% had amputation of all or part of a digit.

Infections in Patients With Human Immunodeficiency Virus

HIV infection that has progressed to acquired immunodeficiency syndrome (AIDS) places the patient at risk for unusual infections, atypical presentations of common hand infections, and opportunistic infections. The course of the infections may also be atypical. Herpetic infections may not resolve spontaneously, and superficial infections may progress to deep infections. Such atypical hand infections may raise the suspicion of HIV infection in the patient at risk.

A study of 24 HIV-positive patients seen on an emergency hand service showed that 14 of these patients who had septic hands spent more time in the hospital and required more operations than did septic patients who were HIV negative. Further, HIV-positive patients with low CD4 counts required the longest hospitalization and the most aggressive management. In the HIV host, the CD4 T-helper cells that activate and mediate specific cell-mediated immunity are suppressed. The severity of the immunocompromise appears to parallel the decreases in CD4 cell count.

The effect that the altered immune status of a patient with HIV has on wound healing is unclear. Limited data indicate that wound healing is not clinically impaired in patients with asymptomatic HIV infection. Wound healing in patients with AIDS may be impaired, but it has not been established whether the cause is the immune disorder itself or secondary issues such as malnutrition.

Infections of Human and Animal Bite Wounds

Bite wounds are responsible for up to 40% of hand infections. Because of the risk of serious complications, these wounds should be treated aggressively with immediate exploration for foreign bodies and joint capsule penetration, collection of fluids or tissue for aerobic and anaerobic cultures, irrigation and debridement, splinting and elevation, tetanus prophylaxis when appropriate, and prophylactic antibiotics. Bite wounds to the hand should not be closed initially. Postoperative follow-up is essential because deep infection such as osteomyelitis may develop even after seemingly adequate debridement.

Human Bites

Although human bite injuries may result from innocent activities such as nail biting, the most common cause by far is violent attack. Injuries resulting from the latter include common full-thickness bites, bite amputation, and injuries incurred from striking the teeth with a clenched fist. The

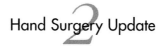

inoculating pathogens reflect the flora of the human mouth. The most commonly isolated aerobic organisms are α- and β-hemolytic streptococci, *S aureus*, *S epidermidis*, *Eikenella corrodens*, and *Neisseria* species. Anaerobic organisms include *Bacteroides*, *Clostridium*, *Fusobacterium*, *Peptococcus*, and *Veillonella*.

In the clenched-fist injury, the injured joint is sealed as the digit is extended, and the tendon that was lacerated by the tooth glides proximally, providing an anaerobic environment for the bacteria that were introduced. For this reason, all patients who have small lacerations over a metacarpophalangeal joint should be considered to have a tooth injury regardless of the history given. The wound should be swabbed for aerobic and anaerobic cultures, with particular attention to *E corrodens*. The antibiotics usually recommended include either penicillin G, ampicillin, carbenicillin, or tetracycline for *E corrodens* and a cephalosporin for *Staphylococcus* organisms. Antibiotic coverage may be targeted more specifically once culture and sensitivity results are obtained.

In a review of 24 cases of osteomyelitis of the hand after a human bite, 2 factors led to the development of these serious infections: a delay of more than 24 hours before debridement or inadequate initial treatment. The mechanism of injury was evenly divided between incisor injuries and clenched-fist injuries. Nine patients required multiple debridements. A case of clenched-fist injury was reported in which the causative organism was methicillin-resistant *S aureus* (MRSA). MRSA is becoming more prevalent in community-acquired infections and should be suspected when empiric antibiotic therapy fails. The case points up the importance of obtaining culture results and antibiotic sensitivity determinations as guides in the choice of antibiotic therapy.

Animal Bites

Dog bites to the hand may appear as puncture wounds or as superficial or deep lacerations, whereas cat wounds more often appear as puncture wounds. Dog-bite wounds are generally considered to be at moderate risk for infection compared with other mammalian bite wounds. Infection rates for all dog bites range from 1.4% to 30%. Dog-bite wounds to the hands present special problems, however, with infection rates around 30% or even up to 80% for contaminated crush injuries or puncture wounds. After cleansing, irrigation, and debridement severe wounds should be left open, but superficial wounds may be closed loosely.

Animal-bite infections are frequently due to anaerobic organisms; thus, empiric antibiotic therapy should cover both aerobic and anaerobic bacteria. In addition to routine pathogens such as *S aureus* and *S pyogenes*, canine oral flora include *Streptococcus viridans*, *Bacteroides* species, and *Pasteurella multocida*. *P multocida* is present in the oral flora of

half of domestic dogs and two thirds of domestic cats and is a frequent cause of infections related to animal-bite wounds. Most of these organisms are sensitive to penicillin, which is the antibiotic of choice.

Infections Associated With Fractures

Infections of the hand after fracture are most commonly associated with the use of percutaneous pins and external fixators. The rate of pin track infection in fractures fixed with pins is around 7% to 8%. External fixators also pose a risk of infection, particularly when larger implants are used for greater strength and stability. Factors associated with pin track infections are motion at the pin–bone interface, pin placement within the cortical bone, necrosis of bone or soft tissue surrounding the pin, and soft-tissue tension where the pin exits the skin. Wound severity, amount of contamination, and delay in presentation also appear to play a role, as do host factors such as presence of systemic disease and noncompliance. Pin track infections may ordinarily be treated with oral antibiotics. If this treatment fails, parenteral antibiotics and possibly pin removal and curettage of any sequestrum in the pin track may be necessary.

Deep infection after internal fixation of hand fractures is rare. Such an infection may occur at 3 stages: in the early postoperative period, at nonunion, and at nonunion with a segmental defect. Treatment goals for an early postoperative infection are to eradicate sepsis, obtain fracture union, and regain satisfactory hand function. Treatment of an infected nonunion may include debridement of all infected bone and fibrous tissue followed by external fracture stabilization and skin coverage. Delayed bone grafting and internal fixation may be performed once the infection has cleared. Goals of treating a segmental defect are to facilitate bone healing and restore normal function. Management includes controlling the infection, restoring bone alignment and length, stabilizing the nonunion, and bone grafting.

Postoperative Infection

The low numbers of infections in hand surgery and the problems of surveillance for outpatient surgery make an accurate determination of the postoperative infection rate difficult. The amount of wound contamination appears to be a significant factor: the infection rates for clean procedures range from 1% to 7%, and those for dirty procedures can be as high as 40%. In clean procedures *S aureus* is the most common pathogen, and *S epidermidis* is often isolated in implant surgery. Pathogens identified less commonly are other gram-positive organisms and *Enterobacteriaceae* and *Bacteroides*. Gram-negative, anaerobic, fungal, and mixed infections can occur, particularly in open, contaminated wounds and in patients whose immune status is altered. Infection generally appears between 3 and 7 days after surgery but can occur as late as 3 to 4 weeks.

Firm recommendations regarding the use of perioperative prophylactic antibiotics do not exist. Perioperative antibiotic use for hand surgery is recommended under the following circumstances: in patients with preexisting conditions predisposing to infection, such as diabetes and rheumatoid arthritis; patients in whom percutaneous Kirschner wires or implants are used; in longer operations; in wounds with more than a 6-hour delay in reaching the operating room; and in open fractures. Their use should also be considered for severe soft-tissue injuries, for injuries involving tendon or joint, for confirmed or suspected human or animal bites, for patients with prosthetic heart valves or mitral valve prolapse, and for noncompliant patients.

Necrotizing Fasciitis

Necrotizing fasciitis is an uncommon soft-tissue infection characterized by widespread fascial necrosis that spreads quickly along fascial planes (Fig. 2). It may be caused by anaerobic or aerobic bacteria. Cases in which only anaerobic organisms are present are rarely seen. More prevalent are cases in which group A streptococci are isolated, either alone or in combination with other species—most commonly *S aureus*. Necrotizing infections are true emergencies that require aggressive surgical and medical treatment to avoid loss of limb or life.

Necrotizing infections may appear relatively benign early on. The patient often presents with an erythematous, hot, exquisitely tender, swollen area of cellulitis accompanied by fever and local pain within about 7 days of the initiating event. Later, blisters and bullae form. These are initially filled with serous fluid but later become hemorrhagic, signaling that the infection has become well established in the subcutaneous plane. Liquefactive necrosis of the subcutaneous fat and fascia, and occasionally of muscle, can progress rapidly along fascial planes until the entire area of undermined skin becomes necrotic. Anesthesia may develop before skin necrosis, providing a clue that the infection is not simply cellulitis. A further clue is provided if a hemostat used to probe the lesion through a limited incision passes easily along the plane just superficial to the deep fascia. Marked systemic toxicity out of proportion to local findings should also cause suspicion.

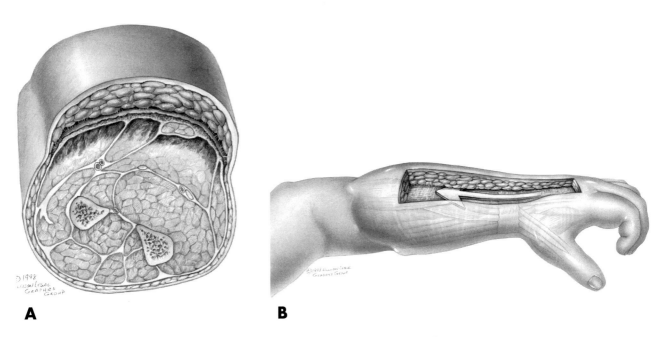

A   **B**

Figure 2

Necrotizing fasciitis of the hand and forearm. **A,** Cross-section at the distal forearm. The area of swollen, darkened skin on the dorsal forearm is clearly demarcated directly over the dorsal fascial compartments. The fascia beneath it has become liquified. **B,** The subcutaneous tissue and fascia are shown in a cut-away view to demonstrate how the infection spreads proximally along fascial planes, as indicated by the arrow. (© Allison Legal Graphics Group, 1998.)

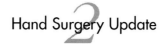

A prompt diagnosis should be followed by immediate surgical debridement and antibiotic therapy that takes into account the mixed organisms generally found in these infections. Long incisions through the skin and subcutaneous tissues should extend well beyond the area of involvement. "Second-look" procedures are often necessary 24 hours later to ensure the adequacy of the debridement. Multiple debridements may be necessary.

Mycobacterial Infection

Mycobacterial infections of the hand are uncommon, but they should be suspected in the chronically painful or swollen hand, particularly if the symptoms are progressive. A persistent or recurring synovitis of the finger or wrist should also lead to suspicion. Certain occupations can increase the risk for infections with specific mycobacterial organisms in healthy workers. Mycobacteria may also cause opportunistic infections in immunocompromised patients.

Mycobacterium tuberculosis in the hand most commonly presents as tenosynovitis, but it may also involve the bones of the fingers and wrist. There are at least 19 species of mycobacteria besides those that cause tuberculosis and leprosy. These "atypical" mycobacteria species, grouped by Runyon classification (Table 1), are increasingly recognized as a cause of hand infections. Approximately 100 cases of deep hand infections caused by these organisms have been reported in the United States in the last 30 years. The species most commonly implicated have been *Mycobacterium marinum, M kansasii,* and *M avium-intracellulare. M marinum* may result from wounds contaminated by marine water, swimming pools, fish tanks, or handling of fish, and infection with this organism may present as a poorly healing ulcer on the hand. It can attack bone, joint, synovium, or skin. *M kansasii* may cause infections in the skin, tenosynovium, and deeper structures. *M avium-intracellulare* has been cultured from fowl, swine, cattle, and birds and inhabits soil and water reservoirs. *M fortuitum* and *M chelonei* have rarely been reported as the cause of hand infections. Infections of the hand due to *M bovis* are very rare and usually are found in those who work with cattle, eg, herders and butchers.

Consultation with an infectious disease specialist may be sought for recommendations regarding diagnosis and treatment of mycobacterial infections. Diagnosis requires surgical debridement and culture of the lesion. Surgical exploration and histopathologic examination of specimens obtained during debridement often reveal granulomatous tenosynovitis typically involving the anterior aspect of a finger or the palm or wrist. Surgical intervention, which frequently includes tenosynovectomy, appears to be important in the management of the infection, and extensive serial debridements may be required.

Empiric antibiotic treatment should be started immediately, because cultures often take as long as 6 to 12 weeks to grow. Acid-fast staining should be done, and the culture should be incubated at both 37° C and 30° C to detect the most common cause of mycobacteriosis in the hand, *M marinum,* because it grows preferentially at the lower temperature. Culture of *M fortuitum* requires incubation at 20° C. The importance of chemotherapy, usually with a combination of bacteriocidal agents, in the treatment of these infections is unclear; it appears to be a necessary adjunctive therapy for some cases but not all.

Gonococcal Infection

Gonorrhea is one of the most common reportable communicable diseases in the United States today. Two distinct forms of disseminated gonococcal infection have been delineated: septic arthritis, which is the more common pattern of dissemination, and another form characterized mainly by tenosynovitis-dermatitis. Gonococcal infection must be considered in any sexually active patient who presents with tenosynovitis or a septic joint.

Gonococcal involvement of the flexor tendons is unusual, but this condition, in the form of a purulent flexor tenosynovitis, has been reported as the single manifestation of a disseminated infection with *Neisseria gonorrhoeae* in an immunosuppressed patient. Prompt surgical response with tendon sheath drainage, culture of the purulent material, and administration of appropriate antibiotics is the recommended treatment. Gram's stain and culture may not be positive until late in the disease, and thus gram-negative stain and culture should not preclude treatment for gonorrhea if it is suspected. Gram's stain of urethral discharge, as well as urethral, pharyngeal, anal, and blood cultures, may help confirm the diagnosis of disseminated gonococcal infection. Penicillin and ceftriaxone are generally the preferred antibiotic agents for treatment of gonorrhea, although other second- and third-generation cephalosporins or β-lactamase inhibitor agents are also used.

Fungal Infection

Three types of fungal infections manifesting in the hand are cutaneous infections caused by dermatophytes, subcutaneous infections, and deep or systemic infections. Onychomycosis is a fungal infection of the nail caused by dermatophytes such as *Trichophyton* species or *Microsporum* species or by *Candida albicans*. Sporotrichosis, a subcutaneous infection, is caused by *Sporothrix schenckii*, which is commonly found in soil and plant matters. At occupational risk are gardeners and farmers, in whom spores may be implanted subcutaneously by penetrating injury from a wood sliver, thorn, or animal bite. Deep or systemic infections are usually caused by sporotrichosis, blastomycosis, coccidioidomycosis, histoplasmosis, or maduromycosis. These rare infections are usually seen in immunocompromised patients. In addition to appropriate medical therapy, surgical debridement may be necessary, particularly for tenosynovitis, fungal arthritis, or fungal osteomyelitis.

Herpetic Infection

Herpetic whitlow is a viral infection caused by the herpes simplex virus. It is usually seen in small children and in medical and dental personnel involved in the care of the oral or respiratory system. It commonly appears over the distal phalanx of a single digit, causing severe throbbing, swelling, and erythema. Vesicles, absence of pus, a soft pulp space, and exposure to the herpes simplex virus help distinguish this lesion from a felon. The infection is self-limited, and medical and surgical treatment usually are not recommended.

Miscellaneous and Unusual Infections

Helminthic Infection
Worm infections contribute significantly to the incidence of infectious diseases worldwide, although most individuals with these infections harbor low worm burdens and are asymptomatic. The major pathogens in this group are roundworms (nematodes), flukes (trematodes), and tapeworms (cestodes). Cysticercosis is an infestation with *Cysticercus cellulosa*, the larval form of the pork tapeworm *Taenia solium*. A case in which cysticercosis involving a deep flexor forearm muscle caused flexion deformity in the fingers has been reported. Although rare, a helminthic etiology should be considered for patients, particularly in tropical areas, who present with a clinical picture of Volkmann's ischemic contracture with insidious onset and progressive deformity but no previous history of injury to the area.

Infection Associated With Compartment Syndrome
Four cases of infection directly associated with compartment syndrome of the upper extremity have been reported. Two patients presented with infection and compartment syndrome, and 2 developed a compartment syndrome 2 to 12 hours after admission. All 4 grew β-hemolytic streptococci on initial culture, and 3 grew group A streptococcus. Fasciotomies and serial debridements were required. The administration of broad spectrum intravenous antibiotics did not prevent the development of a compartment syndrome in 1 patient who ultimately underwent amputation at the elbow.

Infection Following Endoscopic Carpal Tunnel Release
Surgical release of the transverse carpal tunnel has been documented to be a safe and effective therapy for carpal tunnel syndrome. The incidence of overall perioperative complications is low, and infection rates range from 0 to only about 1%. Factors associated with an increased risk of infection are longer procedures, steroid installation at surgery, tenosynovectomy, and the use of drains.

A case of infection following 2-portal endoscopic carpal tunnel release in which the flexor retinaculum was incompletely divided has been reported. The patient developed an *S aureus* tenosynovitis and an infection within the ulnar and radial bursae; an abscess in the middle palmar, thenar, and Parona's space; and a pyogenic wrist arthritis. Aggressive surgical treatment and administration of antibiotics brought this potentially life-threatening infection under control. If a septic complication is suspected after endoscopic carpal tunnel release, early exploration should be performed because the infection is not likely to drain through the small portal incisions.

Another case of serious infection was reported after standard carpal tunnel release in a patient with diabetes. The young woman had undergone a laparoscopic tubal ligation immediately after the carpal tunnel release. On the eighth postoperative day the patient had a swollen, painful hand with mild erythema along the wound margins. The infection progressed and the patient developed fever despite intravenous administration of a broad-spectrum antibiotic. Serial debridements culminating in radical debridement of the entire palmar fascia and overlying skin were required. Debridement revealed microabscesses with widespread necrosis consistent with necrotizing fasciitis. The combining of 2 initial surgical procedures with mixed wound classifications could not be identified as a causative factor in this patient's hand infection. Nevertheless, the practice merits caution in patients with diminished resistance to infection.

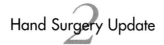
Antibiotic Therapy, Antibiotic Resistance, and Outlook for the Future

Recently, bacterial strains resistant to multiple antibiotics have emerged and spread, limiting the therapeutic options for treatment of many severe bacterial infections. Examples are methicillin-resistant *S aureus* and group A β-hemolytic streptococcus. The emergence of these resistant bacteria has increased the potential seriousness of any infection, even a superficial infection of the hand. The threat of uncontrollable infection is particularly grave in the immunocompromised patient. Antibiotic-resistant infections usually have been encountered in the hospital setting, particularly in intensive care units, but recently reports have revealed a burgeoning of community-acquired cases.

Although there has been a reawakening of interest in anti-infective therapy by research-based pharmaceutical companies, the development of new agents is a long and costly process, and new strains will inevitably emerge that are resistant to these drugs as well. Thus, a time may be approaching in which even healthy patients with clean hand wounds may be at serious risk for an infection that results in permanent loss of function, amputation, or even death.

The treating physician plays an important role in stemming the growth of bacterial resistance by ensuring appropriate antibiotic use and by maintaining appropriate sterile techniques. Once an infection is suspected, initial antibiotic treatment is empiric based on physical examination and Gram's stain. Except for the most superficial infections, wound swabs and/or tissue samples should be sent to the laboratory for culture and sensitivity testing. Once results are obtained, an immediate change to the most specific agent or agents possible should be made. Practitioners prescribing antibiotics need to keep up to date on diagnosis and treatment of infections. Because incorrect use of antibiotics can augment the development of resistance, patients should be provided with sufficient information so that they understand how to take the prescribed drug. Means of ensuring patient adherence to the full treatment should be explored.

At a more basic level, the public needs to be educated about the risks and benefits of antibiotics. Good hygiene and prevention of infection should be the target of a widespread educational campaign. Such practices are essential to reduce the possibility that with the relentless increase in the emergence, evolution, and spread of resistant pathogens, and the inability to produce new drugs rapidly enough, physicians and their patients are truly entering the postantibiotic era.

Annotated Bibliography

Overview

Brown DM, Young VL: Hand infections. *South Med J* 1993; 86:56–66.

This article presents current concepts in the diagnosis and treatment of common hand infections. Topics covered include the anatomy of the hand in relation to infection, etiology, factors predisposing to infection, causative organisms, antibiotic therapy, and general treatment principles.

Moran GJ, Talan DA: Hand infections. *Emerg Med Clin North Am* 1993;11:601–619.

This article reviews the important diagnostic and management issues for infections of the hand. Anatomy is outlined, microbiology and antibiotic use are discussed, and surgical principles are given.

Wright PE II: Hand infections, in Canale ST, Daugherty K, Jones L (eds): *Campbell's Operative Orthopaedics*, ed 9. St Louis, MO, Mosby-Year Book, 1998, vol 4, pp 3735–3747.

This chapter outlines the factors influencing hand infections and presents a general approach to hand infections, including technique for incision and drainage. The following hand infections are discussed, and the surgical technique for each type is described: paronychia, web space infections, deep fascial space infections, tenosynovitis, infections of radial and ulnar bursae, and finger joint infections. Also discussed are osteomyelitis; human bite injuries; and miscellaneous and unusual infections such as herpetic infections, infections in drug addicts, infections in patients with AIDS, mycobacterial infections, and fungal infections.

Infection in Patients With an Altered Immune Status

Ching V, Ritz M, Song C, De Aguir G, Mohanlal P: Human immunodeficiency virus infection in an emergency hand service. *J Hand Surg* 1996;21A:696–699.

Over a 6-month period 504 consecutive patients at the Emergency Hand Service were tested for HIV, and 24 patients tested positive. Fourteen of 121 patients with hand sepsis had HIV, and 10 of 383 patients who had nonseptic hand problems were HIV-positive. Patients with HIV and hand sepsis had a longer delay in seeking medical attention, spent more time in the hospital, and required more operations than did HIV-negative patients with hand sepsis. Furthermore, of all 504 patients, a larger percentage of HIV-positive persons than HIV-negative persons was likely to be seen for infection.

Gunther SF, Gunther SB: Hand infections in patients with diabetes, in Pritchard DJ (ed): *Instructional Course Lectures 45*. Rosemont, IL, American Academy of Orthopaedic Surgeons, 1996, pp 37–43.

The authors estimate that serious hand infections are twice as common in patients with diabetes as in the general population. Patients with the worst complications are those with chronic renal failure, because these patients have the worst protein depletion, neuropathies, and regional ischemia secondary to arterial disease. Surgical dialysis shunts in these patients may steal blood from the hand.

Kour AK, Looi KP, Phone MH, Pho RW: Hand infections in patients with diabetes. *Clin Orthop* 1996;331:238–244.

Twenty-five patients with adult-onset diabetes and hand infections were reviewed. Only 4 patients had open injuries or volunteered a history of trauma before the sepsis. Eighty percent were younger than 60 years of age and had had diabetes mellitus for 5 years or less. Tissue sepsis was confined to the soft tissues in all patients. Multiple organisms were cultured in 55% of patients. Four patients requiring repeated debridements had cultures of multiple gram-negative organisms, and 3 of them required amputation. An aggressive treatment protocol of hospital admission, intravenous combination antibiotics, surgical debridement, appropriate diabetes control, and strict elevation of the hand was important in management of the sepsis.

Pinzur MS, Bednar M, Weaver F, Williams A: Hand infections in the diabetic patient. *J Hand Surg* 1997;22B:133–134.

The authors reviewed 23 patients admitted to a university hospital/Department of Veterans Affairs Medical Center over a 9-year period with a codiagnosis of diabetes mellitus and hand infection. They compared the data with those on 688 patients retrieved from the Department of Veterans Affairs National Database for 5 of the 9 years. Local data agreed with national data and showed that most infections were nonspecific cellulitis, which nearly universally responded clinically to various broad-spectrum parenteral antibiotics. In the national group, only 20% of the 688 patients admitted to the hospital for hand infections had a deep-seated infection requiring surgery, and only 2.2% required amputation.

Infection of Bite Wounds

Berlet G, Richards RS, Roth JH: Clenched-fist injury complicated by methicillin-resistant *Staphylococcus aureus*. *Can J Surg* 1997;40:313–314.

A case of a 51-year-old man with a 2-week-old methicillin-resistant *S aureus* infection of the dorsum of the hand is presented. Successful treatment consisted of 5 weeks of intravenous vancomycin.

Dire DJ, Hogan DE, Riggs MW: A prospective evaluation of risk factors for infections from dog-bite wounds. *Acad Emerg Med* 1994;1:258–266.

A prospective survey was conducted of 769 dog-bite victims who came into a community hospital emergency department over a 2-year period. A standardized wound-cleaning protocol was used. Wound closure and use of antibiotics were left to the discretion of the treating physician. Of the 734 patients who had complete records, 20 (4%) had bites to the hand. Wound infection was diagnosed in 21% of the 734 wounds at follow-up. Wounds that had required surgical debridement had a 7-fold higher infection rate than those not surgically debrided. Patients older than 50 years had an infection rate that was 6 times higher than that in younger patients. Wound depth, patient gender, and wound debridement were clinical variables that best predicted the likelihood of developing infection. Reviewers' comments appended to the article noted that the finding regarding clinical variables should be viewed cautiously. A multicenter bite-wound study was recommended to standardize a wound care protocol and to collect data associated with a high risk of infection, including the additional variable of antibiotic use.

Gonzalez MH, Papierski P, Hall RF Jr: Osteomyelitis of the hand after a human bite. *J Hand Surg* 1993;18A:520–522.

Twenty-four cases of osteomyelitis of the hand after a human bite were reviewed. Two factors led to the development of osteomyelitis: a delay of more than 24 hours before debridement or inadequate initial treatment. The mechanism of injury was evenly divided between incisor injuries and clenched-fist injuries.

Infection Associated With Fractures

Ebraheim NA, Biyani A, Wong FY, Cornicelli S: Management of infected defect nonunion of the metacarpals. *Am J Orthop* 1997;26:362–364.

The authors describe a case of an infected defect nonunion of the metacarpal with shortening secondary to open reduction and internal fixation with Kirschner wires. Aggressive radical debridements, intravenous antibiotics, fracture stabilization, and gradual distraction of the nonunion site with an external minifixator led to an excellent result.

Postoperative Infection

Rieger H, Grünert J, Brug E: A severe infection following endoscopic carpal tunnel release. *J Hand Surg* 1996;21B:672–674.

A case of infection following 2-portal endoscopic carpal tunnel release in which the flexor retinaculum was incompletely divided is reported. The patient developed an *S aureus* tenosynovitis and an infection within the ulnar and radial bursae; an abscess in the middle palmar, thenar, and Parona's space; and a pyogenic wrist arthritis. Aggressive surgical treatment and administration of appropriate antibiotic therapy brought the potentially life-threatening infection under control. The patient regained full hand function and returned to his work as a farmer.

Shapiro DB: Postoperative infection in hand surgery: Cause, prevention, and treatment. *Hand Clin* 1994;10:1–12.

The article presents a comprehensive review of postoperative infection of the hand. Topics covered are epidemiology and etiology of postoperative infection, common pathogens, diagnosis and treatment of infections, and management of complications. Prevention of infection by techniques to decrease wound contamination and by prophylactic antibiotic therapy is discussed. Factors affecting a patient's ability to ward off a postoperative infection, eg, diabetes, rheumatoid arthritis, HIV, and AIDS, are considered.

Necrotizing Fasciitis

Greco RJ, Curtsinger LJ: Carpal tunnel release complicated by necrotizing fasciitis. *Ann Plast Surg* 1993;30:545–548.

A case of a diabetic woman who underwent carpal tunnel release followed by a laparoscopic tubal ligation is described. The procedure was complicated by a severe necrotizing fasciitis infection of the carpal tunnel release incision postoperatively. The patient regained full range of motion. Her long history of insulin-dependent diabetes and a concomitant clean-contaminated procedure are complicating factors.

Swartz MN: Cellulitis and subcutaneous tissue infections, in Mandell GL, Bennett JE, Dolin R (eds): *Principles and Practice of Infectious Diseases*, ed 4. New York, NY, Churchill Livingstone, 1995, pp 909–929.

The chapter considers bacterial and mycotic infections of the skin and subcutaneous tissues. Cellulitis and superficial infections as well as

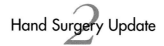
subcutaneous tissue infections and abscesses are covered. Necrotizing fasciitis, which includes streptococcal gangrene as a major subset, is well described, and therapy is outlined.

Mycobacterial Infection

Bagatur E, Bayramicli M: Flexor tenosynovitis caused by *Mycobacterium bovis:* A case report. *J Hand Surg 1996;* 21A:700–702.

A case of flexor tenosynovitis caused by *M bovis* is described. The patient's history of a wrist puncture during a cattle slaughter a few months before the onset of symptoms led authors to suspect the correct diagnosis of this rare condition. Treatment was a combination of chemotherapy and surgical debridement.

Darrow M, Foulkes G, Richmann PN, de los Reyes CL, Floyd WE III: Deep infection of the hand with *Mycobacterium avium-intracellulare:* Two case reports. *Am J Orthop 1995;* 24:914–917.

Two cases of deep hand infections with *M avium-intracellulare* (Runyon group III, nonphotochromogen) occurred in elderly men. Both patients had long histories of progressive swelling, a characteristic of deep mycobacterial hand infections. Aggressive surgical debridement combined with antitubercular chemotherapy led to an excellent outcome in both cases.

Hellinger WC, Smilack JD, Greider JL Jr, et al: Localized soft-tissue infections with *Mycobacterium avium/Mycobacterium intracellulare* complex in immunocompetent patients: Granulomatous tenosynovitis of the hand or wrist. *Clin Infect Dis* 1995;21:65–69.

Six cases of localized soft-tissue infection with *M avium/M intracellulare* complex in immunocompetent hosts are described. These cases were similar to 11 previously reported cases. Sixteen of the 17 cases were characterized by chronic tenosynovitis or synovitis with granuloma formation that involved the anterior aspect of a finger or the palm or wrist. In most cases the infection followed trauma of, surgical treatment of, or corticosteroid injection into the affected extremity. Most patients were in the fifth to seventh decades of life. Surgical intervention with appropriate culture was critical for diagnosis, and surgical debridement appeared to be important for management. The role of antimycobacterial chemotherapy was unclear, but it seemed to be a beneficial adjunctive measure in most cases.

Gonococcal Infection

Krieger LE, Schnall SB, Holtom PD, Costigan W: Acute gonococcal flexor tenosynovitis. *Orthopedics* 1997;20:649–650.

The article describes a case of acute suppurative flexor tenosynovitis of the long finger caused by *N gonorrhoeae.* This was the singular manifestation of a disseminated gonococcal infection. An HIV test obtained on admission was positive. Incision and drainage of the finger and appropriate antibiotic therapy led to a good result.

Helminthic Infection

Anderson GA, Chandi SM: Cysticercosis of the flexor digitorum profundus muscle producing flexion deformity of the fingers. *J Hand Surg* 1993;18B:360–362.

A middle-aged female from a tropical country presented with a selective, gradually worsening flexion deformity of the middle and ring fingers that resembled mild Volkmann's contracture. The cause was *Cysticercus cellulosa* infection within the deep flexor muscles of the forearm. Treatment consisted of mepacrine and filix mas, an extract of male fern. Excision of the fibrotic segment of the muscle and tenodesis of all flexor profundus tendons restored normal range of motion to the affected fingers.

Infection Associated With Compartment Syndrome

Schnall SB, Holtom PD, Silva E: Compartment syndrome associated with infection of the upper extremity. *Clin Orthop* 1994; 306:128–131.

A retrospective review of all admissions to the musculoskeletal infection ward during a 1-year period identified 4 patients with a compartment syndrome directly associated with upper extremity infection. Fasciotomies and serial debridements were performed. Amputation through the elbow was necessary in 1 patient.

Antibiotic Usage

Madsen MS, Neumann L, Andersen JA: Penicillin prophylaxis in complicated wounds of hands and feet: A randomized, double-blind trial. *Injury* 1996;27:275–278.

The study examined the effect of prophylactic penicillin treatment on the infection rate in patients with traumatic wounds to the hands or feet with underlying lesions of bone, tendon, or joint. Patients (599) were randomized to double-blinded treatment with either (A) 1 injection of penicillin G, (B) penicillin V tablets for 6 days, or (C) no antibiotic. The infection rate was 4.9% in group A, 6.7% in group B, and 10.2% in group C. There was no significant difference in infection rates of all 3 groups, but the difference in infection rate between patients given a penicillin injection and patients not given antibiotics was 5.3%. The authors conclude that a single prophylactic injection of penicillin G is advisable for patients with these wounds.

Platt AJ, Page RE: Post-operative infection following hand surgery: Guidelines for antibiotic use. *J Hand Surg* 1995; 20B:685–690.

In a prospective study of 236 adult patients admitted to the hospital for elective or emergency hand surgery over a 4-month period, the infection rate was 10.7% in elective operations and 9.7% in emergency operations. There was no significant reduction in infection rate with the use of antibiotics ($p = 0.5$) in the elective group and an 8.5-fold reduction in infection rate ($p = 0.014$) with perioperative antibiotic administration in the emergency group. The presence of a dirty wound was associated with a 13.4-fold increase in postoperative wound infection rate ($p = 0.002$).

Williams RJ, Heymann DL: Containment of antibiotic resistance. *Science* 1998;279:1153–1154.

The threat posed by the upward trend in the numbers of bacteria resistant to multiple antibiotics is discussed. A broad strategy for reducing selective pressure from the presence of antibiotics is proposed: improve the rational use of antibiotics in human medicine, reduce the global selective pressure of antibiotics by reducing or eliminating uses other than in human medicine, and reduce the spread of resistant organisms by improving hospital hygiene and public health infrastructure.

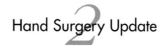

Chapter 42
Injection and Extravasation Injuries

423

Douglas M. Rothkopf, MD

The injection and infusion of a variety of medications and solutions is routine for the care of both outpatients and hospitalized patients of all ages. A fraction of these treatments are complicated by extravasation of intra-arterial or intraneural injection. Outside the health care setting, high-pressure injection injuries of the upper extremity are encountered with an increasing array of substances. Prompt diagnosis and treatment of all injection and extravasation injuries are critical for tissue preservation and limiting morbidity.

Injection Injuries

High-Pressure Injection Injuries

The high-pressure injection of diesel fuel in the hand was first reported in 1937. With the increasing use of high-pressure injectors, a wide variety of substances have been implicated, including grease, paint, paint thinner, hydraulic fluid, molten metal, anti-rust sealant, wax, water, oil, molding plastic, air, mud, and cement. The devices most commonly responsible for injury are grease guns, spray guns, and diesel fuel injectors; defects in high-pressure hoses, veterinary inoculators, and water guns also contribute.

In the typical case, the nondominant index or middle finger of a relatively inexperienced worker is used to clean the nozzle of a high pressure injector. The 2,000 to 10,000 lbs/in^2 of pressure then discharges rapidly, sending a variable amount of fluid through the skin and into the hand. The volume discharged is time- and pressure-related. Small volumes may be retained locally in the digital pulp, whereas large volumes may reach the wrist, elbow, or on rare occasions the chest. Injections have little tendency to spread laterally until they reach resistant structures (tendons, bones, or fibrous tendon sheaths). Injections over the rigid pulleys in the central area of the phalanges spread circumferentially around the digit; injections over the interphalangeal joints penetrate the tendon sheath and travel easily along the tendons. Injections in the thumb and little finger can spread to the radial and ulnar bursae, respectively.

Because high-pressure injection injuries often present with an innocuous puncture wound, a delay in presentation can create complications. Radiographs may be helpful in assessing the extent of spread in the case of lead-based paints, lead-thickened grease, or air. Oil-based solvents (eg, grease, paint, or paint thinner) are especially dangerous, with amputation rates reported as high as 48%. Oil-based paints are more hazardous than water-based products. In a recent review of 23 high-pressure paint gun injection injuries of the hand, the 3 patients requiring amputation were all injected with oil-based paint. Infection was a complicating factor; over 50% of the patients had positive initial debridement cultures. Because the majority of cultures included gram-negative organisms, initial antibiotic coverage for gram-positive and gram-negative organisms is recommended. Tetanus prophylaxis is also important.

Acute pathologic changes caused by oil-based paint injection include immediate tissue necrosis and a necrotizing inflammatory reaction with vascular thrombosis. Grease injections can be more insidious, with chronic draining sinuses and oleogranulomas (Fig. 1). Systemic toxicity—including central nervous system, renal, and hepatic damage—is possible with large injections of toxic solvents.

Initial damage can be complicated by the blast injury component. Increasing inflammation coupled with volume infusion in a closed space can lead to vascular compromise. Prompt surgical intervention is recommended in the majority of cases. Surgical exposure is obtained via midaxial incisions. Digital blocks are avoided as well as Esmarch exsanguination, with its potential for spreading the injected material. All devitalized tissue and injected material should be debrided as soon as possible with careful preservation of the neurovascular bundles. Treatment includes pulsed lavage, drainage, open packing, and dressing changes, with repeat debridement at 24 to 72 hours as necessary. Delayed wound closure or healing via secondary intention is generally practiced. Sterile whirlpools and early active range of motion therapy are critical to optimize functional results. Intravenous antibiotics are important because *Staphylococcus epidermidis* or polymicrobial infections are common. In a recent series of 25 patients treated

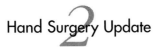

with this protocol, only 4 (16%) required amputation; all patients presented from 3 to 8 days after injury. Furthermore, 64% of the patients regained near-normal hand function. Steroids have been of no proven benefit and are probably contraindicated given their depression of immune function. Early and thorough serial debridement with aggressive hand therapy are the cornerstones of modern care.

In rare circumstances, injury from injection of a low-volume, relatively innocuous substance may be treated conservatively. An injection with Freon-isopropyl alcohol solution, used to clean computers, was successfully treated. Low-volume (0.2 cc) injections with a mineral oil-based chicken vaccine have also been managed nonsurgically without tissue loss. Infections secondary to bacterial contaminants

of the injected substance are possible. *Corynebacterium aquaticum* infection was recently reported in a high-pressure water injection case. In addition, large-volume water injection can cause compartment syndrome.

Nerve Injection Injuries

Although relatively uncommon, injection injuries of peripheral nerves have serious consequences. In the upper extremity, peripheral nerves are most at risk during regional nerve blocks or steroid injections. Once injured, complete nerve recovery is rare. Median, ulnar, radial, posterior interosseous, axillary, and brachial plexus injuries have been reported. The relative neurotoxicity of local anesthetics and steroids, as determined in experimental studies, are listed in Table 1. Intrafascicular injection of a toxic agent is associated with serious nerve injury, while extrafascicular injection can be largely innocuous. Pathologically, injections can vary from mild myelin degeneration to total myelinated and nonmyelinated axonal degeneration.

Clinically, nerve injection injury is associated with severe pain in the distribution of the nerve and the onset of neurologic deficit immediately or within minutes of injury. Severe radiating pain is an important signal to stop injecting and redirect the needle. Because sedated patients or those under general anesthesia cannot provide this signal, they may be

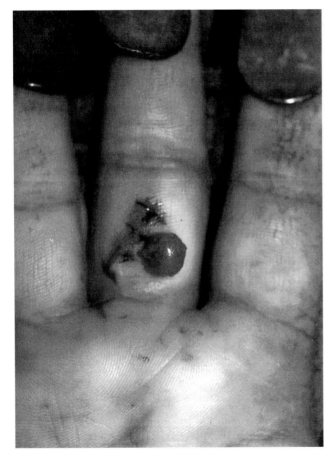

Figure 1

Cystic mass excised 6 months after grease gun injection injury of the left index finger demonstrated acute inflammation, histiocytic infiltrate, foreign material, and marked fibrosis.

Table 1

Relative neurotoxicity of injection substances

Local Anesthetics*	Steroids*
Tetracaine	Triamcinolone
Procaine	Hydrocortisone
Lidocaine hydrocarbonate	Methylprednisolone
Lidocaine hydrogen chloride	Dexamethasone
Bupivacaine (with epinephrine)	
Mepivacaine	
Bupivacaine	
Etidocaine	

*Listed in descending order of toxicity

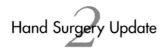
more at risk for injection injury. Once nerve injection injury occurs, recovery should be closely monitored with serial examinations including nerve conduction and electromyographic studies. Some authors recommend immediate nerve decompression. With a motor deficit, inadequate recovery after 3 months is an indication for exploration, neurolysis, and possible nerve grafting. Sensory deficits can be safely monitored for longer periods because reinnervation of sensory receptors is not as time dependent as motor receptors. Prevention of nerve injection injuries is paramount. Careful monitoring of paresthesias in the awake patient is critical, and blocks in the anesthesized patient should be conducted with extreme caution. In the case of steroid injection of the carpal canal for relief of time-limited nerve compression (pregnancy), an ulnar approach deep to the median nerve has been recommended.

Intra-arterial Injection Injuries

Self-inflicted or therapeutic intra-arterial injections are another source of hand and upper extremity injury. The inadvertent intra-arterial injection of vasoconstrictors in the compromised patient can lead to severe vasospasm and tissue loss. Severe limb ischemia secondary to the accidental intra-arterial injection of temazepam in intravenous drug users is a case example. Vascular injury results from particulate obstruction, vasospasm, thrombosis, chemical endarteritis, and direct cytotoxic effects on the endothelium. Reversal of ischemic symptoms—including cyanosis, mottling, swelling, and muscle tenderness—has been reported in a series of patients with iloprost, a prostaglandin analog. Iloprost is a potent vasodilator with anti-aggretory activity on platelets and neutrophils. All 8 patients made dramatic improvement; limited digital amputations were performed in 2 patients, who presented 1 and 2 weeks after injury.

Intra-arterial chemotherapy for sarcoma is also not without complications. Three of 200 patients treated with intra-arterial adriamycin and intravenous FUDR, G-CSF, and leukovorin developed soft-tissue necroses that required skin graft or muscle flap reconstruction. Hand surgeons need be aware of such possibilities, given the increased use of intra-arterial chemotherapy and isolated hyperthermic limb perfusion.

Extravasation Injuries

The extravasation of a wide variety of therapeutic agents and solutions can cause iatrogenic injury, including skin sloughs, compartment syndrome, tendon and nerve injury, joint fibrosis, and amputation. Blood and routinely infused solutions such as Ringer's lactate and 5% dextrose have led to compartment syndrome, typically when manual bulb pump, power injector, or other pressurized systems are used in anesthetized or acutely ill patients. Other agents that can cause skin sloughs include hyperalimention solution; fat emulsions; 10% glucose; radiographic contrast material; urea; sodium bicarbonate; potassium chloride; and calcium salts, including calcium chloride, calcium gluconate, and calcium gluceptate. Extravasated vasoactive drugs, including norepinephrine, dopamine, and doputamine have also been implicated, often in critically ill patients. Various antibiotics have been responsible for soft-tissue loss, including chloramphenicol, cephalothin, gentamycin, oxacillin, and nafcillin. Among antineoplastic agents, those reported to cause ulceration include actinomycin D, cisplatinum, daunorubicin, doxorubicin, fluorouracil, mithramycin, mitomycin C, mitozantrone, mustine hydrochloride, nitrogen mustard, vinblastine, vincristine, vindesine, VP16, and VM26. Daunorubicin and doxorubicin are most often responsible, causing ulcerations secondary to interference with nuclear function related to DNA base binding. Impaired healing results because cell replication is inhibited. Prolonged tissue retention of the agents up to five months after injury can further complicate management.

Timely treatment is essential to prevent or eliminate soft-tissue loss. The application of cold has been shown both clinically and experimentally to help decrease damage. By contrast, heat increases the local metabolic rate and can augment tissue destruction. In one series of 148 patients (approximately 80% doxorubicin extravasations), locally injected hyaluronidase (150 units/1,000 cc saline) within 1 hour of extravasation prevented soft-tissue loss. From 12 to 38 cc of solution were injected locally to disperse the offending agent. Although no patients suffered full-thickness skin loss, many had subcutaneous induration for weeks and some had transient blistering that resolved with conservative treatment.

One recent study has gone a step further, with encouraging results. Forty-four patients seen within 24 hours of an extravasation incident (and before the overlying skin became necrotic) were treated with local hyaluronidase injection combined with saline washout and/or liposuction of the area. In the saline washout patients, 500 cc of saline were flushed through the subcutaneous space that was made more permeable with hyaluronidase preinjection (1,500 units). Four puncture wounds surrounding the site permitted drainage of effluent, which was documented to contain chemotherapeutic agents in 5 test patients. This protocol thus allows for not only dilution, but elimination of the offending agent. This population, treated up to 24 hours after injury, required no surgery. The vast majority (89%) had no soft-tissue damage; 11% exhibited minor blistering or delayed healing.

Given the success of such relatively simple therapy, protocols should be established to promptly treat extravasation injuries. Delayed presentation may still require serial debridement, skin grafting, and/or flap reconstruction (Fig. 2). As soon as an extravasation is recognized, the infusion should be stopped, cold applied, and the saline washout protocol instituted. Other preventive measures include the atraumatic intravenous insertion technique (to avoid venous backwall damage), close monitoring of intravenous sites, avoidance of proximal obstruction with thrombosis or blood pressure cuffs, elimination of high pressure injection techniques, and the development of less locally toxic antineoplastic agents. In the radiology suite, the vast majority of extravasation injuries leading to tissue loss or compartment syndrome have been with high-osmolality contrast agents. Experimental data has confirmed that low-osmolality agents are much safer, supporting clinical work documenting only rare problems with their use. More widespread use of the safer, albeit more costly, low-osmolality contrast agents should further decrease the incidence of serious extravasation injuries.

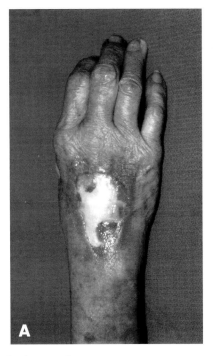
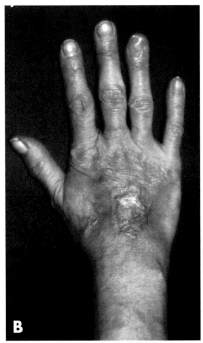

Figure 2

A, Full-thickness eschar dorsum right hand 1 week after extravasation injury from intravenous contrast. **B,** 10 weeks after debridement and successful split-thickness skin grafting on viable paratenon.

Annotated Bibliography

High Pressure Injection Injuries

Behar TA, Anderson EE, Barwick WJ, Mohler JL: Sclerosing lipogranulomatosis: A case report of scrotal injection of automobile transmission fluid and literature review of subcutaneous injection of oils. *Plast Reconstr Surg* 1993;91:352–361.

This work contains a valuable historic review of grease gun injuries.

Couzens G, Burke FD: Veterinary high pressure injection injuries with inoculations for larger animals. *J Hand Surg* 1995; 20B:497–499.

In this excellent review of injection injury, conservative treatment for small volume veterinary inoculations is advocated.

Failla JM, Linden MD: The acute pathologic changes of paint-injection injury and correlation to surgical treatment: A report of two cases. *J Hand Surg* 1997;22A:156–159.

These 2 cases emphasize early pathologic changes after injection injury with oil-based paint, including immediate tissue necrosis and a persistent necrotizing inflammatory reaction.

Harter BT Jr, Harter KC: High-pressure injection injuries. *Hand Clin* 1986;2:547–552.

An historic perspective is provided in this excellent review.

Larsson P, Lundin O, Falsen E: "Corynebacterium aquaticum" wound infection after high-pressure water injection into the foot. *Scand J Infect Dis* 1996;28:635–636.

The authors present an interesting case, raising concern for bacterial contamination of injected fluids.

Pinto MR, Turkula-Pinto LD, Cooney WP, Wood MB, Dobyns JH: High-pressure injection injuries of the hand: Review of 25 patients managed by open wound technique. *J Hand Surg* 1993;18A:125–130.

This important series points out the need for prompt wide debridement, drainage, open packing, and delayed closure in order to achieve superior results.

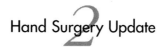
Schnall SB, Mirzayan R: High pressure injection injuries to the hand. *Hand Clin* 1999;15:245–248.

The authors review the history of these injuries, focusing on materials injected, clinical presentation, surgical management, bacteriology, and postoperative management. In a paper on paint gun injection injures, presented at the 1998 ASSH annual meeting, they demonstrated increased severity of injury with oil- versus water-based paints. The paper also documents a high percentage of polymicrobial and gram-negative cultures.

Shea MP, Manoli A II: High pressure water injection injuries of the foot: A report of two cases. *Foot Ankle* 1993;14:104–106.

High-pressure water injection can cause morbidity secondary to blast injury and compartment syndrome.

Nerve Injection Injuries

Fremling MA, Mackinnon SE: Injection injury to the median nerve. *Ann Plast Surg* 1996;37:561–567.

This is an excellent review of nerve injection injuries.

Kasten SJ, Louis DS: Carpal tunnel syndrome: A case of median nerve injection injury and a safe and effective method for injecting the carpal tunnel. *J Fam Pract* 1996;43:79–82.

This important article describes a safe injection method of the carpal canal.

Villarejo FJ, Pascual AM: Injection injury of the sciatic nerve (370 cases). *Childs Nerv Syst* 1993;9:229–232.

This large series supports surgical neurolysis 3 months after nerve injection injury if there is no improvement in physical examination and electromyographic studies.

Intra-arterial Injection Injuries

Bezwada HP, Granick MS, Long CD, Moore JH Jr, Lackman RL, Weiss AJ: Soft tissue complications of intra-arterial chemotherapy for extremity sarcomas. *Ann Plast Surg* 1998;40:382–387.

In this 118-patient series, infrequent (2.5%) complications were noted with the use of intra-arterial chemotherapy; 3 patients experienced soft-tissue necrosis that required excision and reconstruction. A later series was presented at the 1997 annual meeting of the Northeastern Society of Plastic Surgeons; the complication incidence was only 1.5% in 200 patients.

Tait IS, Holdsworth RJ, Belch JJ, McCollum PT: Letter: Management of intra-arterial injection injury with iloprost. *Lancet* 1994;343:419.

Intra-arterial injection injuries in intravenous drug users are successfully treated with iloprost, a prostacyclin analog.

Extravasation Injuries

Elam EA, Dorr RT, Lagel KE, Pond GD: Cutaneous ulceration due to contrast extravasation: Experimental assessment of injury and potential antidotes. *Invest Radiol* 1991;26:13–16.

In a laboratory setting, ulceration occurred only with high-osmolality agents, and improved with cold and hyaluronidase treatment.

Gault DT: Extravasation injuries. *Br J Plast Surg* 1993;46:91–96.

In an excellent article, Gault noted that use of hyaluronidase combined with saline washout within 24 hours of an extravasation injury eliminated skin necrosis.

Goodie DB: The effect of manual bulb pump infusion systems on venous luminal pressure and vein wall integrity. *Anesth Analg* 1995;80:552–556.

In an experimental study of human veins, traumatic venopuncture was shown to decrease the pressure at which veins leak. This pressure can be exceeded with manual bulb pump infusion systems.

Heckler FR: Current thoughts on extravasation injuries. *Clin Plast Surg* 1989;16:557–563.

In a very good review of extravasation injuries, the clinical efficacy of hyaluronidase is demonstrated.

Larson DL: What is the appropriate management of tissue extravasation by antitumor agents? *Plast Reconstr Surg* 1985; 75:397–405.

The use of cold is advocated for extravasation injuries.

Laurie SW, Wilson KL, Kernahan DA, Bauer BS, Vistnes LM: Intravenous extravasation injuries: The effectiveness of hyaluronidase in their treatment. *Ann Plast Surg* 1984;13:191–194.

This experimental study demonstrates the effectiveness of hyaluronidase up to 1 hour after extravasation injury.

MacDonald JR, Pegg DG: Extravasation injury potential of CI-980, a novel synthetic mitotic inhibitor. *Cancer Chemother Pharmacol* 1993;32:365–367.

A new antineoplastic agent proves to be less prone to cause ulceration in an experimental model. The potential for using safer agents is highlighted.

Memolo M, Dyer R, Zagoria RJ: Letter: Extravasation injury with nonionic contrast material. *Am J Roentgenol* 1993;160:203–204.

An unusual case of compartment syndrome with a low-osmolality agent, involving subfascial extravasation and the use of a power injector, is presented.

Pond GD, Dorr RT, McAleese KA: Letter: Skin ulceration from extravasation of low-osmolality contrast medium: A complication of automation. *Am J Roentgenol* 1992;158:915–916.

High-volume extravasation of low-osmolality contrast caused a blistering skin reaction. An inflated blood pressure cuff led to increased venous resistance to flow.

Sistrom CL, Gay SB, Peffley L. Extravasation of iopamidol and iohexol during contrast-enhanced CT: Report of 28 cases. *Radiology* 1991;180:707–710.

428 Injection and Extravasation Injuries

Conservative treatment of extravasation injuries with low-osmolality contrast agents is recommended.

Sneyd JR, Lau W, McLaren ID: Forearm compartment syndrome following intravenous infusion with a manual "bulb" pump. *Anesth Analg* 1993;76:1160–1161.

Bulb pumps generate pressures sufficient to rupture veins and cause an extravasation injury-induced compartment syndrome. Modification of the device is recommended.

Tobias MD, Hanson CW III, Heppenstall RB, Aukburg SJ: Compartment syndrome after pressurized infusion. *Br J Anaesth* 1991;67:332–334.

Pressurized infusions can be complicated by extravasation and compartment syndrome.

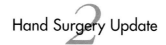

Chapter 43
Cumulative Trauma
and Tendinitis

Peter C. Amadio, MD

Introduction

The term cumulative trauma disorders (CTD) energizes some, who see it as the scourge of modern industrial life, and enrages others, who see it as a vague catchall phrase designed to "medicalize" life's normal aches and pains. Since the first edition of *Hand Surgery Update,* some of the controversies surrounding CTD have been clarified, but many others remain.

Pathophysiology

Much has been learned about the pathophysiology of repetitive trauma as it affects connective tissue in general and the musculoskeletal system in particular. The phenomena of stress fractures and skin blisters related to repetitive, submaximal loading are well known. It is also clear that exercise induces muscle hypertrophy only after an initial phase of muscle inflammation and tissue breakdown. When time is permitted between exercise periods for rest and healing, the muscle can heal and hypertrophy, to better handle future loads. When insufficient rest is permitted between contractions, recovery may be impaired. Future research is aimed at identifying thresholds for injury in humans, better conditioning methods, and the impact of comorbidities such as obesity, smoking, and vascular disease.

Tendons also respond to repetitive loading by remodeling, but to a lesser extent than muscle. Thus, as muscle contractions become more powerful, the risk of tendon rupture increases.

A variety of external factors other than load and rate affect connective tissues, and their risk of developing pathology. Examples include postures and tool size and weight. Exercise increases joint laxity and, thereby, should reduce the risk of injury. Certain techniques may be more beneficial than others; large proximal muscle groups seem to be more resistant to the ill effects of repetitive activity than smaller, distal muscles. Psychomotor capacity (coordination) however, does not appear to be a risk factor.

Exposure to vibration continues to be an issue in some industries. Mechanically dampened grinders, chippers, and chain saws appear to have reduced the incidence of CTD. Neurosensory symptoms often appear within 10 years, cold intolerance within 20 years, and the classic vibration white finger after 20 years of regular exposure to vibration. It is important to remember that, in vibration disease, finger vibration and temperature thresholds are increased, while there is little effect on motor and sensory latencies at the wrist. Patients with a history of vibration exposure and fingertip numbness thus may have vibration neuropathy, and not carpal tunnel syndrome (CTS).

Epidemiology

Studies of the epidemiology of CTD have been plagued by many problems. Because most of the conditions suspected to be CTD are clinically diagnosed musculoskeletal syndromes, with no readily identifiable gold standard for diagnosis, disputes have arisen as to whether epidemiologic surveys are identifying disease or merely cataloging complaints. Most studies have been cross-sectional, so that the effect of work over time usually can be inferred only through the experience of senior workers, who may represent hardier-than-normal survivors and, thus, underestimate the impact of work on pathology. Few studies have looked adequately at confounding variables, such as obesity, smoking, and lack of fitness, all of which may both increase the risk of injury with work and reduce the threshold at which injury occurs. Finally, investigators have argued over basic principles: must CTD be exclusively caused by work, and only work? Most investigators consider CTD to be multifactorial; in that case, under what circumstances should such a condition be designated as work-related? This last issue is much more philosophic than scientific.

Some recent studies reflect these issues. In one study obesity was a major risk factor for CTS. The average body mass index of the CTS patients was 29.59; that of the controls was 25.65, with *p* < 0.0000001 and an odds ratio of 3.9 (95% CI,

2.6 to 5.8). Another epidemiologic study reviewed all cases of nerve compression syndromes in navy personnel from 1980 to 1988. The usual 3:1 female to male ratio was found, but only in Caucasians; in blacks the ratio was 1:1. Overall rates were similar to those found in other epidemiologic studies, but several occupations stood out in both men and women as having increased risk of CTS: maintenance workers, mechanics, and corpsmen. Among women more than men, clerical occupations also had an increased risk of association, but no effort was made to correlate these observations with aspects of body habitus or lifestyle factors.

Several studies have called into question the use of electrodiagnostic studies (EDS) alone as the gold standard for diagnosis of CTS. In these studies, mostly done by using EDS in preemployment screening, large numbers of asymptomatic individuals with abnormal EDS were identified, while only a minority of patients with CTS-like symptoms had abnormal EDS.

CTD in the Workplace

A review of the literature suggests that there are multiple risk factors for at least one CTD—CTS. There have been few studies of the epidemiology of other putative CTD, and none were recent enough to be included in this survey. What evidence there is suggests that the connection between most CTD and any specific work activity is tenuous at best. The most that can be said is that some types of neck, elbow, and shoulder complaints occur more often in certain occupations. For CTS the situation is improved by the fact that there are more studies, but muddied by the fact that these reports differ in the way they define CTS (by symptoms alone, by EDS alone, or by some incomplete combination of symptoms and EDS), by study design (most are cross-sections of active workers), or by limitations in risk factors studied (work alone, comorbidities alone, or some combination of work, comorbidities, lifestyle issues, and/or psychosocial factors). For example, one study compared managers and factory workers. The factory workers had significantly greater EDS evidence of median neuropathy; however, participants were not controlled for obesity or smoking, two known risk factors for CTS.

Another study showed that the prevalence of median nerve slowing is similar in American and Japanese workers, but that the American workers were more likely to complain of symptoms of CTS. The strongest risk factor for the presence of CTS symptoms in this study was body mass index. However, cultural factors and psychosocial issues were not studied. This is relevant, because in another study, patients with work-related (at least by their claim) CTS were more likely to have had multiple surgeries, a shorter work history, anger toward their employer, and greater psychological response to pain than their working peers. Finally, another study showed that costs, time to settlement, and claim rates varied considerably by state, emphasizing the impact of state law and legal climate on the reported incidence of CTDs.

CTD in Musicians

Most musicians have musculoskeletal symptoms while playing. Characteristic patterns relate to specific instruments, with prevalence being highest (nearly 80%) among string players. Women have more problems than men. Although most musicians are self-employed and thus not covered by workers' compensation laws, many report disabling symptoms, usually associated with significant changes or faults in technique or total playing (practice plus performance) time. Unlike the factory workforce, where those with high force, high repetition jobs tend to be obese and to smoke, the ages, general fitness level, and body mass indices of musicians and nonmusicians are similar. Further, although the rate of musculoskeletal symptoms between the 2 groups is similar, instrumentalists have nearly double the rate of upper limb musculoskeletal complaints as noninstrumentalists do. Location of symptoms correlates with type of instrument.

Thus, in musicians, where secondary gain from workers' compensation is usually not an issue, and comorbidity and lifestyle habits appear to be similar to those of matched peer groups, there does appear to be a correlation between specific activities and certain symptom clusters. These conditions, which include specific (CTS, ulnar neuropathy, focal dystonia) and nonspecific (shoulder or hand pain) diagnoses, are aggravated by performance, interfere with virtuosity, and are treated, at least in part, by some modification in technique or duration of performance. As with other types of work, whether something is gained or lost by labeling such problems as "caused by" or "related to" music, remains as much a philosophic issue as a medical one.

Carpal Tunnel Syndrome

Each year the National Center for Health Statistics conducts a questionnaire survey of the US population. In 1988, the survey included an Occupational Health Supplement. Data was collected on health status and job status. The usual 3:1 female to male ratio for CTS was observed. Whites were noted to be more likely to have a diagnosis of CTS than nonwhites, but nonwhites were more likely to be disabled by CTS. Self-reported health status did not differ

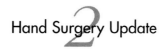
among CTS and non-CTS respondents. Work exposure to more than 2 hours of repetitive hand-wrist bending was associated with a slightly increased risk of diagnosis of CTS (odds ratio 95% confidence limits, 1.2 to 1.4) and, among CTS respondents only, an increased risk of work disability (odds ratio 1.7 for > 2 hr exposure and 2.7 for > 4 hr exposure), although among all respondents (CTS and non-CTS), repetitive hand-wrist movements were not a risk factor for lost work. Self-estimates of repetitive work exposure correlated well with those taken from job descriptions. In a study of workers' compensation claims, the sex distribution of claimants having surgery was nearly equal. After carpal tunnel release (CTR), 60% of those in high-risk jobs returned to their preoperative job, but patients with normal EDS were less likely both to report improvement and to return to their original job.

Patients who have significant occupational exposure to vibration do less well after CTR (59% improved versus 79% improved). Preoperative sensorineural testing, including vibratory and temperature thresholds, should be done in all CTS patients with a significant occupational exposure to pneumatic chippers, grinders, chain saws, and similar tools.

Tendon Entrapment Syndromes

The tendon entrapment syndromes are well characterized. The most common are trigger finger, trigger thumb, and de Quervain's disease. Although tendon entrapment syndromes usually are included in the CTD category, there is little epidemiologic evidence to support their association with specific activities. Nonetheless, the histopathology is consistent with changes seen as a reaction to chronic or repetitive loading. Although usually referred to as stenosing tenosynovitis, rarely is any inflammation noted histologically. The treatment of these conditions is fairly well agreed upon: except in cases of locked finger, an initial steroid injection usually is the first line of treatment, with surgical release reserved for failures. A series of 2 injections provides lasting relief in most patients. Where the injection goes seems not to matter much, so long as it is in the vicinity of the problem. A prospective randomized study of 60 compared intrasheath injection with extrasheath subcutaneous injection. Success rates were identical in the 2 groups. Intrasheath injection may not be necessary to achieve a therapeutic effect.

Less clear are the other aches and pains often loosely labeled as tendinitis. In most cases, these represent cases of tenderness in the region of a tendon, perhaps associated with pain when the limb is moved in a direction opposite to that of tendon pull, presumably stretching the tendon. There is rarely any redness, swelling, or other sign of inflammation.

Treatment is usually empiric. In such cases, it may be preferable to avoid a label that suggests a specific pathology and, instead, to refer simply to pain or tenderness as the problem. Tendinitis, as currently used by most practitioners, may well represent an unwise and misleading medicalization of a common, even everyday, phenomenon.

Epicondylitis

Epicondylitis has not received much attention in the literature lately. Controversies still remain, specifically as to the role and even existence of radial tunnel syndrome as a concomitant or confounding condition. Diagnosis can, at least, be confirmed in severe cases: the characteristic surgical findings of degenerative tendinopathy and tendon tears usually can be predicted on the basis of preoperative magnetic resonance imaging. Treatment is usually nonsurgical. The association of medial and lateral epicondylitis with certain work or sports activities is supported by anecdote but not by any solid epidemiologic data.

Rehabilitation

Rehabilitation of CTD often requires a team approach involving not only health care professionals but also the patient and employer. Effective return to work programs usually require the ability to provide temporary or permanent workplace modifications or accommodations. All should be in agreement as to the goals of therapy, which should include return to gainful work in all but the most extreme cases.

To ensure that these goals are reached, a systematic approach to the patient is beneficial. The multifactorial nature of CTD (or at least musculoskeletal complaints in the context of work) has led some authors to suggest characterizing workers according to 3 axes: musculoskeletal, ergonomic, and psychosocial. In a review of 50 patients, 23 of 25 with objective and/or reasonable subjective findings consistent with a specific musculoskeletal diagnosis returned to work; those who did not return to work had major unresolved psychosocial and ergonomic issues. Among the 25 with vague or nonreproducible physical findings, 16 returned to work. None of the 12 patients who were off work at the time of presentation and had a combination of ill-defined physical findings and major ergonomic (unmodifiable work) and psychosocial (long-standing anger and frustration or chronic pain behaviors) issues could be returned to their original job, and only 6 went back to any job.

Annotated Bibliography

Pathophysiology of CTD

Byl NN, Merzenich MM, Cheung S, Bedenbaugh P, Nagarajan SS, Jenkins WM: A primate model for studying focal dystonia and repetitive strain injury: Effects on the primary somatosensory cortex. *Phys Ther* 1997;77:269–284.

An owl monkey trained to perform repetitive forceful finger squeezing (400 repetitions per day for 5 months) developed dedifferentiation and deterioration of the cerebral motor cortex, while a similar monkey who performed the same task with repetitive arm pulling developed no changes.

Crisco JJ, Chelikani S, Brown RK, Wolfe SW: The effects of exercise on ligamentous stiffness in the wrist. *J Hand Surg* 1997; 22A:44–48.

Exercise increases joint laxity and, thereby, should reduce the risk of injury. This evidence supports the benefit of "warming up" before work or sport.

Gordon SL, Blair SJ, Fine LJ (eds): *Repetitive Motion Disorders of the Upper Extremity.* Rosemont, IL, American Academy of Orthopaedic Surgeons, 1995.

This is an excellent reference, especially for pathophysiology.

Strömberg T, Dahlin LB, Lundborg G: Hand problems in 100 vibration-exposed symptomatic male workers. *J Hand Surg* 1996;21B:315–319.

Neurosensory symptoms often occur within 10 years, cold intolerance within 20 years, and the classic vibration white finger after 20 years of exposure.

Viikari-Juntura E, Hietanen M, Kurppa K, Huuskonen M, Kuosma E, Mutanen P: Psychomotor capacity and occurrence of wrist tenosynovitis. *J Occup Med* 1994;36:57–60.

Psychomotor capacity (coordination) is not a risk factor for wrist tenosynovitis in meatpackers.

Risk Factors/Epidemiology

Bingham RC, Rosecrance JC, Cook TM: Prevalence of abnormal median nerve conduction in applicants for industrial jobs. *Am J Ind Med* 1996;30:355–361.

One thousand job applicants had screening nerve conduction studies (NCS). Seventeen percent were abnormal, but only 10% of those with abnormal NCS had symptoms. Men were more likely to have abnormal NCS than women. The authors question the assumption that CTS and abnormal EDS are one and the same.

Franzblau A, Werner R, Valle J, Johnston E: Workplace surveillance for carpal tunnel syndrome: A comparison of methods. *J Occup Rehab* 1993;3:1–14.

In a survey of 130 workers, 24% had abnormal EDS, 33% had symptoms of CTS, and 15% had both symptoms and EDS findings. This study calls into question the use of EDS alone as the gold standard for diagnosis of CTS.

Garland FC, Garland CF, Doyle EJ Jr, et al: Carpal tunnel syndrome and occupation in U.S. Navy enlisted personnel. *Arch Environ Health* 1996;51:395–407.

This epidemiologic study reviewed all cases of nerve compression syndromes in Navy personnel from 1980 to 1988. The usual 3:1 female/male ratio was found, but only in whites; in blacks it was 1:1.

Himmelstein JS, Feuerstein M, Stanek EJ III, et al: Work-related upper-extremity disorders and work disability: Clinical and psychosocial presentation. *J Occup Environ Med* 1995;37: 1278–1286.

Of 124 consecutive patients, 59 were unable to work because of CTDs. These patients were more likely to have had multiple surgeries, a shorter work history, anger toward their employer, and greater psychological response to pain than their working peers.

Nathan PA, Takigawa K, Keniston RC, Meadows KD, Lockwood RS: Slowing of sensory conduction of the median nerve and carpal tunnel syndrome in Japanese and American industrial workers. *J Hand Surg* 1994;19B:30–34.

The prevalence of median nerve slowing is similar in American and Japanese workers, but American workers were more likely to have symptoms of CTS. The strongest risk factor for CTS symptoms was body mass index.

Rosén I, Strömberg T, Lundborg G: Neurophysiological investigation of hands damaged by vibration: Comparison with idiopathic carpal tunnel syndrome. *Scand J Plast Reconstr Surg Hand Surg* 1993;27:209–216.

In vibration disease, finger vibration and temperature thresholds are increased, while motor and sensory latencies at the wrist are little affected. Patients with a history of vibration exposure with fingertip numbness may have vibration neuropathy and not CTS.

Stallings SP, Kasdan ML, Soergel TM, Corwin HM: A case-control study of obesity as a risk factor for carpal tunnel syndrome in a population of 600 patients presenting for independent medical examination. *J Hand Surg* 1997;22A: 211–215.

Three hundred workers' compensation CTS cases were compared with 300 age and gender matched controls with other upper extremity problems. The average body mass index of the CTS patients was 29.59; that of the controls was 25.65, with $p < 0.0000001$ and an odds ratio of 3.9 (95% CI, 2.6 to 5.8).

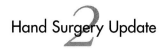

Stetson DS, Silverstein BA, Keyserling WM, Wolfe RA, Albers JW: Median sensory distal amplitude and latency: Comparisons between nonexposed managerial/professional employees and industrial workers. *Am J Ind Med* 1993;24:175–189.

This study compared 105 managers and 103 factory workers. The factory workers had significantly greater EDS evidence of median neuropathy. However, participants were not controlled for obesity or smoking, 2 known risk factors for CTS and median nerve slowing.

Webster BS, Snook SH: The cost of compensable upper extremity cumulative trauma disorders. *J Occup Med* 1994;36:713–717.

This study reports the experience of Liberty Mutual, a large workers' compensation insurance carrier. The mean cost of upper extremity CTD, $8,000, was nearly double that of the average workers' compensation claim. Costs, time to settlement, and claim rates varied considerably by state, emphasizing the impact of state law and legal climate on the reported incidence of CTDs.

Musicians

Brandfonbrener AG: Musicians with focal dystonia: A report of 58 cases seen during a ten-year period at a performing arts medicine clinic. *Med Prob Perf Artists* 1995;10:121–127.

In 58 musicians, dystonia developed most often after a significant change in work intensity or technique.

Larsson LG, Baum J, Mudholkar GS, Kollia GD: Nature and impact of musculoskeletal problems in a population of musicians. *Med Prob Perf Artists* 1993;8:73–76.

A survey of 660 musicians showed that more than half had musculoskeletal symptoms while playing. Characteristic patterns were noted related to specific instruments, with prevalence being highest (nearly 80%) among string players. Women had more problems than men.

Lederman RJ: Treatment outcome in instrumentalists: A long-term follow-up study. *Med Prob Perf Artists* 1995;10:115–120.

One hundred musicians were followed for 5 to 7 years for a variety of CTD, primarily muscular pain and tenderness or nerve compression syndromes. At follow-up only half were still performing regularly, and only a third were symptom-free.

Roach KE, Martinez MA, Anderson N: Musculoskeletal pain in student instrumentalists: A comparison with the general student population. *Med Prob Perf Artists* 1994;9:125–130.

In a random survey of university students, 90 instrumental musicians and 160 nonmusicians were identified. The ages and body mass indices of the 2 groups were similar. There were more men in the instrumentalist group, which was more physically active than the noninstrumentalist group. The rate of musculoskeletal symptoms between the groups was similar, but the instrumentalists had nearly double the rate of upper limb musculoskeletal complaints. Location of symptoms correlated with type of instrument, but not with total hours of play or practice.

Carpal Tunnel Syndrome in the Workplace

Adams ML, Franklin GM, Barnhart S: Outcome of carpal tunnel surgery in Washington State workers' compensation. *Am J Ind Med* 1994;25:527–536.

In this study of workers' compensation claims, the sex distribution of claimants having surgery was nearly equal. Sixty percent of those in high-risk jobs returned to their previous work. Mean lost time was 113 days.

Blanc PD, Faucett J, Kennedy JJ, Cisternas M, Yelin E: Self-reported carpal tunnel syndrome: Predictors of work disability from the National Health Interview Survey Occupational Health Supplement. *Am J Ind Med* 1996;30:362–368.

Each year the National Center for Health Statistics conducts a questionnaire survey of the US population. The 1988 Occupational Health Supplement is discussed.

Boström L, Göthe CJ, Hansson S, Lugnegård H, Nilsson BY: Surgical treatment of carpal tunnel syndrome in patients exposed to vibration from handheld tools. *Scand J Plast Reconstr Surg Hand Surg* 1994;28:147–149.

Patients who have significant occupational exposure to vibration do less well after CTR (59% improved versus 79% improved) and should undergo preoperative sensorineural testing.

Higgs PE, Edwards DF, Martin DS, Weeks PM: Relation of preoperative nerve-conduction values to outcome in workers with surgically treated carpal tunnel syndrome. *J Hand Surg* 1997;22A:216–221.

Patients with normal EDS were less likely to report improvement and less likely to return to their original job after CTR.

Katz JN, Keller RB, Fossel AH, et al: Predictors of return to work following carpal tunnel release. *Am J Ind Med* 1997;31:85–91.

This community-based study evaluated risk factors associated with delayed return to work (> 6 months) after CTS surgery. The major factors were the presence of a workers' compensation claim, involvement of an attorney, preoperative lost work time, and worse mental health. Delayed return to work also correlated well with persisting symptoms.

Trigger Finger

Benson LS, Ptaszek AJ: Injection versus surgery in the treatment of trigger finger. *J Hand Surg* 1997;22A:138–144.

A first injection provided lasting relief in 55%, and a second injection in 44%, in this study of 102 patients.

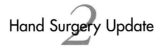

434   Cumulative Trauma and Tendinitis

Taras JS, Raphael JS, Culp RW: Corticosteroid injections in trigger fingers: Is intrasheath injection necessary? *Jefferson Orthop J* 1995;24:20–22.

A prospective randomized study of 60 patients was done, using radioopaque contrast to assure intrasheath injection in 1 group, while confirming extrasheath subcutaneous injection in the other. Success rates were identical in the 2 groups.

Lateral Epicondylitis

Potter HG, Hannafin JA, Morwessel RM, DiCarlo EF, O'Brien SJ, Altchek DW: Lateral epicondylitis: Correlation of MR imaging, surgical, and histopathologic findings. *Radiology* 1995;196:43–46.

The characteristic surgical findings of degenerative tendinopathy and tendon tears can often be predicted on the basis of preoperative magnetic resonance imaging.

Rehabilitation

Bonzani PJ, Millender L, Keelan B, Mangieri MG: Factors prolonging disability in work-related cumulative trauma disorders. *J Hand Surg* 1997;22A:30–34.

These authors suggest characterizing workers with work-related CTD according to musculoskeletal, ergonomic, and psychosocial factors. A review of 50 patients is reported.

Kasdan ML (ed): *Occupational Hand and Upper Extremity Injuries and Diseases*, ed 2. Philadelphia, PA, Hanley & Belfus, 1998.

This is a good general overview of clinical issues, with the last 100 pages covering rehabilitation and return to work programs.

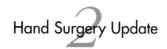
Chapter 44
Amputation

Michael S. Bednar, MD

The goal of amputation in hand surgery is to restore function by preserving length, maintaining sensibility and mobility of the part, minimizing scar and adjacent contractures, and preventing symptomatic neuromas and shortening morbidity. When appropriate, early prosthetic use should be instituted because it has been shown to increase prosthetic wear. Finally, cosmesis should not be ignored; a functional stump will not be used if the patient refuses to accept the way it looks.

Fingertip Amputations

The treatment of fingertip amputations depends on the area, depth, and location of the defect; the contamination and viability of the remaining tissue; and the time since injury. Conservative care is indicated for soft-tissue loss, generally less than 1 cm, with no bone exposed. The type of dressing used on the wound may influence the way the tip heals. Silver sulfadiazine dressings over these wounds have been shown to lead to more comfortable dressing changes and significantly greater finger length preservation as compared to paraffin gauze dressings. However, fingertips treated with paraffin gauze were shown to heal more rapidly and to have earlier resolution of scar sensitivity.

Controversy remains concerning replantation versus completion amputation of traumatic amputations in the distal phalanx. In children, composite flap reattachment of amputations in zone II (Rosenthal classification) gave a normal appearing finger with no cold sensitivity and a 4-mm 2-point discrimination in 12 children whose average age at surgery was 3.5 years. Mild tip asymmetry was noted in 4 patients, but no nail abnormalities were noted although the injury involved the nail in 90% of cases. Composite flap reattachment is the preferred treatment in young patients.

In adults, results of composite flaps are poor. However, the bone and nail bed from the amputated part can be used as a graft and covered with a homodigital neurovascular island flap. Shortening as a result of bone resorption was seen in most patients in 1 study. All fingernails were clawed. Despite the disadvantages, the authors felt this was an alternative to complete loss of the fingertip and nail when replantation was not possible.

Replantation continues to be an option for isolated distal finger amputations. In one study, 11 of 20 distal amputations survived attempted replantation. The site of amputation was distal to the nail fold in 2, between the nail fold and distal interphalangeal (DIP) joint in 4, and between the flexor digitorium superficialis (FDS) insertion and DIP joint in 5. These fingers were compared to a group of 19 fingers that either failed replantation or were not considered candidates for reattachment. The total cost of a successful replant was 3 times greater than that of primary amputation in this study done in the United Kingdom. At follow-up of more than 2 years, hyperesthesia and tenderness were problems in 4 of 9 replanted digitis and 11 of 14 amputated fingers. The patients felt the replanted digit was useful in grasp in 6 of 9 cases, whereas the patients with amputated fingers stated that 11 of 14 treated digits were not helpful in grasp. No patient whose finger was replanted felt his or her grasp was weak, but 10 of 14 patients with an amputated digit complained of a weak grasp.

The greatest technical challenge in replantation of a finger through the distal phalanx is venous repair. In a series of 42 replantations, venous repair was possible in 19. Leech therapy was used for 5 days in all cases. Overall survival rate was 65.5%, increasing to 75% among nonsmokers and decreasing to 53.2% in smokers. Replanted parts regained 2-point discrimination of 11 to 12 mm. Replantation was felt to be a worthwhile procedure in certain patients with distal phalangeal amputations.

Finger Amputation

The basic concepts of performing a digital amputation are to remove bone, especially if the amputation is through a joint, in order to provide a rounded rather than bulbous shape to the stump; to adequately contour the skin flaps to produce a rounded, well padded tip; and to sharply cut the digital nerves under gentle traction to allow retraction from the wound edge. The flexor and extensor tendons should not be sutured together over the end of the tip. However, in amputations through the distal phalanx, the flexor digitorum profundus may be sutured to the A4 pulley to prevent an intrinsic plus deformity.

When the entire small finger must be amputated, controversy remains as to how much of the ray should be left. In 1 study, 17 small finger amputations were done for recurrent Dupuytren's contracture. When the amputation was distal to the metacarpophalangeal (MCP) joint, 9 of 16 patients developed a recurrent contracture of the joint. Five of 7 patients whose fingers were amputated through or proximal to the MCP joint complained of a painful neuroma or phantom limb pain. These authors stated that alternatives to amputation for the treatment of recurrent small finger Dupuytren's disease should be used preferentially. In another study, 21 small finger amputations in 17 patients were examined. Fourteen of 15 of the fingers were amputated through the proximal metacarpal for severe, recurrent Dupuytren's contracture. In contrast to the previous study, all of these older patients were satisfied with the appearance and function of their hand.

Six little fingers were amputated for trauma in younger patients. Three were through the proximal metacarpal and 3 through the MCP joint. Those whose fingers were amputated through the metacarpal complained of a weak grip, even though objectively they performed as well as their counterparts whose fingers were amputated through the MCP joint. The patients with the amputation through the metacarpal also felt the appearance of the hand was poor, in contrast to those with the amputation through the joint who felt the appearance was acceptable. The conclusion was to avoid transmetacarpal amputation of the small finger in young male laborers.

When the middle finger is amputated through the proximal phalanx or MCP joint, the gap left in the hand can be a functional and cosmetic problem. A middle metacarpal ray resection may be performed to close this space. However, when the base of the middle metacarpal is left attached to the capitate, the gap between the fingers may be insufficiently closed by sewing the deep intermetacarpal ligaments of the index and ring fingers. In these patients, an index ray transposition is necessary, with the potential complications of nonunion, malunion, and excessive widening of the first web space. The adverse outcomes of nonunion and digital stiffness were avoided after index transposition for long finger ray resection in 10 patients uniformly managed by soft-tissue flap elevation and metacarpal alignment, T-plate rigid internal fixation, and early active range of motion. Neuromas were not encountered, and cosmetic and functional recovery were timely and satisfactory. In another study, 8 patients underwent a middle ray amputation with excision of the entire metacarpal. The extensor carpi radialis brevis was detached subperiosteally from the bone and attached to the adjacent index and ring metacarpals. Care also was taken to avoid injury to the ulnar motor branch, which lies immediately palmar to the middle metacarpal base. Once the entire bone was removed, the index and ring metacarpals were allowed to migrate together, creating a good 3-finger hand, both functionally and cosmetically.

Development of a painful neuroma after amputation can impair function of the whole hand. A variety of techniques have been tried to prevent this condition. Epineurium may prevent neuroma formation. In 1 study, the shortened fascicles of the free nerve endings were covered with epineurium using 1 of 3 methods. The redundant epineurium was either ligated over the fascicles, sewn to itself to form a flap, or a separate piece of epineurium was removed from the nerve of the amputated part and sewn over the nerve as a graft. At 6 months, those patients in the epineurial graft group had statisically less pain when the neuroma was tapped.

Once a neuroma develops, treatment of the condition is difficult. Seventy patients who had undergone surgical treatment of 112 upper-extremity neuromas by a single surgeon were evaluted for subjective outcome at a mean of 5 years from surgery. The nerve was buried into a muscle bed in 60 patients and transposed into bone and/or dorsal subcutaneous tissue in 10 patients. Forty-five patients stated improvement in pain. If pain relief lasted longer than 1 month after surgery, the pain did not recur. Site of surgery did not influence whether the patient had a good result. However, patients receiving workers' compensation did worse, with 29 of 51 of these patients reporting good pain relief as compared to 16 of 19 patients not receiving workers' compensation.

Even in those patients who do not develop neuromas, changes occur in the way the finger is perceived. Patients examined a mean of 16 years after traumatic amputation of a digit were noted to have no spontaneous pain but did complain of hyperesthesia, usually after bumping against an object. On examination, the skin over the stump had heightened responses to pinprick and cold, which usually was double the intensity of that in corresponding normal fingers. The hypersensitivity usually extended for 0.5 to 1.0 cm proximal to the amputation. Responses to light touch, pressure, and warmth were approximately equal on both sides. Vibration and 2-point discrimination were significantly worse for the amputated finger. On nerve conduction testing, the amplitudes were smaller for the amputated than for the normal side. The authors concluded that retrograde degeneration of the digital nerve is in part responsible for the sensory changes noted in the stump. Other changes include the loss of touch end organs from the palmar skin.

One way of avoiding the potential for neuroma formation in elective amputations is to preserve a neurovascular island flap. If the pulp is uninjured, it is retained with its normal innervation and blood supply and transferred proximally. This is

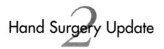
particularly useful for an amputation through the middle phalanx. In the index finger, normal retained sensibility prevented patients from transferring pinch to the long finger tip.

Proximal tissues other than the nerve are also affected by amputation of a distal part. Cortical bone loss occurs in metacarpals of patients who have undergone traumatic amputation of a digit distal to the metacarpal. The average cortical width was significantly reduced by an average of 13% of controls. The pattern of bone loss differed between those who had the amputation before versus after skeletal maturity. In those whose amputation occurred when they were younger than 19 years of age, the loss of cortical width was almost completely attributable to reduction in total metacarpal width. Therefore, the smaller bone was secondary to failure of periosteal bone formation; that is, the bone never grew to its normal size without the appropriate stress applied to it. In the older group, the reduction in cortical width was less marked, but the cortical width was reduced further by an increase in medullary width. In this group, the normal increase in the diameter of aging cortical bone did not occur. In addition, more bone was resorbed from the endosteal cortical surface than in the younger group. The pattern of bone loss in both groups was different than age-related bone loss, which is characterized by endosteal resorption alone.

Hand, Wrist, and Forearm Amputations

Amputations through the hand, wrist, and forearm are devastating injuries. All attempts should be made to salvage viable parts of the amputated limb to help restore some function. When the parts are not salvageable, free-tissue transfer may help to restore some function. In a patient with loss of all 4 fingers, transfer of the second and third toes with a great toe wrap-around flap on 1 vascular pedicle can be used to construct 3 digits in 1 operation. The defect left in the foot is substantial, but acceptable. This technique allows substantial reconstruction of the hand through a single microvascular procedure.

When amputations occur through the forearm, care should be exercised in attempting to maintain length. Although pronation and supination are best preserved with the distal radioulnar joint maintained, the ideal level for a below-elbow amputation is through the junction of the middle and distal thirds of the forearm. This allows for an appropriate length to house the motor of a myoelectric prosthesis.

When the traumatic amputation occurs near the elbow, preservation of the joint should be attempted. Coverage of the remaining radius and ulna has been reported with a free latissmus flap when no other soft tissue is present. The disadvantages of this flap are that it is insensate and the flap takes a significant time to shrink, delaying prosthetic fitting by 6 months. Despite the disadvantages, preservation of the elbow joint significantly improves prosthetic function compared to that of an above-elbow amputation.

Annotated Bibliography

Fingertip Amputations

Dubert T, Houimli S, Valenti P, Dinh A: Very distal finger amputations: Replantation or "reposition-flap" repair? *J Hand Surg* 1997;22B:353–358.

Ten successful distal finger amputations were compared to 6 reposition-flap reconstructions. The reconstruction consisted of replacing the distal phalanx and nail bed and covering the exposed bone with a rotation flap. Reposition-flap repair results were less satisfactory with more finger shortening, nail curvature, and loss of motion at the proximal interphalangeal joint.

Elliot D, Sood MK, Flemming AFS, Swain B: A comparison of replantation and terminalization after distal finger amputation. *J Hand Surg* 1997;22B:523–529.

Isolated digital amputation distal to the FDS insertion was treated by replantation in 11 patients and terminalization in 19. Complaints of tip tenderness, hyperesthesia, and weak grasp were more common in the terminalization group.

Riyat MS, O'Dwyer FG, Quinton DN: Comparison of silver sulphadiazine and paraffin gauze dressings in the treatment of fingertip amputations. *J Hand Surg* 1997;22B:530–532.

Fingertip amputations in 40 patients were treated with silver sulfadiazine or paraffin gauze. Patients stated the silver sulphadiazine dressing was more comfortable. Fingertips treated with a sulfadiazine dressing took longer to heal, but the final fingertip length was greater.

Rosslein R, Simmen BR: Fingertip amputations in children. *Handchir Mikrochir Plast Chir* 1991;23:312–317.

Composite flap reattachment of amputated fingertips in children gave normal appearing fingers, no cold insensitivity, and normal sensation in 12 children, ages 1 to 8 years. No nail deformities were seen.

Finger Amputation

Chu NS: Long-term effects of finger amputation on stump skin sensibility and digital nerve conduction. *Muscle Nerve* 1996;19:1049–1051.

Eleven patients were studied 16 years after digital amputation. Skin over the stump had heightened response to pinprick and cold; normal response to light touch, pressure, and warmth; and decreased response to vibration and 2-point discrimination. Nerve conduction tests showed lower amplitudes. The author concluded that retrograde degeneration of the digital nerve is partially responsible for the sensory changes of the stump.

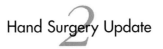
438 Amputation

Cundy T, Grey A: Mechanisms of cortical bone loss from the metacarpal following digital amputation. *Calcif Tissue Int* 1994; 55:164–168.

The metacarpal proximal to a digital amputation undergoes cortical osteoporosis secondary to inhibition of periosteal bone formation.

Hanel DP, Lederman ES: Index transposition after resection of the long finger ray. *J Hand Surg* 1993;18A:271–277.

Index to long finger ray transposition was performed in 10 patients after resection of the long finger ray. There were no nonunions or painful neuromas. Good function was restored in all patients.

Hogh J, Hooper G: Amputation of the little finger. *Arch Orthop Trauma Surg* 1988;107:269–272.

Fourteen little fingers were amputated proximal to the MCP joint for severe, recurrent Dupuytren's disease. All patients were happy with the results. Six small fingers were amputated in young patients for trauma. The 3 patients in whom the amputation was proximal to the MCP joint complained of weaker grip and poorer cosmesis.

Jensen CM, Haugegaard M, Rasmussen SW: Amputations in the treatment of Dupuytren's disease. *J Hand Surg* 1993;18B: 781–782.

Seventeen little fingers and 6 ring fingers were amputated for Dupuytren's disease. Seven patients had the amputation at or proximal to the MCP joint and 16 were distal. Fingers amputated distal to the MCP joint developed a recurrent MCP joint contracture. Those amputated at or proximal to the joint had a higher incidence of pain at the stump.

Lanzetta M, St-Laurent JY: Pulp neurovascular island flap for finger amputation. *J Hand Surg* 1996;21A:918–921.

In 8 patients requiring digital amputation in whom the digital nerves and pulp were uninjured, the palmar pulp was preserved with its neurovascular bundles. The best indication for this technique is amputation through the middle phalanx distal to the flexor superficialis insertion.

Lyall H, Elliot D: Total middle ray amputation. *J Hand Surg* 1996;21B:675–680.

Total excision of the metacarpal in middle-finger ray resection allows migration of the index and ring metacarpals, improving cosmesis and function.

Novak CB, vanVliet D, Mackinnon SE: Subjective outcome following surgical management of upper extremity neuromas. *J Hand Surg* 1995;20A:221–226.

Seventy patients had surgical treatment of 112 upper extremity neuromas by surgical excision and transposition into proximal muscle. Forty-five reported good pain relief at 3 months. Results were poorer in patients receiving workers' compensation.

Yuksel F, Kislaoglu E, Durak N, Ucar C, Karacaoglu E: Prevention of painful neuromas by epineural ligatures, flaps and grafts. *Br J Plast Surg* 1997;50:182–185.

Free nerve ends covered with a graft of epineurium were less painful than those capped by ligating or suturing persisting epineurium.

Hand, Wrist, and Forearm Amputations

Jones ML, Blair WF: Salvage of a below-elbow amputation stump with a free latissimus dorsi muscle flap: A case report. *J Hand Surg* 1995;19A:207–208.

A latissimus dorsi free flap was used to cover the radius and ulna after a proximal forearm traumatic amputation, thereby preserving a below-elbow amputation stump.

Nishijima N, Yamamuro T, Fujio K: Toe-to-finger transfer combined with wrap-around flap: A new technique for four-finger amputation. *J Hand Surg* 1995;20A:213–217.

A great toe wrap-around flap, second toe, and third toe can be harvested on 1 vascular pedicle and transferred following a 4-digit amputation.

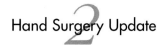
Chapter 45
Restoration of Tetraplegic Hand Function With a Functional Electrical Stimulation Neuroprosthesis

Michael W. Keith, MD

One of the most exciting developments in upper extremity functional restoration in the last 5 years is the first clinically implantable neuroprosthesis, now in multicenter clinical trials with tetraplegic patients. We elected to devote an entire chapter to this work, and asked Dr. Keith to share the important research he and his colleagues have undertaken.

—TR Light, MD

Introduction

Paralysis of upper extremities is profoundly disabling. Patients with tetraplegia require attendants, assistive equipment, devices, splints, and reconstructive surgery to restore some degree of personal independence and enhance their self-esteem. Those with strong character and will can use residual verbal and personal skills to achieve a high quality of life despite the physical challenges of paralysis. Hand surgeons play a critical role in patient rehabilitation by reducing the impairment and functional loss in their hands.

Because of limitations in the donor muscles and control provided by traditional tendon transfer procedures and surgical management, my colleagues and I focused on new technologies that could help control and stabilize paralyzed muscles, and new strategies for reconstruction that build upon traditional knowledge and methods. We developed a motor systems neuroprosthesis, which was approved for public use by the Food and Drug Administration in 1997 as a class III device. The device incorporates the basic science knowledge of functional electrical stimulation (FES) as applied for safe stimulation of muscle and nerve inside the body. The device is intended for the most significantly paralyzed (C5 or C6 motor levels in the American Spinal Injury Association classification or O:0 to Ocu:3 in the international classification), who have the least potential for surgical reconstruction.

Functional Electrical Stimulation Neuroprosthesis (Freehand®)

The neuroprosthesis uses 8 channels of electrical stimulation under voluntary control to excite forearm and hand muscles. The implanted and external components of the neuroprosthesis are shown in Figure 1. Voluntary movements of the contralateral shoulder are detected by an externally mounted sensor. Protraction, retraction, and upward and downward movements are sensed, as well as the velocity of the movements. The protraction-retraction axis is typically used for control of opening and closing of the hand, while vertical movements control lock and hold functions. Because most patients do not have pure orthogonal control of these axes, the software must use offsets or opposite preferred axes for control. An external cable leads these signals to an external control unit (ECU). The ECU contains all of the upgradable electronic components, the program that synthesizes lateral and palmar prehension, and microprocessors and memory to log the patient's activity and hand use. The sensed shoulder movements are converted using muscle recruitment curves

This chapter has been adapted with permission from Keith MW: Restoration of tetraplegia hand function using an FES neuroprosthesis, in Hunter JM, Schneider LH, Mackin EJ (eds): *Tendon and Nerve Surgery in the Hand: A Third Decade.* Philadelphia, PA, Mosby, 1997, pp 226–232.

The author or the department with which he is affiliated has received something of value from a commercial or other party related directly or indirectly to the subject of this chapter.

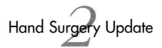

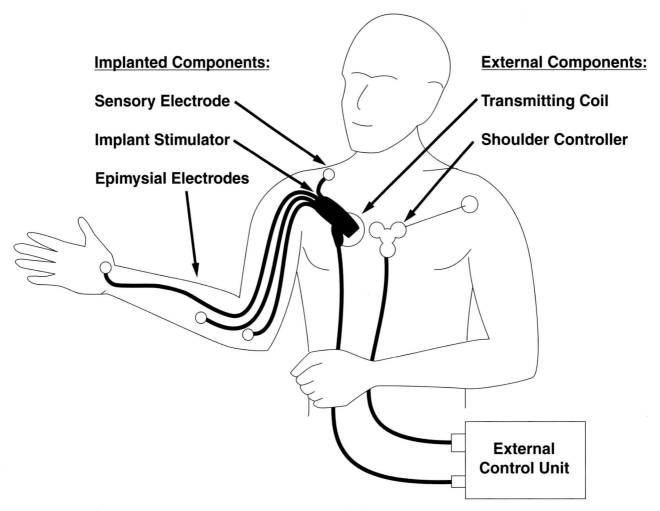

Implanted Components:

Sensory Electrode

Implant Stimulator

Epimysial Electrodes

External Components:

Transmitting Coil

Shoulder Controller

External Control Unit

Figure 1

Components of the implantable functional neuroprosthesis. External components consist of the shoulder position controller, external control unit, and transmitting coil/antenna. Internal components are the receiver-stimulator, leads, and electrodes. (Adapted with permission from Keith MW: Restoration of tetraplegia hand function using an FES neuroprosthesis, in Hunter JM, Schneider LH, Mackin EJ (eds): *Tendon and Nerve Surgery in the Hand: A Third Decade.* Philadelphia, PA, Mosby, 1997, pp 226–232.)

and patterned to coordinate thumb, finger, wrist, and elbow movement. Another cable leads to an antenna coil that is affixed by tape to the chest over the implanted stimulator-receiver. The commands are transmitted by encoded radiofrequency signals from a surface mounted antenna to the implanted receiver-stimulator. The carrier power of the transmitted signal is absorbed by circuitry in the receiver and stored to power the muscles. The stimulator creates waveforms of balanced charge to prevent corrosion of the electrodes and supply safe current that will not harm muscle or nerve. The output is fixed constant current with modulated pulse width. The stimulation waveforms generated are carried by leads and applied by platinum electrodes to the epimysial surface to excite intramuscular nerve branches.

Sensory force feedback may be applied to the subcutaneous nerve branches in the intact C5 sensory dermatome over the shoulder. The stimulus is perceived as rhythmic taps on the shoulder above the clavicle; the taps vary in rate and correspond to the applied command. Published reports have demonstrated that perception of this stimulus is improved when applied below the skin surface.

Surgical Strategy

Standard surgical procedures are combined with FES neuroprosthesis implantation in a single stage to reduce cost and anesthetic risk. Contractures must be corrected first. When

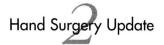

contractures are severe, they may have to be released or combined with serial cast immobilization and stretching before reconstructive surgery can be considered. Contractures of the fingers, especially proximal interphalangeal (PIP) joint flexion contractures or a tight flexor digitorum sublimis, are best prevented rather than released. From the first days of injury, the hands of tetraplegic patients must be classified and evaluated. A program is developed to prevent contractures. Although some centers believe that the development of "functional" finger contractures is desirable, we have found the residual claw posturing finger flexion and adductor tightness difficult to release; reversal requires prolonged and expensive therapy. Furthermore, motor recovery is more common and partial injuries more frequent with improved acute management of spinal cord injuries; a pessimistic outlook toward hand use is no longer warranted. More centers than ever before are prepared to deal with hand weakness. Voluntary tendon transfers, such as posterior deltoid transfer for elbow extension, are always considered both to provide elbow extension and to stabilize the elbow in the workspace. Voluntary brachioradialis transfer to augment wrist extension in the C5 patient will allow tenodesis patterns to develop, obviating wrist bracing. In principle, FES replaces the remaining involuntary muscle groups. FES tendon transfers replace denervated muscle groups or supply extra motors to enhance wrist extension. Arthrodeses or tenodeses replace absent functional movements or simplify grasp.

The receiver-stimulator is placed on the chest wall through a transverse incision over the pectoralis fascia. The leads are tunneled to the middle of the upper arm, where they will be connected (Fig. 2). The limb is warmed throughout the procedure with a heating blanket to maintain nerve excitability.

Programming Grasp Patterns

Recruiting the thenar intrinsics to position the thumb opposite the long finger creates palmar prehension. The stimulating electrode must recruit both the abductor pollicis brevis and the opponens pollicis to achieve this position. The fingers start in full extension by recruiting extensor digitorum communis. The fingers move at the metacarpophalangeal (MCP) and PIP joints from full extension to flex into contact with the thumb. Increasing command then increases the grasp force. The muscle patterns used for palmar grasp are depicted in Figure 3.

Lateral prehension is initiated by extending the thumb and fingers. Extensor pollicis longus (EPL) extends the thumb. If EPL is weak, extensor pollicis brevis can be recruited, but with less excursion. Extensor digitorum communis extends the fingers. The fingers are flexed by flexor digitorum pro-

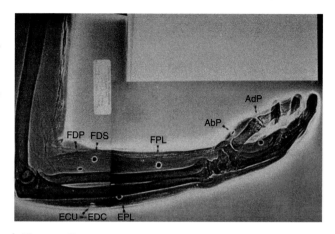

Figure 2

Seven electrodes are dispersed at the motor points of the forearm and hand muscles. A tendon transfer of extensor carpi ulnaris (ECU) to extensor digitorum communis (EDC) is present. AbP = abductor pollicis brevis, AdP = adductor pollicis, FPL = flexor pollicis longus, EPL = extensor pollicis longus, FDP = flexor digitorum profundus, FDS = flexor digitorum superficialis. (Reproduced with permission from Keith MW: Restoration of tetraplegia hand function using an FES neuroprosthesis, in Hunter JM, Schneider LH, Mackin EJ (eds): *Tendon and Nerve Surgery in the Hand: A Third Decade*. Philadelphia, PA, Mosby, 1997, pp 226–232.)

Palmar Grasp

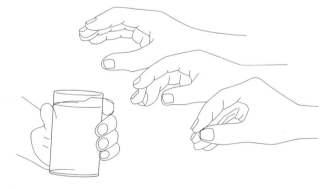

Figure 3

Muscle patterns used for palmar grasp. (Reproduced with permission from Keith MW, Peckham PH, Kilgore K, Wuolle K, Grill J: Multi-channel functional electrical stimulation in spinal cord injury and stroke, in Ito H, Yamashita K (eds): *Brain Hemorrhage '97*. Tokyo, Japan, Neuron Publishing, 1997, vol 2, pp 35–44.)

fundus or flexor digitorum sublimis. The thumb closes against the positioned PIP joints with additional command, adding more pinch force (Fig. 4).

Total active motion improves after surgery in both lateral and palmar prehension (Fig. 5). For example, the total active range of motion (sum of the range of motion of the MCP,

Lateral Grasp

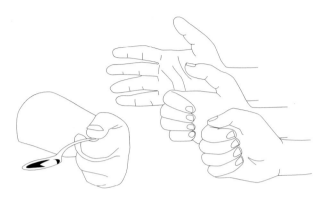

Figure 4

Muscle patterns used in lateral pinch. (Reproduced with permission from Keith MW, Peckham PH, Kilgore K, Wuolle K, Grill J: Multi-channel functional electrical stimulation in spinal cord injury and stroke, in Ito H, Yamashita K (eds): *Brain Hemorrhage '97*. Tokyo, Japan, Neuron Publishing, 1997, vol 2, pp 35–44.)

Median Total Active Motion

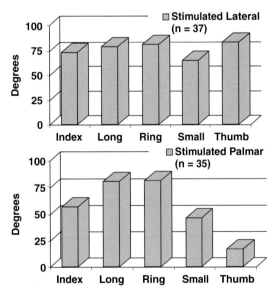

Figure 5

Total active motion in lateral prehension is absent preoperatively. Range of motion of each digit increases, although not to normal due to the absence of intrinsic muscle force and residual flexor tone and the presence of adhesions. There is no movement preoperatively in the palmar grasp pattern. The thumb is positioned in palmar abduction and accordingly shows little active range of motion. Fingers flex until in contact with the thumb. (Adapted with permission from Keith MW, Peckham PH, Kilgore K, Wuolle K, Grill J: Multi-channel functional electrical stimulation in spinal cord injury and stroke, in Ito H, Yamashita K (eds): *Brain Hemorrhage '97*. Tokyo, Japan, Neuron Publishing, 1997, vol 2, pp 35–44.)

PIP, and distal interphalangeal joints of each of the digits) is approximately 75° in lateral grasp, compared to 0° without the neuroprosthesis. The thumb range of motion in palmar prehension is low because the thumb is positioned in a fixed grasp pattern. Full total active motion cannot be achieved, because there is no intrinsic muscle excitation in this version of the neuroprosthesis. In vivo experiments have shown that intrinsic replacement can increase finger extension. There is an interphalangeal extension deficit that varies with antagonist tone, flexion contracture, and extensor muscle amplitude. The degree of contracture varies from patient to patient and is a product of maintenance therapy and overall muscle stiffness. Addition of intrinsic control in the next generation of the device may improve finger posture and range of motion.

The median pinch force attainable in lateral prehension, palmar prehension, or 5-fingertip pinch exceeds preoperative or tenodesis pinch force and surpasses the threshold for functional pinch based on common object masses. Median pinch was 12 N in lateral prehension, 6.4 N in palmar prehension, and 6.7 N in the 5-finger grasp pattern. Without the neuroprosthesis, median postoperative pinch force was 1.6 N in lateral, 0.7 N in palmar, and 0.8 N in 5-finger.

Preliminary Results of Standard Tests

The grasp-release test is a standardized series of single-hand transfer and movement tests. The series emphasizes the impairment of tetraplegic patients attempting to use 1 hand for activities that able-bodied individuals can perform with only 1 hand. As most tetraplegics do not have a second able hand, or even one with modest motor function, the second hand is often an assisting post. In addition, the patient's strategy for object acquisition and movement often involves use of the mouth as a prehensile appendage, with sensation and dexterity exceeding the impaired hand. Although functional, the transfer of saliva, limitation of conversation, and awkwardness of manipulation, are problematic. While this method is acceptable among the disabled and their families by necessity, more normal hand function is preferred. The neuroprosthesis is currently provided only for 1 hand, with the exception of 1 individual with an experimental bilateral device. Patients with neuroprostheses demonstrate greater success in acquiring and transferring the peg, fork, and weight in the lateral prehension test (Fig. 6). The objects are oriented so that they can be grasped and used with slight pronation of the forearm. The "weight" is 264 g of smooth metal; few surgical reconstruction patients with Moberg tenodesis or

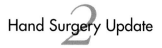

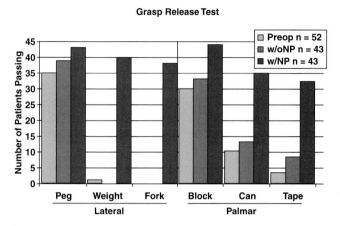

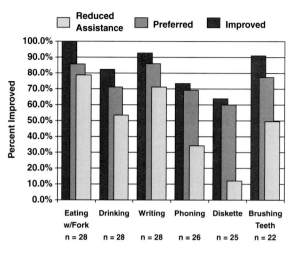

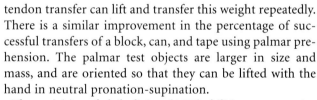

Figure 6

Patients passed the grasp release test items more often with the neuroprosthesis. Small light objects, such as the peg or block, can be grasped without motor control or active force. (Adapted with permission from Keith MW, Peckham PH, Kilgore K, Wuolle K, Grill J: Multichannel functional electrical stimulation in spinal cord injury and stroke, in Ito H, Yamashita K (eds): *Brain Hemorrhage '97*. Tokyo, Japan, Neuron Publishing, 1997, vol 2, pp 35–44.)

Figure 7

Reliance on assistance, preference, and overall improvement of patients in various activities of daily living. (Adapted with permission from Keith MW, Peckham PH, Kilgore K, Wuolle K, Grill J: Multichannel functional electrical stimulation in spinal cord injury and stroke, in Ito H, Yamashita K (eds): *Brain Hemorrhage '97*. Tokyo, Japan, Neuron Publishing, 1997, vol 2, pp 35–44.)

tendon transfer can lift and transfer this weight repeatedly. There is a similar improvement in the percentage of successful transfers of a block, can, and tape using palmar prehension. The palmar test objects are larger in size and mass, and are oriented so that they can be lifted with the hand in neutral pronation-supination.

The activities of daily living (ADL) abilities test contains functional models for eating, drinking, writing, using a telephone, handling a computer diskette, brushing teeth, and other common tasks; results of this test are shown in Figure 7. Our subjects showed the greatest improvement in performance of heavy object transfers and high-force tasks. ADL assessment showed reduced dependence on self-assistance from the mouth or opposite hand, assistive devices such as braces, or an attendant. A high percentage of patients indicate a strong preference for the control afforded by the neuroprosthesis compared to other methods of performing the same function.

Complications

In the first series of over 140 patients treated at 30 centers and followed through the perioperative period, 3 complete systems were removed due to infection after skin breakdown. Three of 1120 electrodes (0.03%) were removed for skin erosion or infection. There were 11 examples of sensory or muscle stimulation that required reduction of stimulation level in the target muscle, but grasp patterns remained func-

tional. Investigation is focused on the device-tissue interface. The electronic components remained reliable.

Outcome Survey

In interviews 1 year after device installation, patients predominantly agreed with statements concerning improvement in hand appearance, system reliability, system function, willingness to undergo the surgical procedure again, personal benefit, life impact, and an increase in the number of activities performed. Questions on device impact related to their ability to function independently; feel more comfortable in the community; perform activities faster, more easily, and more "normally"; perform more activities; and maintain an improved quality of life. Questions on external assistance related to their need for less adaptive equipment and reduced assistance from others.

Conclusion

At this stage of the multicenter clinical trial, we believe that an FES neuroprosthesis is effective in reducing impairment by improving hand strength and range of motion. Functional outcome measures show improvement in independence. The device is safe and reliable; the problems of adhesions and potential infection are similar to those seen in tendon transfer surgery and other implanted devices.

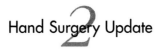
Annotated Bibliography

Keith MW: Restoration of tetraplegia hand function using an FES neuroprosthesis, in Hunter JM, Schneider LH, Mackin EJ (eds): *Tendon and Nerve Surgery in the Hand: A Third Decade.* Philadelphia PA, Mosby, 1997, pp 226–232.

This chapter provides an expanded description of the first multicenter clinical trial preliminary data. It includes greater detail on study findings and surgical placement.

Keith MW, Kilgore KL, Peckham PH, Wuolle KS, Creasey G, Lemay M: Tendon transfers and functional electrical stimulation for restoration of hand function in spinal cord injury. *J Hand Surg* 1996;21A:89–99.

Expanded indications for reconstruction based on neurologic deficiencies by spinal injury level are presented.

Keith MW, Lacey SH: Surgical rehabilitation of the tetraplegic upper extremity. *J Neurol Rehabil* 1991;75–87.

The authors summarize surgical procedures favored at their center.

Keith MW, Peckham PH, Thrope GB, et al: Implantable functional neuromuscular stimulation in the tetraplegic hand. *J Hand Surg* 1989;14A:524–530.

The authors outline details of system design and philosophy of implementation.

Kilgore KL, Peckham PH: Grasp synthesis for upper extremity FNS: Part 2: Evaluation of the influence of electrode recruitment properties. *Med Biol Eng Comput* 1993;31:615–622.

The authors present a physiologic study of muscle properties and electrode placement.

Kilgore KL, Peckham PH, Keith MW, et al: An implanted upper-extremity neuroprosthesis: Follow-up of five patients. *J Bone Joint Surg* 1997;79A:533–541.

Details of early outcomes are presented.

Riso RR, Ignagni AR, Keith MW: Cognitive feedback for use with FES Upper extremity neuroprostheses. *IEEE Trans Biomed Eng* 1991;38:29–38.

The authors discuss the importance of sensory feedback and describe a method of delivery of sensory information via cutaneous FES.

Wuolle KS, VanDoren CL, Thrope GB, Keith MW, Peckham PH: Development of a quantitative hand grasp and release test for patients with tetraplegia using a hand neuroprosthesis. *J Hand Surg* 1994;19A:209–218.

New outcome measures for impairment in patients with tetraplegia are described.

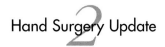
Index

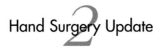

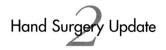

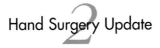

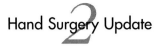

Free-tissue reconstruction
and congenital hand anomalies, 395–398
and hand/wrist/forearm amputation, 437
indications, 287–289
psychology of congenital anomalies and, 400–401
recent advances, 292–293
reconstruction by location, 289–292

Freeman-Sheldon syndrome, 397
fetal ultrasound and, 395

Frykman fracture classification system, 77

Full-thickness skin grafts (FTSG), 250

Fungal infection, 417–418

Fusion of metacarpophalangeal (MCP) joints and, 32

G

Gamekeeper's deformity (rheumatoid arthritis), 321

Ganglion mass, 194

Gangrene
infection and, 413
and ischemia of the hand, 277

Garrod's nodes, Dupuytren's disease and, 269

Gate theory of pain perception, 223

Germinal matrix grafts, nail-bed injuries and, 259

Giant cell tumor of bone, 371–372

Gigantism, 392

Glial-derived neurotrophic factor (GDNF), 179

Glycosaminoglycan (GAG) analysis, 325–326

Gonococcol infection, 417

Gout, 342–343
and carpal tunnel syndrome (CTS), 186
MRI imaging and, 71

Grafts, 204
and brachial plexus injuries, 215–217
donor nerve grafts, 206–207
and Dupuytren's disease, 269
electrical injuries and, 245
extravasation injuries and, 426
and extremity reconstruction, 381
fingertip injuries and, 257–258
full-thickness skin grafts (FTSG), 250
hemodialysis access, 277
infection and, 415
metacarpal synostosis and, 399–400
and metacarpophalangeal (MCP) joint defects, 39
and nail-bed injuries, 259
nerve, 200
nerve repair results, 208–209
osteochondral, 388
peripheral nerve injury and, 203–207
polytetrafluoroethlyene (PTFE), 293
and replantation, 282
and rheumatoid arthritis, 315
scaphoid fractures and, 110–111
soft tissue hand coverage and, 249–250
split-thickness skin grafts (STSG), 241–242, 250
sural nerve, 206–207
tendon, 136, 145–146
using polytetrafluoroethylene (PTFE) in tendon repair, 133
of vascularized bone, 47–48

Grayson's ligaments, Dupuytren's disease and, 267

Grip. See also Thumb injuries, restoration of opposition
and carpal tunnel syndrome (CTS), 189

Grossman classification system II, 136–137

Gunshot wounds, 291–292. See also Wound healing

Guyon canal problems. See Hypothenar hammer syndrome; Ulnar tunnel syndrome

H

Hamate fractures (carpal), 115

Hand diagram test, 187

Hand volume stress test, 187

Hansen's disease, 164–165

Healing process. See Wound healing

Heberden's nodes, 327

Helminthic infection, 418

Hemangiomas
pediatric, 297–299
treatment, 303

Hematoma block, 5

Hemodialysis
and carpal tunnel syndrome (CTS), 186
and ischemia of the hand, 277

Herbert's classification of scaphoid fractures, 109

Herpetic infection, 418

High dose methotrexate (HDMTX), osteosarcoma and, 379–380

High pressure injection injuries, 423–426

Highet's sensory rating scale, 209

Holt-Oram syndrome, 392

Hook nail deformity, 260

Horner's sign, obstetric palsy and, 218

Human immunodeficiency virus (HIV)
and Dupuytren's disease, 264
infection and, 411–412, 414

Humerus prosthetics, 381

Hyaline cartilage disorder. See Osteoarthritis (OA)

Hydrofluoric acid burns, 245

Hydrostatic pressure, carpal tunnel syndrome (CTS) and, 187

Hyperesthesia after amputation, 436

Hypertrophic scarring, 235

Hyphecan, 258

Hypoplasia, 392

Hypothenar hammer syndrome, 276

Hypothyroidism, 183–184

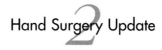

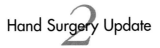

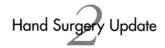

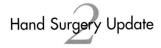

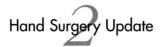

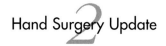

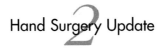